# Cytokine Regulation of Humoral Immunity

# Cytokine Regulation of Humoral Immunity

## BASIC AND CLINICAL ASPECTS

*Edited by*
**CLIFFORD M. SNAPPER**
*Uniformed Services University of the Health Sciences, Bethesda, Maryland, USA*

JOHN WILEY & SONS
Chichester · New York · Brisbane · Toronto · Singapore

National 01243 779777
International (+44) 1243 779777





*Other Wiley Editorial Offices*

John Wiley & Sons, Inc., 605 Third Avenue,
New York, NY 10158-0012, USA

Jacaranda Wiley Ltd, 33 Park Road, Milton,
Queensland 4064, Australia

John Wiley & Sons (Canada) Ltd, 22 Worcester Road,
Rexdale, Ontario M9W 1L1, Canada

John Wiley & Sons (SEA) Pte Ltd, 37 Jalan Pemimpin #05-04,
Block B, Union Industrial Building, Singapore 2057

*Library of Congress Cataloging-in-Publication Data*

Cytokine regulation of humoral immunity: basic and clinical aspects / edited by Clifford M. Snapper.
p. cm.
Includes bibliographical references and index.
ISBN 0–471–95953–7 (hardbound : alk. paper)
1. Cytokines. 2. Immune response Regulation. I. Snapper, Clifford M.
QR185.8.C95C9817 1996.
616.07′9—dc20 95–23822
CIP

*British Library Cataloguing in Publication Data*

A catalogue record for this book is available from the British Library

ISBN 0 471 95953 7

Typeset in 10/12pt Times by Mackreth Media Services
Printed and bound in Great Britain by Biddles Ltd, Guildford, Surrey

This book is printed on acid-free paper responsibly manufactured from sustainable forestation, for which at least two trees are planted for each one used for paper production.

# Contents

**Contributors** vii

**Preface** xi

**Part I General Concepts**

1 **Overview** 3
*Clifford M. Snapper*

2 **T-cell-independent and T-cell-dependent Humoral Immunity** 23
*Jon D. Laman and Eric Claassen*

3 **B-cell Subpopulations and Microenvironments** 73
*Thomas J. Waldschmidt*

4 **B-cell Activation and Maturation to Immunoglobulin Secretion** 99
*David C. Parker and Jeffrey M. Purkerson*

5 **Immunoglobulin Class Switching** 109
*Matthias Lorenz and Andreas Radbruch*

**Part II Cytokines**

6 **Cellular Sources and Regulation of Cytokine Production** 139
*William C. Gause and Pin Lu*

7 **Interleukin-2** 159
*Melissa J. McIlraith and Peter E. Lipsky*

8 **Interleukin-4 and Interleukin-13** 195
*Jan E. de Vries and Juha Punnonen*

9 **Interleukin-5** 217
*Kiyoshi Takatsu*

10 **Interleukin-6** 251
*Toshio Tanaka, Yoshinori Katada, Masaki Suemura and Tadamitsu Kishimoto*

11 **Interleukin-10** 273
*Francine Briere, Florence Malisan, Christine Servet-Delprat and Jacques Banchereau*

**12 Transforming Growth Factor Beta** 289
*Janet Stavnezer*

**13 Interferon-Gamma** 325
*Clifford M. Snapper*

**14 Neuropeptides** 347
*Hajime Kimata*

**Part III Pathophysiology**

**15 IgE Regulation in Allergy and Helminth Parasite Infections** 379
*Robert L. Coffman*

**16 Regulation of Mucosal Immunity** 391
*K. W. Beagley, C. A. Black, M. L. Dunkley and J. R. McGhee*

**17 Abnormalities in Cytokine Production and Responsiveness in Autoimmune Disease** 409
*Eri Hagiwara and Dennis M. Klinman*

**Index** 431

# Contributors

**Jacques Banchereau**
*Schering-Plough, Laboratory for Immunological Research, Dardilly, France*

**K. W. Beagley**
*Discipline of Pathology, Faculty of Medicine, University of Newcastle, Newcastle, NSW 2300, Australia*
*and*
*Australian Institute for Mucosal Immunology, Newcastle, NSW 2300, Australia*

**C. A. Black**
*Discipline of Pathology, Faculty of Medicine, University of Newcastle, NSW 2300 Australia*
*and*
*Australian Institute for Mucosal Immunology, Newcastle, NSW 2300, Australia*

**Francine Brière**
*Schering-Plough, Laboratory for Immunological Research, Dardilly, France*

**Eric Claassen**
*Department of Immunological and Infectious Diseases, TNO Prevention and Health, 2301 CE Leiden, The Netherlands*

**Robert L. Coffman**
*Human Immunology Department, DNAX Research Institute of Molecular and Cellular Biology, 901 California Avenue, Palo Alto, CA 94304-1104, USA*

**M. L. Dunkley**
*Australian Institute for Mucosal Immunology, Newcastle, NSW 2300, Australia*

**William C. Gause**
*Department of Microbiology, B3106, Uniformed Services University of the Health Sciences, 4301 Jones Bridge Road, Bethesda, MD 20814, USA*

**Eri Hagiwara**
*Division of Viral Products, Center for Biologics Evaluation and Research, Food and Drug Administration, 29 Lincoln Drive, Bethesda, MD 20892-4555, USA*

**Yoshinori Katada**
*Department III of Internal Medicine, Osaka University Medical School, 2-2 Yamada-oka, Suita, Osaka 565, Japan*

**Hajime Kimata**
*Department of Pediatrics, Faculty of Medicine, Kyoto University Hospital, 54 Kawahara-cho, Shogoin, Sakyo-ku, Kyoto 606, Japan*

**Tadamitsu Kishimoto**
*Department III of Internal Medicine, Osaka University Medical School, 2-2 Yamada-oka, Suita, Osaka 565, Japan*

**Dennis M. Klinman**
*Division of Viral Products, Center for Biologics Evaluation and Research, Food and Drug Administration, 29 Lincoln Drive, Bethesda, MD 20892-4555, USA*

**Jon D. Laman**
*Department of Immunological and Infectious Diseases, TNO Prevention and Health, 2301 CE Leiden, The Netherlands*

**Peter E. Lipsky**
*Harold C. Simmons Arthritis Research Center and the Molecular Microbiology Graduate Program, University of Texas Southwestern Medical Center at Dallas, 5323 Harry Hines Boulevard, Dallas, TX 75235-8884, USA*

**Matthias Lorenz**
*Institute for Genetics, Weyertal 121, 50931 Cologne, Germany*

**Pin Lu**
*Department of Microbiology, B3106, Uniformed Services University of the Health Sciences, 4301 Jones Bridge Road, Bethesda, MD 20814, USA*

**Florence Malisan**
*Schering-Plough, Laboratory for Immunological Research, Dardilly, France*

**Jerry R. McGhee**
*Department of Microbiology, Immunobiology Vaccine Center, Medical Center, University of Alabama at Birmingham, UAB Station BHS 392, Birmingham, AL 35294-0005, USA*

**Melissa J. McIlraith**
*Harold C. Simmons Arthritis Research Center and the Molecular Microbiology Graduate Program, University of Texas Southwestern Medical Center at Dallas, 5323 Harry Hines Boulevard, Dallas, TX 75235-8884, USA*

**David C. Parker**
*Department of Molecular Microbiology and Immunology, Oregon Health Sciences University, 3181 S.W. Sam Jackson Park Road, Portland, OR 97201-3098, USA*

**Juha Punnonen**
*Human Immunology Department, DNAX Research Institute of Molecular and Cellular Biology, 901 California Avenue, Palo Alto, CA 94304-1104, USA*

**Jeffrey M. Purkerson**
*Department of Molecular Microbiology and Immunology, Oregon Health Sciences University, 3181 S.W. Sam Jackson Park Road, Portland, OR 97201-3098, USA*

**Andreas Radbruch**
*Institute for Genetics, Weyertal 121, 50931 Cologne, Germany*

**Christine Servet-Delprat**
*Schering-Plough, Laboratory for Immunological Research, Dardilly, France*

**Clifford M. Snapper**
*Department of Pathology, Uniformed Services University of the Health Sciences, 4301 Jones Bridge Road, Bethesda, MD 20814, USA*

**Janet Stavnezer**
*Department of Molecular Genetics and Microbiology, University of Massachusetts Medical School, 55 Lake Avenue N, Worcester, MA 01655-0001, USA*

**Masaki Suemura**
*Department III of Internal Medicine, Osaka University Medical School, 2-2 Yamada-oka, Suita, Osaka 565, Japan*

**Kiyoshi Takatsu**
*Department of Immunology, Institute of Medical Science, University of Tokyo, 4-6-1 Shirokanedai Minato-ku, Tokyo 108, Japan*

**Toshio Tanaka**
*Department III of Internal Medicine, Osaka University Medical School, 2-2 Yamada-oka, Suita, Osaka 565, Japan*

**Jan E. de Vries**
*Human Immunology Department, DNAX Research Institute of Molecular and Cellular Biology, 901 California Avenue, Palo Alto, CA 94304-1104, USA*

**Thomas J. Waldschmidt**
*Department of Pathology, University of Iowa College of Medicine, Iowa City, IA 52242, USA*

# Preface

In 1985 I began my scientific career as a post-doctoral fellow in Bill Paul's laboratory at the NIH. At the time that I arrived, Junichi Ohara had recently succeeded in purifying IL-4 from the crude culture supernatant of the murine EL-4 thymoma line and raising a monoclonal antibody that neutralized IL-4 function. This paved the way for the cloning of the IL-4 gene and its receptor, establishing a firm foundation for building a comprehensive understanding of IL-4 biology. Few of us at that time imagined that this general paradigm of discovery would be repeated many times over the next ten years, revealing a virtual treasure trove of new cytokines. Early on, the simple view was in vogue that each immune cell type coevolved with a single cytokine partner that would serve as its key regulator of growth and differentiation. Today we now appreciate the existence of a complex cytokine network with a rich level of pleiotropy and redundancy. We see how each immune cell type integrates distinct signals delivered by combinations of cytokines as well as other soluble and cell surface-associated activators to determine the ultimate quantity, quality and timing of its response. Intrinsic features of the cell itself are further seen to temper its functional reactivity to a given set of stimuli. Most impressively, in response to a complex pathogen, all the participating immune cell types typically manage to act in a temporally coordinated fashion to make the overall immune response an effective one. Many of the parameters that underlie the precise staging of this performance remain unknown.

It has been my privilege and pleasure to see the field of cytokine biology rapidly evolve over the past 10 years from infancy to young adulthood. I have great sympathy, however, for the young scientists and physicians who must now assimilate this overwhelming body of information. I thus accepted, with enthusiasm, the opportunity to assemble one aspect of this field, the role of cytokines in regulating B-lymphocyte function and humoral immunity, on which I have focused my own research efforts. With introductory, specialized and applied chapters, comprising the three sections of this book, it was my intent to facilitate the formation of a comprehensive body of information and an extensive list of references that would be of value to both beginning and established, basic and clinical scientists. I have taken immense satisfaction in having been able to recruit an outstanding group of leading investigators to write the various chapters that comprise this volume. I am of the opinion that they have amply succeeded in their collective effort to reveal a meaningful and current image of 'the big picture', depicting this aspect of humoral immunity. Nevertheless, it is prudent to keep in mind that this vision is still a fluid one and that great effort will be required in the coming years before we see the final masterpiece.

Clifford M. Snapper, MD
*Bethesda, Maryland*
*June, 1995*

Dedication

To Iris, Jessica, and Dustin with love

# Part I

# GENERAL CONCEPTS

# 1 Overview

**CLIFFORD M. SNAPPER**
*Uniformed Services University of the Health Sciences, Bethesda, Maryland, USA*

A meaningful appreciation of how cytokines regulate the humoral immune response must begin with an understanding of the cellular events which transpire upon the host encountering a microorganism, in the context of the ongoing 'dialogue' between the host and its own antigenic milieu. In *Chapter 2*, Jon D. Laman and Eric Claassen bring together our current understanding of these events. They begin our exploration of the humoral immune system by elucidating the fundamental structural differences between the antigens themselves within the context of three broad categories: T-cell-dependent type 1 (TI-1), TI-2, and T-cell-dependent (TD). The reader is advised at the outset to discriminate between phenomena which emerge from artificial encounters of the immune system with relatively large amounts of pure antigen, and the more dynamic and physiological responses that ensue when the host responds to a live multi-antigenic organism.

The parameters which shape the quality and quantity of the humoral immune response are indeed complex. We must first appreciate the significance of the microbe's route of entry into the host, for the immune system has evolved distinct structural and functional paradigms integrated within the tissue in which it resides. This will in turn determine the initial physicochemical, cellular and molecular events which will guide the emerging pattern of subsequent responses. We thus learn about the detailed functional organization of the major secondary lymphoid organs, the spleen and lymph node, including their panoply of resident and circulating immune cell types. Further detailed insight into the structure of the mucosal immune system, notably the Peyer's patch, can be obtained in Chapter 16. A finer analysis of B-cell subsets ensues in Chapter 3. With this information in hand, we proceed to follow the 'fate of antigen *in vivo*'. We learn the implications underlying the immunization route, use of adjuvants, dose of antigen and whether the antigen exists in a soluble or particulate form, and the role of complement and other interacting serum proteins.

We are then ready to grapple with the mechanistic underpinnings governing the relative requirement for T cells, and the participation of non-T-cell types, in induction of a humoral immune response. We learn that this is

*Cytokine Regulation of Humoral Immunity: Basic and Clinical Aspects.* Edited by Clifford M. Snapper.

based in large part on the physicochemical nature of the antigens within the context of other parameters intrinsic to the living microbe that has perturbed the immune system. This leads to engagement, and a characteristic trafficking of distinct groupings of cells and cytokines to form a particular integrated response, that hopefully will contain and eliminate the inciting pathogen with minimal damage to host tissue. In order for cytokines to manifest their adaptive effects they must be delivered, with appropriate concentration and timing, to particular cells that have also received a correct set of non-cytokine signals from a large potential menu of membrane-bound and soluble ligands. In particular, we learn of the especial importance of B-cell activation through CD40, by T cells expressing the inducible CD40 ligand. A major role for signaling through the antigen receptor is also revealed, as well as the role of numerous B-cell membrane proteins serving additional signaling and/or adhesion functions. A complementary and more detailed discussion of these events will follow in Chapter 4. We also come to appreciate the dynamic crosstalk between the B cell and, in particular, the T cell, and see how their mutual communication effects increasing states of B- and T-cell activation. Throughout this volume the reader should come to appreciate that the nature of the activational signals delivered to the B cell will ultimately determine its functional response to a given set of cytokines.

Another theme developed in this chapter, and further complemented in Chapter 6, is that cytokines are elicited in distinct patterns, determined both by the particular immune cells which become activated, and induction of distinct differentiation events within the T-cell compartment leading to formation of T-cell subsets producing characteristic sets of cytokines. The authors address the question: what are the key parameters that guide the immune system towards particular cytokine synthesis response patterns? In later chapters we will learn the consequences to the host inherent in making the correct or incorrect choice of cytokines in response to a given pathogen.

Finally, we come to appreciate that the host typically benefits by its first encounter with a particular pathogen and its antigenic repertoire, by enhancing its state of readiness for its next encounter with that pathogen. This is accomplished through the generation of 'memory', including the expansion of specific B-cell clones possessing antigen receptors with higher affinity for antigen ('somatic hypermutation and affinity maturation') and a new, specialized effector function ('Ig class switching'—see Chapter 5), accomplished in large part through the 'germinal center reaction'.

Although much of this book details the various mechanisms and functional consequences of diverse stimuli in regulating the B-cell response to antigenic and/or microbial stimulation, in *Chapter 3* Thomas Waldschmidt discusses the substantial complexity of the B-cell compartment itself and how various B-cell subpopulations display heterogeneity in their functional responses to a given set of stimuli. Distinct B-cell subsets are subdivided into two broad families: one subsumed under 'maturational state' and including pro-B, pre-

B, immature, mature and memory B cells, and the other either consequent to development along distinct lineage pathways or perhaps reflecting a characteristic activation state in response to a particular type of antigenic stimulus. These latter subpopulations include B1 (B1a = $CD5^+$ and B1b = $CD5^-$), and B2 (follicular and marginal zone) B cells. In particular, a potential role for the B1 cell in autoimmunity is introduced here, and further expanded upon in Chapter 17.

The microenvironments, including spleen, lymph node, peritoneum, bone marrow, Peyer's patch and fetal liver and omentum, in which various B-cell subpopulations reside, are discussed, and this complements the information provided in Chapter 2 on histologic compartments in the context of T-cell-dependent and -independent humoral immunity. A particular emphasis on the role of the Peyer's patch in mucosal immunity is found in Chapter 16. Substantial information is given on defining B-cell subsets on the basis of their expression of surface markers, cytoplasmic proteins, and Ig gene rearrangements. These characteristic as well as shared phenotypic attributes in part also define their functional potentials. Extensive data are provided on multiparameter flow cytometric analyses of B-cell subpopulations, giving the reader sufficient information on how to isolate these cells for further study as well as following their development during immune responses *in vivo*. In the subsequent chapters it should become apparent to the reader that the nature of the B cell itself will often play a determining role in its response to a given set of stimuli. As Dr Waldschmidt concludes, the diversity within the B-cell population has no doubt evolved to provide adaptability of the humoral immune system to challenges by diverse groups of pathogenic organisms on the one hand, and the maintenance of tolerance to self on the other.

In *Chapter 4* David Parker and Jeffrey Purkerson proceed from, and complement, the concepts developed in Chapters 2 and 3 to weave a general picture of how B cells become activated, proliferate, and mature into Ig-secreting cells. This conceptual track is then completed in Chapter 5 with an in-depth discussion of the parameters which regulate Ig isotype switching. The G0, resting B-cell population is seen to have the potential to realize a variety of ultimate fates in response to various immunizing agents. These include various combinations of clonal expansion, maturation to Ig synthesis, Ig class switching, somatic hypermutation with affinity maturation, memory cell formation, tolerance, apoptosis, and the ability to present antigen to, and receive help from, T cells. The authors bring into focus the central and organizing concept that the functional readout of a particular B cell will reflect its integration of a wide array of potential signals mediated through its antigen, cytokine and other membrane receptors, and delivered within a particular temporal pattern. The response of the B cell will further reflect a filtering of these signals through the intracellular milieu of the responding B cell, as determined by its status as a member of a particular subpopulation or lineage, and/or its initial activation state upon its encounter with such stimuli.

The role of cytokines in humoral immunity must be appreciated within the broader view that the specific response of the B cell to a particular cytokine or group of cytokines will often depend upon the precise manner by which the resting B cell becomes activated in order to become responsive to those cytokines. Such modes of activation include antigen receptor crosslinking, activation through CD40 and perhaps other members of the tumor necrosis factor (TNF) receptor family on B cells, stimulation by bacterial cell wall components such as lipopolysaccharide (LPS), and perhaps to a lesser extent signals delivered through MHC class II and adhesion molecules, as well as other defined and as yet undefined membrane structures.

The authors conclude by stating: 'To contribute to an effective antibody response, the B cell must not only receive the appropriate activating signals through its antigen and cytokine receptors, but also avoid those signals and combinations of signals that kill or inactivate it. Ultimately, a satisfactory explanation of the various B cell responses to activating signals will require an intimate knowledge of how various extracellular signals are integrated through cytoplasmic signal transduction pathways to regulate the transcriptional, cell cycle progression, and programmed cell death machinery inside the cell'. The very beginnings of this goal are starting to be realized, as will be seen in the subsequent chapters.

In *Chapter 5* Matthias Lorenz and Andreas Radbruch discuss the cellular and molecular biology of the Ig class switch, a process whereby B cells expressing IgM and/or IgD of a particular antigen specificity (encoded by a rearranged VDJ heavy chain and VJ light chain gene) switch upon activation to the expression of IgE, IgA or one of four IgG subclasses, each encoded by a particular constant heavy ($C_H$) gene. In this manner, the B cell confers a new effector function upon the antibody it expresses while maintaining the original specificity for the antigen which elicited it. As discussed here, the Ig class switch is a directed process in which the instructions that determine the particular $C_H$ gene that will ultimately be expressed can be delivered to the B cell via a number of distinct cytokines acting in concert with various activational stimuli; both the cytokine and the activator play determining roles in the selectivity of the response. The Ig class switch is thought to serve the host mainly through the generation of functional diversity, to allow for maximal adaptation of the humoral immune response to pathogens of widely differing biologies. The evidence to support this intuitively compelling notion, however, is still incomplete, perhaps in part due to functional overlap among the various Ig isotypes.

The functional properties of various Ig classes and subclasses, as well as the cellular parameters which lead to their induction, are discussed. Our current understanding of the molecular basis for the Ig class switch, including the role of cytokines in this process, is presented here in detail. Cytokines, such as interleukin-4 (IL-4), interferon gamma (IFN-$\gamma$), and transforming growth factor beta (TGF-$\beta$), are shown to act as switch factors through their ability, via induction of regulatory proteins prior to class switch recombination, to selectively activate (and suppress) $C_H$ gene promoters leading to changes in $C_H$ gene transcription and synthesis of corresponding germline $C_H$ RNA transcripts. A major recent advance is revealed by the demonstration that transcription alone is insufficient to target $C_H$ genes for recombination, and that the processed germline $C_H$ RNA transcript itself may play an active role.

The weight of evidence favors switch recombination with looping out and deletion as the primary mechanism by which B cells change their Ig isotype expression, although potential alternative mechanisms such as processing of long transcripts and trans-splicing are discussed. Through looping out and deletion, B cells that have switched to one Ig isotype have been found capable of switching, in a sequential manner, to another downstream $C_H$ gene. An additional requirement for DNA synthesis to allow for switch recombination to occur is suggested but the mechanistic basis for this remains a mystery. Finally, the structure–function relationship of the switch regions themselves, the site of $C_H$ DNA recombination, is discussed, and data suggesting that the rearrangement event itself is targeted to particular sequences within the switch region are presented.

In *Chapter 6,* William Gause and Pin Lu introduce the second section of the book, which deals with the effect of individual cytokines on B-cell function. Central to our understanding the biological, *in vivo* meaning that underlies any particular *in vitro* property of a cytokine on the B-cell functional program is an appreciation of the context in which a particular cytokine is released during the course of an immune response. Thus, the ultimate contribution of a particular cytokine to the humoral immune response will depend in part upon the overall qualitative make-up of the cytokine milieu and other activational influences exerted on the responding B cell, the timing, duration and intensity of cytokine action, as well as other parameters. In turn, the B-cell response must be appreciated within the context of the entire network of responding and interacting immune elements.

As in Chapter 2, the authors begin by underscoring the importance of studying cytokine induction in response to living, whole pathogens, and not simply isolated antigens, since conclusions based on the latter may not adequately reflect the more physiological response of the former. We have recently come to appreciate that a predictable and distinct pattern of cytokines is released early (within hours) after a particular pathogen first confronts the immune system (the ‘innate’ or ‘antigen non-specific’ response) which then determines the pattern of cytokines released later in the immune response (days) as part of an ‘adaptive’ or ‘antigen-specific’ response. The innate response, which is mediated by such ‘front-line’ cells as macrophages, natural killer (NK) cells, and perhaps T-cell receptor (TCR)-$\gamma/\delta^+$ T cells, neutrophils, mast cells and eosinophils, represents the immune system’s initial and rapid mobilization towards containment of the invading pathogen.

The adaptive response which is mediated primarily by TCR-α/β⁺ CD4⁺ T cells serves to augment and refine these initial events.

Families of pathogens possessing distinct biologies require qualitatively different responses from the immune system in order to effect their containment or elimination. This is reflected by the predictable elicitation of cytokine synthesis response patterns. Overall, two broad response patterns have been defined: (1) the type 1 or IFN-γ-dominant response, which also includes IL-2, IL-12, IFN-α/β, TNF-β, TNF-α, and often IL-6 and IL-10; and (2) the type 2 or IL-4-dominant response, which also includes IL-5, IL-6, IL-9, IL-13, and sometimes IL-10. Both type 1 and type 2 profiles may also include IL-3 and granulocyte/macrophage colony-stimulating factor (GM-CSF). Less is known to make a clear assignment for TGF-β, although as will be seen in Chapters 12 and 17 its inclusion as a component of both type 1 and type 2 responses might be anticipated. Type 1 and type 2 responses are appreciated for both the innate and adaptive phases of an immune reaction, where the presence of a type 1 response during the innate phase predicts the emergence of an adaptive type 1 profile, with an analogous relationship holding true for the type 2 response. As will be discussed in some detail, bacteria and viruses tend to elicit type 1 responses, whereas the much larger multicellular nematode parasites elicit responses defined as type 2. This is seen to be based in part on these organisms possessing conserved structures which induce distinct stereotypical cytokine profiles during the innate phase of the response. However, type 1 and type 2 cytokine profiles are not rigidly fixed, as evidenced by particular instances where significant variations from this consensus paradigm are observed. In regard to the humoral immune response, substantial Ig secretion is observed in the context of both type 1 and type 2 responses, although the Ig isotypic profile is different. The cellular basis for these observations will be revealed or suggested in the subsequent chapters.

In *Chapter 7,* Melissa McIlraith and Peter Lipsky discuss the role of IL-2 in regulating B-cell activation, growth, differentiation to Ig secretion, and possibly Ig class switching in murine and/or human B cells. Overall, IL-2 is revealed as a positive regulator of these B-cell functions and appears to act in this context directly at the level of the B cell. Although IL-2 by itself is often seen here as sufficient to induce activated B cells to secrete Ig, data presented in Chapter 13 also indicate that, under certain conditions, IL-2 must act in concert with other cytokines, such as IL-3, GM-CSF and IFN-γ, in order to promote maturation to Ig secretion by activated murine B cells. A role for IL-2 in the induction of Ig class switching in activated B cells is suggested. Unlike the isotype-specific effects of IL-4/IL-13 (Chapter 8), IL-10 (Chapter 11), TGF-β (Chapter 12) and IFN-γ (Chapter 13), the effects of IL-2 appear to be relatively isotype-non-specific. This is supported by the observation that IL-2 can induce multiple germline $C_H$ RNA transcripts in activated human B cells (see also Chapter 5). Although IL-2 exerts direct effects on B cells, it also plays a key positive role in T-cell and NK cell activation and may thus exert additional effects on B cells, indirectly through its effects on these cells.

Resting murine and human B cells express low or undetectable levels of IL-2 receptor and thus are unresponsive to the actions of IL-2. A diverse group of activation stimuli have been shown to be sufficient for inducing IL-2 receptor expression on normal resting B cells, and this is correlated with responsiveness of the activated B cell to the growth and differentiation effects of IL-2. The nature of the IL-2 receptor is discussed in some detail, and it is shown to consist of three distinct polypeptides. One of these, the $\gamma$ chain, has also been implicated as a key signaling component of the receptors for IL-4, IL-7, IL-9 and IL-15. Indeed, IL-15 has recently been shown to mimic many of the functional effects of IL-2. In Chapter 8 we see further the striking functional overlap between IL-4 and IL-13, at least in part due to their sharing of an as yet undefined common receptor component. As discussed in Chapter 9, another common receptor chain has been described for IL-3, IL-5 and GM-CSF, cytokines which also elicit a number of common functional outcomes on hematopoietic cells. These observations may shed light on the mechanisms underlying some of the overlapping functions of these cytokines on lymphoid cells.

Although IL-2 exerts direct and positive effects at multiple stages of the B-cell functional program, the authors point out that *in vivo* studies in mice made genetically deficient in IL-2 gene expression by the process of homologous recombination (IL-2 knockout mice) reveal that, whereas IL-2 may play some direct or indirect role in B-cell development and function, it is not necessary for induction of humoral immune responses. With certain exceptions, for example IL-4/IL-13 induction of IgE class switching (see Chapters 8 and 15), this reflects a more general principle that most events which collectively constitute the humoral immune response can be induced independently by more than one cytokine. However, the activational milieu and the B-cell subpopulation in which these events occur, as well as the cellular sources and induction characteristics of the various cytokines (see Chapter 6), may differ somewhat for each cytokine, thus conferring 'unique' aspects to their redundant properties. As will become apparent during the reading of this book, and as discussed in some detail in this chapter on IL-2, the signal transduction pathways which mediate cytokine-induced changes in lymphocyte function comprise a related family of signaling molecules (the Jak–STAT pathway) with both distinct and overlapping features among the various cytokines, that may shed light on both the unique and redundant features of cytokine action.

An understanding of IL-2 action on B cells may prove to be of clinical importance. In particular, the authors point out that its intravenous administration to patients with hypogammaglobulinemia can induce long-term production of protective Ig, consistent with its B-cell-, as well as T-cell-stimulating properties. IL-2, when incorporated as part of a fusion protein or co-administered with antigen, has also demonstrated significant adjuvant properties for humoral immune responses to the immunizing protein.

IL-4 and IL-13 are the main subjects discussed by Jan E. de Vries and Juha Punnonen in *Chapter 8*. The inclusion of these cytokines together in the same chapter reflects the fact that, with certain notable exceptions, they possess nearly identical biological effects on cells of the immune system; while human IL-4 and IL-13, for example, share only 30 per cent homology at the protein level, they appear to utilize a shared, though undefined, receptor component involved in signal transmission. It is reasonable, on the basis of their known differences, to speculate that IL-4 and IL-13 operate in a somewhat complementary fashion during immune responses, but the nature of this adaptation remains obscure.

IL-4 and IL-13 are both Th2-derived cytokines whose major, and certainly unique, role in the humoral arm of the immune system appears to be the induction of switching to, and secretion of, IgE, an antibody class implicated in the pathogenesis of immediate hypersensitivity reactions. In regard to their effects on B cells, IL-4 and/or IL-13 promote B-cell survival, upregulate MHC class II, CD23, membrane IgM and CD40 expression, induce B7-1 (a ligand for CD28/CTLA4 on T cells), costimulate proliferation, synergize with other cytokines such as IL-5 for differentiation to Ig secretion, and selectively induce germline transcription of the $C_H$ genes for IgE (murine and human), IgG1 (murine), and IgG4 (human), thus targeting them for switch recombination (see Chapter 5). IL-4 itself has been shown to be a key cytokine for directing the evolution of an immune response towards a Th2 pattern of cytokine synthesis, including the production of IL-4. Thus, for the B cell, a coordinated IL-4-mediated signaling program is revealed which appears to have evolved for the purpose of using IL-4 and/or IL-13 for directly costimulating the resting B cell for clonal expansion, switching to and synthesis of IgE, and for facilitating the focusing of cytokine- and contact-mediated Th2-type help onto the B cell for this purpose, in part through modulation of B-cell membrane proteins and in part through directing Th2 differentiation.

Consistent with the theme followed for discussions of each of the cytokines in this book, the authors in this chapter summarize the molecular characteristics of IL-4 and IL-13, their receptors, and the manner in which and cell types from which they are produced. In addition, as will be seen throughout this book, cytokines such as IL-4 and IL-13 are shown to exert their effects not in isolation, but in the context of a cytokine network. Specifically, the functional consequences coincident with a given cytokine's actions will depend upon the presence of other cytokines, as well as activators, that may deliver signals which are additive, synergistic or inhibitory to those imparted by that particular cytokine. Thus, in regard to one major effect of IL-4 and IL-13 on B cells, induction of IgE synthesis, we find that costimulation with IL-5, IL-6 or TNF-α will enhance IL-4-

dependent IgE synthesis, whereas the actions of IL-10, IL-12, IFN-γ, IFN-α and TGF-β can be inhibitory. In this regard, not all of the effects of these cytokines are mediated directly at the level of the B cell, but instead are accomplished through actions on other cell types. Similarly, IL-4 has been shown to induce IgE class switching in murine B cells stimulated with certain activators, such as CD40 ligand or LPS, but not in B cells activated through multivalent membrane Ig crosslinking, despite its ability to stimulate murine IgG1 class switching with any of the three modes of activation.

In a final section, the authors describe an exciting model, the SCID-hu mouse, in which human T and B cells and macrophages are grafted into a T- and B-cell-deficient (SCID) mouse. This model allows for the study of human immune responsiveness, including IL-4-dependent IgE synthesis, in an *in vivo* environment that can be manipulated experimentally. Using the SCID-hu mouse and a novel human IL-4 mutant protein, which binds to the IL-4 receptor without signaling it, and thus acts as an inhibitor of natural IL-4 action, the authors describe data showing the ability of this mutant protein to significantly inhibit ongoing human IgE responses *in vivo*. The potential for this novel protein antagonist to be used therapeutically for human allergic disease is thus revealed, as well as a system for studying other potential therapeutic modalities.

In *Chapter 9* Kiyoshi Takatsu develops our current view of IL-5 as a positive regulator of B-cell proliferation, maturation to Ig secretion, and class switch recombination *in vitro*. In these capacities, IL-5 can act in concert with the murine 'switch factors', IL-4 (Chapter 8), TGF-β (Chapter 12) and IFN-γ (Chapter 13) to costimulate the synthesis of and/or switching to the respective Ig isotypes targeted for expression by these latter cytokines (see Chapter 5). Evidence is presented that IL-5 can also prevent apoptosis of B cells and eosinophils, as well as support the development of early B cells. The selective, constitutive expression of IL-5 receptors on a substantial percentage of Ly-1$^{+}$ (B1) B cells (see Chapter 3), and the ability of IL-5 to stimulate Ly-1 B cells in the absence of additional stimuli, suggests a special role for IL-5 in the development and/or function of this B-cell subpopulation. Nevertheless, upon appropriate activation conventional B cells also respond to IL-5. These functional effects of IL-5 are readily demonstrated in a variety of *murine* cellular systems, but effects of IL-5 on human B-cell function have been more difficult to demonstrate, being observed only under a narrow set of conditions. Thus, as will be seen for certain other cytokines, such as IL-10 and IFN-γ, it appears that a significant functional dichotomy has evolved between the mouse and human in how IL-5 is utilized by the immune system. Of note is the fact that a critical *in vivo* role for IL-5 for either mouse or human B-cell responses has not as yet been demonstrated. IL-5, by contrast, appears to be a *key* positive regulator of *in vitro* and/or *in vivo* eosinophil growth and differentiation in both mouse and humans. Indeed, the IL-5 knockout mouse is markedly defective in its induction of eosinophils after an appropriate immune challenge, whereas humoral immunity in the absence of IL-5 appears to be intact, at least under the limited conditions so far studied.

Takatsu develops in some depth a wealth of recent data concerning IL-5 and IL-5 receptor (IL-5R) structure and the signal transduction pathway(s) engaged after IL-5 binding to its receptor. Specific IL-5 binding is shown to be mediated by an IL-5R α chain, but signal transduction occurs only upon interaction of this α chain with a β chain, the latter being common (βc) to IL-3R and GM-CSFR as well. It has been suggested that this βc accounts for the similar, though not identical, functional effects of IL-5, IL-3 and GM-CSF, especially on eosinophils, but, as seen in Chapter 13, on B cells as well.

As with other cytokines, IL-5 appears to act, at least in part, through the Jak–STAT signaling pathway. Like IL-3, IL-6, GM-CSF, G-CSF and IFN-γ, IL-5 induces activation, through tyrosine phosphorylation, of a number of cellular proteins, including the Jak-2 kinase. Tyrosine phosphorylation of proteins containing *Src*-homology 2 (SH2) and/or *Src*-homology 3 (SH3) domains, including PI-3 kinase, the HS-1 protein, Vav protooncogene product, and Shc, have also been implicated in the IL-5 signaling pathway. It is suggested that IL-5Rα contributes to signal transduction by promoting, through its cytoplasmic proline-rich regions, the dimerization of the βc, perhaps leading to cross-phosphorylations of associated Jak-2 kinases. IL-5 binding to its receptor also leads to induction of the growth-regulating oncogenes c-*fos*, c-*jun* and c-*myc*.

Genetic abnormalities in IL-5 signaling may have clinical implications. Thus, recent evidence indicates that the Bruton's tyrosine kinase, Btk, which has been identified as the molecule involved in X-linked human agammaglobulinemia (XLA), is a key component in the IL-5 signaling pathway. A mutation in the *btk* gene has also been identified in XID mice and appears to account for the defective responses of XID B cells to IL-5. Evidence suggests that the *btk* mutation may also account for the striking reduction of peritoneal Ly-1 B cells, and perhaps the reduced serum levels of IgM and IgG3, in XID mice. The normal responsiveness of eosinophils from XID mice to IL-5 strongly suggests that the IL-5 signaling cascade in eosinophils and B cells diverges. A natural soluble form of IL-5Rα has been identified and can be detected in the sera of aged NZB and NZW mice, but not in normal mouse sera, also suggesting a possible role for IL-5 in certain autoimmune diseases (also see Chapter 17). Finally, given the primary role of eosinophils in mediating tissue damage in bronchial asthma, developing the means for selectively inhibiting *in vivo* IL-5 synthesis or action holds great promise as an effective new treatment for this disease.

Tadamitsu Kishimoto and Toshio Tanaka and colleagues detail our current understanding of IL-6 biology in *Chapter 10*, with particular emphasis on its effect on B cells. IL-6 as a central mediator of the early immune/inflammatory response appears to exhibit the broadest range of functions, target cells and cell sources for its synthesis among the major B-cell-active cytokines. In regard to normal B-cell function, the major role of IL-6 appears to be the stimulation of *in vitro* and *in vivo* terminal maturation to Ig secretion, including B cells which have switched to downstream Ig isotypes, whereas IL-6 is revealed as a key autocrine growth factor for B-cell tumors, both *in vitro* and *in vivo*. Although data obtained from IL-6 knockout mice suggest a key role for endogenous IL-6 in mucosal IgA production and demonstrate an effect of IL-6 on a TD antiviral antibody response, it is clear that additional cytokine pathways for maturation of the humoral immune response also exist *in vivo*. Thus, IL-6 appears to be both selective and redundant in its effects on Ig secretion. As might be expected, IL-6, like other cytokines discussed in this book, acts in concert with B-cell-activation stimuli and other cytokines. In particular, the authors reveal an important role for IL-6 in stimulating CD40 plus IL-4-dependent human IgE secretion *in vitro*, by enhancing the levels of productive, secretory $\epsilon$ mRNA in B cells that have already switched to IgE.

The structure of IL-6, its receptor and the nature of IL-6-mediated signal transduction are discussed in detail and shed additional light on the redundancy and pleiotropy of cytokine action. As with most of the other cytokine receptors, including IL-2R$\beta$, IL-2R$\gamma$ ($\gamma$c), IL-3R, IL-4R, IL-5R, IL-7R, IL-9R, G-CSFR, GM-CSFR and IL-6-signal transducer (gp130), IL-6R is a member of the *type 1 cytokine receptor family*. IL-6-mediated signaling involves an interaction of IL-6R with gp130, a signal transducer common to other cytokine receptors, with induction of both the Jak–STAT signaling pathway and the Ras-dependent MAP kinase signaling cascade. Thus, we now see that, on one level, cytokine redundancy segregates into three broad families encompassing the common signal transducers gp130 (IL-6, Oncostatin-M, leukemia inhibitory factor, ciliary neurotrophic factor and perhaps IL-11R), $\beta$c (IL-3, IL-5 and GM-CSF) and $\gamma$c (IL-2, IL-4, IL-7 and perhaps IL-9 and IL-13). By contrast, we will see that IFN-$\gamma$ and IL-10 mediate their effects through receptors comprising the *type 2 cytokine receptor family*.

The molecular mechanism through which IL-6 stimulates Ig secretion is discussed and seen to lie in part with the ability of IL-6 to induce both the Oct-2 and NF-IL-6 transcription factors which bind to a ATGCAAAT octomer and E box motif, respectively both present in the Ig promoters and enhancers. The finding of C/EBP sites, which are homologous to NF-IL-6, in the germline $C_H\epsilon$ and $C_H\gamma1$ promoters suggests a possible role for IL-6 in germline $C_H$ transcription, although no data are provided in this regard.

The multiplicity of IL-6 action in immune and inflammatory responses forms a basis for understanding its demonstrated and presumed role in such disease states as: (1) multiple myeloma; (2) autoimmune phenomena and hypergammaglobulinemia associated with cardiac myxoma, Castleman's disease, and rheumatoid arthritis; (3) mesangial proliferative glomerulonephritis; and (4) paraneoplastic syndromes associated with a number of malignancies. The therapeutic potential of neutralizing IL-6 in such conditions is discussed. The ability of IL-6 to stimulate cytotoxic T-cell function and antibody-dependent cellular cytotoxicity (ADCC) by peripheral blood mononuclear cells (PBMC) suggests a role for IL-6 administration in the treatment of malignancy. IL-6 stimulation of multilineage hematopoiesis and maturation of megakaryocytes also suggests a role for IL-6 delivery in a number of additional clinical settings.

In *Chapter 11* Francine Briere *et al.* underscore a key role for IL-10, a cytokine originally defined by its ability to act on macrophages to suppress cytokine production by $CD4^+$ T cells of the Th1 type, as an important regulator of B-cell function. Perhaps more than those of other cytokines that act on B cells, the effects of IL-10 on murine versus human B cells appear to be substantially different. In humans, unlike in mice, IL-10 appears to be a major positive regulator of proliferation, Ig secretion, and perhaps Ig class switching. Thus, Chapters 7, 8 and 11 reveal IL-2, IL-4 and IL-10, respectively, as key positive regulators of both proliferation and Ig secretion in human B cells, but, as the authors point out, IL-10 stands out among these cytokines for its particular ability to strongly stimulate Ig synthesis. This point is highlighted by the recent demonstration of a major role for IL-10 in stimulating autoantibody production in patients with systemic lupus erythematosus (SLE) and suggests future therapeutic strategies for this relatively common condition. IL-10 may also be important in the induction of switching to human IgG1 and IgG3. This observation, in addition to a lack of any demonstrated effect of IFN-$\gamma$ for induction of switching to the various IgG subclasses in the human (see Chapter 13), suggests significant divergent evolution between mouse and human in cytokine regulation of switching to various IgG subclasses, consistent with the distinct structural differences of the $C_H\gamma$ locus between these two species (see Chapter 5).

In constrast to human B cells, limited murine studies indicate a negative influence of IL-10 for both B-cell proliferation and Ig secretion, although recent unpublished data from our laboratory demonstrate that IL-10 augments the percentage of murine B cells switching to IgG3, while inhibiting the switch to IgA, in LPS-activated cells. IL-10 production is clearly upregulated during at least some murine humoral immune responses *in vivo*, although its physiological role in regulating B-cell function under these circumstances is unclear. Nevertheless, IL-10 does not appear to be critical for humoral immunity, in that mice made genetically deficient in IL-10 expression have normal B-cell development and display normal levels of serum Ig isotypes. Since IL-10 downregulates IFN-$\gamma$ production by T cells, it could also act indirectly to regulate both human and murine B-cell function.

IL-10 may have clinical relevance in disease states involving perturbations in B-cell function and humoral immunity. Thus, in addition to its potential importance in mediating autoantibody production in autoimmune diseases such as SLE, IL-10 may be of importance in regulating the course of B-cell transformation and neoplasia, IgA deficiency, and perhaps common variable immunodeficiency (CVI).

In *Chapter 12* Janet Stavnezer discusses the role of TGF-β in B-cell proliferation, Ig secretion and Ig class switching. TGF-β is revealed to possess both suppressive and inductive effects on B cells. In both murine and human systems TGF-β exerts antiproliferative effects on B cells by preventing or slowing their progress from late G1 to the S phase of the cell cycle in a reversible fashion without inducing apoptosis. This antiproliferative effect, however, can be modulated by the presence of additional cytokines or activators. The signaling events underlying TGF-β regulation of the cell cycle are discussed. Specifically, TGF-β-induced changes in the expression or activity of the oncogene c-*myc*, the anti-oncogene Rb, the transcription factor E2F, and members of the family of cyclin-dependent kinases (CDKs) are implicated in TGF-β action. TGF-β is made by a multitude of cell types, including B cells, and its production as an active molecule is revealed to have many regulatory levels. Autocrine TGF-β is shown to regulate proliferation, differentiation and/or class switching by normal or neoplastic human and murine B cells. Evidence is presented that TGF-β may also play a role in B-cell, as well as thymocyte, development. TGF-β is typically observed to inhibit B-cell differentiation to Ig secretion in both murine and human B cells, independent of its antiproliferative effects, although this also can be modulated by the presence of additional activators and/or cytokines. A possible role for the transcription factors Oct-2 and AP-1 in TGF-β-induced downregulation of B-cell differentiation is discussed.

A key role for TGF-β in directing the class switch to IgA in both murine and human B cells is discussed in some detail both at the cellular and molecular levels. Indeed, human IgA deficiency is discussed as possibly resulting from a defect in the production of active TGF-β. Optimal IgA class switching is shown to result from the cooperative action of TGF-β with a combination of several B-cell activators and/or cytokines. The mechanism for TGF-β induction of IgA switching is shown to involve the transcriptional activation of the Cα gene prior to its switch rearrangement, through TGF-β induction of a specific 5′ α promoter. Promoter activity is shown to depend at least in part upon the binding of several transcription factors, including Ets and ATF/CRE family members, to a unique sequence within the α promoter. Finally, TGF-β is also shown to be a switch factor for murine IgG2b, as well as IgA in appropriately activated B cells. Little is known regarding the role of TGF-β in regulating humoral immunity *in vivo*, but its importance, especially in mucosal immunity, is strongly suspected.

In *Chapter 13*, I discuss the ability of IFN-γ to regulate B-cell function *in vitro*, and Ig secretory responses *in vivo*. Much like TGF-β (see Chapter 12), IFN-γ can be either inductive or suppressive of B-cell function, depending upon the attendant activational milieu and the parameter being studied. Like IL-10 (see Chapter 11), IFN-γ, especially in regard to Ig isotype expression, and perhaps B-cell maturation to Ig secretion, appears to demonstrate significant functional differences when the murine and human immune systems are compared. The molecular nature of IFN-γ, its receptor and signal transduction pathway and the cellular sources for its production are discussed. Similar to certain cytokines such as IL-2, IL-3, IL-4 and IL-5, where the cellular sources for their production are relatively limited, and *unlike* IL-6, IL-10, TGF-β and GM-CSF, which are produced by a wide array of cell types, IFN-γ synthesis is restricted, predominantly, to two cell types, T cells and NK cells, although its production by macrophages has been recently described.

Like a number of other cytokines, IFN-γ mediates its functional effects through the selective use of members of the Jak–STAT signaling pathway. In both the murine and human system IFN-γ shares the ability to inhibit IL-4-mediated IgE responses under certain, but not all, conditions, although the mechanisms through which this occurs may differ. By contrast, whereas IFN-γ induces IgG2a and IgG3 switching in the mouse, there are no convincing data implicating an inductive role for IFN-γ in human Ig class switching, and indeed this role in humans may have been adopted by IL-10 (see Chapter 11). Thus, we see that to date the evidence indicates that only IL-4 (for IgE) and TGF-β (for IgA) are clearly conserved between mouse and human for their ability to induce Ig class switching.

In the mouse, *in vivo* studies have confirmed a physiological role for endogenous IFN-γ in stimulating and inhibiting IgG2a and IgE synthesis, respectively. In particular, IFN-γ appears to be the mediator of the virus-induced shift toward IgG2a production *in vivo* observed during many, though not all, viral infections, and can also account for the selective production of IgG2a in response to certain bacteria. Its role in mediating murine IgG3 responses *in vivo* is less certain.

In the mouse IFN-γ has been found to be either inductive or suppressive for B-cell maturation to Ig secretion, depending upon the manner in which the B cell is activated, the timing of IFN-γ action, and the presence of other cytokines. By contrast, human studies have typically failed to implicate IFN-γ as an Ig-inducing cytokine, although IL-10 (see above) demonstrates this property. IFN-γ is highly stimulatory for Ig secretion by murine B cells activated through multivalent membrane Ig crosslinkage, but is either ineffective or inhibitory for Ig secretion in response to T cells or CD40 signaling, and LPS. The inductive effect of IFN-γ further appears to require costimulation with IL-2, and is augmented in the presence of IL-3 and/or GM-CSF. The more stringent requirements thus necessary to allow for Th1-mediated, as opposed to Th2-mediated, induction of Ig secretion may account in part for the experimental data to date, which emphasize the Th2 cytokine profile for induction of humoral immunity. However, substantial Ig secretion is often also observed during immune responses dominated by Th1 cytokines. Further, despite extensive *in vitro* data on the B-cell-activating properties of cytokines, and a number of *in vivo* associations between the synthesis of certain cytokines and Ig secretion (see below), the cytokines responsible for stimulating maturation to Ig secretion during most *in vivo* humoral immune responses have not as yet been established.

This chapter also includes recent data from my laboratory establishing a novel role for IL-3 and GM-CSF in stimulating murine B-cell maturation to Ig secretion. Like that observed for IFN-γ, the IL-3 and GM-CSF induction also requires multivalent membrane Ig crosslinkage, must act in concert with IL-2, and fails to stimulate Ig secretion by B cells activated through CD40 alone. Collectively, the data indicate at least several potential cytokine pathways which can lead to the elicitation of an Ig secretory response, under varying conditions.

Hajime Kimata brings to a close the second section of this book with *Chapter 14*, discussing the role of neuropeptides in regulating B- and T-cell proliferation, Ig synthesis and Ig class switching in mice and humans. The ability of vasoactive intestinal peptide (VIP), somatostatin (SOM), and substance P (SP) to either directly or indirectly (through monocytes and T cells) regulate *in vitro* B-cell function suggests a key link between the nervous and immune systems, especially during allergic and inflammatory processes. The finding that VIP, SOM and SP are also released by neutrophils, eosinophils and mononuclear cells, and in turn regulate the release of other cytokines such as IL-1, IL-2, IL-6, IFN-γ and TNF-α, further suggests that the immune/inflammatory system itself has incorporated these mediators as part of its own repertoire.

Consistent with a theme developed throughout this book, the effects of neuropeptides, be they stimulatory or inhibitory for a given B-cell function, will depend upon the manner in which the B cell is activated, the particular B-cell function being studied, such as the production of specific Ig isotypes, the presence of other cell types, especially monocytes and T cells, and the additional influence of other cytokines. Three major areas are discussed in detail, the effect of neuropeptides on: (1) Ig secretion by human B-cell tumors; (2) IL-4-induced Ig isotype production, especially synthesis of IgE and IgG4; and (3) spontaneous production of IgE and IgG4 by B cells from atopic individuals.

VIP is found to directly enhance Ig synthesis by B-cell tumors. In IL-4-stimulated cultures the effects of neuropeptides on Ig isotype production are found to require the presence of both monocytes and T cells. Neuropeptides regulate IL-4-induced IgE and IgG4 synthesis at the level of Ig class switching; VIP and SOM inhibit IgE production, whereas SOM and SP enhance the synthesis of IgG4. By contrast, neuropeptide enhancement of IgG2 and inhibition of IgG3 synthesis in these IL-4-dependent cultures is at the level of the post-switched cell. Finally, in atopic patients, VIP, SOM and SP inhibit the spontaneous *in vitro* synthesis of both IgE and IgG4. This effect also appears to require monocytes and T cells, but appears to act at the level of the post-switched cell. The overall pattern of Ig isotype regulation effected by neuropeptides appear unique to this class of mediators, and indeed neuropeptides do not appear to exert their effects through well-characterized endogenous factors. The ability of neuropeptides to stimulate proinflammatory cytokines, induce histamine secretion from mast cells and promote eosinophil infiltration suggests that they play an augmenting role in allergic and inflammatory responses. The observation, however, that neuropeptides inhibit IL-4-induced and spontaneous IgE production suggests that neuropeptides may additionally limit the intensity of such allergic and inflammatory reactions, in a negative feedback loop.

In *Chapter 15* Robert Coffman summarizes the key parameters which govern *in vivo* IgE responses in allergy and helminth parasite infections. As the author points out, more is known about the physiological regulation of this Ig isotype than any of the others. This reflects, in part, its extremely low basal level of production and its dramatic induction by, and absolute dependence upon, a single cytokine in the mouse, IL-4, and the closely related cytokine pair in humans, IL-4 and IL-13. Thus, this chapter complements the material discussed in Chapter 8. The particularly tight regulation of IgE production probably reflects its unique, but potentially harmful, property of mediating mast cell degranulation upon crosslinkage with allergen or antigen. Clearly, an understanding of IgE regulation has major implications for designing therapeutic strategies for control of allergic disease in humans. Indeed, the observation that IL-4 is absolutely necessary for a primary IgE response, and plays a significant role in a secondary IgE response, suggests that sustained IgE production requires ongoing IL-4-dependent IgE switching. Thus controlling established IgE-dependent clinical disease at the level of IL-4 production or action would appear feasible.

In addition to IL-4 and/or IL-13 as the key IgE-inductive cytokines, we appreciate the role of a number of cytokines, including IFN-$\gamma$ (see Chapter 13), IFN-$\alpha$ and IL-12, as directly or indirectly inhibiting IL-4-induced IgE production. This is accomplished through their antagonizing IL-4 action on B cells and/or shifting an immune response from the IgE-inductive Th2 to the IgE-suppressive Th1 pattern of $CD4^+$ T-cell cytokine production (see Chapter 6). We also see from other chapters that TGF-$\beta$ may also play a role in downregulating IL-4-dependent IgE switching. In addition, the B cell must be activated in an appropriate fashion in order for IL-4 to induce the IgE class switch. CD40L, which is expressed transiently on activated T cells, appears to be the key physiological trigger for IL-4-dependent IgE switching *in vivo*. By contrast, murine B cells activated through multivalent membrane Ig crosslinking, as might occur with TI-2 (polysaccharide) antigens, fail to switch to IgE in response to IL-4, while being capable of switching to and synthesizing all other Ig isotypes, except IgG2b. Finally, we see that whereas *in vitro* studies, especially in the human, suggested a key role for CD23

(FcεRII) in IgE regulation, CD23 transgenic and knockout mice fail to reveal a critical role for CD23 in IgE regulation *in vivo*.

Overall, an appealing model for induction of human allergy has emerged involving cytokine produced by the CD4+ Th2 subset. Thus, IL-4 and/or IL-13 are the key stimulators of IgE, IL-5 appears essential for induction of eosinophilia, and IL-3, IL-4 and IL-10 participate in the outgrowth of mast cells. The CD4+ Th1 subset may in turn downregulate IgE through production of IFN-γ.

Beagley *et al.* discuss in *Chapter 16* the role of cytokines in regulating the humoral immune response at mucosal surfaces. In particular, because mucosal microenvironments are highly enriched for the expression and synthesis of IgA, attention is focused on the parameters that selectively induce the class switch to IgA and the subsequent differentiation of membrane IgA+ cells into IgA-secreting plasma cells. To some extent this material complements that discussed in the previous chapter on TGF-β, a switch factor for the IgA class. The structure–function relationship of the mucosa-associated lymphoreticular tissues (MALT) is discussed in detail and is seen to divide between inductive sites, such as the Peyer's patch where IgA switching occurs, and effector sites, for example the lamina propria, where large numbers of IgA-secreting plasma cells are found. No doubt the regulatory influences at these two functionally distinct sites, including the cytokine profile that is elaborated, will differ.

Unlike other lymphoid sites, the MALT, especially that found in the gastrointestinal tract (i.e. GALT), is unique by virtue of its close proximity to a rich and varied microbial/antigenic milieu, and its possessing mechanisms through which lymphoid cells can constitutively sample and respond to such stimuli. Thus it is no surprise to learn that both the inductive and effector sites are constitutively and highly active, independent of the presence of any pathogenic organisms. This implies in turn that mechanisms to limit these responses must be in place, and indeed a system for inducing tolerance to particular antigens, including food antigens, is revealed, and appears to involve a number of cytokines, including TGF-β. The GALT is also shown to be distinct in its possession of a unique regulatory T cell, the intraepithelial lymphocyte (IEL); the characteristics of the IEL are discussed in detail.

A number of studies on induction of humoral immunity in the MALT have shown a strong positive association between Ig secretory responses at this site and the elaboration of an essentially 'Th2' pattern of cytokine secretion, including IL-4, IL-5, IL-6 and IL-10. Indeed, mice made genetically deficient in either IL-4 or IL-10 expression were shown to have functional abnormalities in IgA expression in the GALT. An association between induction of an Ig secretory response and elaboration of Th2 cytokines is also revealed in the discussion in the next chapter on autoimmunity. Whereas the MALT may 'tend' towards Th2 immune responses, it is nevertheless capable of mounting a Th1 response, as evidenced, for example, by its predominant synthesis of IFN-γ after infection with *Salmonella typhimurium* (see Chapter 6). Thus, similar to that observed in certain autoimmune states, the elaboration of IFN-γ, which has been shown in other circumstances to stimulate Ig secretion under appropriate conditions (see Chapter 13), suggests that it could play an inductive role in the MALT, as well as downregulate IL-4-mediated responses. As discussed in Chapter 12, although no direct role for TGF-β in regulating IgA responses *in vivo* has yet been demonstrated, its importance in regulating mucosal immune responses is strongly suggested on the basis of *in vitro* studies. The implications of these observations for the rational design of mucosal vaccines, including those engineered for induction of protective immunity, or for limiting certain autoimmune phenomena through establishment of tolerance to the inciting antigen, are discussed.

In *Chapter 17*, Eri Hagiwara and Dennis Klinman detail our current knowledge concerning dysregulations in cytokine production and/or responsiveness, and their potential roles in the pathogenesis of murine models, and human disease states associated with autoimmune-mediated B-cell hyperactivity and hypergammaglobulinemia. The authors discuss *in vitro* and/or *in vivo* studies exploring the mechanisms of immune dysfunction in SLE and experimental SLE-like states (i.e. NZB, B/W and MRL/lpr mice), rheumatoid arthritis (RA), experimental $HgCl_2$-induced autoimmunity and neonatal graft versus host disease, Castleman's disease and cardiac myxoma. Throughout the book we will come to appreciate the ability of Th2 cytokines such as IL-4, IL-5, IL-6 and IL-10 to promote B-cell growth and/or differentiation to Ig secretion. As the authors point out, the most notable perturbations in cytokine production associated with hypergammaglobulinemia, especially SLE, appear to involve overproduction of Th2 cytokines. We will read, however, both in Chapter 7 and Chapter 13, that Th1 cytokines such IL-2 and IFN-γ, respectively, as well as IL-3 and GM-CSF, under appropriate conditions, are also capable of strongly stimulating Ig secretion, and learn here, for example, that the overproduction of IgG autoantibodies observed in MRL/lpr mice is associated with a shift towards a Th1 pattern of cytokine production, and that long-term administration of IFN-γ to NZB mice accelerates their production of autoantibodies.

The authors devote substantial effort towards critically assessing the 'complexity and pitfalls of ascribing disease manifestations to specific cytokine abnormalities'. This should constitute sound advice to both basic and clinical scientists when formulating study design and drawing conclusions from the data obtained. Unfortunately, although we have come to appreciate a fair degree of phenomenology regarding abnormalities in cytokine synthesis and responsiveness in B-cell hyperactivity states, the authors conclude that compelling models of etiology and pathogenesis which need to incorporate these observations remain to be formulated. As the authors state, this experimental resolution is, in part, frustrated by the fact that 'perturbation of the cytokine milieu has multiple effects on the immune system', making direct cause and effect assessments difficult. Nevertheless, even our current understanding may allow for the consideration of therapeutic strategies encompassing cytokine administration and/or blockade of cytokine action for ameliorating the Ig overproduction and immune complex formation which underlie much of the tissue damage observed in these conditions.

# 2 T-cell-independent and T-cell-dependent Humoral Immunity

**JON D. LAMAN and ERIC CLAASSEN**
*TNO Prevention and Health, Leiden, The Netherlands*

## INTRODUCTION

This chapter deals with the antibody response against T-cell-independent (TI) versus T-cell-dependent (TD) antigens. How do their different structural properties determine the way in which these antigens engage distinct cell types of the immune system, ultimately resulting in a specific antibody response? How does the nature of the antigen determine the quality of the antibody response as defined by isotype profile, affinity maturation and memory formation? How does the functional organization of spleen and lymph nodes dictate which antigens, cell types and cytokines can interact during an *in vivo* response? Which signals (i.e. cognate interactions, induction of accessory molecules, cytokines) are required to initiate the humoral response, and how do TI and TD antigens differ in this respect?

We will attempt to shed light on these questions by first detailing the characteristics of TI and TD antigens, followed by a brief description of the anatomy of spleen and lymph nodes with emphasis on features relevant to the humoral immune response. Next, routing of antigens into secondary lymphoid tissues and handling by different cell types in the intact animal will be touched upon. This will set the stage for discussion of the mechanisms operational in TI and TD B-cell activation, with a proposed sequence of events for TI and TD responses *in vivo*. Special attention will be given to the aspect of B-cell memory formation. Finally, we formulate a number of questions which in our eyes are in urgent need of an answer to improve the understanding of lymphocyte activation and the requirements for efficient induction of specific antibody. Such understanding is instrumental in the rational development of new vaccine technology and treatment of antibody-mediated autoimmune disease. Examples of TI and TD antigens have been listed in Table 2.1 and some of their properties in Table 2.2.

*Cytokine Regulation of Humoral Immunity: Basic and Clinical Aspects.* Edited by Clifford M. Snapper.

**Table 2.1** Thymus-independent and -dependent antigens

| | |
|---|---|
| **Thymus-independent Type 1** | |
| Soluble | LPS and haptenated derivatives |
| | *Nocardia* water-soluble mitogen and haptenated derivatives |
| | *Neisseria meningitidis* outer membrane proteins |
| | Dextran sulfate |
| Particulate | *Brucella abortus* and haptenated derivatives |
| | *Neisseria meningitidis* heat-killed bacteria |
| | Streptococci |
| | High epitope density acrylamide beads and haptenated derivatives |
| **Thymus-independent Type 2** | |
| Soluble | Capsular polysaccharides from pneumococcal bacteria |
| | Streptococcal carbohydrates |
| | *Haemophilus influenzae* polysaccharides |
| | *Neisseria meningitidis* polysaccharides |
| | Phosphorylcholine |
| | Detoxified LPS |
| | Haptenated Ficoll |
| | Haptenated HES |
| | Haptenated dextran |
| | Dextrane levane |
| | Bacterial levane and haptenated derivatives |
| | Polyvinylpyrrolidone |
| | R36A |
| | Polynucleotides [poly (I:C)] |
| | Dextran-coupled anti-IgD or anti-IgM antibodies |
| | Synthetic polymers of D-isomer amino acids |
| Particulate | Low epitope density acrylamide beads |
| | Liposomes without protein |
| | Haptenated liposomes |
| **Thymus-dependent** | |
| Soluble | Proteins, such as KLH, OVA, BSA, CGC, myoglobin |
| | Haptenated protein derivatives |
| | Bacterial proteins such as tetanus toxoid and diphtheria toxoid |
| | Synthetic peptide conjugated protein derivatives |
| | Synthetic peptides containing at least one B-cell and one T-cell epitope |
| | RαIgD, GαIgD |
| Particulate | Sheep red blood cells |
| | Nucleated cells |
| | Viruses |
| | Parasites |
| | TNP-*Lactobacillus* |

Compiled from: Stein[4]; Subbarao and Garg[5]; Laman *et al.*[6]

**Table 2.2** Properties of thymus-independent and -dependent antigens

| Antigen type | Examples | Handling by | Presentation by B cells direct | Mitogenic activity | Memory formation |
|---|---|---|---|---|---|
| **Thymus-independent type 1** | | | | | |
| Soluble | LPS | MZM, RPM | B cells direct | + | – |
| | Dextran sulfate | ? | B cells direct | + | ± |
| Particulate | *Brucella abortus* | MZM, F | MZM, B cells | + | ± |
| **Thymus-independent type 2** | | | | | |
| Soluble | Dextran | MZM, B cells, FDC | FDC, B cells (MZ/F) | – | – |
| | TNP-Ficoll/HES | MZM, B cells, FDC | FDC, B cells (MZ/F) | – | – |
| | Detoxified LPS | MZM, B cells, FDC | FDC, B cells (MZ/F) | – | – |
| Particulate | Liposomes (no protein) | MZM | B cells (MZ/F), FDC | – | – |
| | Haptenated liposomes | MZM | B cells (MZ/F), FDC | – | – |
| **Thymus-dependent** | | | | | |
| Soluble | Globular proteins | RPM, IDC | IDC, B cells | – | + |
| | RαIgD, GαIgD | B cells | B cells | + | + |
| Particulate | Liposomes with protein | MZM (RPM) | IDC, B cells | – | + |
| | SRBC | MZM (RPM) | IDC, B cells | – | + |
| | TNP-*Lactobacillus* | MZM (RPM), FDC | FDC, IDC, B cells | – | + |

This table is mostly based on studies in the mouse.
RαIgD and GαIgD are globular protein antigens, but in addition to that they have mitogenic properties by virtue of their sIgD-crosslinking capacity.
F, follicle; RP, red pulp; MZ, marginal zone; M, macrophage; RPM, red pulp macrophages.
Compiled from Laman *et al.*[6] Van den Eertwegh *et al.*[7]

Because the matter of this chapter has been the subject of several extensive reviews in the past, we aim to limit our discussion of basic concepts, and to focus on recent developments, including new insights provided by the application of targeted disruption of immunologically relevant genes (reviewed in reference 1).

## T-CELL-INDEPENDENT AND -DEPENDENT ANTIGENS

### TI ANTIGENS

TI antigens were originally defined as the class of substances able to induce a specific antibody response without the requirement for T cells. TI antigens in general are large molecules with repeating determinants, which enable them to crosslink receptors on B cells for activation without T-cell involvement (see p. 39 for discussion of mechanisms).

TI antigens are poorly degradable and are able to generate responses in nude mice lacking T cells[2,3]. Physiologically, the TI antibody response is extremely important in providing protection against bacterial infections by pathogens like *Streptococcus pneumoniae, Neisseria meningitidis* and *Hemophilus influenzae*. The polysaccharides of the bacterial capsule with their repeating oligosaccharides are TI antigens, inducing specific antibodies leading to complement-mediated lysis, opsonization, and phagocytosis of the bacteria. However, if rigorous attention is given to complete depletion of T cells in experiments, the concept of T-cell independence does not hold up. More recent data have shown that accessory cells and T cells can definitely contribute to the magnitude and quality of the TI antibody response through cytokines or cell-bound stimuli. TI responses have evolved to deal with bacterial pathogens, but several synthetic model antigens have been shown to mimic such naturally occurring antigens. Ficoll, a neutral synthetic polysaccharide, and the Gram-negative bacterial capsule component lipopolysaccharide (LPS), are widely used as standard TI antigen models (see Table 2.1). In addition, haptenated dextran and dextran-coupled antibodies to IgM and IgD (anti-μ-dextran, anti-δ-dextran) on the B-cell surface have been used extensively.

Immunization with TI antigen does not require the use of an adjuvant. Both IgM and IgG are produced in humans and mice, both in relatively low amounts, and in a one-to-one ratio that changes very little upon secondary immunization. In contrast to TD responses, there is some significant subclass restriction: mice have high levels of IgG3 after immunization with polysaccharides. The restriction is less marked in humans, but more IgG2 is produced[4].

TI antigens can be endowed with TD characteristics by coupling them to protein carriers, which has obvious implications for vaccine development and probing of lymphocyte activation mechanisms. TI antigen–protein conjugates induce isotype profiles which are a mixture of those induced by either component alone and can generate memory[4]. In general, TI antigens are unable to induce the formation of B-cell memory, germinal centers or affinity maturation.

Murine and human neonates are deficient in their response against TI antigens, which presents a challenge for development of bacterial vaccines protecting children after their maternal antibodies disappear. The cause for this defect is not known at present.

Within the group of TI antigens two subtypes have been defined. TI-1 antigens such as haptenated LPS and *Brucella abortus* are naturally occurring antigens which activate B cells directly. TI-1 antigens can induce antibody responses in neonatal mice and CBA/N mice[2,3]. Neonatal mice have impaired antibody responses and CBA/N (*xid*) mice have an X-linked recessive immunodeficiency, leading to abnormal humoral immunity. Many TI-1 antigens have mitogenic capacity. The lipid-A component in LPS, for instance, is responsible for its mitogenicity. Detoxification of LPS can be achieved by removing the lipid-A component. However, mitogenic capacity is not a distinctive property of TI-1 antigens, as there are also some TI-2 antigens with mitogenic capacity, e.g. levan and poly(I:C). Antigens of the TI-2 subtype are, for example, pneumococcal polysaccharide and Ficoll, the latter being a synthetic model TI-2 antigen. In contrast to the TI-1 subtype, antigens of the TI-2 subtype do not induce antibodies in neonatal or CBA/N mice.

More detail on the properties and classification of TI antigens can be found in the systematic and elaborate review by Subbarao and Garg[5].

## T-CELL-DEPENDENT ANTIGENS

By definition, presence of functional T cells is indispensable for specific antibody formation against TD antigens, as was shown by classical experiments using thymectomy, thymic transplants and nude mice. Typically, TD antigens are protein antigens (for example KLH, BSA, OVA, BGG, CGG), protein–hapten conjugates or protein–synthetic peptide conjugates (see Table 2.1). Proteins in general do not contain repeating B-cell epitopes which would allow them to engage multiple antigenic receptors on the same individual B cell in the way that TI antigens can. Instead, protein antigens are taken up by specialized cell types serving as antigen-presenting cells (APC), i.e. dendritic cells/interdigitating cells (IDC), macrophages, or B cells themselves. Antigens are digested by the proteolytic machinery of the APCs, and peptides are displayed on the surface anchored in the MHC class II molecule. $CD4^+$ T-helper cells (Th) carrying the appropriate T-cell receptor (TCR) can interact with the peptide plus MHC and become activated. For subsequent B-cell activation, cell–cell contact (cognate interaction) between

T and B cells is required, as well as production of cytokines by the T cell. The requirement for cell–cell contact indicates that membrane ligand–receptor interactions form an essential part of the activation mechanism. This process will be discussed in detail on p. 44. The activation of B cells for antibody production by TD antigens is therefore fundamentally different from that by TI antigens.

Another important difference is that TD antigens induce B-cell memory, i.e. upon second exposure to the same TD antigen the ensuing antibody response is more rapid, reaches higher titers and has a different isotype profile. Primary immunization with a TD antigen leads to a short-lived rise in specific IgM titer and some IgG coming up later. In contrast, secondary immunization leads to an accelerated response of both IgM and IgG, with IgG titers reaching sustained high levels. In addition, as a result of affinity maturation, the antibodies of the secondary response have higher affinity. In both mice and humans, the predominant isotype elicited by TD antigens is IgG1. IgG2 is also present. Relatively little IgG3 is produced in the mouse, while IgG3 and IgG4 are low in humans[4]. Memory B cells are generated in the germinal centers present in lymph nodes and spleen. Both the formation of germinal centers and reactivation of memory B cells are dependent on T-cell help. This will be discussed in more detail on p. 57.

## FUNCTIONAL ORGANIZATION OF SPLEEN AND LYMPH NODES

### THE SPLEEN

We here concisely review the organization of spleen and lymph nodes as relevant to this chapter. More detailed discussions and primary references on the architecture and function of the spleen can be found in references 6–8. The properties of different cell types in the marginal zone have been extensively reviewed by Kraal[9]. A schematic representation of the mouse spleen is given in Figure 2.1.

#### General Architecture

The spleen is the largest single secondary lymphoid organ in the body and it has often been likened to an immunologic filter. Its functional organization with respect to blood flow and localization of specialized cell types makes it particularly suitable for monitoring the blood, allowing recognition and phagocytosis of antigens, and generation of specific antibody responses. In the spleen, the blood actually leaves the system of endothelium-lined blood vessels, allowing optimal contact between phagocytic cells and foreign particles in the bloodstream.

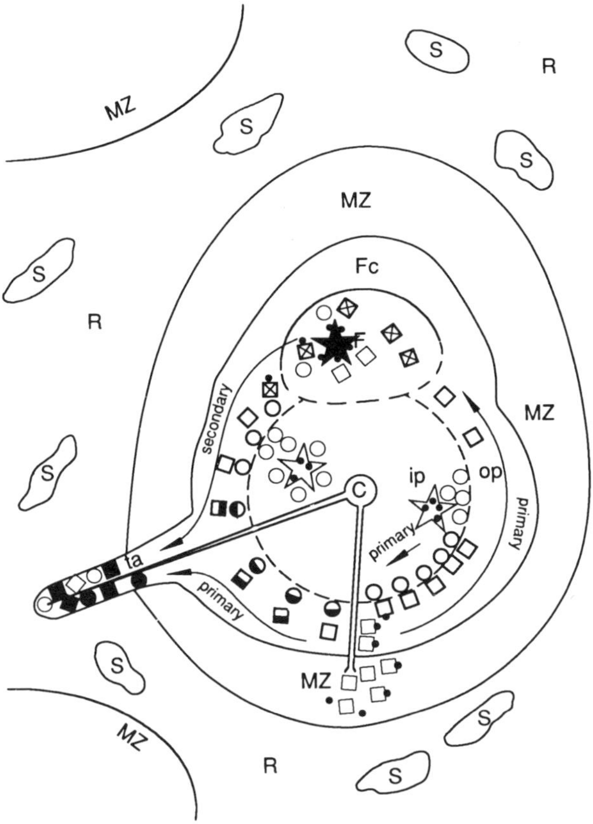


**Figure 2.1** Diagrammatic representation of the murine spleen. In addition, events occurring during primary and secondary immune responses against TD antigens are shown. For discussion, see text. Arrows indicate the migration patterns of B and T cells. Structural elements: MZ, marginal zone; S, sinus; R, red pulp; Fc, follicle corona; F, follicle; C, central arteriole; ip, inner periarteriolar lymphocyte sheath (PALS); op, outer PALS; ta, terminal arteriole. Symbols: small closed circles, antigen; open squares, resting B cells; half-filled squares, differentiating antigen-specific B cells; closed squares, antibody-forming B cell; open circles resting T cells; bold open circles, activated antigen-specific T cells expressing CD40 ligand; filled stars in follicles, follicular dendritic cell; open stars in inner PALS, interdigitating cell

The spleen is morphologically divided into red and white pulp. The red pulp contains large numbers of erythrocytes, lymphocytes, megakaryocytes and macrophages. The red pulp receives the bulk of the blood flow through the spleen, filtering particulate matter and damaged erythrocytes from the circulation.

The white pulp has three compartments: the periarteriolar lymphocyte sheath (PALS), the follicles, and the marginal zone. The PALS is a cuff of cells around the central arteriole. The inner PALS consists mainly of T cells and IDCs, while the outer PALS contains T cells, B cells and macrophages.

Primary follicles are globular structures of resting ($IgM^+/IgD^+$) B cells, attached to the PALS. After stimulation by TD antigen, primary B blasts can migrate into the primary follicle and undergo intense proliferation. This expanding structure is called a germinal center, and together with the rim of $mIgM^+/mIgD^+$ resting B cells being pushed outward, is called a secondary follicle (see p. 57). Tingible body macrophages are present in germinal centers and they are thought to endocytose apoptosing germinal center B cells.

The marginal zone forming the border with the red pulp is the anatomical compartment endowing the spleen with some unique immunologic properties, most notably the efficient removal of foreign particles and the effective generation of B-cell responses against TD, TI-1 and TI-2 antigens. The marginal zone surrounds the PALS and the primary and secondary follicles. B cells and specialized macrophage subsets are the predominant cell types of the marginal zone, while T cells are relatively rare.

## Vascularization of the Spleen

The splenic artery enters the spleen via the hilus. Smaller arteries then follow the trabeculae, the supporting structural elements of the spleen, and branch into the even smaller central arterioles. It is these arterioles which are encompassed by the PALS. Some branches from the central arteriole form a capillary meshwork, while others traverse the white pulp into the red pulp. The latter are called terminal arterioles, and some of them empty into channels formed by cytoplasmic processes of reticular cells. The blood is then collected in venous sinuses. Other terminal arterioles end directly in the marginal zone, either in open sinuses lined by reticular cells, or between the cells. A third type of terminal arteriole provides a direct connection with the venules and this shunt forms the closed circulation of the spleen.

## Cell Types in the Spleen

### *T cells*

About 26 per cent of nucleated cells in the mouse spleen are $CD4^+$ T cells and 8 per cent are $CD8^+$ T cells. Most of the T cells are located in the PALS. In primary and secondary follicles, low numbers of $CD4^+$ T cells are present (1–10 per cent)[7]. $CD8^+$ T cells are found in the follicles only by exception, although in some pathological conditions, like HIV-1 infection, dramatic infiltration of the germinal centers is found (cf. 10). Both CD4 and $CD8^+$ T cells can be found scattered throughout the marginal zone.

*B cells*

B cells are present in the marginal zone, the follicles and the outer PALS. Marginal zone B cells are strongly $mIgM^+$ and $mIgD^-$ (or $mIgD^{\pm}$). In addition, they express IL-2R and complement receptors. They are sessile unless activated by antigen. These characteristics indicate that they are memory B cells. There are also resting marginal zone B cells.

As mentioned, primary follicles contain small resting $mIgM^+/mIgD^+$ B cells. Germinal center B cells are $IgD^-$ and IgG or $IgA^+$. After antigenic challenge, specific B cells proliferate in the PALS and differentiate into plasma cells. It was previously demonstrated that for both TD and TI antigens the specific plasma cells are found in the outer PALS and in the sheaths of lymphoid tissue surrounding the terminal arterioles[11]. Low numbers of plasma cells are found in the red pulp, representing the specific B cells leaving the spleen headed for the bone marrow, the major site of antibody production.

Detailed discussion of phenotype and function of B-cell subpopulations and their microenvironments can be found in Chapter 3.

*Macrophages*

Eleven different macrophage subsets can be defined by phenotypic and functional criteria. The best defined subsets are the red pulp macrophages, marginal zone macrophages and marginal metallophilic macrophages. The function of red pulp macrophages is thought to be restricted to the scavenging of antigen, immune complexes and damaged erythrocytes. Marginal zone macrophages are positioned throughout the marginal zone, from the marginal sinus to the border area with the red pulp. They display high phagocytic activity and have the ability to take up neutral polysaccharides, e.g. TI-2 antigens used as a model for infection with capsular bacteria. Although this is highly suggestive for a function in antigen presentation, a plethora of studies argues otherwise. For instance, marginal zone macrophages do not express MHC class II molecules. *In vivo* elimination of macrophages with a liposome-encapsulated drug followed by differential repopulation of macrophage subsets in time showed that the absence of marginal zone macrophages did not affect the antibody response against soluble TI or TD antigens[12]. Similar conclusions were reached using splenic autotransplants, which also have differential macrophage repopulation. It was concluded that the marginal zone macrophages are highly efficient in taking up and digesting TI-2 antigens, without presenting the antigen (see also p. 35). In contrast, soluble TD antigens are probably processed and presented by IDC and/or B cells, while the soluble TI-2 antigens activate B-cells directly (reviewed in detail in reference 9). However, Delemarre *et al.*[13] showed that marginal zone macrophages are indeed crucial for the response against a particulate haptenated TD antigen, TNP-SRBC (see also p. 35).

*Marginal metallophilic macrophages* This macrophage subset was originally identified by silver impregnation. They are located at the periphery of the white pulp following the inner border of the marginal zone. Hence, moving outward from the central arteriole one finds the inner PALS, outer PALS with follicles, a ring of marginal metallophilic macrophages and a ring of marginal zone macrophages. The role of the marginal metallophilics is obscure, but it has been suggested (reviewed in reference 9) that their high non-specific-esterase activity may be related to degradation of incoming material (for example endotoxin), while their expression of sialic acid-containing glycoconjugates is indicative of a role in lymphocyte homing.

*Follicular dendritic cells (FDC)*

FDCs are found in the follicles and are cells with extensive cellular dendrites, forming a network closely interwoven with follicular B cells. They can trap and retain immune complexes by means of the C3b and Fc receptors on their membrane. This reservoir of persistent antigen is thought to be involved in the induction, maintenance and regulation of the secondary/memory humoral response (see p. 58).

*Interdigitating cells (IDC)*

IDCs are present scattered in the inner PALS, with their dendrites in close contact with the T cells. It has been suggested that Langerhans cells in the skin, veiled cells in the lymph and IDCs in the spleen and lymph node are all the same cell type, seen at different points in migration. *In vitro* studies have suggested that IDGs are highly effective as APFs in primary immune responses against TD antigens and in alloresponses.

*Natural killer (NK) cells*

NK cells are found in the mouse and rat spleen in the red pulp in significant numbers (± 12 per cent), whereas few of these cells are present in the white pulp (± 0.2 per cent). The marginal zone contains ± 2 per cent of NK cells. They are large granular lymphocytes which can lyse neoplastic or virally infected target cells, as well as certain microorganisms, without previous sensitization or MHC restriction. There is some evidence for a role of NK cells in the development of humoral responses (see p. 42).

## The Lymph Node: General Architecture and Cell Types

Lymph nodes are bean-shaped structures clustering in certain areas of the body. The lymph collected locally by the lymphatic capillaries is transported through the afferent lymphatic vessels, which empty in the convex side of the node. Multiple afferent vessels contact the node and after transit of the lymph through the node, where phagocytic filtering and immune responses take place, efferent lymphatics exit from the hilus of the lymph node, eventually leading to the thoracic duct. The hilus is also the site where the nodal arteries go in, and the nodal veins exit.

The afferent lymph enters into the subcapsular or marginal sinus. Here mostly macrophages, dendritic cells and stromal cells are present, as well as some lymphocytes. The lymph then follows the radial sinuses through the cortex, which consists of highly organized regions of lymphocytes, and reaches the medulla. The medulla is made up of connecting compartments of stromal cells and fibers. These are separated by medullary sinuses containing large numbers of plasma cells and macrophages.

The cortex contains B-cell areas with primary and secondary follicles, as described for the spleen, with FDCs, some $CD4^+$ T cells and tingible body macrophages. The $CD4^+$ T cells in the germinal center mostly have a CD45RA-$RO^+$ memory/effector phenotype. In between the follicles are the T-cell areas (paracortex). Postcapillary high endothelial venules (HEV) allow lymphocytes expressing appropriate homing receptors to exit the bloodstream and gain access to the paracortex. Many IDCs are found in the paracortex, but not in the other areas of the lymph node, consistent with their role in T-cell activation.

## FATE OF ANTIGEN *IN VIVO*

### ANTIGEN ADMINISTRATION AND CHARACTERISTICS

Antigen routing and handling *in vivo* is determined by a multitude of parameters related to the immunization/infection and the characteristics of the antigen. Although some of these parameters seem quite obvious, we do mention them here, because if overlooked they may lead to erroneous interpretation of data.

#### Immunization Route

Experimental intraperitoneal (i.p.) immunization will stimulate the spleen, peritoneal macrophages and the mesenteric lymph nodes. Subcutaneous (s.c.) immunization will stimulate the local draining lymph nodes first, but may also reach the spleen by the lymph flow and the thoracic duct. Intravenous (i.v.) immunization is a very effective route to deposit antigen in the spleen, because blood vessels actually open into this organ, and antigen is effectively filtered from the blood (see p. 28). Oral immunization will activate the lymphoid organs of the gastrointestinal tract: specialized epithelial cells (M cells) can take up both particulate and soluble antigens from the lumen and transport them to the underlying lymphoid tissue of the Peyer's patch. There is evidence that differences exist in the capacity of secondary lymphoid tissues (i.e. spleen versus lymph nodes, mesenteric versus peripheral lymph nodes) to mount antibody responses[5,14].

Obviously, the situation is much more complex during natural immunization/infection. Antigen usually gains access to the body through mucosal surfaces (respiratory tract, gastrointestinal tract, genitourinary tract), and often the antigen will be actively replicating. In the case of a wound or during sepsis, antigen can also enter the bloodstream, activating splenic phagocytosis and immune responses. As another example, HIV-1 infection by both sexual transmission and sharing of infected needles is thought to occur by means of infected lymphocytes and macrophages, effectively sequestering the pathogen away from antibodies and complement.

## Use of Adjuvant

TI antigens do not require mixing with an adjuvant to generate good responses, but many researchers do use adjuvants for TD antigens. Although the reason for using adjuvant is clear, i.e. to generate higher titers of antibody, and may be totally acceptable for some purposes, there are several practical and scientific disadvantages:

1. Emulsifying TD antigens in oil-in-water and water-in-oil adjuvants may disrupt discontinuous B-cell epitopes.
2. The mechanism of action of most adjuvants is poorly known: some of them induce cytokine secretion independent of antigen. In addition, antigen–adjuvant micelles will be handled by different cell types (i.e. macrophages) than soluble antigen (i.e. IDCs, B cells). This may distort the physiological picture of the humoral response.
3. Many adjuvants have a depot function, ensuring slow release of antigen over longer periods of time. As a consequence, the distinction between primary and subsequent antibody responses can no longer be made.
4. The commonly used Freund's complete adjuvant (mycobacterium emulsified in mineral oil) provokes severe discomfort in experimental animals. Mechanisms of action of adjuvants, as well as alternatives to the use of Freund's complete adjuvant, have been recently reviewed[15].

In our hands, i.v. immunization with 100 μg of TNP-keyhole limpet hemocyanin (TNP-KLH) (TD) generates excellent immune responses as evaluated by immunocytochemistry and ELISA, thereby obviating the need for adjuvant. For TNP-Ficoll (TI-2), 20 μg given i.v. or i.p. without adjuvant works quite effectively.

## Dose of Antigen

Commonly used doses of purified antigen are in the range of 10–250 μg per injection. Very little is known about the quantities of antigen/pathogen entering the body during a natural immunization/infection, but it can be safely assumed that several log-fold less antigen will be available to the immune system. At this point, we can only begin to suspect how activation processes may operate at such physiological antigen levels, and simply hope the current models reflect this accurately.

In general, minimal doses of antigen will not induce detectable antibody responses. Over the subsequent range of antigen doses, the response will gradually increase, reaching a maximum level. Depending on the antigen, this maximum level and plateau may persist over a wide dose range. At very high doses, the response may decrease and eventually disappear. For *in vivo* immunomodulation studies, it is vital to perform measurements in the dose range comprising the climbing part of the curve. Modulation during the plateau phase is unlikely to yield measurable effects. Figures 2.2 and 2.3 illustrate the points made here about antigen dose. Many of the

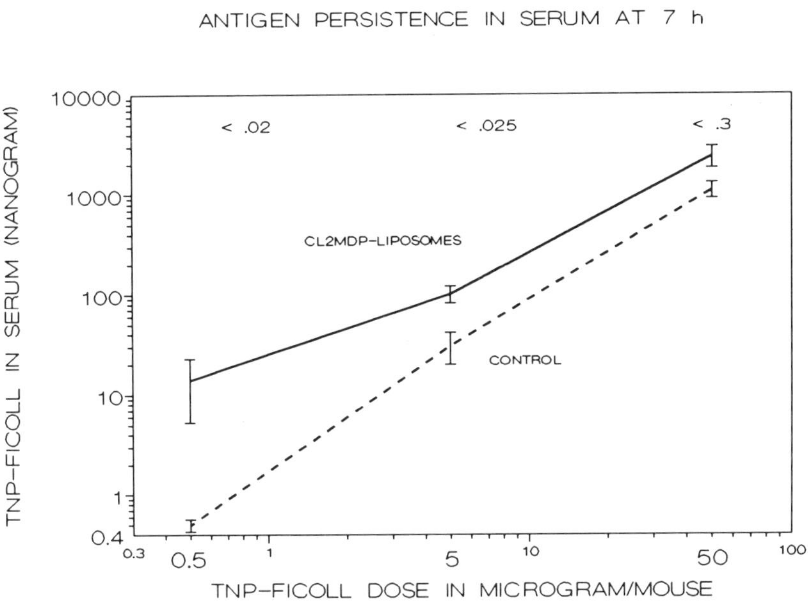


**Figure 2.2** Role of splenic macrophages in scavenging of TI-2 antigens. The figure shows persistence of TNP-Ficoll (TI-2) after i.v. administration in the serum of control animals (dotted line), or animals treated with liposomes containing a drug eliminating splenic macrophages *in vivo* (solid line). At high doses of antigen (>5 μg), differences between groups were minimal. However, at lower doses, a clear separation of the groups was found, with much higher levels of antigen persisting in the animals lacking macrophages. The antigens also persisted for longer periods (not shown here). These data show that at low antigen dose, the scavenging role of macrophages, and thereby the obscuring of TI-2 antigen for generation of specific antibody responses, becomes apparent

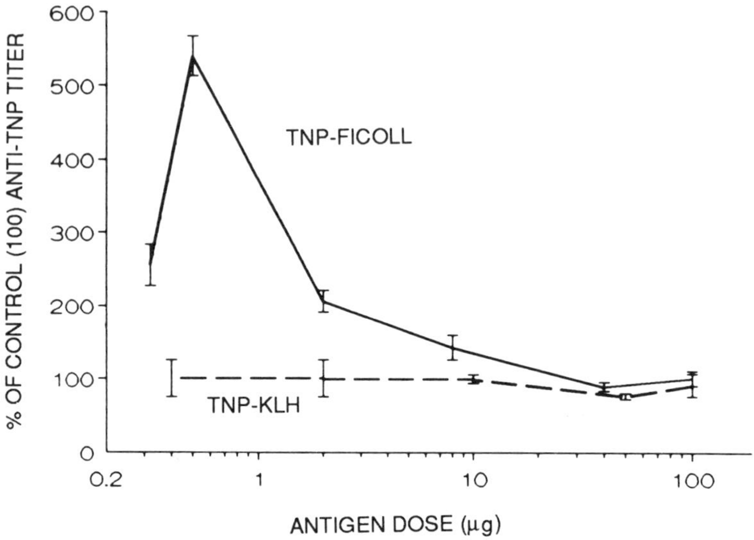


**Figure 2.3** Role of splenic macrophages in antibody responses against TI and TD antigens. The figure shows the percentage of the antibody response of animals treated with liposomes containing a drug eliminating macrophages, followed by i.v. antigen administration, compared to the response in control animals (100 per cent). Mice were immunized with either TNP-Ficoll (TI-2) or TNP-KLH (TD). Over a wide dose range, the response against TNP-KLH is not affected by macrophage elimination, compared to dose-matched control animals, consistent with the view that not macrophages but IDCs and B cells present TD antigen. In contrast, at low doses (<10 μg) of TNP-Ficoll, *in vivo* elimination of macrophages leads to a dramatic increase in specific antibody titer compared to dose-matched control animals. These data demonstrate that at low dose, the role of macrophage scavenging of TI-2 antigen for the antibody response becomes apparent. These data also emphasize that *in vivo* immunomodulation studies should be performed over a range of doses, to prevent erroneous conclusions based on measurements in the plateau range of the response only

immunomodulation studies in the literature, including autoimmunity models, are performed with high antigen doses only. It would be advisable in such studies to include a very low antigen dose eliciting a barely measurable response, and a dose leading to a half-maximal signal. This approach may yield new useful insights.

### Soluble versus Particulate Nature of the Antigen

Within the categories of TD and TI antigens, it is useful to distinguish antigens based on their soluble or particulate nature. This parameter has a decisive influence on the localization of the antigen *in vivo* and the cell type(s) that will eventually handle the antigen (see Tables 2.1 and 2.2). Macrophages will be the first cells to phagocytose particulate antigen. In general, a major fraction of the antigen will thus be degraded without leading to an antibody response. Macrophages are also thought to transfer processed antigen to other cell types, such as marginal zone B cells, which can subsequently present it to T cells. Finally, macrophages can directly present antigenic fragments to T cells in a MHC class II restricted fashion.

Soluble antigen can be taken up by macrophages or by IDCs, leading to T-cell presentation. In addition, soluble antigen can directly stimulate B cells in the case of TI antigens, or antigen can be taken up by the specific mIg of B cells, processed and presented to T cells.

### Other Factors

Complement-activating capacity of antigens impacts upon their localization and handling. TI-2 antigens, TNP-Ficoll and TNP-hydroxyethyl starch (TNP-HES) are able to activate complement, leading to rapid localization (within 1 h) in the follicles of the spleen[16] (see p. 38). This complement activation may also promote ingestion by macrophages.

Some antigens can interact with serum proteins. For example, LPS binds to lipopolysaccharide-binding protein (LBP) and this complex binds to CD14 on macrophages and monocytes, inducing secretion of several different cytokines (see below). In a secondary response against TD antigen, circulating antibody will complex the antigen, leading to increased uptake by phagocytes on the one hand, and to follicular localization in the form of immune complexes on the other hand (see p. 57).

Finally, if live pathogens are used, their tissue and cell tropism, as well as their possible capability to replicate in cells of the immune system (e.g. *Listeria monocytogenes*, HIV-1), will profoundly influence the nature of the humoral response.

## ANTIGEN HANDLING *IN VIVO*

Most studies on antigen handling *in vivo* have been done using mouse spleen, and consequently the emphasis in the discussion below will be on that organ.

### Particulate Antigens

After i.v. injection, carbon particles used as an indigestible endocytic tracer localize in the marginal zone of the spleen and are taken up by macrophages[17]. Subsequently, these macrophages transport the 'antigen' to the follicles and the inner PALS. Sheep red blood cells (SRBC) injected i.v.

are trapped in the red pulp and the marginal zone. After 48 h, SRBC-containing macrophages are found in the inner PALS. The localization of various particulate antigens after i.v. injection was compared (TD: TNP-SRBC, bovine serum albumin (BSA)-liposomes; TI-2: TNP-liposomes; TI-1: *Brucella abortus*)[18,19]. Two hours after injection, for all types of antigen, the major fraction was found at sites where the blood vessels open up into the organ, i.e. in the marginal zone, taken up by marginal zone macrophages and marginal metallophilics. At 24 h after injection, some particulate antigen is found in the macrophages of the white and the red pulp. Apparently, the differences in immune responses between particulate TI and TD antigens cannot be explained by different localization patterns after administration.

Both *in vitro* and *in vivo* studies have provided evidence that macrophages are indispensable for pre-processing of particulate TD antigens. The processed antigen is then transferred to other APCs. In the spleen, the marginal zone B cells, which possess high MHC expression and are in close contact with the marginal zone macrophages, are likely to accept this pre-processed antigen. These B cells then migrate to the PALS and interact with $CD4^+$ Th cells to receive appropriate T-cell help for TD responses, and ultimately differentiate into specific plasma cells. Although this explanation is consistent with most existing data, more experimental detail regarding the how and when of pre-processing and transfer is needed. It has been shown that B cells, although able to endocytose and present soluble TD antigens, cannot present particulate antigens if larger than approximately 200 nm (see reference 20 and references therein).

### Soluble TI Antigens

Classically, TI-2 antigens have been thought to locate mainly in marginal zone macrophages of the spleen. Using a sensitive anti-TNP monoclonal antibody (MAb), the localization of TNP-Ficoll and TNP-HES was examined. Minutes after i.v. injection, these TI-2 antigens were found in the marginal zone, associated with marginal zone macrophages and B cells. A new finding was that 20 min after injection, antigen was detected in the follicles, accumulating there up until 7 h. Thereafter, the amount of antigen trapped in the follicle decreased, but antigen remained detectable for up to 14 days. This follicular localization is complement-mediated, as complement depletion with cobra venom factor abrogated the follicular localization, did not affect localization in macrophages, and reduced the antibody response against these TI-2 antigens[16]. These data suggest that the TI-2 antigens trapped in follicles may activate B cells circulating through this site, and that complement-complexed antigen can bind and activate the CR2-carrying B cells of the marginal zone.

### Soluble TD Antigens

Studies using isotope-labeled soluble TD antigens showed they are discharged from the bloodstream in the marginal zone. Later, antigen can be detected in the follicles in the form of immune complexes. By immunohistochemistry, haptenated TD antigens TNP-KLH and TNP-BSA were found to localize exclusively in the red pulp macrophages during the first few days after injection[16]. This probably represents the bulk of antigen that is degraded by macrophages without contributing to the initiation of the antibody response. Probably the amount of antigen present in APCs is too low to be detected using these techniques. Using functional *in vitro* studies, Crowley *et al.*[21] showed that IDCs are the principal cells in the mouse spleen bearing immunogenic fragments of TD antigens after i.p. or i.v. administration.

As soon as specific antibody appears in the circulation, or when it is already present at the time of secondary immunization, it will form immune complexes with the antigen. Immune complexes can be taken up and digested by macrophages, and uptake is facilitated by the opsonization of the antigen and the Fc and C3 receptors on the macrophage membrane. A fraction of the immune complexes is trapped in the follicles, on the dendrites of the FDCs. These immune complexes are retained for long periods, and they are involved in the formation of B-cell memory, the presentation of antigen to B cells, and the regulation of circulating antibody titers[22].

In conclusion, antigen routing and handling of soluble TD antigens is different for primary and secondary immunization challenge. Macrophages take up and digest most of the (antibody-complexed) antigen in both situations, but after primary immunization antigen localizes in IDCs in the inner PALS and in marginal zone B cells to initiate the primary antibody response.

# T-CELL INDEPENDENT B-CELL ACTIVATION

## MECHANISM OF T-CELL INDEPENDENT B-CELL ACTIVATION

### TI Antigens do not Bind to Class II MHC

The following factors contribute to the fact that TI antigens generally cannot bind class II MHC, which is a prerequisite for MHC-restricted presentation to T cells and subsequent cognate T–B interactions: (1) TI antigens are poorly degradable, so the proteolytic processing occurring for TD antigens is not effective here; (2) binding of antigenic peptides derived from proteins to class II MHC is based on Van der Waals forces, hydrophilic–hydrophobic and charge interactions between specific amino acid residues in the peptide and pockets formed by the appropriate class II molecule. TI antigens do not meet these specific structural requirements for interaction[23]. In keeping with the notion that TI antigen–MHC class II interactions are not possible, and are not required for TI responses, treatment of neonatal mice with anti-class II did not affect TI-2 responses, although TD responses were ablated as expected[24].

However, Zisman *et al.*[25] have described an exception to this rule. Synthetic polypeptide antigens of L-amino acids are TD, although they have repeating sequences. In contrast, the D-amino acid form of these antigens is TI, probably due to a slower rate of metabolism. Interestingly, the D-form does stimulate T cells *in vitro*, binds to class II MHC on APCs and was used to establish TI-specific T-cell hybridomas. These findings demonstrate that class II restricted presentation and specific T cells are involved in the response against a subset of TI antigens.

### TI Antigens Crosslink the mIg Receptor

TI antigens activate B cells by means of appropriately spaced repeated haptens/epitopes on the backbone of a large molecule, like a polysaccharide. The repeated haptens crosslink the mIg receptor. This notion was confirmed by the classic experiments of Dintzis *et al.*[26], who used haptenated polyacrylamide to study number and spacing of haptens for strong TI responses. They concluded that 12–16 properly spaced epitopes provided optimal stimulation. The crosslinking of the mIg receptor is sufficient to induce B-cell proliferation, but does not induce Ig secretion or isotype switching. Apparently, a second signal is required. The nature of this second signal has been the subject of much debate, and a multitude of studies has now provided evidence that the second signal is provided by cytokines (see below).

In addition, it has been shown that mice lacking the CD45 exon6, encoding the B-cell form of CD45 (B220), have normal numbers of B-cell precursors and peripheral B cells. Activation of these B cells by LPS was normal, but triggering through the mIg receptor by anti-IgM was abrogated. This indicates that B-cell CD45 is dispensable for B-cell development, but that the molecule is required for triggering by anti-mIg[27].

### Do TI Antigens Activate Specific B-cell Subsets?

It has been suggested that TI-antigens activate specific B-cell subsets within the spleen, either the Lyb-3,5,7$^+$ subset or the CD5$^+$ B-cell subset. CD5 is expressed on a subset of B cells, and on T cells. CD5-deficient mice are healthy, have normal populations of T and B cells, and can mount effective immune responses against TI and TD antigens[28]. The authors suggest that although CD5 is dispensable for T- and B-cell development and antibody responses, its presence could be involved in fine tuning the sensitivity of thymocytes to various stimuli. The Lyb-3,5,7$^{+}$ subset represents mature B cells, which comprise the B-cell population responsive to TI-2 antigens. This subset of B cells is lacking in CBA/N mice (reviewed in references 5 and 9).

### Contributions of T Cells and Accessory Cells to TI Responses and Isotype Switching

TI responses are influenced by cytokines produced by T cells, NK cells, mast cells and accessory cells. These cytokines act either on the initial clonal expansion of B cells, on isotype switching, on the differentiation of B cells into plasma cells, and on the level of antibody production. Mond and Brunswick[29] demonstrated that IFN-γ and NK cells are involved in responses to TI antigens. TI antigens with mitogenic properties are not influenced by IFN-γ, while the response to TI antigens lacking mitogenic activity (mostly TI-2) is downregulated by IFN-γ. Elkins and co-workers[30] showed that depletion of CD4$^{+}$ T cells reduced the magnitude of the splenic IgM antibody response to a panel of TI antigens, including both mitogenic and non-mitogenic antigens.

Isotype switching from IgM and/or IgD to production of one of the other isotypes requires a B-cell activator and the presence of a cytokine to direct switching. The known roles of cytokines in isotype switching are summarized in Table 2.3. IL-4, IFN-γ and TGF-β have crucial roles in this process in the mouse. IL-4 is produced by T cells and mast cells, IFN-γ is secreted by T cells and NK cells, while TGF-β is produced by T cells, B cells and macrophages (reviewed in reference 31).

TI-2 antigens stimulate production mainly of IgM and IgG3 isotypes. What cell types and factors are involved in this isotype switch? Several studies have been performed with anti-δ-dextran: this is a soluble TI-2-like antigen, which efficiently crosslinks mIgD at ng/ml concentrations. This leads to high levels of B-cell proliferation, comparable to those induced by LPS. In the presence of cytokines, anti-δ-dextran induces secretion of a number of Ig isotypes, but it is different from LPS in that it cannot induce secretion of IgE. Stimulation of B cells with membranes from CD4$^{+}$ clones in the presence of cytokines also induces secretion of Ig isotypes. Consequently, three different mechanisms of Ig secretion could be compared.

Pecanha *et al.*[32] showed that TNP-Ficoll and anti-δ-dextran only induced Ig secretion by resting B cells in the presence of IL-2 or IL-5. IL-10 inhibited IL-5-, but not IL-2-induced Ig secretion by TI antigens. However, IL-10 did not inhibit proliferation of B cells, and did not work through suppression of IFN-γ production. Because activated B cells secreted IL-10, the authors suggested that this may represent a suppression mechanism of bystander-mediated B-cell activation stimulated by autoantigens or cytokines. Anti-δ-dextran effectively induced secretion of most Ig isotypes, but not IgE. However, when added to LPS-activated B cells, anti-δ-dextran inhibited

**Table 2.3** Roles of cytokines in antibody responses

| Cytokine | Cell type | Isotype switching | Growth/ differentiation | Inhibits |
|---|---|---|---|---|
| IL-2 | T, M, NK | — | + | IgG1, IgE[b] |
| IL-3 | NK, eo | — | + | — |
| IL-4 | T, M, eo, mast, NK | IgG1, IgE, hIgE, hIgG4 | + | IgG2a, IgG2b, IgG3, IgM |
| IL-5 | mast, eo | — | + | — |
| IL-6 | B, M, NK | — | + | — |
| IL-10 | M | IgM, IgG, hIgG1, hIgG3 | + | — |
| IL-13 | T | IgM, $IgG_{total}$, hIgE, hIgG4 | − | — |
| IFN-γ | T, NK, M | IgG2a, IgG3[a] | + | IgG1, IgG2b, IgG3[a], IgE (IL-4 and IL-5 antagonist) |
| TGF-β | T, B, M, NK | IgA, IgG2b | + | IgE |
| TGF-β + IL-10 | T, B, M | IgAh | + | — |
| ? | | IgG2h | − | — |
| GM-CSF | T, NK, B | — | + | |

M, macrophage; T, T cell; B, B cell; NK, natural killer cell; mast, mast cell; eo, eosinophil; h, human.
[a]The type of B-cell activator determines the switching or suppressive role of the cytokine.
[b]IL-2 inhibits IgG1 and IgE switching induced by IL-4, independent of IFN-γ[121]
? indicates that switch factor has not been identified yet.
Table is based on references 7, 31 and 159 and individual references cited in this chapter.

production of all isotypes. In contrast, when T-cell-activated B cells were used in combination with IL-4 and IL-5, anti-δ-dextran stimulated IgM and IgG1 secretion, but IgE production was blocked[33]. Although unconjugated anti-IgM can also inhibit LPS-induced B-cell maturation, much higher concentrations are needed, and IgM does not induce secretion of cytokines.

Snapper *et al.*[34] showed that addition of IFN-γ to resting murine B cells activated by anti-δ-dextran plus IL-5 resulted in production of IgG3. IL-4 inhibits production of IgG3. IFN-γ is probably produced by NK cells *in vivo* to bring about this isotype switch. It was demonstrated that *in vitro* activated NK cells can stimulate large marginal zone B cells, but not follicular B cells, to secrete Ig in the absence of exogenous stimuli. Preactivated NK cells can also induce Ig secretion from anti-δ-dextran-stimulated small B cells even in the absence of any added stimuli. These studies identify NK cells as an important accessory cell type in TI responses, point out the differences between small and large B cells, and confirm the special role of marginal zone B cells[35].

In conclusion, the mode of B-cell activation acts in concert with the stimulating cytokines to determine the profile of secreted isotypes. T cells,

NK cells, B cells, mast cells and macrophages can all produce cytokines influencing the isotype profile.

## TI-2 Responses in Spleen versus Lymph Nodes

Goud, Kaplan and Subbarao have published several studies showing differences in the response of various lymph node types and the spleen against TI and TD antigens. Whereas splenic B cells respond well to both TI-1 and TI-2 antigens, TI-2 antigens are unable to induce antibody formation in the popliteal and inguinal lymph nodes[36], and in the lungs and hilar lymph nodes[37]. The antibody response could be restored by mixing TNP-Ficoll with unconjugated *Brucella abortus*. However, addition of *Brucella abortus* did not result in an antibody response against the TI-2 antigen PVP (polyvinylpyrrol idone) in the inguinal or popliteal lymph nodes. On the other hand, TI-2 antigens elicited excellent responses from the mucosa-associated lymphoid organs (i.e. mesenteric lymph nodes and Peyer's patches). Because co-administration of *Brucella abortus* and addition of irradiated lymph node cells *in vitro* can restore the response to (some) TI-2 antigens, it was concluded that a quantitative defect in lymph node accessory cells is responsible for the absence of an antibody response (reviewed in reference 5).

Van den Eertwegh *et al.*[38] examined the same issue using immuno-cytochemical techniques for detection of antigen-specific B cells and cytokine-producing cells. High numbers of TNP-specific-antibody-containing B cells were found in the popliteal lymph nodes after s.c. TNP-Ficoll immunization. However, these B cells were unable to secrete antibody, and low numbers of activated T cells and cytokine-producing cells were found. These findings demonstrate that TNP-Ficoll does prime B cells in peripheral lymph nodes, but that the microenvironment of the lymph node lacks the cytokines to permit final maturation into antibody-secreting cells. Although this can be interpreted as a defect, it may also be argued that there is a physiological advantage in postponing the final maturation of the B cells until they migrate to a microenvironment where they can most efficiently deal with the infection, probably at the site of infection or in the spleen.

## The Role of CD14 in TI Responses

LPS has been found to bind to LBP. This complex as well as free LPS binds to CD14 on macrophages, inducing production of TNF-α, IL-1, IL-6, IL-8, IFN-α and some other non-cytokine biological response modifiers. TNF-α (cachectin) is involved in toxic shock syndrome. Recently, a potent inhibitor of TNF processing has been described which protects mice from a lethal dose of endotoxin[39], which has obvious important clinical implications. The presence of circulating CD14 has been suggested to be involved in neutralizing circulating endotoxin[40], and conversely as a mechanism to reduce the sensitivity of cells to LPS[41]. The cytokines released by macrophages after CD14 engagement may influence B-cell responses (see below for the involvement of CD14 in TD responses).

## T-CELL-DEPENDENT B-CELL ACTIVATION

Although perhaps superfluously, the reader is reminded that the concepts of 'activated' and 'resting' cells are just convenient terms of speech. There are multiple levels of activation for both B and T cells, as reflected by DNA and RNA synthesis, expression of inducible cell surface markers, and production and secretion of molecules like cytokines and antibodies. Below we attempt to clarify cellular correlates of activation stages during three different phases of T-cell-dependent B-cell activation, as modified from Noelle and Snow[42], i.e. recognition, induction of T-cell help and progression of B cells.

### THE RECOGNITION PHASE: CLASS II RESTRICTED, ANTIGEN-SPECIFIC INTERACTIONS

TD antigens (typically proteins) are not able to stimulate B cells directly but require intracellular proteolytic processing in endosomal compartments of APCs, followed by display of antigenic peptides in the peptide-binding cleft of MHC class II molecules (reviewed in reference 43). Subsequently, specific $CD4^+$ Th cells bind to the class II–peptide complex by means of the appropriate T-cell receptor and CD4, and are activated as a result of this interaction. Several cell types can function as APCs *in vitro*, i.e. macrophages, IDCs and B cells (reviewed in references 44 and 45), but the relative contribution of each of these APCs in primary and secondary TD responses is an unresolved question.

#### Antigen Organization and mIg Characteristics

Important features of the recognition phase are the organization of the antigen and the characteristics of the mIg receptor. Recent studies on antigen organization showed that viral antigen (vesicular stomatitis virus (VSV) glycoprotein) found in highly repetitive form on viral particles induces a TI response of IgM isotype in mice within 3–5 days[46]. When mice were injected with infected cells expressing the glycoprotein on their surface in poorly organized form, much lower titers of IgM were induced. Transgenic mice expressing the glycoprotein on the surface of cells were refractory to immunization with soluble glycoprotein, reflecting B-cell unresponsiveness. However, they did respond to wild-type or inactivated VSV by producing IgM antibodies, independently of T-cell help. These data suggest that the organization of foreign antigen or self-antigen determines immunogenicity and responsiveness of B cells. Apparently, membrane-bound proteins at low density induce anergy rather than deletion of B cells[46].

George *et al.*[47] revisited the role of mIg density and affinity in B-cell signaling by antigen binding. Using B-cell lines transfected with H and L chain constructs of different affinity for phosphocholine and calcium mobilization as a readout, it was shown that small changes in receptor number affected the calcium response greatly. Antigen-specific signaling requires only a few thousand receptors per cell (normal range for antigen receptor is 50 000 to 150 000/cell). As would be expected, higher sIgM affinity allows B-cell lines to respond more quickly, and to yield a maximal response at lower receptor density. However, at high antigen concentration, the affinity of the receptor is of much lesser importance. In addition, receptor density plays only a small role once the receptor affinity is high enough to mediate antigen-specific stimulation. The authors conclude that receptor density and receptor affinity work in concert to bring about antigen-driven selection of B-cell clones *in vivo*. TI antigens, being large with repeated determinants, can induce stable receptor cross-linking and activation, over a wide range of receptor density and affinity. This then, can contribute to the fact that most TI antigens do not seem to induce affinity maturation.

In elegant experiments, Luxembourg and Cooper[48] used 100-nm fluorescent latex beads coated with anti-IgD or anti-IgM antibodies to mimic particulate antigens, immune complexes and viruses. These beads bind specifically to resting human tonsillar B cells. Both anti-IgM and anti-IgD induce homotypic B-cell aggregation and increased transcription of c-*fos* and c-*myc*. Both types of beads are mitogenic, but unlike in other models for B-cell mitogenesis, the presence of either IL-2 or IL-4 is required, implying T-cell dependency. Only anti-IgM-coated beads are taken up by the B cells, dependent on IL-4 but not IL-2. No differentiation of the B cells into IgM- or IgG-secreting cells was induced. What factors are important in making these particles act like TD antigens, while the quite similar anti-δ/μ-dextran model has TI characteristics? An obvious point is the local epitope/hapten (in this case anti-IgD) density: the small latex beads carry 24–39 antibody molecules, comparable to dextran, which has 17–33. However, the latex beads are larger, leading to lower epitope density. Other factors are the shape of the molecule (round versus linear for latex beads versus dextran), curvature (greater for 100-nm particles than for large latex beads and polyacrylamide beads) and flexibility (presumably none for latex and considerable for soluble dextran). It will be of interest to see how these 100-nm latex beads activate B cells when coated with mixtures of oligosaccharides and peptides, more accurately mimicking naturally occurring pathogens. Of course, the differences between the two experimental systems should be kept in mind: murine B cells activated with anti-Ig-dextran versus human B cells activated with latex beads.

Velupillai and Harn[49] described oligosaccharides on schistosome eggs and schistosomula that induced proliferation of B cells. One of the sugars (LNFP-III) also induced B cells of infected mice to produce large amounts of IL-10 (but not IL-4) and protaglandin $E_2$, mediators which downregulate Th1 cells. This could represent a mechanism by which parasites skew the Th1/Th2 ratio. The mechanisms of B-cell activation for proliferation and IL-10 production are as yet unclear: either a non-Ig receptor performs both functions, or LNFP-III induces proliferation by binding to the mIgM receptor and a second signal is required for IL-10 production.

### Molecules Involved in Conjugate Stabilization

If Th cells recognize class II–peptide on macrophages or IDC, they migrate subsequently to contact B cells displaying the same class II–peptide combination. If a B cell functions as the first APC, no migration is required for the next interactions. Following peptide-specific interaction of T and B cells, an array of constitutively expressed membrane adhesion molecules assist in stabilization of the cell conjugate (e.g. LFA-1/CD11a-18; LFA-2/CD2; LFA-3/CD58; ICAM-1/CD54; VCAM/CD106; VLA-4/CD49d-29)(reviewed in reference 50).

The role of MHC class II was examined in mice lacking MHC class II genes. These animals displayed normal numbers of B cells. They could not mount TD responses, or generate germinal centers, and showed reduced but detectable basal IgG1 levels. In contrast, IgM and IgG production in response to TI antigens was not affected, indicating that T-cell help but not the functional capacities of B cells was impaired[51].

A number of molecules on the B-cell surface further assist in the interaction and signal transduction (reviewed in reference 52). The B-cell antigen receptor complex consists of IgM associated with two disulfide-linked heterodimers of Ig-$\alpha$ and Ig-$\beta$ (or Ig-$\gamma$), which bind to cytoplasmic effectors for signal transduction. CD45, although probably not part of the receptor complex, is essential for mIgM-mediated signaling, probably through controlling phosphorylation of Ig-$\alpha$ and Ig-$\beta$. CD22, which is present on mature B cells, particularly in the marginal zone, has been reported to be involved in the T–B-cell interaction as an adhesion molecule and in signal transduction. A direct interaction of CD22 with different isoforms of CD45 has been demonstrated[53], as has association of CD22 with the B-cell antigen receptor complex. It has also been argued that CD54 (ICAM-1) and MHC class II signaling complement CD40–CD40L interactions by inducing expression of IL2R on B cells[54].

After crosslinking of the B-cell receptor, CD19 and CD21 (complement receptor CR2) associate with the receptor complex. The role of CD19 is not clear yet, but Carter and Fearon[55] have demonstrated that co-immobilization of CD19 and mIg leads to increased antigen-induced B-cell proliferation.

They concluded that CD19 lowers the antigen threshold for B-cell activation.

Van Noesel *et al.*[56] have suggested that dual binding of the antigen occurs: the B-cell receptor specifically recognizes antigen, while CR2 (CD21) interacts with complement bound to the antigen. This dual binding would improve the stability of the interaction and allows activation of B cells at lower antigen concentrations.

Several other molecules whose function is poorly defined as yet are involved in B-cell activation (CD5, CD6, CD20, CD43 and CD59) (see reference 50 for discussion).

In an intriguing study, Förster *et al.*[57] analyzed the distribution of the G-protein-coupled receptor BLR1 in human peripheral blood and lymphoid tissue. G-protein-coupled receptors are classically activated by hormones or neurotransmitters, but evidence is accumulating for a role of these receptors in immunologic responses. BLR1 has high homology to receptors of the chemokine family. BLR1 is expressed on mature recirculating B cells ($CD19^+$ $IgD^+$ $IgM^+$) and a subpopulation of Th memory cells ($CD45RO^+$, CD44 high, $IL2R^-$, L-selectin low). In tonsils, BLR1 staining is most pronounced in mantle zone cells ($IgD^+$ B cells), and there are some positive cells within the follicles. $CD4^+BLR1^+$ cells are located in both the T-cell zones and the follicles. In the T-cell zones of human spleen, BLR1-positive cells are restricted to the PALS. These findings suggest a functional role for this receptor in mature B cells and memory T cells which merits further analysis.

With respect to the B-cell receptor complex, it is important to note that immunoglobulin D-deficient mice respond normally to TI and TD antigens, can switch isotype production and are able to form germinal centers. They do, however, show a reduced B-cell compartment in the F1 mice, and a reduction in total lymphoid cells in the F2 mice. This indicates that IgD is not required for antibody responses, but may instead be involved in B-cell homeostasis, through as yet unknown mechanisms[58]. Roes and Rajewsky[59] described similar findings for IgD knockout mice, but in addition they found evidence that IgD is involved in affinity maturation early, but not late, in the antibody response.

## INDUCTION OF TH-CELL EFFECTOR FUNCTION AND EFFECTOR PHASE OF HELP

### T-helper Cell Subsets

Murine Th cell clones are classified into two subsets (Th1 and Th2) based on the types of cytokines they produce. Th1 secrete IL-2, IL-3, tumor necrosis factor alpha (TNF-$\alpha$) and IFN-$\gamma$. Th2 clones secrete IL-3, IL-4, IL-5, IL-6, IL-10 and some TNF-$\alpha$. In addition, a Th0 type has been described, capable of secreting all these cytokines. Although the presence of distinct Th1 and Th2 subsets *in vivo* has not been unequivocally proven in humans, the principle of Th1- and Th2-like pathways has been proven to be a useful concept for analysis of humoral and cell-mediated immunity. Aspects of Th cell subsets are discussed in depth in Chapter 6.

## Important Receptor–Ligand Pairs

Two receptor–ligand systems on CD4+ T lymphocytes have prominent roles in the interaction between antigen-specific T and B cells, i.e. CD40–CD40L (gp39, TBAM, TRAP) and CD28/CTLA4-Ig with B7-1/B7-2. Both systems have been extensively reviewed recently (CD40L in references 60 and 61, CD28 in reference 62). They are outlined below with an emphasis on CD40L as related to some of our own work.

### *CD28/CTLA4-Ig with B7-1/B7-2*

CD28 is constitutively expressed on almost all CD4+ and CD8+ peripheral T cells. The ligands for CD28 are B7-1 (BB1/CD80)[62] and B7-2[63,64]. When T cells are activated, they express a second receptor for B7-1 and B7-2, CTLA4, which has a higher binding avidity. Consequently, there are two receptors (CD28 and CTLA4) and two ligands (B7-1 and B7-2) that crossbind and signal each other. B7-1 and B7-2 (also dubbed B7-0) are present on APCs like IDCs and macrophages. Resting B cells do not constitutively express significant levels of B7-1 and B7-2, and as a consequence their ability to act as APCs is poor, but not totally absent ('non-professional' APC). Appropriate activation of B cells leads to expression of B7-1 and B7-2, and these activated B cells are efficient APCs.

Using TCR transgenic T cells, Roy *et al.*[65] showed that antibodies against B7-1 and B7-2 did not inhibit antigen-induced expression of CD40L on T cells *in vitro*. Conversely, anti-CD40L antibody blocked upregulated expression of B7-1 on B cells, and partially blocked B7-2. When anti-IL-4 was added, complete blocking of B7-2 expression was found. Soluble CD40L upregulated B7-1 and B7-2 expression. This indicates that expression of CD40L is dependent on TCR-derived signals, but independent of CD28/CTLA4 costimulatory signals. In addition, B7-2, and B7-1 to a lesser extent, depend on CD40–CD40L interaction for their expression.

Treatment of small splenic B cells with IL-4 induces expression of B7-1 and B7-2[66]. In this study, B7-2 could be detected after 6 h, whereas B7-1 was not seen until 48 h. Yellin *et al.*[67] showed that CD40L induces B7 expression on B cells. These data show that CD40L is involved not only in the more distal differentiation of B cells into plasma cells, but also in enabling B cells to present antigens to T cells, leading to clonal expansion (see below). On the other hand, anti-CD28 antibodies enhance CD40L expression[68]: apparently, interacting T and B cells mutually increase each other's costimulatory capacities.

A soluble form of the CTLA4 molecule suppresses T-cell-dependent antibody responses *in vitro*[69]. Mice transgenic for CTLA4-Hγl also show reduced TD antibody responses. However, $CD4^+$ Th cells showed normal primary activation and enhanced *in vivo* expansion after secondary or tertiary immunization. They were not anergic, although they were unable to provide cognate help to B cells[70]. This was interpreted to mean that, in contrast to previous hypotheses, soluble CTLA4 does not inhibit T-cell responses, but instead prevents the delivery of activation signals to B cells.

Using the same model, Lane *et al.*[14] showed that the impaired TD antibody response is associated with a defect in class switching, with low total IgG and antigen-specific Ig being produced. In addition, no germinal centers are formed and there is a reduction in the degree of somatic mutation. The TI-2 antibody response is normal. In contrast to spleen and lymph nodes, gut-associated tissue did show normal development of germinal centers. Thus far, the mechanism by which CTLA4-Hγl blocks B-cell responses is obscure.

Using CD28-deficient mice, Shahinian *et al.*[71] demonstrated that CD28 is not required for development of cytotoxic cells and delayed-type hypersensitivity responses, but that this molecule is essential for humoral responses. Basal Ig titers were reduced 5-fold, with low IgG1 and IgG2b concentrations, but increased IgG2a levels. Although protective IgM responses were raised against infectious VSV, isotype switching was impaired.

Based on the kinetics of appearance of B7-1 and B7-2, the affinities for their receptors, and recent genetic knockout studies, the current view is that the requirement for B7-1 and/or B7-2 expression in costimulation may depend on the activation stimulus used[72].

### *CD40–CD40L*

CD40 is expressed on B cells, IDCs, FDCs, thymic epithelium and some carcinomas. Human CD40 has a size of 50 kDa and is a member of the nerve growth factor receptor family, together with OX-40, CD27 and 4-1BB. *In vitro* studies using pharmacologic B-cell activators such as phorbol ester (PMA) and ionomycin in combination with anti-CD40 antibodies revealed an essential role for this marker in B-cell activation and isotype switching. It was shown that *in vitro* culture with anti-CD40 antibodies and IL-4 permitted long-term culture of human B-cell lines[73]. CD40L was subsequently identified for the mouse[74,75] and for humans[76]. A hamster monoclonal antibody (mAb) (MR1) against murine CD40L blocks TD B-cell proliferation *in vitro*[77]. Used *in vivo*, it is also able to inhibit primary and secondary antibody responses against the TD antigens SRBC and TNP-KLH, but not the TI antigen TNP-Ficoll[78]. Administration of the mAb *in vivo* during a TD (SRBC) response prevents the formation of B-cell memory and germinal centers[79], demonstrating a role for CD40L in the generation of memory B cells (see

p. 59). A mAb (5C8) has been generated against human CD40L[77] which can block T-cell-mediated B-cell activation *in vitro*.

In both mouse and human, CD40L is a type II membrane protein of approximately 33 kDa (reviewed in reference 80) belonging to a new superfamily of ligand genes involved in activation and cell death, including TNF-α and -β, and the ligands for FAS, CD27, CD30 and 4-1BB[81]. Saeland *et al.*[82] provided data implicating a role for CD40 in proliferation and high expression of CD23. IL-3 was required for this effect, and the combination of IL-10 and IL-7 enhanced the response. B cells cultured in the presence of IL-4 and triggered through CD40 lose their germinal center features[83]. Long-term proliferating cells are mIgD$^+$ mIgM$^+$ derived B cells, showing that mIgD$^+$ cells preferentially proliferate in response to CD40 signaling. Consequently, mIgD$^+$ lymphocytes constitute the long-term IL-4-dependent proliferating B-cell pool[83].

Alderson *et al.*[84] have shown that human monocytes can be induced to express CD40 by stimulation with granulocyte/macrophage colony stimulating factor (GM-CSF), IL-3 or IFN-γ. CD40 ligand-transfected cells induced production of TNF-α and IL-6 if GM-CSF, IL-3 or IFN-γ was present. In addition, IL-8 production was enhanced by GM-CSF or IL-3. CD40 ligand-transfected cells could also enhance tumoricidal activity of monocytes. These are intriguing findings, pointing towards interactions of CD40L$^+$ Th cells with monocytes/macrophages leading to macrophage activation. This considerably extends the potential array of functions that CD40 and CD40L may have besides those in B-cell responses. Finally, CD40L has been shown to act as a costimulatory signal for neonatal thymic γδT cells[85].

### *CD40L expression* in vitro *and* in vivo

Expression of murine CD40L has been observed on normal activated CD4$^+$ Th cells from peripheral blood, activated lymph node cells, and activated Th1 and Th2 clones[86]. CD40L can be induced on CD8$^+$ T cells with PMA/ionomycin but not with anti-CD3. *In vitro*, expression of CD40L on a T-cell clone and on splenic CD4$^+$ T cells was detectable 4 h after activation, peaking between 6 and 8 h post-activation, and returning to near resting levels between 24 and 48 h. IFN-γ inhibits expression of CD40L on activated Th1, Th2 and normal CD4$^+$ T cells. TGF-β inhibited CD40L expression only on the Th2 clone. The short peak of CD40L expression may be a means of safeguarding antigen specificity, i.e. CD40L$^+$ Th will only activate the appropriate conjugal B-cell partner and not B cells of unrelated specificity[86].

Data on *in vivo* expression of CD40L paint quite a different picture. Using immunohistochemistry, Van den Eertwegh *et al.*[87] showed that after i.v. immunization with TNP-KLH or TNP-Ficoll, CD40L expression was induced on murine splenic CD4$^+$ Th cells. CD40L expression *in vivo* appeared on day 3, increasing over the following days, with a peak on day 4, and rapidly dropping off to a little over background levels on days 5 and 6. These kinetics were identical for primary and secondary immunization with TNP-KLH, but absolute numbers of CD40L$^+$ Th cells were high in the secondary response. The kinetics of appearance of CD40L$^+$ cells coincided with the appearance of hapten- and carrier-specific B cells, in a ratio of approximately one CD40L$^+$ cell per 12 plasma cells.

The expression of CD40L was restricted to Th cells in the outer PALS and around the terminal arterioles. No CD40L expression was found in the germinal centers during primary TD responses, and only occasionally were positive cells found during secondary responses. Staining for cytokine production revealed that IL-2-, IL-4- and IFN-γ-producing cells developed with similar kinetics as seen for CD40L$^+$ Th cells. Dual immunohistochemical analysis showed that CD40L- and antigen-specific antibody-forming B cells were localized in close proximity, forming cellular conjugates[87].

The fact that normal numbers of cytokine-producing CD40L$^+$ Th cells are found after treatment with CD40L-specific antibody[79] convincingly refutes the argument that T cells are deleted by *in vivo* administration of this antibody[88].

To investigate whether CD40L is expressed *in vivo* during spontaneous development of autoimmune disease, SNF1 mice were studied. This strain develops lupus as a result of autoantibody formation, forming a model for human lupus. CD40L is spontaneously (i.e. without experimental immunization) expressed in the spleen of SNF1 mice, positively correlated with the development of lupus. This is indicative of ongoing T-cell-mediated B-cell activation. Short-term treatment of animals with anti-CD40L mAb resulted in long-term delay of disease[89].

Using the antibody against human CD40L, Lederman *et al.*[90] found CD40L on CD4$^+$ Th cells in the mantle and centrocytic zones of lymphoid follicles and the PALS of the spleen, in association with CD40$^+$ B cells. The discrepancies between the data of Van den Eertwegh *et al.*[87] and those of Lederman *et al.*[90] may be explained by the fact that the human tissues used are by definition from pathological conditions. Chronic stimulation and inflammation may alter the localization and/or levels of CD40L expression, compared to the tissues of SPF mice immunized with purified proteins. An alternative explanation is a species difference. It is also possible that soluble CD40 obscures CD40L, or that CD40L is locally down-modulated, in part by receptor-mediated endocytosis[91]. Why human and mouse tissues would differ in this respect is unclear. It cannot be formally excluded that the level of murine CD40L expression is too low in the germinal center to be detected immunohistochemically, but this seems unlikely as anti-CD40L antibody staining in tissue sections is quite bright at 10 μg/ml. *In situ* hybridization, *in situ* polymerase chain reaction (PCR), or micromanipulation of individual germinal center cells followed by PCR for CD40L sequences[92,93] can resolve this issue.

*CD40–CD40L in human immune deficiency*

Compelling evidence for the pivotal role of CD40–CD40L in B-cell activation and isotype switching comes from studies of the human X-linked hyper-IgM syndrome (HIGM1), which is characterized by elevated IgM levels and absence of other isotypes. This defect in isotype switching is the result of mutations in the human CD40L gene[94–99]. Point mutations abolish proper CD40–CD40L interactions, and apparently there is no redundancy in the mechanisms for isotype switching, i.e. no other molecule or soluble factor can substitute for CD40L.

Evidence has also been presented that defective CD40–CD40L interactions contribute to clinical signs of some patients suffering from common variable immunodeficiency (CVI)[100].

Interestingly, Chirmule *et al.*[101] have shown that the envelope glycoprotein of HIV-1, gp160, induces B-cell activation in a T-cell-dependent fashion. gp160 induces moderate expression of CD40L on cloned $CD4^+CD45RO^+$ T cells *in vitro*, and expression of IL-2R and CD23 on B cells. IL-6, but not IL-2 or IL-4, was found to be required for gp160-induced IgG secretion.

The role of defective CD40–CD40L interactions in human immunodeficiency has been reviewed by Laman *et al.*[102].

*CD40–CD40L gene targeting models*

Experiments with genetic knockout mice lacking either CD40[103,104] or CD40L[105] have confirmed nearly all conclusions regarding the role of CD40–CD40L interactions for B-cell responses reached with *in vitro* studies and *in vivo* blocking studies with anti-CD40L. Some questions remain as to the requirement for CD40L in TD responses of IgM isotype. Although Kawabe *et al.*[103] found intact specific IgM responses in CD40-deficient mice, Castigli *et al.*[104] demonstrated abolition of specific IgM in another CD40-deficient mouse strain.

The availability of knockout models offers exciting new opportunities to unravel the functions of CD40 and CD40L. In this respect, it is of note that CD40–CD40L interactions seem operational in immunologic mechanisms generally regarded as being T-cell mediated. Treatment with anti-CD40L antibody can prevent collagen-induced arthritis[106], acute and chronic forms of graft versus host disease[107], and development of PLP peptide-induced experimental allergic encephalomyelitis (EAE) in a mouse model[108].

## Incomplete B-cell Activation

It is thought that incomplete activation of B cells leads to anergy or apoptosis, as a protection mechanism against production of antibodies in the absence of an antigenic stimulus, or the production of antibodies against self-antigens. Tsubata *et al.*[109] showed that anti-IgM-induced apoptotic death of a B-cell lymphoma line could be blocked by CD40L. Using a T-cell line expressing CD40L and a B-cell line representative for germinal center B cells, Lederman *et al.*[110] could confirm that CD40L is important for clonal selection of isotype switched B cells. Renschler and colleagues[111] reported experiments in which a human B-cell lymphoma underwent apoptosis after incubation with dimeric or trimeric peptides specifically binding the mIg receptor, which stimulated intracellular tyrosine phosphorylation. Newell *et al.*[112] reported that ligation of MHC class II with specific antibody results in apoptosis of resting B lymphocytes, while treatment with immobilized anti-mIg antibody plus IL-4 protects them. B cells activated *in vivo* are refractory to class II ligation. This suggests that apoptotic death prevents non-specific B-cell activation in the event that ligation of the MHC class II by the T-cell receptor and/or CD4 occurs in the absence of antigen. In this respect it is also of note that CD40 stimulation by anti-CD40 antibodies or soluble CD40L inhibits human lymphoma growth[113], providing further evidence that the result of a specific stimulus is dependent on the activation state of the B cell.

Eris *et al.*[114] analyzed the mechanisms responsible for B-cell tolerance to hen egg lysozyme (HEL) in HEL/anti-HEL double-transgenic mice. B cells from these animals were refractory to carrier-primed T cells, but this defect could be overcome *in vivo*. The efficiency of antigen uptake and processing was reduced, probably due to a 4–10-fold decrease in mIgM. However, re-expression of normal levels of IgM was not accompanied by restoration of the response. Failure of B cells to upregulate CD28 ligands is most probably responsible for these findings. B-cell anergy can be reversible, and two mechanisms for production of autoantibodies can be envisaged[114]: (1) high levels of self-antigen associated with foreign carrier epitopes may compete effectively with self-antigen *per se* on anergic B cells, leading to presentation to carrier-primed T cells; (2) Bona fide T-cell activation may break down anergy of self-reactive B cells by expression of CD40L and cytokines.

### Net Effect of Expression of Activation Markers

As a result of the class II restricted antigen-specific interactions, expression of CD40L and CTLA4 is induced on the T cell, which is now sufficiently activated for the effector phase of help. The interaction between T cells equipped with these activation molecules and B cells induces the B cells to progress from the G0 to the G1 stage of the cell cycle.

## CYTOKINE-DEPENDENT PHASE, B-CELL PROGRESSION

### Role of Cytokines in B-cell Progression

Several cytokines aid in further development of B cells into plasma cells. They function in differentiation and proliferation, and they direct isotype switching as well as the quantity of antibody produced. In Table 2.3 cytokine involvement in antibody responses is summarized. Only some recent studies pertaining to cytokine-induced class switching are discussed here. More detailed information can be found elsewhere in this volume.

To progress from the G1 to S phase of the cell cycle, the B cell requires the presence of cytokines, either singly or in combination. Punnonen *et al.*[115] reported experiments showing that IL-13 induces IL-4-independent production of IgG4 and IgE synthesis, as well as CD23 expression and enhanced CD72, mIgM and class II MHC expression, by highly purified human B cells. This indicates that IL-13 can perform functions identical to, but independent of, IL-4. The levels of IgG4 and IgE induced by IL-13 are lower than for IL-4, and IL-13 does not seem to act on T cells. IL-10 has been identified as the switch factor for IgG1 and IgG3 secretion by human B cells[116]. The switch factor for human IgG2 production has not been identified yet.

T-cell contact-dependent signals (CD40L) and IL-4 can also induce differentiation of human B-cell precursors (pre-B cells) into plasma cells, including isotype switching[117,118]. A number of cytokines (IL-2, IL-3, IL-7 and IL-10) contribute to the efficiency of the *in vitro* systems used, but cannot replace CD40L[118]. This indicates a role for CD40L and these cytokines in B-cell ontogeny.

Boussiotis *et al.*[119] have shown that TNF-α is an autocrine growth factor for human splenic B cells. TNF-α is produced after stimulation through the CD40 and IL-4 pathways and promotes B-cell growth in a fashion similar to IL-2.

IL-3 and GM-CSF induce Ig secretion of murine B cells when these are activated through the membrane Ig, but not when activated through CD40[120]. Nakanishi *et al.*[121] have demonstrated that IL-2 can inhibit IL-4-dependent IgE and IgG1 production *in vitro* and *in vivo*.

## Role of APC Type

The pattern of cytokine secretion determining the isotype switch is influenced by the type of APC operational in the response. Studying a TD response in mice, De Becker *et al.*[122] found that i.v. injecticn with antigen-pulsed dendritic cells (i.e. IDCs) induces synthesis of specific IgG1 and IgG2a. However, peritoneal macrophages induce similar titers of IgG1, much lower IgG2a levels and elevated levels of IgE. Apparently, IDCs activate Th1 cells, whereas peritoneal macrophages activate Th2 cells.

## Local Secretion of Cytokines

There is some *in vitro* evidence for highly localized secretion of cytokines at the interaction site between T and B cells. This polarized delivery has several advantages: (1) only interacting cells take up the cytokine and respond, and not nearby lymphocytes of irrelevant specificity; (2) high cytokine concentrations can be achieved at the site of interaction; (3) the labile cytokines are sequestered away from decay-inducing agents. Recent studies by Kupfer *et al.*[123] using cloned T cells and small splenic B cells showed that all mitotic B cells were bound to Th cells. They faced the microtubule organizing center in the Th cells, where IL-4 was highly concentrated. B cells that bound to the Th cells not near the microtubule organizing center remained in interphase. These data suggest that polarized lymphokine secretion may contribute to the efficiency and specificity of T–B-cell interactions. It should be kept in mind that even when using cloned T cells, significant variability is found in the molecular and cellular properties of T–B-cell interactions[123].

### The Role of CD14 in TD Responses

Engagement of CD14 results in activation of human monocytes, which then release a number of cytokines. Also, it delivers a negative signal terminating T-cell proliferation. In addition, it has been shown that binding of selected mAb to CD14 inhibits IgM, IgG and IgE synthesis acting on a late event in B-cell activation, both in TD and TI systems. This inhibition could not be attributed to effects of IL-10, TGF-β or prostaglandin, and neither could it be overcome by addition of IL-6 or TNF-α. These data imply that CD14 plays a regulatory role in B-cell responses[124]. These authors suggest that both B and T cells have a CD14L, which may or may not be the same molecule.

### Cytokine Gene Targeting Models

Analyzing IL-2 knockout mice, Kündig *et al.*[125] found that Th cell responses were delayed, but intact. VSV-specific IgG responses were consequently delayed, but the quantity and isotype distribution of antibodies was normal. This implies that, at least in the mouse, IL-2 is dispensable for class switching and antibody production.

Disruption of the IL-4 gene has been shown to block Th2 cytokine responses as expected[126]. Serum Ig in IL-4 $^{-/-}$ mice showed a 20-fold decrease in IgG1, and IgE was not detectable. Neither anti-IgD treatment nor infection with *Nippostrongylus brasiliensis* induced detectable IgE levels, and the IgG1 response was still 12-fold lower than in control animals. Immunization of these animals with the TD antigen DNP-OVA resulted in 10-fold lower IgG1 responses in the IL-4 $^{-/-}$ animals, whereas IgG2 and IgG3 levels were 100–500-fold higher. This confirms the dependency of IgE on IL-4, but also proves that some IgG1 can be produced in the absence of IL-4.

### Induction of IgE Synthesis

IgE is the isotype primarily involved in allergic disease, although anaphylactic responses can also be found in IgE knockout mice[127]. IgE binds to the high-affinity FcεRI on mast cells and basophils. Subsequent crosslinking by allergens leads to the release of inflammatory mediators and the clinical signs of allergy. Synthesis of IgE requires T–B-cell interactions leading to an isotype-specific signal provided by IL-4 or IL-13 and a switch signal through CD40. The cytokines are produced by T cells, mast cells and basophils. Linkage analysis in human populations has provided evidence that total IgE levels (i.e. IgE not reactive in a multi-allergen assay) are linked to one or more polymorphisms in a gene or genes within human chromosome 5q31.1. The most likely candidate in this region is the IL-4 gene, but other relevant genes cannot be excluded (IL-5, IL-13, IRF1, IL-12B and ADRB2)[128]. The authors suggest that this is evidence for non-cognate production of IgE, resulting in non-allergen-specific IgE, but this claim needs to be further substantiated.

Gauchat *et al.*[129] have demonstrated that in the presence of IL-4, mast cells and basophils express CD40L and can provide the contact-dependent interactions to drive B cells to IgE secretion. Thus, there would be no absolute requirement for T cells in IgE production during allergic disease. Another implication of these data is that isotype switching, at least for IgE, may occur outside the secondary lymphoid organs. In another study, Gauchat *et al.*[130] provided evidence that IL-4-induced germline ε RNA synthesis in human B cells can be modulated by TNF-α, anti-CD40 monoclonal antibodies and TGF-β.

It has been proposed that FcεRII (CD23), the low-affinity receptor for IgE, is an important regulator of IgE, synthesis in humans. This type II transmembrane lectin is present on B cells and FDCs. Gustavsson *et al.*[131] showed that specific IgE can enhance the murine IgM, IgG1, IgG2a and IgE response. Evidence was provided that binding of antigen complexed with specific IgE to CD23 on B cells is responsible for this enhancement through increased CD23-mediated antigen uptake.

Studies using CD23 gene-targeted mice revealed that normal development of T and B cells takes place[132]. Serum levels of IgM, IgG3 and IgA were not affected, but IgG1 and IgG2b were twofold lower, whereas IgE levels were twofold higher, than controls. Antibody responses to the helminth *Nippostrongylus brasiliensis*, a strong inducer of IgE, were unaffected. Germinal center formation was also normal. However, IgE responses against TD antigens were increased and sustained in the CD23-deficient mice when compared to control littermates. Immunization with the TD antigen DNP-OVA led to comparable IgM, Ig2b and IgG3 titers. However, specific IgG1 was twice as high, and specific IgE was increased 6–12-fold. In addition, the total IgE titer was raised and IgE levels were sustained for longer. Although CD23 was not expressed on FDCs, IgE was present in the germinal centers, binding directly, or being complexed with complement proteins and their receptors. Apparently, expression of CD23 is not a necessary requirement for induction or maintenance of antibody response. The authors suggest that CD23 instead functions in negative feedback control of IgE responses: binding of IgE-containing immune complexes (but not monomeric IgE) renders the B cell unresponsive to further stimulation.

Fujiwara *et al.*[133] found markedly different results in CD23-deficient mice: animals displayed normal lymphocyte differentiation and antibody responses against TD antigens and *Nippostrongylus brasiliensis*. No increased IgE responses were reported. Germinal center formation and *in vitro* proliferation of B cells were also intact. The only difference between deficient mice and controls was an impairment of the antigen-specific IgE-mediated enhancement of the antibody responses. Currently, there is no satisfactory explanation for the discrepancies between these studies.

Kimata *et al.*[134] reported that IL-8 inhibits IL-4-induced IgE secretion by human B cells. This antagonistic effect is independent of IFN-$\gamma$, IFN-$\alpha$ and prostaglandin $E_2$, and IL-8 seems to affect the B cells directly.

## TI AND TD RESPONSES AND MEMORY FORMATION *IN VIVO*

The general aspects of the B-cell responses as described below are based on references 6,7,11,135,136,137 and 138.

### ANTIGEN PRESENTATION AND B-CELL PROLIFERATION

After primary immunization with a soluble TD antigen, B cells in the marginal zone and IDCs in the inner PALS (or the paracortex for the lymph node) process and present the antigen to T cells. Specific T cells cluster around the IDCs and proliferate. For particulate antigens, macrophages in the marginal zone will pre-process the antigen and transfer it to B cells in the marginal zone, or they will migrate into the white pulp and transfer antigen to IDCs in the inner PALS. Specific B cells migrate from the marginal zone and into the adjacent outer PALS. Within the PALS, T and B cells move in opposite directions, increasing the chance of specific cells meeting. T and B cells interact in the T-cell areas, entailing extensive crosstalk by lymphokines and membrane molecules as described on pp. 44–52. In the spleen, B cells proliferate in the PALS and then locally develop into foci of antibody-forming cells, or migrate to the primary follicles, where they participate in the germinal center reaction[92,139,137]. Primary follicles consist of $IgM^+IgD^+$ recirculating B cells and FDCs.

Liu *et al.*[137] have shown that primary immunization with both TD and TI-1 antigens leads to proliferation of hapten-specific B cells around IDCs, in the FDC network and in association with macrophages in the red pulp. For TD antigens, the proliferation in the PALS is low for primary responses, but high for secondary responses. There are massive responses to TI-1 antigens in the PALS, both in the primary and the secondary response, and hapten-specific B blasts are found in the red pulp. In response to TNP-LPS, proliferation is seen in some follicles after both primary and secondary immunization. Specific memory B cells colonized the marginal zone for both TD and TI antigens.

## FORMATION OF GERMINAL CENTERS

In the germinal center, four important B-cell events take place, i.e. clonal expansion of B cells; somatic hypermutation leading to rearranged Ig-variable regions of higher affinity; selection of B cells of appropriate antigen specificity[93]; and the differentiation into memory B cells or plasma cells. Hypermutation and affinity maturation seem to occur mainly during the primary response.

Gray[140] has shown that the B cells giving rise to germinal centers are activated outside the follicle, probably in the T-cell-rich PALS. Germinal centers are oligoclonal: about three B blasts ($CD39^-$, $IgD^-$, but weakly positive for other isotypes) give rise to a germinal center by massive proliferation[141]. The majority of the cells within the germinal center are B cells, while 5–10 per cent are T cells, 1 per cent are FDCs, and some scattered macrophages are present. Fuller *et al.*[142] have provided evidence that the T cells found within germinal centers are specific for the antigen used for immunization. They are positive for CD4, CD3 and CD45RO. The germinal center reaction becomes apparent around three days after immunization, peaks at about 12 days and declines gradually over the next week. Proliferation of the founding B blasts yields a progeny of centroblasts, which carry CD38 and CD10, but no Ig. These centroblasts divide rapidly and give rise to centrocytes, which come out of cell cycle and express low levels of IgGs or IgA. These are the memory B cells, which leave the germinal center and colonize the marginal zone, residing there as a sessile population. In addition, they form the population of recirculating memory B cells. Renewed challenge with antigen induces proliferation of both populations, with the recirculating memory B cells now proliferating in follicles without inducing new germinal centers. The marginal zone memory B cells migrate to the PALS, where they proliferate, presumably after interaction with specific Th cells[136].

*In vitro*, different signals can rescue germinal center B cells from undergoing apoptosis: crosslinking with anti-Ig antibody bound to SRBC may mimic interaction of the antigen receptor with antigen present in immune complexes on FDCs (although it has to be kept in mind that anti-Ig-SRBC has characteristics of TI antigens). Anti-CD40 antibody or soluble CD40L rescue centrocytes, and the resulting B cells have the phenotype of memory B cells. Conversely, the combination of soluble CD23 and IL-1α induces differentiation of tonsillar B cells into IgG-secreting plasmablasts. *In vivo*, the CD23 signal is presumably provided by the FDCs. Presence or absence of expression of the protooncogene *bcl-2* is thought to be an important factor in determining susceptibility to apoptosis of germinal center B-cell subsets[138].

## ROLE OF CD40L IN MEMORY FORMATION

Foy *et al.*[79] showed that anti-CD40L mAb can prevent secondary immune responses to TD antigens *in vivo*. Adoptive transfer experiments confirmed that blocking of CD40–CD40L interactions *in vivo* prevents the secondary immune response[79]. In addition, treatment of mice undergoing a TD response against SRBC with anti-CD40L antibody completely abrogated formation of germinal centers in the spleen[79].

Studies using CD40L gene targeted mice[105] and CD40 knockouts[103,104] confirmed the importance of CD40–CD40L for primary and secondary B-cell responses as well as germinal center formation. Partly contrasting results were obtained by Gray *et al.*[88], who found reduced IgG levels and enhanced IgM titers in the primary response against TD antigen. In these animals, B memory responses were grossly impaired, but germinal centers were formed normally. This led the authors to conclude that CD40 ligation is required to guide B cells into the memory pathway, but that clonal expansion in the germinal center is independent of a CD40 signal. A less appealing explanation is that treatment with the recombinant fusion protein CD40-γl is not fully effective *in vivo*. This would be supported by the data of Lane *et al.*[14], who demonstrated that mouse CD40-γl binds CD40 less effectively than human CD40-Hμ. This group actually used CD40-γl transgenic mice as a negative control in their studies with CTLA4-Ig.

Based on the present data, we favor the view that CD40–CD40L interactions are indispensable for germinal center formation. Whether they are also required for maintenance of memory and germinal centers is currently being investigated by us and others. The issue of where CD40L expression might be required *in vivo* for germinal center formation was discussed on p. 51.

## TI VERSUS TD ANTIGENS IN MEMORY FORMATION

As mentioned above, the inability of TI antigens to induce memory B cells, germinal center formation and affinity maturation can be explained on the basis of their structural characteristics. Because of their poor degradability *in vivo* and inability to bind to class II MHC molecules, no class II restricted presentation of (fragments of) these antigens can take place[23]. In addition, George *et al.*[47] have argued that the potent B-cell-activating abilities of TI antigens preclude receptor density and receptor affinity from working in concert to induce affinity maturation. In other words, TI antigens are so effective in activating B cells that the more subtle process of affinity maturation is not started. Finally, the inability of TI antigens to induce formation of germinal centers is probably crucial. The highly specialized microenvironment of the germinal center apparently is a *sine qua non* for memory formation and affinity maturation. As specific T-cell help is required for germinal center formation, the absence of Th cell induction by TI antigens accounts for the absence of these structures in TI responses. In this respect, it would be predicted that the exceptional TI-antigen-inducing T-cell responses as identified by Zisman *et al.*[25] will also induce B-cell memory and germinal centers.

However, the dogma that TI-2 antigens do not induce germinal centers, memory formation and affinity maturation may be too rigid, and has to be modified when the experiments reported by Wang *et al.*[143] are taken into account. These investigators found that the bacterial polysaccharide $\alpha(1>6)$dextran, a TI-2 antigen, induces a B-cell response at day 4 as expected, but also leads to localization of dextran–anti-dextran immune complexes in the splenic follicles. In addition, dextran-specific germinal centers are formed and affinity maturation occurs to a certain extent. However, the isotype distribution is typical for TI-2 antigens with predominantly IgM and IgA and little IgG. In contrast, the related polysaccharide $\alpha(1>3)\alpha(1>6)$dextran does not induce germinal centers. This study identifies $\alpha(1>6)$dextran as an exceptional TI-2 antigen, allowing further dissection of events required for formation of germinal centers and memory. The fact that no isotype switching is found can be explained by the absence of CD40L-mediated signal and/or the absence of T-cell-derived cytokines. Apparently, the mere presence of the germinal center *per se* is not sufficient to accomplish isotype switching.

## *IN VIVO* CYTOKINE EXPRESSION DURING ANTIBODY RESPONSES

In response to TNP-Ficoll (TI-2) immunization, high frequencies of IFN-$\gamma$-producing cells are found in the murine spleen, produced by CD4 and CD8 positive cells, and by NK cells. These cells were found in direct contact with TNP-specific B cells, in the outer PALS and around the terminal arterioles, confirming the role for IFN-$\gamma$ in regulating TI-2 responses[144]. Cells producing IL-2, IL-4 and IL-5 were found in the same location[38].

As discussed on p. 38, TNP-Ficoll does induce formation of specific B cells in the peripheral lymph nodes, but a local deficiency in cytokine production prevents final maturation of these B cells into actively secreting cells[38].

In response to TNP-KLH (TD) immunization, IgG1 is the principal isotype induced. In agreement with this, high numbers of IL-2- and IL-4-producing cells and lower numbers of IFN-$\gamma$-producing cells are found in the spleen located close to KLH- or TNP-specific B cells[87]. Co-localization of IgM-producing B cells and IL-2- or IL-4-producing cells preceded emergence of IgG-producing B cells, suggesting a role of these cytokines in isotype switching. Bogen *et al.*[145] performed comparable experiments yielding essentially similar results. After TD antigen immunization in complete Freund's adjuvant, IFN-γ-producing NK cells were found at the injection site at day 3. T cells producing IL-2, IL-4 and IFN-γ were detected in the draining lymph nodes and spleen at day 7. IL-2-producing cells were still present several weeks after immunization, which may be explained by the use of adjuvant.

Another TD antigen response which was analysed *in vivo* is the one induced by GαIgD. Binding directly to B cells, this antigen and polyclonal stimulator induces high numbers of IL-2- and IL-4-producing cells, and high titers of IgG1 and IgE (reviewed in reference 146). *In vivo*, IL-2- and IL-4-producing cells were found in contact with IgM-producing B cells 2–5 days after immunization. Production of IgE and IgG1 was found from day 5 onwards. This again is consistent with a role of IL-2 and IL-4 in antibody production and isotype switching, respectively, and confirms *in vitro* studies[147].

Thus, simultaneous *in vivo* detection of cytokine-producing cells, specific B cells and CD40L-expressing cells allows dissection of the antibody response and independent confirmation of *in vivo* studies.

## CYTOKINE PRODUCTION BY GERMINAL CENTER CELLS

Germinal center T cells, B cells and FDCs isolated from human tonsil have been analyzed for the presence of cytokine mRNA. The T cells consistently expressed IL-4 mRNA, and occasionally produced mRNA for IL-10, TNF-α and IFN-γ. The B cells and FDCs did not produce mRNA for any of 10 cytokines evaluated[148]. Based on these findings, only IL-4 mRNA is consistently expressed in germinal centers. By immunocytochemical techniques, no cytokine-producing cells were detected in the follicles of murine spleens or human tonsils[87,144,149,150]. Using similar immunocytochemical procedures, but distinct fixation procedures, Andersson *et al.*[151] found expression of 19 different cytokines in human tonsils. Also in this study, presence of cytokine-producing cells in the germinal centers was rare (IL-5 and TGF-β1, 2 and 3). Cells were mainly found in the epithelial areas of the crypts and the extrafollicular T-cell-rich areas, and were mostly $CD4^+$ T cells.

Corcione *et al.*[152] found that human tonsillar B cells with germinal center B-cell characteristics ($CD38^+$, $CD10^+$ and $sIgG^+$) produced granulocyte colony-stimulating factor (G-CSF) spontaneously in culture. However, cells had to be cultured for at least 2 h before G-CSF transcripts were detectable, which may explain the discrepancy with the data of Butch *et al.*[148].

## LOCALIZATION OF ANTIBODY-FORMING CELLS AND CYTOKINE-PRODUCING CELLS *IN VIVO*

It has been repeatedly and consistently found that antibody-forming cells are only present in the follicles by exception. This was true for antibody-forming cells of known specificity elicited by TD and TI immunization of rabbits and mice[11,87,144,149], but also for antibody-forming cells of unknown specificity in human tonsils[150]. In addition, almost all HIV-1 protein-specific antibody-forming cells were found in the paracortex and medulla of human lymph nodes[153]. It was also demonstrated that cytokine-producing cells are found in the same location as antibody-forming cells, i.e. in the outer PALS and around terminal arterioles of the mouse spleen[87,144] and the extrafollicular areas of human tonsil[150]. Although evidence exists that continuous antigen release favors the intrafollicular development of antibody-forming cells[154], this notion is not supported by data from analysis of human tissue, which was either chronically inflamed in the case of tonsils, or which was undergoing continuous B-cell responses against a locally replicating pathogen in the case of HIV-1-infected lymph nodes.

These findings can be interpreted to mean that the signals required for actual production of considerable quantities of specific antibody are supplied outside the germinal centers, i.e. by the T cells of the paracortex in lymph node and the PALS of the spleen. This does not exclude the possibility that events required for isotype switching and activation of recirculating memory B cells do occur in the germinal centers, but significant antibody synthesis does not take place here.

Figure 2.1 summarizes the sequence of events taking place in murine spleen during the primary antibody response against TD antigens. After i.v. injection, the antigen enters the marginal zone. Particulate antigen will be taken up and pre-processed by the marginal zone macrophages, which transfer it to marginal zone B cells. Alternatively, the marginal zone macrophages may migrate to the inner PALS and transfer the antigen to IDCs. Antigen-specific T cells are activated by IDCs or directly by antigen-presenting B cells, which migrate from the marginal zone into the PALS. Here, antigen-specific B cells and T cells interact. Activation of the T cells leads to expression of CD40L and the cascade of T–B-cell interactions, including cytokine production, and upregulation of B7-1 and B7-2 takes place (see p. 44–54). These interactions lead to full differentiation of B cells to specific plasma cells, found in the outer PALS and around the terminal arterioles.

Antibodies present after primary immunization will complex with antigen after secondary immunization. Immune complexes formed as a result are trapped on the dendrites of FDCs in the follicles, and these complexes aid in the generation of B memory cells. Also in the secondary response, there is a predominance of plasma cells, CD40L positive cells and cytokine-producing cells in the PALS and around the terminal arterioles, indicating that T–C-cell interactions take place here (see, for a more extensive discussion, Van den Eertwegh *et al.*[155]).

## CONCLUSION

In this chapter, we have focused on the cellular interactions and cytokines required for TI and TD responses. However, TI and TD responses also differ in their utilization of signaling pathways, although they both induce expression of ICAM-1 and NFκB. TI antigens extensively crosslink mIg with their repeating epitopes, triggering a mitogenic signal via a protein kinase C (PKC) and a protein tyrosine kinase (PTK) dependent pathway. Some controversy exists with regard to the signaling pathways activated by T-cell-mediated B-cell activation in response to TD antigen (reviewed by Marshall and Noelle in reference 156). Using activated Th membranes, Marshall *et al.*[157] showed that signaling of resting B cells is PTK dependent, but does not require increased intracellular calcium mobilization or PKC activation. This implies that CD40L-induced signaling is distinct from anti-mIg or anti-class II MHC-mediated signaling. Kato *et al.*[158] showed that PTK and PKA pathways are induced by CD40–CD40L interactions. Current knowledge of intracellular B-cell signaling events is reviewed in detail by Cambier *et al.*[52]

Important questions that are currently being addressed by some groups are as follows. Is maintenance of germinal centers dependent on CD40–CD40L interactions? Is CD40L expression within the germinal center required for generation and maintenance of B-cell memory? How can the CD40–CD40L axis be manipulated to induce tolerance? What are the contributions of B7-1 and B7-2 to T–B-cell interaction in response to different stimuli, and what kinetics of expression are operational? In addition, the differential contribution of different APC types in primary and secondary responses against TI and TD antigens needs to be further explored. The mechanism of transfer of processed antigen from macrophages to B cells also needs to be elucidated. How do B cells interact with antigen on FDCs, either in the form of immune complexes or in MHC class II molecules? Finally, despite all the recent new insights the question remains how the specificity of the antibody response is maintained in spite of the fact that the distal phases of B-cell activation are not antigen specific.

A wholly different issue worth pursuing further is what signals determine downregulation and termination of the humoral immune response. An obvious factor is degradation and clearance of the antigen, simply precluding activation of new B cells. Other parameters are the inducible and temporary expression of T- and B-cell accessory molecules, the action of inhibitory cytokines such as IL-10 and TGF-β, the short half-life of cytokines, induction of B-cell anergy or apoptosis by signaling in the absence of antigen, and molecules like CD23 which assist in downregulation.

In conclusion, our understanding of T-cell-independent and T-cell-dependent antibody responses has progressed rapidly in the last few years aided by new technology (e.g. novel molecules mimicking TI and TD antigens, targeted gene disruption), and the functional characterization of novel accessory molecules for cognate T–B-cell interaction (CD40L, B7-1/B7-2) and cytokines. One can safely assume that additional cytokines and receptor–ligand pairs contributing to TI and TD responses will be identified soon. Careful *in vivo* analysis performed in parallel to functional *in vitro* assays and molecular biological approaches will further refine our understanding of TI and TD responses, and will reveal new opportunities for manipulation of the antibody response in vaccination and disease.

## ACKNOWLEDGMENTS

This work was in part supported by a TALENT-stipend from The Netherlands Organization for Scientific Research (NWO) to JDL. Thanks are due to the members of the Division of Immunological and Infectious Disease (TNO Prevention and Health) and the members of the Noelle Laboratory (Department of Microbiology, Dartmouth Medical School, Lebanon NH, USA), who were instrumental in obtaining many of the data described in this chapter. We especially thank Drs Randolph J. Noelle, Michael A. Coppola and Teresa M. Foy for critical reading of the manuscript.

## REFERENCES

1. Pfeffer K, Mak TW. Lymphocyte ontogeny and activation in gene targeted mutant mice. Ann Rev Immunol 1994; 12: 367–412.
2. Scher I. The CBA/N mouse strain: an experimental model illustrating the influence of the X-chromosome on immunity. Adv Immunol 1982; 33:1–71.
3. Chused TM, Kassan SS, Mosier DE. Macrophage requirement for the in vitro response to TNP-Ficoll: a thymic independent antigen. J Immunol 1976; 116:1579–1584.
4. Stein KE. Thymus-independent and thymus-dependent response to polysaccharide antigens. J Infect Dis 1992; 165:S49–S52.
5. Subbarao B, Garg M. Thymus-independent antigens. In: Snow C (ed.) Handbook of T and B lymphocytes. San Diego: Academic Press 1994, pp. 343–370.
6. Laman JD, Van den Eertwegh AJ, Claassen E, van Rooijen N. Cell–cell interactions: in situ studies of splenic humoral immune response. In: Fornusek L, Vetvicka V (eds) Immune System Accessory Cells. Boca Raton: CRC Press Inc. 1992, pp. 201–231.
7. Van den Eertwegh AJM, Boersma WJA, Claassen E. Immunological functions and in vivo cell–cell interactions of T cells in the spleen. Crit Rev Immunol 1992; 11:337–380.

8. Claassen E (ed). Histological organization of the spleen: implications for immune functions in different species. Forum in Immunology, Res Immunol 1991; 142:315–372.
9. Kraal G. Cells in the marginal zone of the spleen. Int Rev Cytol 1992; 132:31–74.
10. Laman JD, Van den Eertwegh AJM. Cytotoxic potential of CD8+ T cells in lymphoid follicles during HIV-1 infection. AIDS 1992; 6:333–334.
11. Van Rooijen N, Claassen E, Eikelenboom P. Is there a single differentiation pathway for all antibody forming cells in the spleen? Immunol Today 1986; 7:193–196.
12. Claassen E, Vos Q, Ott A *et al.* Role of the splenic marginal zone in the removal of, and immune response against, neutral polysaccharides. In: Imhof B, Berrih-Aknin S, Ezine S (eds) Lymphatic Tissues and Immune Responses. New York: Marcel Dekker 1991, pp. 855–862.
13. Delemarre FGA, Kors N, Van Rooijen N. Elimination of spleen and of lymph node macrophages and its difference in the effect on the immune response to particulate antigens. Immunobiology 1990; 182:70–78.
14. Lane P, Burdet C, Hubele S *et al.* B cell function in mice transgenic for mCTLA4-Hγl: lack of germinal centers correlated with poor affinity maturation and class switching despite normal priming of CD4+ T cells. J Exp Med 1994; 179:819–830.
15. Claassen E, Boersma WJA (eds). Characteristics and practical use of new-generation adjuvants as an acceptable alternative to Freund's complete adjuvant. Forum in Immunology, Res Immunol 1992; 143:475–582.
16. Van den Eertwegh AJM, Laman JD, Schellekens MM *et al.* Complement-mediated follicular localization of T-independent type 2 antigens: the role of marginal zone macrophages revisited. Eur J Immunol 1992; 22:719–726.
17. Witmer-Pack MD, Crowley MT, Inaba K, Steinman RM. Macrophages, but not dendritic cells, accumulate colloidal carbon following administration in situ. J Cell Sci 1993; 105:965–973.
18. Buiting AMJ, De Rover Z, Claassen E, Van Rooijen N. In vivo distribution of particulate antigens and liposomes in the murine spleen. A possible role in the humoral immune response. Immunobiology 1992; 188:13–22.
19. Claassen, E. Detection, localisation and kinetics of immunomodulating liposomes in vivo. Forum in Immunology, Res Immunol 1992; 143:235–241.
20. Galelli A, Charlot B, Deriaud E, Leclerc C. B cells do not present antigen covalently linked to microspheres. Immunology 1993; 79:69–76.
21. Crowley M, Inaba K, Steinman RM. Dendritic cells are the principal cells in the mouse spleen bearing immunogenic fragments of foreign proteins. J Exp Med 1990; 172:383–386.
22. Van Rooijen N. The role of the FDC-retained immune complex network and its dynamics in the activity of germinal centres. Res Immunol 1993; 144:545–552.
23. Harding CV, Roof RW, Allen PM, Unanue ER. Effects of pH and polysaccharides on peptide binding to class II major histocompatibility molecules. Proc Natl Acad Sci USA 1991; 88:2740–2744.
24. Fultz M, Carman J, Finkelman FD, Mond JJ. Neonatal suppression with anti-Ia antibody. III. In vivo responses to the type 2 antigen TNP-Ficoll. J Immunol 1989; 143:403–406.
25. Zisman E, Dayan M, Sela M, Mozes E. Ia-antigen–T cell interactions for a thymus-independent antigen composed of D amino acids. Proc Natl Acad Sci USA 1993; 90:994–998.
26. Dintzis HM, Dintzis RZ, Vogelstein B, Molecular determinants of immunogenicity: the immunon model of the immune response. Proc Natl Acad Sci USA 1976; 73:3671–3675.

27. Kishihara K, Penninger J, Wallace VA *et al.* Normal B lymphocyte development but impaired T cell maturation in CD45-exon6 protein tyrosine phosphatase deficient mice. Cell 1993; 74:143–156.
28. Tarakhovsky A, Muller W, Rajewsky K. Lymphocyte populations and immune responses in CD5-deficient mice. Eur J Immunol 1994; 24:1678–1684.
29. Mond JJ, Brunswick M. A role for IFN-γ and NK cells in immune responses to T-cell regulated antigens types 1 and 2. Immunol Rev 1987; 99:105–118.
30. Elkins, KL, Buller RML, Stashak PW, Baker PJ. CD4+ T cells regulate the magnitude of the antibody response to several helper T cell independent antigens. Immunobiology 1991; 183:69–78.
31. Snapper CM, Mond JJ. Towards a comprehensive view of immunoglobulin class switching. Immunol Today 1993; 14:15–17.
32. Pecanha LMT, Snapper CM, Lees A, Mond JJ. Lymphokine control of type 2 antigen response. IL-10 inhibits IL-5- but not IL-2-induced secretion by T-cell independent antigens. J Immunol 1992; 148:3427–3432.
33. Pecanha LMT, Yamaguchi H, Lees A *et al.* Dextran-conjugated anti-IgD antibodies inhibit T cell mediated IgE production but augment the synthesis of IgM and IgG. J Immunol 1993; 150:2160–2168.
34. Snapper CM, McIntyre TM, Mandler R *et al.* Induction of Ig3 secretion by interferon γ: a model for T cell-independent class switching in response to T cell-independent type 2 antigens. J Exp Med 1992; 175:1367–1371.
35. Snapper CM, Yamaguchi H, Moorman MA, Mond JJ. An in vitro model for T cell-independent induction of humoral immunity. A requirement for NK cells. J Immunol 1994; 152:4884–4892.
36. Goud SN, Kaplan AM, Subbarao B. Priming of peripheral lymph node B cells with TNP-Ficoll: role of lymphokines in B cell differentiation. Cell Immunol 1992; 144:407–416.
37. Goud SN, Kaplan AM, Subbarao B. Primary antibody responses to thymus-independent antigens in the lungs and hilar lymph nodes of mice. Infect Immun 1990; 58:2035–2041.
38. Van den Eertwegh AJM, Laman JD, Van Meurs M *et al.* Differential in vivo appearance of activated T cells, cytokine producing cells and antibody-forming cells in peripheral lymph nodes and the spleen after immunization with thymus independent type 2 antigens. Submitted.
39. Mohler KM, Sleath PR, Fitzner JN *et al.* Protection against a lethal dose of endotoxin by an inhibitor of tumour necrosis factor processing. Nature 1994; 370:218–220.
40. Maliszewski CR. CD14 and immune response to lipopolysaccharide. Science 1991; 252:1321.
41. Wright SD. CD14 and immune response to lipopolysaccharide. Science 1991; 252:1321–1322.
42. Noelle RJ, Snow EC. Cognate interactions between helper T cells and B cells. Immunol Today 1990; 11:361–368.
43. Germain RN, Margulies DH. The biochemistry and cell biology of antigen processing and presentation. Annu Rev Immunol 1993; 11:403–450.
44. Grey HM, Chesnut R. Antigen processing and presentation to T cells. Immunol Today 1985; 6:101–105.
45. Lanzavecchia A. Receptor-mediated antigen uptake and its effect on antigen presentation to class-II-restricted T lymphocytes. Annu Rev Immunol 1990; 8:773–794.
46. Bachmann MF, Hoffman Rohrer U, Kündig TM *et al.* The influence of antigen organization on B cell responsiveness. Science 1993; 262:1448–1451.

47. George J, Penner SJ, Weber J *et al.* Influence of membrane Ig receptor density and affinity on B cell signaling by antigen. Implications for affinity maturation. J Immunol 1993; 151:5955–5965.
48. Luxembourg AT, Cooper NR. T cell-dependent, B cell-activating properties of antibody-coated small latex beads. J Immunol 1994; 153:604–614.
49. Velupillai P, Harn DA. Oligosaccharide-specific induction of interleukin 10 production by B220+ cells from schistosome infected mice: a mechanism for regulation of CD4+ T cell subsets. Proc Natl Acad Sci USA 1994; 91:18–22.
50. Clark EA, Ledbetter JA. How B and T cells talk to each other. Nature 1994; 367:425–428.
51. Cosgrove D, Gray D, Dierich A *et al.* Mice lacking MHC class II molecules. Cell 1991; 66:1051–1066.
52. Cambier JC, Pleiman CM, Clark MR. Signal transduction by the B cell antigen receptor and its coreceptors. Annu Rev Immunol 1994; 12:457–486.
53. Aruffo A, Kanner SB, Sgroi D *et al.* CD22-mediated stimulation of T cells regulates T-cell receptor/CD3-induced signaling. Proc Natl Acad Sci USA 1992; 89:10242–10246.
54. Poudrier J, Owen T. CD54/intercellular adhesion molecule 1 and major histocompatibility complex II signaling induces B cells to express interleukin 2 receptors and complements help provided through CD40 ligation. J Exp Med 1994; 179:1417–1427.
55. Carter RH, Fearon DT. CD19: lowering the threshold for antigen receptor stimulation of B lymphocytes. Science 1992; 256:105–107.
56. Van Noesel CJM, Lankester AC, Van Lier RAW. Dual antigen recognition by B-cells. Immunol Today 1993; 14:8–11.
57. Förster R, Emrich T, Kremmer E, Lipp M. Expression of the G-protein-coupled receptor BLR1 defines mature, recirculating B cells and a subset of T-helper memory cells. Blood 1994; 84:830–840.
58. Nitschke L, Kosco MH, Kohler G, Lamers MC. Immunoglobulin D-deficient mice can mount normal immune responses to thymus-independent and -dependent antigens. Proc Natl Acad Sci USA 1993; 90:1887–1891.
59. Roes J, Rajewsky K. Immunoglobulin D (IgD) deficient mice reveal an auxiliary receptor function for IgD in antigen-mediated recruitment of B cells. J Exp Med 1993; 177:45–55.
60. Durie FH, Foy TM, Masters SR *et al.* The role of CD40 in the regulation of humoral and cell-mediated immunity. Immunol Today 1994; 15:406–411.
61. Banchereau J, Bazan F, Blanchard D *et al.* The CD40 antigen and its ligand. Annu Rev Immunol 1994; 12:881–922.
62. Linsley PS, Ledbetter JA. The role of the CD28 receptor during T cell responses to antigen. Adv Immunol 1993; 11:191–212.
63. Hathcock KS, Laszlo G, Dickler HB *et al.* Identification of an alternative CTLA-4 ligand costimulatory for T-cell activation. Science 1993; 262:905–909.
64. Azuma M, Ito D, Yagita H *et al.* B70 antigen is a second ligand for CTLA-4 and CD28. Nature 1993; 366:76–79.
65. Roy M, Aruffo A, Ledbetter JA *et al.* Studies on the interdependence of gp39 and B7 expression during antigen-specific immune responses. Eur J Immunol 1995; 25:596–603.
66. Stack RM, Lenschow DJ, Gray GS *et al.* IL-4 treatment of small splenic B cells induces costimulatory molecules B7-1 and B7-2. J Immunol 1994; 152:5723–5733.
67. Yellin MJ, Sinnig, J, Covey LR *et al.* T lymphocyte T cell–B cell-activating molecule/CD40L molecules induce normal B cell or chronic lymphocytic

leukemia B cells to express CD80 (B7/BB1) and enhance their costimulatory activity. J Immunol 1994; 153:666–674.

68. Klaus SJ, Pinchuk LM, Ochs HD *et al.* Costimulation through CD28 enhances T-cell dependent B cell activation via CD40–CD40L interaction. J Immunol 1994; 152:5643–5652.
69. Linsley PS, Wallace PM, Johnson J *et al.* Immunosuppression in vivo by a soluble form of the CTLA-4 T cell activation molecule. Science 1992; 257:792–795.
70. Ronchese F, Hausmann B, Hubele S, Lane P. Mice transgenic for a soluble form of murine CTLA-4 show enhanced expansion of antigen-specific CD4+ T-cells and defective antibody production in vivo. J Exp Med 1994; 179:809–817.
71. Shahinian A, Pfeffer K, Lee KP *et al.* Differential T cell costimulatory requirements in CD28-deficient mice. Science 1993; 261:609–612.
72. Hathcock KS, Laszlo G, Pucillo C *et al.* Comparative analysis of B7-1 and B7-2 costimulatory ligands: expression and function. J Exp Med 1994; 180:631–640.
73. Banchereau J, de Paoli P, Valle A *et al.* Long-term human B cell lines dependent on interleukin-4 and antibody to CD40. Science 1991; 251:70–72.
74. Armitage RJ, Fanslow WC, Strockbine L *et al.* Molecular and biological characterization of a murine ligand for CD40. Nature 1992; 357:80–82.
75. Hollenbaugh D, Grosmaire L, Kullas CD *et al.* The human T cell antigen gp39, a member of the TNF gene family, is a ligand for the CD40 receptor; expression of a soluble form of gp39 with B cell co-stimulatory activity. EMBO J 1992; 11:4313–4321.
76. Lederman S, Yellin MJ, Krichevsky A *et al.* Identification of a novel surface protein on activated CD4+ T cells that induces contact-dependent B cell differentiation (help). J Exp Med 1992; 175:1091–1101.
77. Noelle RJ, Roy M, Shepherd DM *et al.* A novel ligand on activated T helper cells binds CD40 and transduces the signal for the cognate activation of B cells. Proc Natl Acad Sci USA 1992; 89:6550–6554.
78. Foy TM, Aruffo A, Ledbetter JA, Noelle RJ. In vivo CD40–gp39 interactions are essential for thymus-dependent immunity. II. Prolonged in vivo suppression of primary and secondary humoral immune responses by an antibody targeted to the CD40 ligand, gp39. J Exp Med 1993; 178:1567–1575.
79. Foy TM, Laman JD, Ledbetter JA *et al.* gp39–CD40 interactions are essential for germinal center formation and the development of B cell memory. J Exp Med 1994; 180:157–163.
80. Hollenbaugh D, Ochs HD, Noelle RJ *et al.* The role of CD40 and its ligand in the regulation of the immune response. Immunol Rev 1994; 148:23–37.
81. Beutler B, van Huffer C. Unraveling function in the TNF ligand and receptor families. Science 1994; 264:667–668.
82. Saeland S, Duvert V, Moreau I, Banchereau J. Human B cell precursors proliferate and express CD23 after CD40 ligation. J Exp Med 1993; 178:113–120.
83. Galibert L, Durand I, Bancherau J, Rousset F. CD40-activated surface IgD-positive lymphocytes constitute the long term IL-4 dependent proliferating B cell pool. J Immunol 1994; 152:22–29.
84. Alderson MR, Armitage RJ, Tough TW *et al.* CD40 expression by human monocytes: regulation by cytokines and activation of monocytes by the ligand for CD40. J Exp Med 1993; 178:669–674.
85. Ramsdell F, Seaman MS, Clifford KN, Fanslow WC. CD40 ligand acts as a costimulatory signal for neonatal $\gamma\delta$ T cells. J Immunol 1994; 152:2190–2197.
86. Roy M, Waldschmidt T, Aruffo A *et al.* Regulation of gp39 expression on normal and cloned CD4+ T cells. J Immunol 1993; 151:2497–2510.

87. Van den Eertwegh AJM, Noelle RJ, Roy M *et al.* In vivo CD40–gp39 interactions are essential for thymus-dependent immunity. I. CD40–gp39 interactions are essential for thymus dependent humoral immunity and identify sites of cognate interactions in vivo. J Exp Med 1993; 178:1555–1565.
88. Gray D, Dullforce P, Jainandunsing S. Memory B cell development but not germinal center formation is impaired by in vivo blockade of CD40–CD40 ligand interaction. J Exp Med 1994; 180:141–155.
89. Mohan C, Shi Y, Laman JD, Datta SK. Interaction between CD40 and its ligand in the development of murine lupus nephritis. J Immunol 1995; 154:1470–1480.
90. Lederman S, Yellin MJ, Inghirami G *et al.* Molecular interactions mediating T–B lymphocyte collaboration in human lymphoid follicles. Roles of T cell–B-cell-activating molecule (5c8 antigen) and CD40 in contact-dependent help. J Immunol 1992; 149:3817–3826.
91. Yellin MJ, Sippel K, Inghirami G *et al.* CD40 molecules induce down-modulation and endocytosis of T cell surface T cell–B cell activating molecule CD40L. Potential role in regulating helper effector function. J Immunol 1994; 152:598–608.
92. Jacob J, Kelsoe G. In situ studies of the primary immune response to (4-hydroxy-3-nitrophenyl) acetyl. II. A common clonal origin for periarteriolar lymphoid sheath-associated foci and germinal centers. J Exp Med 1992; 176:679–687.
93. Küppers R, Zhao M, Hansmann M-L, Rajewsky K. Tracing B cell development in human germinal centers by molecular analysis of single cells picked from histological section. EMBO J 1993; 12:4955–4967.
94. Aruffo A, Farrington M, Hollenbaugh D *et al.* The CD40 ligand, gp39, is defective in activated T cells from patients with X-linked hyper-IgM syndrome. Cell 1993; 72:291–300.
95. DiSanto JP, Bonnefoy JY, Gauchat JP *et al.* CD40 ligand mutations in X-linked immunodeficiency with hyper-IgM. Nature 1993; 361:541–543.
96. Allen RC, Armitage RJ, Conley ME *et al.* CD40 ligand gene defects responsible for X-linked hyper-IgM syndrome. Science 1993; 259:990–993.
97. Fuleihan R, Ramesh N, Loh R *et al.* Defective expression of the CD40 ligand in X chromosome-linked immunoglobulin deficiency with normal or elevated IgM. Proc Natl Acad Sci USA 1993; 90:2170–2173.
98. Körthauer U, Graf D, Mages HW *et al.* Defective expression of T-cell CD40 ligand causes X-linked immunodeficiency with hyper-IgM. Nature 1993; 361:539.
99. Ramesh N, Fuleihan R, Ramesh V *et al.* Deletions in the ligand for CD40 in X-linked immunoglobulin deficiency with normal or elevated IgM (HIGMX-1). Int Immunol 1993; 5:769–773.
100. Farrington M, Grosmaire LS, Nonoyama S *et al.* CD40 ligand expression is defective in a subset of patients with common variable immunodeficiency. Proc Natl Acad Sci USA 1994; 91:1099–1103.
101. Chirmule N, Kalyanaraman VS, Lederman S *et al.* HIV-gp160 induced T cell-dependent B cell differentiation. Role of T cell–B cell activation molecule and IL-6. J Immunol 1993; 150:2478–2486.
102. Laman JD, Claassen E, Noelle RJ. Immunodeficiency due to a faulty interaction between T cells and B cells. Curr Opin Immunol 1994; 6:636–641.
103. Kawabe T, Naka T, Yoshida K *et al.* The immune responses in CD40-deficient mice: impaired immunoglobulin class switching and germinal center formation. Immunity 1994; 1:167–178.
104. Castigli E, Alt F, Davidson L *et al.* CD40 deficient mice generated by RAG-2

deficient blastocyst complementation. Proc Natl Acad Sci USA 1994; 91:12135–12139.

105. Xu J, Foy TM, Laman JD *et al.* Mice deficient for the CD40 ligand. Immunity 1994; 1:423–431.

106. Durie FH, Fava RA, Foy TM *et al.* Prevention of collagen-induced arthritis with an antibody to gp39, the ligand for CD40. Science 1993; 261:1328–1330.

107. Durie FH, Aruffo A, Ledbetter JA *et al.* Antibody to the ligand of CD40, gp39, blocks the occurrence of the acute and chronic forms of graft-vs-host disease. J Clin Invest 1994; 94:1333–1338.

108. Gerritse K, Laman JD, Noelle RJ, *et al.* CD40-CD40 ligand interactions in experimental allergic encephalomyelitis and multiple sclerosis. Proc Natl Acad Sci USA, in press.

109. Tsubata T, Wu J, Honjo T. B-cell apoptosis induced by antigen receptor crosslinking is blocked by a T-cell signal through CD40. Nature 1993; 364:645–648.

110. Lederman S, Yellin MJ, Cleary AM *et al.* T-BAM/CD40-L on helper T lymphocytes augments lymphokine-induced B cell Ig isotype switch recombination and rescues B cells from programmed cell death. J Immunol 1994; 152:2163–2171.

111. Renschler MF, Bhatt RR, Dower WJ, Levy R. Synthetic peptide ligands of the antigen binding receptor induce programmed cell death in a human B-cell lymphoma. Proc Natl Acad Sci USA 1994; 91:3623–3627.

112. Newell MK, VanderWall J, Beard KS, Freed JH. Ligation of major histocompatibility complex class II molecules mediates apoptotic death in resting B lymphocytes. Proc Natl Acad Sci USA 1993; 90:10459–10463.

113. Funakoshi S, Longo DL, Beckwith M *et al.* Inhibition of human B-cell lymphoma growth by CD40 stimulation. Blood 1994; 83:2787–2794.

114. Eris JM, Basten A, Brink R *et al.* Anergic self-reactive B cells present self antigen and respond normally to CD40-dependent T-cell signals but are defective in antigen-receptor-mediated functions. Proc Natl Acad Sci USA 1994; 91:4392–4396.

115. Punnonen J, Aversa G, Cocks BJ *et al.* Interleukin 13 induces interleukin 4-independent IgG4 and IgE synthesis and CD23 expression by human B-cells. Proc Natl Acad Sci USA 1993; 90:3730–3734.

116. Brière F, Servet-Delprat C, Bridon J-M *et al.* Human interleukin 10 induces naive sIgD+ B cells to secrete IgG1 and IgG3. J Exp Med 1994; 179:757–762.

117. Punnonen J, Aversa G, de Vries JE. Human pre-B cells differentiate into Ig-secreting plasma cells in the presence of interleukin-4 and activated CD4+ T cells or their membranes. Blood 1993; 82:2781–2789.

118. Renard N, Duvert V, Blanchard D *et al.* Activated CD4+ T cells induce CD40-dependent proliferation of human B cell precursors. J Immunol 1994; 152:1693–1701.

119. Boussiotis VA, Nadler LM, Strominger JL, Goldfeld AE. Tumor necrosis factor α is an autocrine growth factor for normal human B cells. Proc Natl Acad Sci USA 1994; 91:7007–7011.

120. Snapper CM, Moorman MA, Rosas FR *et al.* IL-3 and granulocyte-macrophage colony-stimulating factor strongly induce Ig secretion by sort-purified murine B cells activated through the membrane Ig, but not the CD40, signaling pathway. J Immunol 1995: 154:5842–5850.

121. Nakanishi K, Yoshimoto T, Chu CC *et al.* IL-2 inhibits IL-4-dependent IgE and IgG1 production in vitro and in vivo. Int Immunol 1995; 7:259–268.

122. De Becker G, Sornasse T, Nabavi N *et al.* Immunoglobulin isotype regulation by antigen-presenting cells in vivo. Eur J Immunol 1994; 24:1523–1528.

123. Kupfer H, Monks CRF, Kupfer A. Small splenic B cells that bind to antigen-specific T helper (Th) cells and face the site of cytokine production in the Th cells selectively proliferate: immunofluorescence microscopic studies of Th–B antigen-presenting cell interactions. J Exp Med 1994; 179:1507–1515.
124. Jabara HH, Vercelli D. Engagement of CD14 on monocytes inhibits the synthesis of human Igs, including IgE. J Immunol 1994; 153:972–978.
125. Kündig TM, Schorle H, Bachmann MF *et al.* Immune responses in interleukin-2-deficient mice. Science 1993; 262:1059–1061.
126. Kopf M, Le Gros G, Bachmann M *et al.* Disruption of the murine IL-4 gene blocks Th2 cytokine responses. Nature 1993; 362:245–248.
127. Oettgen HC, Martin TR, Wynshaw-Boris A *et al.* Active anaphylaxis in IgE-deficient mice. Nature 1994; 370:367–370.
128. Marsh DG, Neely JD, Breazeale DR *et al.* Linkage analysis of IL4 and other chromosome 5q31.1 markers and total serum immunoglobulin E concentrations. Science 1994; 264:1152–1156.
129. Gauchat J-F, Henchoz S, Mazzei G *et al.* Induction of human IgE synthesis in B cells by mast cells and basophils. Nature 1993; 365:340–343.
130. Gauchat J-F, Aversa G, Gascan H, de Vries JE. Modulation of IL-4 induced germline $\epsilon$ synthesis in human B cells by tumor necrosis factor-$\alpha$, anti-CD40 monoclonal antibodies or transforming growth factor-$\beta$ correlates with levels of IgE production. Int Immunol 1992; 4:397–406.
131. Gustavsson S, Hjulström S, Tianmim L, Heyman B. CD23/IgE-mediated regulation of the specific antibody response in vivo. J Immunol 1994; 152:4793–4800.
132. Yu P, Kosco-Vilbois M, Richards M *et al.* Negative feedback regulation of IgE synthesis by murine CD23. Nature 1994; 369:753–756.
133. Fujiwara H, Kikutani H, Suematsu S *et al.* The absence of IgE antibody-mediated augmentation of immune responses in CD23-deficient mice. Proc Natl Acad Sci USA 1994; 91:6835–6839.
134. Kimata H, Yoshida A, Ishioka C *et al.* Interleukin 8 (IL-8) selectively inhibits immunoglobulin E production induced by IL-4 in human B cells. J Exp Med 1992; 176:1227–1231.
135. Van Rooijen N. Antigen processing and presentation in vivo: the microenvironment as a crucial factor. Immunol Today 1990; 11:436–439.
136. Gray D. Immunological memory. Annu Rev Immunol 1993; 11:49–77.
137. Liu Y-J, Zhang J, Lane PJL *et al.* Sites of specific B cell activation in primary and secondary response to T cell-dependent and T cell-independent antigens. Eur J Immunol 1991; 21:2951–2962.
138. MacLennan ICM. Germinal centers. Annu Rev Immunol 1994; 12:117–139.
139. Jacob J, Kassir R, Kelsoe G. In situ studies of the primary immune response to (4-hydroxy-3-nitrophenyl)acetyl. I. The architecture and dynamics of responding cell populations. J Exp Med 1991; 173:1165–1175.
140. Gray D. Recruitment of virgin B cells into an immune response is restricted to activation outside of follicles. Immunology 1988; 65:73–80.
141. Kroese FGM, Wubbena AS, Seijen HG, Nieuwenhuis P. Germinal centers develop oligoclonally. Eur J Immunol 1987; 17:1069–1077.
142. Fuller KA, Kanagawa O, Nahm MH. T cells within germinal centers are specific for the immunizing antigen. J Immunol 1993; 151:4505–4512.
143. Wang D, Wells SM, Stall AM, Kabat EA. Reaction of germinal centers in the T-cell-independent response to the bacterial polysaccharide $\alpha(1>6)$dextran. Proc Natl Acad Sci USA 1994; 91:2502–2506.
144. Van den Eertwegh AJM, Fasbender MJ, Schellekens MM *et al.* In vivo kinetics

and characterization of IFN-γ producing cells during a thymus independent immune response. J Immunol 1991; 147:439–446.

145. Bogen SA, Fogelman I, Abbas A. Analysis of IL-2, IL-4 and IFN-γ-producing cells in situ during immune responses to protein antigens. J Immunol 1993; 150:4197–4205.
146. Finkelman FD, Holmes JM, Katona IM *et al.* Lymphokine control of in vivo immunoglobulin isotype selection. Annu Rev Immunol 1990; 8:303–334.
147. Finkelman FD, Urban JF, Beckman MP *et al.* Regulation of murine in vivo IgG and IgE responses by a monoclonal anti-IL-4 receptor antibody. Int Immunol 1991; 6:599–607.
148. Butch AW, Chung GH, Hoffman JW, Nahm MH. Cytokine expression by germinal center B cells. J Immunol 1993; 150:39–47.
149. Claassen E, Gerritse K, Laman JD, Boersma WJA. New immunoenzyme-cytochemical stainings for the in situ detection of epitope specificity and isotype of antibody forming B cells in experimental and natural (auto)immune responses in animals and man. J Immunol Methods 1992; 150:207–216.
150. Hoefakker S, van't Erve EHM, Deen C *et al.* Immunohistochemical detection of co-localizing cytokine and antibody producing cells in the extrafollicular area of human palatine tonsils. Clin Exp Immunol 1993; 93:223–228.
151. Andersson J, Abrams J, Björk L *et al.* Concomitant in vivo production of 19 different cytokines in human tonsils. Immunology 1994; 83:16–24.
152. Corcione A, Baldi L, Zupo S *et al.* Spontaneous production of granulocyte colony-stimulating factor in vitro by human B-lineage lymphocytes is a distinctive marker of germinal center cells. J Immunol 1994; 153:2868–2877.
153. Laman JD, Rácz P, Tenner-Ràcz K *et al.* Immunocytochemical determination of antigen and epitope specificity of HIV-1 specific B cells in lymph node biopsies from HIV-1 infected individuals. AIDS 1991; 5:255–262.
154. Van Rooijen N. Direct intrafollicular differentiation of memory B cells into plasma cells. Immunol Today 1990; 11:154–157.
155. Van den Eertwegh AJM, Laman JD, Noelle RJ *et al.* In vivo T–B cell interactions and cytokine production in the spleen. Semin Immunol 1994; 6:327–336.
156. Marshall LS, Noelle RJ. Distinctive signalling pathways for TI versus TD B cell responses. In: Snow C (ed.) Handbook of T and B Lymphocytes. San Diego: Academic Press 1994, pp. 371–387.
157. Marshall LS, Shepherd DM, Ledbetter JA *et al.* Signaling events during T cell dependent B cell activation. I. Analysis of the signal transduction pathways triggered by activated helper T cells in resting B cells. J Immunol 1994; 152:4816–4825.
158. Kato T, Kokuho T, Tamura T, Nariuchi H. Mechanisms of T cell contact-dependent B cell activation. J Immunol 1994; 152:2130–2138.
159. Burke F, Naylor MS, Davies B, Balkwill F. The cytokine wall chart. Immunol Today 1993; 14:165–170.

# 3 B-cell Subpopulations and Microenvironments

**THOMAS J. WALDSCHMIDT**
*University of Iowa College of Medicine, Iowa City, Iowa, USA*

## INTRODUCTION

For a number of years, immunologists have appreciated significant diversity within the T-cell compartment. In addition to the well-established CD4+ and CD8+ populations, subsets are also defined by their T-cell receptor usage ($\alpha\beta$ versus $\gamma\delta$), cytokine secretion profiles (Th1 versus Th2), and site of origin (thymic versus extrathymic). When considering the B-cell compartment however, few acknowledge a similar range of diversity. The intent of this chapter is to review the available data which demonstrate the existence of histologically, phenotypically, and functionally distinct B-cell subsets. The present chapter will focus on murine B cells, with particular emphasis on surface marker expression. Specific information on the histologic distribution of B cells is found in Chapter 2. Also, excellent reviews have recently appeared which discuss the complexity of the human B-cell compartment in great detail[1,2].

## B-CELL SUBSETS DURING MATURATION

It is well established that during their maturation, B cells go through a series of highly regulated steps. Many of these maturational steps can be defined by combinations of surface and cytoplasmic markers, along with assessment of immunoglobulin (Ig) heavy and light chain genes. Accordingly, the environment where B cells mature is a rich source of B-cell subsets, defined in this case by the ontogenic stage. The site of murine B-cell lymphopoiesis differs depending upon the age of the organism. In the fetus, the major site of B-cell maturation is clearly the liver (reviewed in reference 3), with additional sites, such as the omentum, being reported[4]. After birth, B-cell maturation moves to the spleen for a period ranging from days[5] to weeks[6], with the bone marrow being the primary site of maturation in the adult[3].

By combining molecular and flow cytometric approaches, a number of

*Cytokine Regulation of Humoral Immunity: Basic and Clinical Aspects.* Edited by Clifford M. Snapper.

**Table 3.1** B-cell maturational stages

| | A | B | C | C′ | D | E | F |
|---|---|---|---|---|---|---|---|
| DJ—heavy chain | +/− | + | + | + | + | + | + |
| VDJ—heavy chain | − | +/− | + | + | + | + | + |
| VJ—kappa | − | +/− | +/− | +/− | + | + | + |
| B220 | Low | Low | Low | Low | Low | Int.[a] | High |
| HSA | Low | Int. | High | Bright | Bright | Bright | Int. |
| CD43R (S7) | + | + | + | + | − | − | − |
| BP1 | − | − | + | + | + | +/− | − |
| c-kit | − | + | + | +/− | − | − | − |
| IL-7R | − | + | + | + | + | − | − |
| TdT | +/− | + | + | + | − | − | − |
| RAG 1/2 | + | + | +[b] | | + | − | − |
| Bcl-2 | + | + | + | | − | − | + |
| $V^{pre\text{-}B}/\lambda 5$ | − | + | + | | + | − | − |
| IgM | − | − | − | − | − | High | Low |
| IgD | − | − | − | − | − | −/Low | High |
| Igα,B | − | − | + | | + | + | + |
| CD25 | − | − | − | − | + | + | − |
| pan CD43 (S11) | + | + | + | + | + | + | − |
| MHC class II | − | − | − | − | Int. | Int. | High |
| FcγRII (CD32) | + | + | + | + | + | + | + |
| CR2 (CD21) | − | − | − | − | − | +/− | + |
| CD22 | − | − | − | − | − | +/− | + |
| FcεRII CD23 | − | − | − | − | − | +/− | + |

[a]Intermediate levels.
[b]Boxed areas indicate that C and C′ stages were analyzed together[8].

groups have been able to identify marker combinations which clearly demarcate the various stages of murine B-cell maturation. These studies have correlated the recombination status of the Ig heavy and light chain variable region genes with the presence of cytoplasmic and surface markers[7–10]. Using such an approach, Hardy and co-workers defined seven maturational B-cell stages present in the bone marrow[7]. As summarized in Table 3.1, these stages are referred to as A, B, C, C′, D, E and F, and are listed with their variable region, cytoplasmic and surface characteristics. Other investigators have likewise studied the maturational sequence of murine B cells, and have offered alternative schemes[11,12].

## MATURATIONAL SUBSETS DEFINED BY IMMUNOGLOBULIN GENE REARRANGEMENT AND EXPRESSION

Central to discussing the maturational progression of B cells is an understanding of heavy and light chain variable region gene rearrangement (reviewed in reference 13). The complete heavy chain variable region is constructed by a D to J rearrangement, followed by a V to DJ rearrangement.

The light chain variable region requires only a V to J recombination. The earliest identifiable B-lineage cell is that which has both its heavy and light chain variable region genes in germline configuration. These cells exist in the A population[7–10]. This cell proceeds to undergo heavy chain D to J joining (populations A–C), followed by V to DJ rearrangements (populations B–C[7–10]). Upon productive recombination of a complete heavy chain variable region, μ heavy chain protein can now be found in the cytoplasm, as well as on the cell surface in combination with the surrogate light chain complex (population D[8,11]). This latter complex consists of the $V^{pre\text{-}B}$ and λ5 proteins (reviewed in reference 11). Light chain V to J rearrangements, detectable already in population B, come to completion in population D, and allow for the production of light chain proteins[7–10]. The presence of both μ heavy chains and either κ or λ light chains allows for assembly and surface expression of a complete IgM molecule (population E). The $IgM^+$ immature B cell progresses to display high levels of IgM, followed by concomitant expression of IgM and low levels of IgD, and finally low levels of IgM and high levels of IgD. This $IgM^{lo}/IgD^{hi}$ B cell is considered to be a mature, naive, immunocompetent B cell (population F). Evidence suggests that B cells leave the bone marrow at the immature $IgM^{hi}/IgD^{lo}$ stage, seed the secondary lymphoid organs, and complete their maturational sequence in the periphery[14,15].

## MATURATIONAL SUBSETS DEFINED BY CYTOPLASMIC PROTEINS

As the B cell progresses through its maturational sequence, proteins required for this process can be found in the cytoplasm at defined stages. Terminal deoxynucleotidyl transferase (TdT) and the recombinase-associated gene products RAG-1 and RAG-2 are proteins involved in coding joint modification and variable region assembly respectively. TdT appears early in population A and is present through the C and C′ stages[8,10]. Its absence in population D is consistent with the paucity of N region insertions in light chain V–J coding joints. RAG-1 and RAG-2 are also detectable in population A, consistent with the onset of D–J rearrangement, and remain present through light chain variable region assembly (population D[8,10]). Bcl-2 is another cytoplasmic protein whose presence is tightly correlated with maturational stage[8,10]. Bcl-2 is found in populations A–C, is absent in populations D and E, and reappears in the mature B cell (stage F). Given its apparent role in maintaining cell viability, the pattern of Bcl-2 expression is predictable. During the early stages, maintenance and expansion of clones is desired (populations A–C), whereas once B cells have the capacity to display their newly formed antigen receptors (population E), purging of self-reactive clones requires susceptibility to programmed cell death[16]. Subsequent to the tolerance-susceptible stage, mature B cells (population F) reacquire Bcl-2 to aid in extending peripheral lifespan[8,10].

## MATURATIONAL SUBSETS DEFINED BY SURFACE MARKERS

### Pan-B Cell Markers

In addition to surface markers which allow for definition of subsets, it is essential to have markers which can identify the B-cell lineage in total. In the mouse, antibodies directed against the B220 form of the CD45 antigen, such as 6B2[17] or 14.8[18] have been most utilized. Other markers broadly expressed on B cells include Fc$\gamma$RII (CD32[6]), heat-stable antigen (HSA[19]), and Lyb-2 (CD72[20]). B220 has been the marker of choice, given the wide availability of rat antibodies and its minimal expression on cells of other lineages.

### Early B-cell Markers

A number of surface markers are useful in defining the early stages of B-cell maturation. The most useful of these is the CD43 isoform defined by the S7 antibody[21]. CD43, or leukosialin, is a heavily glycosylated protein which exists in at least three isoforms in the mouse (C. Best, J. Kemp and T. Waldschmidt, unpublished). Compared to the pan CD43 form (see below), the S7 or CD43R form is restricted in its expression on B cells. This isoform is present on populations A–C′, as it is the defining marker of these subsets, and is absent on later stages[7]. Also present during the early phases of B-cell maturation are the receptors for steel factor (c-kit) and IL-7[10,22–24]. These receptors are most prominently expressed during the B and C stages, with the IL-7 receptor still detectable in the D population. Although the pan B cell markers B220 and HSA are broadly expressed, their surface density is regulated according to maturational stage. Throughout the early phases B220 is characteristically displayed at low levels, whereas HSA progressively increases from low expression in the A population to high levels in the C′ population[7].

### Intermediate B-cell Markers

During the late pro-B, pre-B and early immature B-cell stages (populations C–E), the metallopeptidase ectoenzyme defined by the antibodies BP-1 and 6C3[25,26] is readily detectable. In maturing B cells of the adult bone marrow, MHC class II also appears at stage D in moderate levels, and continues increasing its expression until the B cell is mature[27–29]. CD25, the $\alpha$ chain of the IL-2 receptor complex, also appears on population D cells and is maintained through the E or immature B-cell stage[30,31]. Upon final maturation of the B cell, CD25 is lost. Whereas the S7 form of CD43 is restricted to early B cells, the pan form, defined by the antibody S11, is present from the earliest stage (population A) to the immature stage (population E (C. Best, J. Kemp and T. Waldschmidt, unpublished)).

### Late B-cell Markers

In addition to the acquisition of IgD, a number of other markers define the murine B cell as mature. These markers include CD21 (complement receptor 2 (T. Waldschmidt, personal observation)), CD22 (Lyb-8[32]) and CD23 (the low-affinity FcεR[33,34]). As described later, CD23 is only useful in defining mature conventional B cells. Also characteristic of mature B cells is the high expression of B220, and moderate levels of heat-stable antigen (HSA).

## B-CELL SUBSETS IN THE PERIPHERAL LYMPHOID ORGANS

### ANATOMICALLY DEFINED SUBSETS

In the periphery, B-cell diversity can be defined by a number of criteria. Using histologic means, investigators have long recognized a number of distinct B-cell populations[2,35,38] (reviewed in Chapter 2). These anatomically defined subsets vary according to lymphoid organ, and whether the B-cell compartment is activated or in a basal state.

#### Resting B-cell Subsets

In the secondary lymphoid organs of adult mice, lymphoid follicles contain most of the resting peripheral B-cell pool. Mature resting conventional B cells compose the majority of primary follicles, and reside in the mantle of secondary follicles, or those which have active germinal centers. In the spleen, resting B cells are also found in another discrete anatomical location, that of the marginal zone. As discussed below, marginal zone and follicular B cells are functionally and phenotypically distinct. Other B-cell subsets also exist in the peripheral lymphoid organs; however, these typically do not have discrete histologic locations, or their locations are poorly defined. These latter subsets include immature B cells, $CD5^+$ (B1a) B cells, and switched memory B cells.

#### Activated B-cell Subsets

Upon immune challenge, and the induction of a humoral response, distinct anatomical loci of activated B cells are observed. As detailed by Kelsoe and co-workers, loci of activated B cells are found early in the immune response in the outer region of the splenic periarteriolar lymphatic sheath (PALS[36,37]). Subsequent to the formation of these loci, germinal centers appear in neighboring follicles, apparently seeded from activated B cells in nearby loci. Germinal centers are sites where class switching, somatic mutation and affinity maturation occur (reviewed in references 2, 35, 38 and 39). Within the germinal center itself, histologically defined subsets of B cells are also found.

These subsets include the centroblasts in the dark zone, and the centrocytes in the light zone[2,35,38] (Chapter 2). The centroblasts within the dark zone are large cycling cells which divide at a high rate. These cells give rise to the medium-sized, non-cycling centrocytes. This latter population is highly sensitive to programmed cell death, with survival depending upon the continued presence of signals provided by germinal center T cells and dendritic cells. Centrocytes which survive selection within the germinal center can undergo terminal differentiation and form plasma cells. Histologically, plasma cells can be found in the red pulp of the spleen, the medullary cords of the lymph nodes, and the bone marrow[35,40].

## PHENOTYPICALLY DEFINED B-CELL SUBSETS

As discussed above, the peripheral lymphoid organs contain a rich mixture of B-cell subsets. Among the resting populations, immature B cells, follicular or mantle B cells, marginal zone B cells and $CD5^+$ B cells can be defined using a mixture of cell surface markers.

### Follicular or Mantle B Cells

Follicular or mantle B cells constitute the majority of the B-cell pool in the peripheral lymphoid organs. Follicular B cells are thus found in the spleen, lymph nodes and Peyer's patches. These B cells, also termed conventional B cells, have a number of phenotypic characteristics which distinguish them from other B-cell populations (Table 3.2). In particular, follicular B cells are $IgM^{lo}$ and $IgD^{hi}$, and express a high density of CD23[41–43]. They also bear high levels of B220, intermediate levels of HSA, and intermediate levels of CD22[32]. Table 3.2 further shows that follicular B cells express intermediate levels of

**Table 3.2** Splenic B-cell subsets

| | Follicular | Marginal zone | Immature |
|---|---|---|---|
| IgM | Low | High | High |
| IgD | High | Low | Low |
| CD21 | Int.[a] | High | Low |
| CD22 | Int. | Int. | Low |
| CD23 | + | − | − |
| HSA (CD24) | Int. | High | Bright |
| pgp-1 (CD44) | Int. | High | High |
| LFA-1 (CD11a) | Int. | High | Low |
| Mel 14 (CD62-L) | High | Low | −/Low |
| CD5 | − | − | − |

Balb/c or C3H spleen cells were stained in a four-color protocol using antibodies directed against B220, HSA, CD23 and the markers listed in the table.
[a]Intermediate levels.

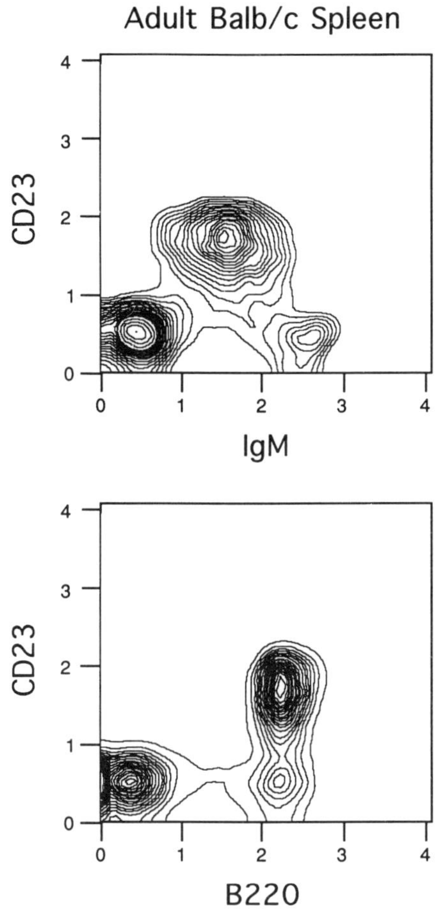


**Figure 3.1** Spleen cells from adult Balb/c mice were stained with FITC–goat anti-IgM, cyanine 5.18–anti-B220 (6B2) and biotin–anti-CD23 (B3B4) plus PE (phycoerythrin)–avidin. Stained cells were analyzed on a dual laser FACS 440 interfaced with a Vaxstation 3200 computer equipped with DESK software

adhesion and homing molecules. When attempting to identify follicular B cells with surface markers, either for enumeration or sort purification, the use of CD23 with either IgM or B220 typically gives a clean separation. As shown in Figure 3.1, the $IgM^{lo}$, $B220^{+}$, $CD23^{+}$ B-cell subset is easily identified.

## Marginal Zone B Cells

Marginal zone B cells are found in the spleen, and vary in frequency from strain to strain[42]. Some strains, such as Balb/c, exhibit low marginal zones, while others, such as C3H, contain high marginal zones and hence have a higher percentage of these B cells. Marginal zone B cells characteristically display high levels of IgM and low levels of IgD, and fail to express CD23[41–43]. Marginal zone B cells also have high levels of B220, high levels of HSA, and intermediate levels of CD22[32]. Compared to follicular B cells, marginal zone B cells have slightly higher amounts of the major adhesion molecules and lower levels of the homing receptor L-selectin. To identify the compartment which contains the marginal zone B cells with surface markers, one can again utilize CD23 in combination with either IgM or B220 (Figure 3.1). Additional markers must be used, however, to distinguish marginal zone from immature B cells in the spleen (see below).

## Immature B Cells

Late in their maturational sequence, immature B cells leave the bone marrow to seek space in peripheral lymphoid tissues, predominantly in the spleen. Phenotypically, these cells are similar to marginal zone B cells in that they are primarily $CD23^-$ $IgM^{hi}$, and $IgD^{lo}$ [33–34]. Given this shared phenotype, and the presence of nearly mature levels of B220, additional markers are required to distinguish immature from marginal zone B cells. As shown in Figure 3.2A, a three-color protocol using antibodies to B220, CD23 and HSA is useful in discriminating between marginal zone and immature B cells. When gating on the $B220^+$ splenic compartment, three populations are seen. The $CD23^+$, HSA intermediate cells are the follicular B cells, as described above. The CD23− compartment is now split into HSA-high and HSA-bright subsets. Based on several lines of evidence, we would suggest that the $CD23^-$, HSA-high B cells are the marginal zone population, with the $CD23^-$, HSA-bright cells representing immature B cells[32]. First, as shown in Figure 3.2B, young mice exhibit an excess of the immature B-cell population, consistent with a higher level of maturational activity in adolescent animals. Figure 3.2B also shows a transitional population which is gaining CD23 and reducing its levels of HSA. Second, in strains which contain a high marginal zone B-cell content (e.g. C3H), the $B220^+$, $CD23^-$, HSA-high population is greatly increased. Also, in mice treated long term with an anti-IL-7 antibody, a regimen which blocks B-cell maturation[44], the splenic $B220^+$, $CD23^-$, HSA-bright subset is missing[32]. This conclusion is consistent with the work of Cancro and colleagues, who demonstrated HSA-bright B cells to comprise the recent bone marrow émigrés, and further demonstrated the maturation of these cells into HSA-intermediate cells[14,15]. Additional markers reveal further differences between the marginal zone and immature B cells. When adding a fourth color to the B220, CD23 and HSA protocol, flow cytometric analysis demonstrates that marginal zone B cells express mature levels of CD22 and high levels of CD21 and LFA-1, whereas the immature B cells display low levels of CD21, CD22 and LFA-1 (Table 3.1).

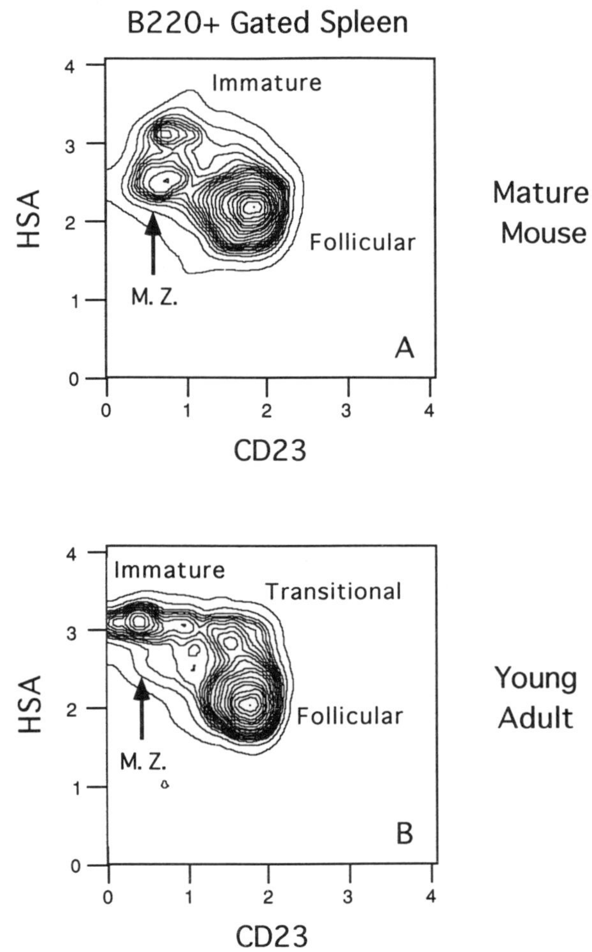


**Figure 3.2** Spleen cells from young and mature Balb/c mice were stained with FITC–anti-HSA (M1/69), cyanine 5.18–anti-B220 (6B2), and PE–anti-CD23 (B3B4). Stained cells were analyzed as described in the legend to Figure 3.1. The CD23 versus HSA contour plots are derived from the B220$^{+}$ gated spleen cells

**CD5+ B cells**

As discussed on pp. 85–87, CD5$^{+}$ (or B1a) B cells are a major constituent of the peritoneal cavity (reviewed in references 45 and 46). Although found at low frequency in the spleens of normal mice, they can be distinguished phenotypically. In certain autoimmune strains, CD5$^{+}$ B cells are found in greater numbers in both the spleen and peritoneal cavity[47]. In addition to the expression of low levels of CD5, these B cells display low amounts of B220.

Splenic CD5+ B cells are IgM-positive and typically IgD-low. Similar to marginal zone and immature B cells, CD5+ B cells are CD23-negative[42,43]. Thus, in order to reliably identify these cells, one again needs to utilize a multicolor flow cytometric approach. As shown in Figure 3.3, one can use

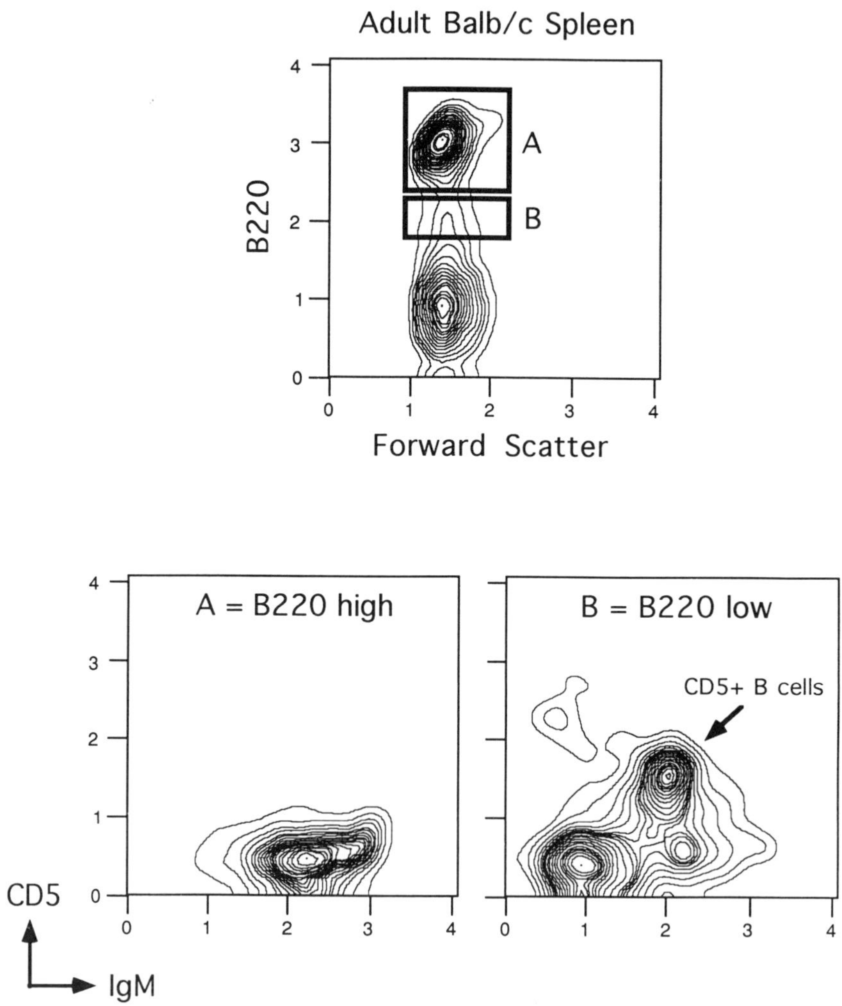


**Figure 3.3** Spleen cells from adult Balb/c mice were stained with FITC–goat anti-IgM, PE–anti-CD5 (53.7.313), and biotin–anti-B220 (6B2) plus cyanine 5.18–avidin. Stained cells were analyzed as described in the legend to Figure 3.1. The IgM versus CD5 contour plots in the lower panel are derived from the designated B220 high and low gates in the upper panel

antibodies directed against B220, CD5 and IgM. By gating on the B220$^{lo}$ compartment, one can enrich for the small percentage of CD5$^{+}$ B cells found in the spleen, and hence visualize them with the IgM versus CD5 contour plot. Since other cell types (such as T cells and NK cells) can express the B220 form of CD45, it is important to utilize a marker such as IgM to unequivocally identify the CD5$^{+}$ cells as B cells. Splenic CD5$^{+}$ B cells also express CD43 (both S7 and S11 forms). This marker is not found on resting follicular and marginal zone B cells in the spleen, and thus can also serve to delineate peripheral CD5$^{+}$ B cells[48] (C. Best, J. Kemp and T. Waldschmidt, unpublished). Although splenic CD5$^{+}$ B cells are phenotypically similar to their peritoneal counterparts, two exceptions are noteworthy. The first is that splenic CD5$^{+}$ B cells do not normally express Mac1 (CD11b), a molecule prominently displayed on peritoneal B1 B cells. The second is that whereas peritoneal B1 cells typically display high levels of IgM, splenic CD5$^{+}$ B cells bear intermediate levels.

### Activated B Cells

Upon activation, B cells undergo a programmed series of events leading to proliferation and differentiation. During this sequence, B cells markedly change their surface phenotype by upregulating or downregulating existing surface markers, or expressing new molecules. Given the mixture of B-cell subsets in the periphery, however, the issue of defining activated cells can be problematic. Specifically, the activated phenotype of one subset can mimic the resting phenotype of another. Upon activation of conventional or follicular B cells, it is well described that surface IgM increases, whereas IgD decreases[49,50]. Upon further stimulation, CD23 is also downregulated[51]. This phenotype now resembles that of a resting marginal zone or immature B cell. Accordingly, care must be taken when choosing markers to delineate activated B cells. Perhaps the best early and intermediate activation markers are those which are newly expressed, or expressed in high amounts only upon activation. Molecules of this type would include receptors necessary for increased metabolic activity, such as the transferrin receptor[52], receptors for cytokines such as the $\alpha$ chain of the IL-2R (CD25[53]), costimulation molecules such as B7.2[54], and the markers Ly-6A[55] and CD69[56]. During the later stages of activation, B cells will display peanut agglutinin (demarcating germinal center B cells[40,57,58]), and re-express both the pan and restricted forms of CD43[21]. B cells which have been activated *in vivo* can constitute a sizeable proportion of freshly harvested splenic B cells, especially those obtained from conventionally housed (non-specific pathogen-free) mice. These cells have been shown to have different *in vitro* activation requirements than resting cells[59–61], an important consideration when assessing the response of B cells to polyclonal stimulators and/or cytokines.

## Memory B Cells

Of the various B-cell subsets, the most difficult to identify and isolate are memory B cells. Functionally, memory B cells are those which give rise to rapid high-affinity responses upon challenge with a recall antigen. These cells are generated in germinal centers, and require the participation of T-helper cells (reviewed in references 2, 35 and 38). The recall antibodies are typically of a switched isotype, and consist of variable regions which have been somatically mutated (reviewed in reference 39). Accordingly, the best approach to identify the memory B-cell pool with surface markers is to focus on the $IgM^-$, $IgD^-$ B-cell compartment (those B cells expressing IgG, IgA or IgE). In non-immunized mice kept in specific pathogen-free conditions, this population typically accounts for less than 3 per cent of the B-cell population[62,63]. In a study by Hayakawa and Hardy, splenic $IgM^-$, $IgD^-$ memory B cells were shown to express B220, MHC class II, and low levels of the switched isotype[62]. Our laboratory also showed that resident $IgA^+$ B cells in Peyer's patches had lost expression of CD23[33], but retain mature levels of CD32[6] and CD22[32]. In order to verify the $IgM^-$, $IgD^-$, $B220^+$ and switched $Ig^+$ B cells as memory cells, several groups have demonstrated this population to produce high levels of switched antibody to recall antigen[62–64] and contain variable regions which have been subjected to extensive somatic mutation[63,64]. $IgM^+$, $IgD^+$ B cells, on the other hand, do not contain variable regions with mutations[63].

In a series of studies reported by Klinman and co-workers, data were presented suggesting that separate peripheral B-cell subsets give rise to primary antibody-forming cell (AFC) responses and secondary or memory responses[65,66]. Specifically, B cells displaying the highest levels of HSA were shown to give rise to primary AFC responses when tested in either the splenic fragment assay, or when co-transferred with T cells into SCID mice. In the latter experiment, $HSA^{hi}$ cells also failed to form germinal centers, a key event for secondary or memory responses. B cells expressing low levels of HSA served as potent precursors for secondary responses in both the splenic fragment and SCID transfer systems, and allowed for the formation of germinal centers. On the basis of these and other findings[67,68], the proposal was put forth that precursors for primary and memory responses are not only phenotypically distinct (based on HSA levels), but are products of distinct lineages[65]. The conclusion of separate lineages is not consistent, however, with the work of Kelso and colleagues, who determined that B-cell clones seeding germinal centers are primarily derived from nearby PALS loci of activated B cells[36,37]. The B cells in the loci were shown to produce low-affinity, unmutated antibodies characteristic of a primary response, whereas the germinal center B cells produced high-affinity, somatically mutated B cells characteristic of a secondary response. Since the primary and secondary responding B cells were clonally related, these data suggest a direct relationship between B cells involved in primary AFC production and memory cell formation. Also, Allman *et al.* showed that splenic $HSA^{hi}$ B cells were competent to reconstitute both primary and secondary responses when transferred with primed T cells into SCID mice[15]. Although both groups used nearly identical systems, it is not clear why the $HSA^{hi}$ cells responded differently in the two studies.

As shown by Allman *et al.*[14,15], and by our laboratory (pp. 80–81, Figure 3.3), $HSA^{lo}$ cells represent follicular B cells, whereas those expressing the highest levels of HSA are immature B cells. Marginal zone B cells display HSA at levels intermediate between follicular and immature B cells. Based on this information, therefore, it is likely that studies analyzing the responses of B cells with high and low levels of HSA are actually assessing the properties of immature and follicular B cells respectively. This does not rule out the possibility, however, that more than one lineage of B cell is produced in the bone marrow, and co-exists in the immature fraction in the spleen. Careful developmental analysis will be required to formally demonstrate the existence of these multiple lineages.

## B-CELL SUBSETS IN THE PERITONEAL CAVITY

### B1 AND B2 CELLS

In the mouse, the peritoneal cavity is also a rich source of B-cell subsets. In particular, this location contains small numbers of B2 or conventional B cells and a larger population of B1 or CD5/sister B cells (reviewed in references 45 and 46). The B2 B cells are phenotypically and functionally identical to follicular B cells found in the peripheral lymphoid organs, and are likely to be 'floating' counterparts of these cells in the peritoneum. The B1 population has been the subject of intense study for a number of years. As described below, this population has a distinct phenotype, and can be further divided into the B1a and B1b subsets. What has focused attention on the B1 population, is a series of functional attributes which distinguish this B-cell subset from other B-cell populations. B1 cells constitute the majority of the B-cell compartment early in life, but comprise only a small proportion in the adult[47]. B2 (or follicular) cells begin to accumulate after birth, and, with maturation, eventually dominate in the peripheral lymphoid organs (as described on pp. 78–79). Consistent with this pattern, precursors for B1 cells (specifically B1a cells) are dominant in sites of B-cell lymphopoiesis early in life, but are infrequent in the bone marrow upon maturation of the mouse. This has been demonstrated using adoptive transfer protocols[69–71]. What appears to allow for the perpetuation of the B1 population in adult mice is the capacity of these cells to undergo self-renewal. Hence, transfer of purified mature B1 cells into an appropriate host results in expansion and maintenance of the B1 B-cell pool[72]. It is of interest that, when purified and transferred, mature B1a and B1b cells will only give rise to cells of the original phenotype; cross-replenishment is not observed[45]. When examining the antigen receptor repertoire of B1 cells, it is clear that variable region utilization is restricted, and is likely to be antigen selected[46,73–76]. In addition, the antigen receptors primarily consist of germline sequences, with a nominal level of N region insertion[46]. Together, this translates into an antibody response which is low affinity, polyreactive, and often exhibits reactivity towards self[46,49]. These characteristics of the B1 repertoire are clearly different from those of the B2 population, and indicate a fundamentally different role for B1 and B2 cells in the humoral immune response.

## PHENOTYPIC CHARACTERISTICS OF PERITONEAL B CELLS

Based on the expression of surface markers, the peritoneal subsets are easily distinguished (Table 3.3). B1 cells display high levels of IgM and little or no IgD, with B2 cells expressing high levels of IgD and intermediate levels of

**Table 3.3** Peritoneal B-cell subsets

| | B1a | B1b | B2 |
|---|---|---|---|
| IgM | High | High | Low |
| IgD | −/Low | −/Low | High |
| CD5 | + | − | − |
| CD11b | + | + | − |
| CD23 | − | − | + |
| pan CD43 (S11) | + | +/− | − |

IgM[45,46]. Further distinguishing B1 and B2 cells is the differential expression of Mac1 (CD11b), CD23, IL-5 receptor and B220. B1 cells are Mac1 positive, CD23 negative and IL-5 receptor positive, and display low levels of B220, whereas B2 cells are Mac1 negative, CD23 positive, IL-5 receptor negative, and B220$^{hi}$ [42,43,45,46,77,78]. The B1 population can be further divided into the B1a and B1b subsets based upon CD5 expression. B1a cells (formerly CD5$^{+}$ B cells) are CD5 positive, with B1b cells (formerly sister B cells) being CD5 negative. Similar to splenic CD5$^{+}$ B cells, the peritoneal B1a cells also express CD43 (both S7 and S11 forms), with B1b cells displaying lower levels[48]. (C. Best, J. Kemp and T. Waldschmidt, unpublished). In order to distinguish the B1 and B2 populations, one can again utilize a flow cytometric strategy which employs CD23 in combination with either IgM or B220. Figure 3.4 illustrates the clear demarcation between the CD23-positive and -negative B-cell subsets.

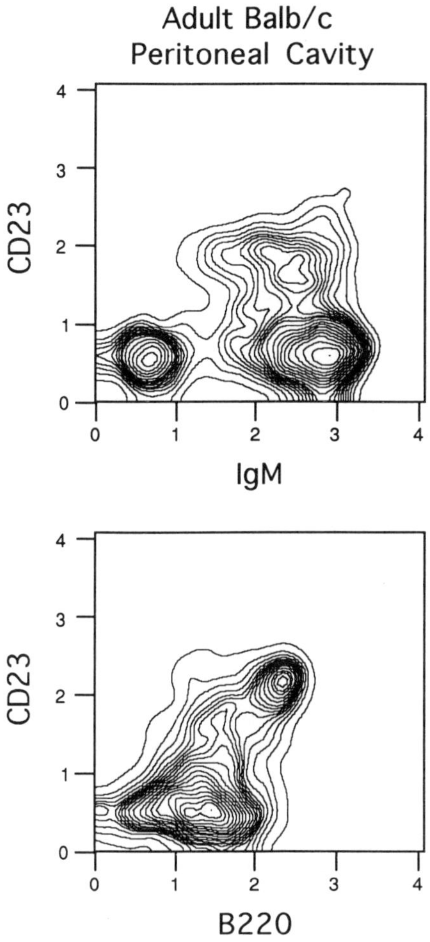


**Figure 3.4** Peritoneal lavage cells from Balb/c mice were stained with FITC--goat anti-IgM, cyanine 5.18–anti-B220 (6B2) and biotin–anti-CD23 (B3B4) plus PE–avidin. Stained cells were analyzed as described in the legend to Figure 3.1

## DERIVATION OF B1 CELLS: NATURE OR NURTURE?

At present, one of the most contested issues regarding B1 and B2 cells is the question of their derivation. One argument holds that B1 and B2 cells represent products of distinct maturational lineages, whereas another proposes that B1 cells arise from a mature B cell subsequent to a particular type of antigenic encounter. Given the capacity of B-cell precursors from fetal omentum to give rise exclusively to $CD5^+$ B cells[4], and the propensity of

B-cell precursors from adult bone marrow to produce predominantly B2 cells[69–71], the first model argues that different precursors must exist for the two B-cell types[79]. This interpretation thus implies that B1 (or at least B1a) cells and B2 cells arise from divergent developmental programs. Although the transfer experiments provide strong evidence for this model, further support will require the identification of markers which unequivocally define precursors for B1 versus B2 cells, or define a branch point for the two proposed lineages. Towards this end, Hardy and co-workers have demonstrated that pro-B cells from adult bone marrow (B2 precursors) contain abundant levels of mRNA for TdT and a myosin-like light chain termed PLRLC, whereas fetal liver pro-B cell (B1 precursors) do not[8,46]. Whether this is inherent to the B cells, or a result of the microenvironment, remains to be determined.

Based on studies from the laboratories of Wortis[80,81] and Haughton[82], an alternative hypothesis proposes a precursor–product relationship between the $IgD^{hi}$, $CD23^+$ B cell and the $CD5^+$ (B1a) B cell. In this model, a single type of B cell emerges from the maturational process, with the potential to take on a new form should it engage a specific type of antigen. These investigators propose that upon stimulation with a thymus-independent type 2 (TI-2) antigen, an $IgD^{hi}$, $CD23^+$ B cell can acquire the characteristics of a $CD5^+$ B cell. In support of this, Ying-zi *et al.* have demonstrated that anti-IgM, thought to be a model of TI-2 antigens, induced the expression of CD5 on splenic $IgD^{hi}$, $CD23^+$ cells, especially in the presence of IL-6[80]. Further support comes from the study of mice carrying the XID defect. These mice are unable to respond to TI-2 antigens, and exhibit a corresponding paucity of $CD5^+$ B cells[83]. Hence, this latter model suggests that $CD5^+$ B cells do not arise from a distinct developmental program, but accumulate as the B-cell compartment encounters TI-2 antigens[81,82]. If indeed the diversity within the B-cell compartment results from antigenic challenge, one would have to further propose that the marginal zone and B1b (sister) B cells likewise appear subsequent to particular types of stimulation. At present, these investigators have not reported conditions which allow for the conversion of an $IgD^{hi}$, $CD23^+$ B cell into these latter two subsets.

## FUNCTIONAL CHARACTERISTICS OF B-CELL SUBSETS

### IMMATURE B CELLS

Within the context of the humoral immune response, B cells can be viewed as potentially functional once they have expressed their surface antigen receptors. As outlined on pp. 74–75 B cells first express a complete antigen receptor subsequent to successful heavy and light chain variable region gene rearrangement. This corresponds with stage E, and a B cell which is IgM positive and IgD negative. The question arises as to whether these cells can respond to thymus-dependent and -independent stimuli. A number of groups have clearly demonstrated (reviewed in reference 84) that engagement of surface Ig with either antigen or anti-IgM reagents fails to stimulate immature B cells. This holds true whether the immature B cells are isolated from bone marrow[85], neonatal spleen[86–88] or adult spleen[14]. Further work has demonstrated that crosslinking of surface Ig in the absence of other signals leads to programmed cell death[87]. This response is consistent with models of B-cell tolerance, given the need to eliminate self-reactive clones. Upon T-cell-dependent stimulation, however, immature B cells can respond vigorously[14,87]. Thus, under conditions of cognate interaction, stage E B cells can proliferate and differentiate.

## MATURE B-CELL SUBSETS

In order to effectively study the functional characteristics of mature B-cell subsets, it is necessary to first isolate the various populations. Our laboratory has undertaken a series of experiments whereby B-cell subsets were purified based on CD23 expression, and their functional characteristics analyzed. The results of these experiments are summarized in Table 3.4.

**Table 3.4** Functional responses of B-cell subsets

| | Spleen | | Peritoneum | |
|---|---|---|---|---|
| | $CD23^+$ | $CD23^-$ | $CD23^+$ | $CD23^-$ |
| LPS[a] | ++ | +++ | ++ | +++ |
| Anti-IgM[b] | ++ | − | ++ | − |
| Anti-IgM + Anti-class II[c] | ++ | +++ | NT | NT |
| IgM production[d] | + | + | + | + |
| IgG1 production[e] | + | + | + | + |
| IgE production[e] | + | + | + | [−] |
| IgA production[f] | + | + | + | + |
| Th membranes[g] | + | + | + | [−] |
| rCD40L[h] | ++ | ++ | ++ | [±] |
| Th2 clone[i] | +++ | +++ | +++ | +++ |

Spleen cells from C3H/Hen mice, or peritoneal lavage cells from Balb/c mice, were sort purified into $CD23^+$ and $CD23^-$ fractions.
[a]Proliferation in response to 40 μg/ml of lipopolysaccharide (LPS) (48 h).
[b]Proliferation in response to 10–25 μg/ml of b-7-6 (48 h).
[c]Proliferation in response to 10 μg/ml of bet 2, 10 μg/ml of 34-5-3S, and 100 U/ml of rIL-4.
[d]Secretion in response to 40 μg/ml of LPS (6 days).
[e]Secretion in response to 40 μg/ml of LPS plus 10 000 U/ml rIL-4 (6 days).
[f]Secretion in response to 40 μg/ml of LPS plus rIL-4 and rIL-5 ((5% v/v Cos cell supernatant) 6 days).
[g]Proliferation in response to 1 μg of membranes from anti-CD3 activated D1.6 Th1 cells (72 h).
[h]Proliferation in response to 200 ng/ml of rCD40 ligand trimer (48 h).
[i]Proliferation in response to anti-CD3 activated and irradiated CDC35 Th2 cells (72 h).
NT, not tested.

### Follicular B Cells

When staining cells with antibodies to B220 and CD23, as shown in Figure 3.1, one can easily identify the follicular B-cell population, and isolate it with electronic cell sorting. These sort-purified B cells can then be tested for their response to thymus-independent and -dependent stimuli, as well as their capacity for isotype switching. As summarized in Table 3.4, CD23$^+$ B cells isolated from the spleens of C3H/Hen mice proliferated well in response to the polyclonal stimulators lipopolysaccharide (LPS) and anti-IgM[43]. When tested for their capacity to differentiate and isotype switch, C3H/Hen follicular B cells were shown to produce a full range of isotypes[89]. LPS stimulation resulted in the secretion of high levels of IgM, with LPS and IL-4 producing significant levels of IgG and IgE[89]. Using purified splenic CD23$^+$ B cells from Balb/c mice, Snapper and colleagues obtained identical results[90]. In their studies, follicular B cells likewise responded to LPS and anti-Ig treatment, and produced IgG and IgE when stimulated with LPS and cytokines. In further studies, our laboratory has examined the capacity of CD23$^+$ splenic B cells to proliferate in response to T-helper cell activity[91]. These cells proliferated well when incubated with membranes isolated from activated T-helper cell clones, or recombinant CD40 ligand trimer. As expected, the CD23$^+$ B cells also responded vigorously when stimulated with an intact anti-CD3 stimulated T-helper cell clone (CDC35). Together, these studies demonstrate that follicular B cells are fully programmed to respond to both thymus-independent and CD40 ligand-directed T-cell-dependent stimulation.

### Marginal Zone B Cells

In conjunction with studying the responses of follicular B cells, we similarly tested the functional properties of marginal zone B cells. B220$^{hi}$, CD23$^-$ B cells were therefore sort purified from the spleens of C3H/Hen mice. C3H mice were used for these studies on account of their large marginal zones, and hence better cell recovery. In addition, purification of CD23$^-$ B cells from strains with high marginal zones substantially decreases the number of immature B cells which are co-purified with this two-marker approach. (As discussed on pp. 80–81 immature B cells are also found in the B220$^{hi}$, CD23$^-$ B-cell compartment.) Similar to follicular B cells, stimulation of the splenic CD23$^-$ subset revealed a strong proliferative response to LPS, as well as proliferation to T-cell membranes, recombinant CD40 ligand, and intact activated CDC35 Th2 cells[43,91]. These cells also produced IgM, IgG and IgE when appropriately stimulated[89,90]. CD23$^-$ B cells differed, however, in that they failed to respond to a mitogenic anti-IgM[43]. This lack of response appears to be due to a negative signal delivered to the B cells. Curiously, splenic CD23$^-$ B cells responded vigorously to surface IgM engagement when anti-MHC class II and IL-4 were added to the culture[92]. Snapper *et al.*

likewise observed a poor response of Balb/c-derived splenic CD23$^{-}$ B cells to dextran-conjugated anti-IgD and anti-IgM[90]. Thus, marginal zone B cells are fully competent to respond to LPS and CD40 ligand-directed stimulation. However, similar to neonatal B cells, marginal zone B cells are not programmed to positively respond to surface antigen receptor crosslinking in the absence of other signals. Since marginal zone B cells represent a mature B-cell subset, the meaning of this unresponsiveness is presently unclear.

### Peritoneal B1 Cells

As summarized on pp. 85–86, peritoneal B1 cells clearly display a number of traits which set them apart from B2 or conventional B cells. In addition to a distinct phenotype, these cells exhibit a restricted antigen receptor repertoire and have the unique property of self-renewal. This leads to the question as to whether these B cells display other functional attributes which distinguish them from the B2 population. Our laboratory has therefore purified peritoneal B1 and B2 cells based on CD23 expression, and tested their response to a series of stimuli. As with the splenic B-cell studies, peritoneal lavage cells were sorted into B220$^{+}$, CD23$^{-}$ (B1), and B220$^{+}$, CD23$^{+}$ (B2) populations, and tested for their response to LPS and a mitogenic anti-IgM. Similar to the marginal zone B cells, the peritoneal B1 cells proliferated well in response to LPS, but again failed to register a positive response upon surface IgM crosslinking (T. Foy and T. Waldschmidt, unpublished). This result has also been obtained by Rothstein and co-workers[93], who further demonstrated that B1 cells fail to fully activate the enzymatic activity of their PLCγ2[94], and subsequently fail to induce the expression of nuclear NFκB[95]. When testing for the response of peritoneal B cells to T-cell-dependent stimulation, our laboratory found that B1 cells did not respond to membranes from activated T cells, either with proliferation or differentiation, and proliferated poorly when cultured with recombinant CD40 ligand and cytokines[91]. In comparison, CD23$^{+}$ peritoneal B cells responded normally to both T-cell-membrane and recombinant CD40 ligand stimulation[91]. Curiously, when cultured with intact activated CDC35 Th2 cells, the peritoneal B1 population demonstrated a strong response comparable to that of their CD23$^{+}$ peritoneal counterparts. Hence, B1 cells appear unable to register a vigorous proliferative response to a CD40 ligand-dependent signal, although they respond well to T-helper cells. The meaning of this observation is presently unclear, although several explanations can be offered. Since peritoneal CD23$^{+}$ and CD23$^{-}$ B cells display similar levels of CD40 (T. Waldschmidt, unpublished observation), it is possible that engagement of CD40 on B1 cells fails to invoke an appropriate intracellular response, similar to the muted activation of PLCγ2 upon anti-IgM stimulation. Given the strong response to the intact T-helper-cell clone, it is further possible that B1 cells might preferentially use a receptor–ligand pair other than the CD40–CD40 ligand, in order to receive signals from T cells.

In further experiments, we tested the capacity of peritoneal $CD23^-$ and $CD23^+$ B cells to differentiate and isotype switch[89]. As expected, the conventional $CD23^+$ B2 subset produced IgM when stimulated with LPS, and IgG1 and IgE when treated with LPS plus IL-4. $CD23^-$ B1 cells likewise produced high levels of IgM upon LPS stimulation, and switched to IgG1 when IL-4 was added. Interestingly, peritoneal B1 cells did not make IgE when cultured with LPS plus IL-4 ($\pm$ IL-5), although they produced IgA, an isotype located downstream of the $\epsilon$ locus. The inability to secrete IgE may be consistent with the poor response of B1 cells to CD40-directed stimulation. It is well established that IgE responses are dependent upon signals generated through the CD40 molecule. In CD40 ligand-deficient mice, where downstream IgG and IgA isotypes are still detectable, there is a striking absence of IgE production[96,97]. If, as suggested above, B1 cells preferentially respond to T-cell help through a non-CD40 ligand-dependent mechanism, is it possible that the residual antibody response in these knockout mice is derived from the B1 subset.

## CONCLUSIONS

It is clear that the B-cell compartment is a complex mixture of subsets distinguished by a number of criteria. Although all B cells have the same ultimate differentiative outcome, that of secreting Igs, it would be a mistake to assume that these subsets play similar roles in the humoral immune response. It is likely that, similar to the T-cell compartment, the diversity within the B-cell population is designed to respond to the diverse nature of pathogenic insults, as well as aid in regulating its own antibody response. Hence, different populations may be better poised to respond to thymus-independent versus thymus-dependent antigens, primary versus recall antigens, and even self- versus non-self-antigens. As summarized in the present chapter, the diversity is well characterized in terms of histology, phenotype and function. The major challenge to B-cell biologists in forthcoming years will be to resolve key issues regarding the derivation of the various subsets. Are these subsets a result of inherent developmental programs, or do they arise subsequent to encounters with the vast array of external and internal antigens? This issue is key to our understanding not only of B1a and B2 cells, and precursors of primary and secondary responding cells, but also of the origins of B1b and marginal zone B cells. Resolution of these questions will contribute to our understanding not only of lymphopoiesis, but also of the origin of B-cell tumors. Additional studies will be required to fully understand the various activation requirements of the B-cell subsets. It is clear that some subsets are negatively regulated by surface antigen receptor engagement, whereas others are triggered into cell cycle. Further evidence suggests that T-helper cells may engage and activate the subsets through different means. Accordingly, it will be critical to document the various signal transduction pathways operative in the different subsets. This knowledge should further efforts to design vaccines which optimally invoke protective and long-lasting humoral responses.

## ACKNOWLEDGMENTS

The author thanks L. Tygrett, Dr T. Foy, Dr Karen Snapp, Dr C. Best, and L. Erickson for contributing key results, Dr R. Noelle for the activated T-cell membranes, Dr W. Fanslow for the rCD40 ligand, Dr M. Howard for the anti-CD40 antibody, Dr M. Holers for the anti-CD21 antibodies, and T. Swartzendruber for preparation of the manuscript. Supported by NIH AI 31265 and by a grant from the Council for Tobacco Research.

## REFERENCES

1. Banchereau J, Rousset F. Human B lymphocytes: phenotype, proliferation, and differentiation. Adv Immunol 1992; 52:125–162.
2. MacLennan ICM. Germinal centers. Annu Rev Immunol 1994; 12:117–139.
3. Kincade PW, Gimble JM. B lymphocytes. In: Paul WE (ed.) Fundamental Immunology. New York: Raven Press, 1993, pp. 43–73.
4. Solvason N, Lehuen A, Kearney JF. An embryonic source of Ly1 but not conventional B cells. Int Immunol 1991; 3:543–550.
5. Velardi A, Cooper MD. An immunofluorescence analysis of the ontogeny of myeloid, T, and B lineage cells in mouse hemopoietic tissues. J Immunol 1984; 133:672–677.
6. Foy TM, Lynch RG, Waldschmidt TJ. Ontogeny and distribution of the murine B cell FcγRII. J Immunol 1992; 149:1516–1523.
7. Hardy RR, Carmack CE, Shinton SA *et al.* Resolution and characterization of pro-B and pre-pro-B cell stages in normal mouse bone marrow. J Exp Med 1991; 173:1213–1225.
8. Li Y-S, Hayakawa K, Hardy RR. The regulated expression of B lineage associated genes during B cell differentiation in bone marrow and fetal liver. J Exp Med 1993; 178:951–960.
9. Ehlich A, Schaal S, Gu H *et al.* Immunoglobulin heavy and light chain genes rearrange independently at early stages of B cell development. Cell 1993; 72:695–704.
10. Löffert D, Schaal S, Ehlich A *et al.* Early B-cell development in the mouse: insights from mutations introduced by gene targeting. Immunol Rev 1994; 137:135–153.
11. Melchers F, Haasner D, Grawunder U *et al.* Annu Rev Immunol 1994; 12:209–225.
12. Osmond DG. B cell development in the bone marrow. Semin Immunol 1990; 2:173–180.

13. Alt FW, Oltz EM, Young F *et al.* VDJ recombination. Immunol Today 1992; 13:306–314.
14. Allman DM, Ferguson SE, Cancro MP. Peripheral B cell maturation. I. Immature peripheral B cells in adults are heat-stable antigen$^{hi}$ and exhibit unique signaling characteristics. J Immunol 1992; 149:2533–2540.
15. Allman DM, Ferguson SE, Lentz VM, Cancro MP. Peripheral B cell maturation. II. Heat-stable antigen$^{hi}$ splenic B cells are an immature developmental intermediate in the production of long-lived marrow-derived B cells. J Immunol 1993; 151:4431–4444.
16. Hartley SB, Cooke MP, Fulcher DA *et al.* Elimination of self-reactive B lymphocytes proceeds in two stages: arrested development and cell death. Cell 1993; 72:325–335.
17. Morse III HC, Davidson WF, Yetter RA, Coffman RL. A cell-surface antigen shared by B cells and Ly2$^{+}$ peripheral T cells. Cell Immunol 1982; 70:311–320.
18. Kincade PW, Lee G, Watanabe T *et al.* Antigens displayed on murine B lymphocyte precursors. J Immunol 1981; 127:2262–2268.
19. Bruce J, Symington FW, McKearn TJ, Sprent J. A monoclonal antibody discriminating between subsets of T and B cells. J Immunol 1981; 127:2496–2501.
20. Nakayama E, von Hoegen I, Parnes JR. Sequence of the Lyb-2 B-cell differentiation antigen defines a gene superfamily of receptors with inverted membrane orientation. Proc Natl Acad Sci USA 1989; 86:1352–1356.
21. Gulley ML, Ogata LC, Thorson JA *et al.* Identification of a murine pan-T cell antigen which is also expressed during the terminal phases of B cell differentiation. J Immunol 1988; 140:3751–3757.
22. Rico-Vargas SA, Weiskopf B, Nishikawa S-I, Osmond DG. c-*kit* expression by B cell precursors in mouse bone marrow. Stimulation of B cell genesis by in vivo treatment with anti-c-*kit* antibody. J Immunol 1994; 152:2845–2852.
23. Sudo T, Nishikawa S, Ohno N *et al.* Expression and function of the interleukin 7 receptor in murine lymphocytes. Proc Natl Acad Sci USA 1993; 90:9125–9129.
24. Era T, Nishikawa S, Sudo T *et al.* How B-precursor cells are driven to cycle. Immunol Rev 1994; 137:35–51.
25. Wu Q, Lahti JM, Air GM *et al.* Molecular cloning of the murine BP-1/6C3 antigen: a member of the zinc-dependent metallopeptidase family. Proc Natl Acad Sci USA 1990; 87:993–997.
26. Wu Q, Tidmarsh GF, Welch PA *et al.* The early B lineage antigen BP-1 and the transformation-associated antigen 6C3 are on the same molecule. J Immunol 1989; 143:3303–3308.
27. Tarlinton D. Direct demonstration of MHC class II surface expression on murine pre-B cells. Int Immunol 1993; 5:1629–1635.
28. Lam K-P, Stall AM. Major histocompatibility complex class II expression distinguishes two distinct B cell developmental pathways during ontogeny. J Exp Med 1994; 180:507–516.
29. Hayakawa K, Tarlinton D, Hardy RR. Absence of MHC class II expression distinguishes fetal from adult lymphopoiesis in mice. J Immunol 1994; 152:4801–4807.
30. Rolink A, Grawunder U, Winkler TH *et al.* IL-2 receptor α chain (CD25, TAC) expression defines a crucial stage in pre-B cell development. Int Immunol 1994; 6:1257–1264.
31. Chen J, Ma A, Young F, Alt FW. IL-2 receptor α chain expression during early B lymphocyte differentiation. Int Immunol 1994; 6:1265–1268.
32. Erickson L, Tygrett L, Bhatia S *et al.* The ontogeny and distribution of murine CD22 (Lyb8). Submitted.

33. Waldschmidt TJ, Conrad DH, Lynch RG. The expression of B cell surface receptors. I. The ontogeny and distribution of the murine B cell IgE Fc receptor. J Immunol 1988; 140:2148–2154.
34. Waldschmidt TJ, Conrad DH, Lynch RG. Expression of B cell surface receptors. II. IL-4 can accelerate the developmental expression of the murine B cell IgE Fc receptor. J Immunol 1989; 143:2820.
35. Tew JG, DiLosa R, Burton GF *et al.* Germinal centers and antibody production in bone marrow. Immunol Rev 1992; 126:99–112.
36. Jacob J, Kassir R, Kelsoe G. In situ studies of the primary immune response to (4-hydroxy-3-nitrophenyl)acetyl. I. The architecture and dynamics of responding cell populations. J Exp Med 1991; 173:1165–1175.
37. Jacob J, Kelsoe G. In situ studies of the primary immune response to (4-hydroxy-3-nitrophenyl)acetyl. II. A common clonal origin for periarteriolar lymphoid sheath-associated foci and germinal centers. J Exp Med 1992; 176:679–687.
38. Liu Y-J, Johnson GD, Gordon J, Maclennan ICM. Germinal centres in T-cell-dependent antibody responses. Immunol Today 1992; 13:17–21.
39. Kocks C, Rajewsky K. Stable expression and somatic hypermutation of antibody V regions in B-cell developmental pathways. Annu Rev Immunol 1989; 7:537–559.
40. DiLosa RM, Maeda K, Masuda A *et al.* Germinal center B cells and antibody production in the bone marrow. J Immunol 1991; 146:4071–4077.
41. Gray D, MacLennan ICM, Bazin H, Khan M. Migrant $\mu^+\delta^+$ and static $\mu^+\delta^+$ B lymphocyte subsets. Eur J Immunol 1982; 12:564–569.
42. Waldschmidt TJ, Kroese FGM, Tygrett LT *et al.* The expression of B cell surface receptors. III. The murine low-affinity IgE Fc receptor is not expressed on Ly 1 or 'Ly 1-like' B cells. Int Immunol 1991; 3:305–315.
43. Waldschmidt T, Snapp K, Foy T *et al.* B-cell subsets defined by the Fc$\epsilon$R. Ann N Y Acad Sci 1992; 651:84–98.
44. Grabstein KH, Waldschmidt TJ, Finkelman FD *et al.* Inhibition of murine B and T lymphopoiesis in vivo by an anti-interleukin 7 monoclonal antibody. J Exp Med 1993; 178:257–264.
45. Kantor AB, Herzenberg LA. Origin of murine B cell lineages. Annu Rev Immunol 1993; 11:501–538.
46. Hardy RR, Carmack CE, Li YS, Hayakawa K. Distinctive developmental origins and specificities of murine CD5+ B cells. Immunol Rev 1994; 137:91–118.
47. Hayakawa K, Hardy RR, Parks DR, Herzenberg LA. The 'Ly-1 B' cell subpopulation in normal, immunodefective, and autoimmune mice. J Exp Med 1983; 157:202–218.
48. Wells SM, Kantor AB, Stall AM. CD43 (S7) expression identifies peripheral B cell subsets. J Immunol 1994; 153:5503–5515.
49. Hayakawa K, Hardy RR, Honda M *et al.* Ly-1 B cells: functionally distinct lymphocytes that secrete IgM autoantibodies. Proc Natl Acad Sci USA 1984; 81:2494–2498.
50. Monroe JG, Havran WL, Cambier JC. B lymphocyte activation: entry into cell cycle is accompanied by decreased expression of IgD but not IgM. Eur J Immunol 1983; 13:208–213.
51. Snapper CM, Hooley JJ, Urban JF Jr, Finkelman FD. Lack of Fc$\epsilon$RII expression by murine B cells after in vivo immunization is directly associated with Ig secretion and not Ig isotype switching. J Immunol 1991; 146:2161–2168.
52. Futran J, Kemp JD, Field EH *et al.* Transferrin receptor synthesis is an early event in B cell activation. J Immunol 1989; 143:787–792.
53. Ortega G, Robb RJ, Shevach EM, Malek TR. The murine IL-2 receptor. I.

Monoclonal antibodies that define distinct functional epitopes on activated T cells and react with activated B cells. J Immunol 1984; 133: 1970–1975.
54. Hathcock KS, Laszlo G, Pucillo C *et al.* Comparative analysis of B7-1 and B7-2 costimulatory ligands: expression and function. J Exp Med 1994; 180:631–640.
55. Ortega G, Korty PE, Shevach EM, Malek TR. Role of Ly-6 in lymphocyte activation. I. Characterization of a monoclonal antibody to a nonpolymorphic Ly-6 specificity. J Immunol 1986; 137:3240–3246.
56. Yokoyama WM, Koning F, Kehn PJ *et al.* Characterization of a cell surface-expressed disulfide-linked dimer involved in murine T cell activation. J Immunol 1988; 141:369–376.
57. Butcher EC, Rouse RV, Coffman RL *et al.* Surface phenotype of Peyer's patch germinal center cells: implications for the role of germinal centers in B cell differentiation. J Immunol 1982; 129:2698–2707.
58. Weinstein PD, Schweitzer PA, Cebra-Thomas JA, Cebra JJ. Molecular genetic features reflecting the preference for isotype switching to IgA expression by Peyer's patch germinal center B cells. Int Immunol 1991; 3:1253–1263.
59. Ratcliffe MJH, Julius MH. H-2-restricted T–B interactions involved in polyspecific B cell responses mediated by soluble antigen. Eur J Immunol 1982; 12:634–641.
60. Thompson CB, Scher I, Schaefer ME *et al.* Size dependent B lymphocyte subpopulations: relationship of cell volume to surface phenotype, cell cycle, proliferation response and requirements for antibody production to TNP-ficoll and TNP-BA. J Immunol 1984; 133:2333–2342.
61. Pecanha LMT, Snapper CM, Finkelman FD, Mond JJ. Dextran-conjugated anti-Ig antibodies as a model for T cell-independent type 2 antigen-mediated stimulation of Ig secretion in vitro. I. Lymphokine dependence. J Immunol 1991; 146:833–839.
62. Hayakawa K, Ishii R, Yamasaki K *et al.* Isolation of high-affinity memory B cells: phycoerythrin as a probe for antigen-binding cells. Proc Natl Acad Sci USA 1987; 84:1379–1383.
63. Schittek B, Rajewsky K. Natural occurrence and origin of somatically mutated memory B cells in mice. J Exp Med 1992; 176:427–438.
64. McHeyzer-Williams MG, Nossal GJV, Lalor PA. Molecular characterization of single memory B cells. Nature 1991; 350:502–505.
65. Linton P-J, Decker DJ, Klinman NR. Primary antibody-forming cells and secondary B cells are generated from separate precursor cell subpopulations. Cell 1989; 59:1049–1059.
66. Linton P-J, Lo D, Lai L *et al.* Among naive precursor cell subpopulations only progenitors of memory B cells originate germinal centers. Eur J Immunol 1992; 22:1293–1297.
67. Wu P, Ward R. Ig repertoire expression of BALB/c primary and secondary B cell precursors specific for phosphorylcholine. J Immunol 1993; 150:3862–3872.
68. Yin X-M, Vitetta ES. The lineage relationship between virgin and memory B cells. Int Immunol 1992; 4:691–698.
69. Hayakawa K, Hardy RR, Herzenberg LA, Herzenberg LA. Progenitors for Ly-1 B cells are distinct from progenitors for other B cells. J Exp Med 1985; 16:1554–1568.
70. Hardy RR, Hayakawa K. A developmental switch in B lymphopoiesis. Proc Natl Acad Sci USA 1991; 88:11550–11554.
71. Kantor AB, Stall AM, Adams S *et al.* Differential development of progenitor activity for three B-cell lineages. Proc Natl Acad Sci USA 1992; 89:3320–3324.
72. Hayakawa K, Hardy RR, Stall AM *et al.* Immunoglobulin-bearing B cells

reconstitute and maintain the murine Ly-1 B cell lineage. Eur J Immunol 1986; 16:1313–1316.
73. Hardy RR. Variable gene usage, physiology and development of Ly-1$^+$ (CD5$^+$) B cells. Curr Opin Immunol 1992; 4:181–185.
74. Pennell CA, Maynard E, Arnold LW *et al.* High frequency expression of S107 $V_H$ genes by peritoneal B cells of B10.H-2$^a$H-4$^b$P/WTS mice. J Immunol 1990; 145:1592–1597.
75. Pennell CA, Mercolino TJ, Grdina TA *et al.* Biased immunoglobulin variable region gene expression by Ly-1 B cells due to clonal selection. Eur J Immunol 1989; 19:1289–1295.
76. Clarke SH, McCray SK. $V_H$ CDR3-dependent positive selection of murine $V_H$12-expressing B cells in the neonate. Eur J Immunol 1993; 23:3327–3334.
77. Wetzel GD. Interleukin 5 regulation of peritoneal Ly-1 B lymphocyte proliferation, differentiation and autoantibody secretion. Eur J Immunol 1989; 19:1701–1707.
78. Hitoshi Y, Yamaguchi N, Mita S *et al.* Distribution of IL-5 receptor-positive B cells. Expression of IL-5 receptor on Ly-1 (CD5)+ B cells. J Immunol 1990; 144:4218–4225.
79. Herzenberg AL, Kantor AB. B-cell lineages exist in the mouse. Immunol Today 1993; 14:79–83.
80. Ying-zi C, Rabin E, Wortis HH. Treatment of murine CD5$^-$ B cells with anti-Ig, but not LPS, induces surface CD5: two B-cell activation pathways. Int Immunol 1991; 3:467–476.
81. Wortis HH. Surface markers, heavy chain sequences and B cell lineages. Int Rev Immunol 1992; 8:235–246.
82. Haughton G, Arnold LW, Whitmore AC, Clarke SH. B-1 cells are made, not born. Immunol Today 1993; 14:84–87.
83. Hayakawa K, Hardy RR, Herzenberg LA. Peritoneal Ly-1 B cells: genetic control, autoantibody production, increased lambda light chain expression. Eur J Immunol 1986; 16:450–456.
84. Waldschmidt TJ. B cell tolerance. In: Snow EC (ed.) T-Cell Dependent and Independent B-Cell Activation. Boca Raton: CRC Press 1991, pp. 231–253.
85. Seyfert VL, McMahon SB, Glenn WD *et al.* Methylation of an immediate-early inducible gene as a mechanism for B cell tolerance induction. Science 1990; 250: 797–800.
86. Brines RD, Klaus GGB. Effects of anti-immunoglobulin antibodies, interleukin-4 and second messenger agonists on B cells from neonatal mice. Int Immunol 1991; 3:461–466.
87. Chang T-L, Capraro G, Kleinman RE, Abbas AK. Anergy in immature B lymphocytes. Differential responses to receptor-mediated stimulation and T helper cells. J Immunol 1991; 147:750–756.
88. Yellen AJ, Glenn W, Sukhatme VP *et al.* Signaling through surface IgM in tolerance-susceptible immature murine B lymphocytes. Developmentally regulated differences in transmembrane signaling in splenic B cells from adult and neonatal mice. J Immunol 1991; 146:1446–1454.
89. Foy TM, Waldschmidt TJ. Switching capacity of FcεRII-positive and -negative murine B cells. Eur J Immunol 1993; 23:3208–3216.
90. Snapper CM, Yamada H, Smoot D *et al.* Comparative in vitro analysis of proliferation, Ig secretion, and Ig class switching by murine marginal zone and follicular B cells. J Immunol 1993; 150:2737–2745.
91. Waldschmidt T, Erickson L, Foy T *et al.* Murine B cell subsets differentially respond to CD40 ligand-directed signaling. FASEB J 1994; 8:A470.

92. Bishop GA, Ramirez LM, Waldschmidt TJ. Differential responses to Ig and class II-mediated signals in splenic B cell subsets from normal and autoimmune mice. Int Immunol 1994; 6:1049–1059.
93. Rothstein TL, Kolber DL. Anti-Ig antibody inhibits the phorbol ester-induced stimulation of peritoneal B cells. J Immunol 1988; 141:4089–4093.
94. Morris DL, Rothstein TL. Decreased surface IgM receptor-mediated activation of phospholipase C$\gamma$2 in B-1 lymphocytes. Int Immunol 1994; 6:1011–1016.
95. Morris DL, Rothstein TL. Abnormal transcription factor induction through the surface immunoglobulin M receptor of B-1 lymphocytes. J Exp Med 1993; 177:857–861.
96. Xu J, Foy TM, Laman JD *et al.* Mice deficient for the CD40 ligand. Immunity 1994; 1:423–431.
97. Renshaw BR, Fanslow WC, Armitage RJ *et al.* Humoral immune responses in CD40 ligand-deficient mice. J Exp Med 1994; 180:1889–1900.

# 4 B-cell Activation and Maturation to Immunoglobulin Secretion

**DAVID C. PARKER and JEFFREY M. PURKERSON**
*Oregon Health Sciences University, Portland, Oregon, USA*

## INTRODUCTION

In this chapter, we will summarize the largely shared basic assumptions about B-cell activation and maturation as an introduction to the more specialized chapters in this book in which many of these assumptions are challenged or qualified. First we lay out the signals that activate B lymphocytes and drive B-cell responses, and then we discuss the branching differentiation pathways that result from these signals.

The adaptive immune response is regulated at the level of proliferation and differentiation of individual lymphocyte clones, each committed to making a particular molecular species of antigen receptor[1]. By combining with the antigen receptor on a B cell, the antigen selects those rare clones committed to making antibodies against it. Without its antigen, the B cell abides as a small, resting lymphocyte, a G0 cell with just enough cytoplasm to maintain itself. After selection by antigen, the B cell becomes 'activated', a process that can result in cellular proliferation and differentiation to produce a clone of antibody-secreting effector cells. Years ago, B-cell activation was described as a linear process. The small B cell was poised to produce a clone of antibody-secreting cells, and one or two of a small number of signals could trigger the program. The small B lymphocyte enlarges, RNA content increases, activation antigens are expressed on the cell surface, and the cell begins to replicate its DNA and becomes a clone of rapidly proliferating cells. The dividing cells differentiate into antibody-secreting cells, and eventually become non-dividing, terminally differentiated plasma cells.

But even in the early years of cellular immunology, it was clear that initial signals needed to be followed by further signals which could determine the timing of terminal differentiation and so regulate clone size. Also, we knew that not all clones and not all members of a clone shared the same fate: some switched to make antibodies of other classes, and others reverted to long-lived small lymphocytes to await a second encounter with antigen as memory cells. The more we learn about B cells and B-cell activation, the more fates

*Cytokine Regulation of Humoral Immunity: Basic and Clinical Aspects.* Edited by Clifford M. Snapper.

and signals we find. At each stage along a branching pathway of differentiation, the activated, proliferating B cell integrates multiple signals from its environment into an appropriate response. The signals include various patterns and duration of aggregation of membrane immunoglobulin (Ig) in the antigen receptor complex, a dozen or more cytokines acting in various combinations, and cell contact-dependent signals from adhesion molecules and membrane-bound cytokines like CD40 ligand (CD40L). Appropriate responses include small or large clones of cells secreting different classes of antibodies with different biological activities, clones secreting mucosal antibodies in special sites, somatic mutation, maintenance or loss of antigen-presenting cell functions such as costimulation, reversion to memory cells, anergy, or cell death.

## ACTIVATION AND MATURATION SIGNALS

### MEMBRANE Ig, THE ANTIGEN RECEPTOR

The key event in the specific antibody response is the combination of antigen with the antigen receptor complex on the B-cell surface. If the antigen is multivalent, complexed with antibody, or membrane-bound, the resulting aggregation, or crosslinking, of the antigen receptor delivers an activating signal to the cell that has many consequences. *In vitro*, strong signals through the antigen receptor are directly mitogenic for small B cells in the absence of exogenous help or cytokines, but the dependence of this response on high B-cell culture densities *in vitro*, together with the tendency for B cells to grow as clumps of aggregated cells, suggests that B cells may provide some helper signals to one another. For some T-cell-independent antibody responses (those against the type 2 antigens such as some polysaccharides that lack intrinsic mitogenic activity for B cells), a strong signal through the antigen receptor is a necessary first step for an antibody response. Proliferation and maturation to antibody secretion depends on additional signals that can be delivered by soluble cytokines, which can act in this way on antigen-activated but not resting B cells. The nature and sources of these cytokines or other helper signals for T-cell-independent responses *in vivo* remain to be discovered; the natural killer (NK) cell is a good candidate[2]. But for other T-cell-independent antigens, the antigen receptor serves a different, passive role as an address for another activating signal. These are the type 1 antigens such as lipopolysaccharide (LPS) that have an intrinsic ability to activate B cells through the more primitive receptors for microbial products that regulate innate immunity. At low concentrations of these antigens, only antigen-specific B cells respond, because only they can gather an activating dose of the antigen with their antigen receptors[3].

In T-cell-dependent antibody responses, the antigen receptor functions both to deliver an activating signal and as an address for T-cell help. B cells get help in the antibody response by presenting antigen to helper T cells[4]. Since antigens bound to the antigen receptor are processed and presented on MHC class II very efficiently, B cells act as antigen-specific antigen-presenting cells. When the antigens are at low concentrations, only antigen-specific B cell can present them. Crosslinking or aggregation is not required for efficient antigen processing and presentation to a differentiated helper effector T cell, such as a helper T-cell line that makes T-helper type 2 (Th2) cytokines upon activation[5]. But with less avid or less differentiated helper cells, a signal through the B-cell antigen receptor may be necessary for effective antigen presentation[6]. Even weak signals through the antigen receptor prepare the B cell for a more effective interaction with a helper T cell by activating adhesion molecules, increasing MHC class II expression, and turning on costimulatory activities such as B7-2[7] that enable the B cell to induce help from the T cell. In addition, signals through the B-cell antigen receptor can enhance the B-cell response to T-cell help, as shown by the synergistic response to simultaneous signals through membrane Ig and CD40, the receptor for cell contact-dependent help on the B cell[8].

## CONTACT-DEPENDENT T-CELL HELP

T-cell help is mediated by secreted and membrane-bound cytokines that are made transiently by antigen-activated T cells. The key membrane-bound cytokine in the delivery of help is CD40L, a member of the tumor necrosis factor (TNF) family, which engages CD40, a member of the TNF receptor family, on the B cell[9,10]. It accounts for the cell contact dependence of T-cell help for the antigen-presenting B cell[11]. This kind of help is also called cognate help, or MHC-restricted help, because it is linked to T-cell recognition of antigen on the B-cell surface. Some immunologists believe that B cells also get signals directly through MHC class II molecules as a consequence of antigen recognition by a helper T cell. There is no convincing evidence for this[12,13], although antibodies to class II molecules can certainly deliver positive and negative signals[14,15]. The key role of CD40L–CD40 in T-cell help is underscored by the dramatic effects of CD40 and CD40L deficiency on T-cell-dependent antibody responses *in vivo* in mice and humans[16–20]. All that is left in the absence of the CD40L–CD40 interaction is a primary IgM antibody response in some experiments. There is no class switching in response to T-dependent antigens, no B-cell memory, no germinal centers, and no affinity maturation. It is not known whether the residual IgM antibody response depends on cognate help rather than bystander help mediated by soluble cytokines. The striking phenotype of the CD40- and CD40L-deficient animals contrasts with the less impressive defects in antibody formation in IL-2- and IL-4-deficient mice[21,22].

Aggregation of the antigen receptor complex by antigen and ligation of

CD40 by CD40L can each deliver initial activating signals to small, resting B cells. They result in superficially similar activation sequences, with enhancement of antigen presentation functions and the ability to respond to cytokines by proliferation and maturation to Ig secretion. Although the signals are synergistic when received together, they can substitute for one another in the antibody response. The T-cell-independent type 2 antigens induce antibody responses and class switching, except to IgE, in the absence of a CD40L–CD40 interaction[18]. Likewise, a Th2 cell line can induce a maximal antibody response from resting B cells in the absence of a signal through the antigen receptor[5]. Nevertheless, it is becoming apparent that different activating signals have major effects on the ability of B cells to respond to particular cytokines and the resulting profile of Ig isotypes that are made[23]. They also induce a different cell surface phenotype: signals through the antigen receptor induce expression of CD5, while signals through CD40 induce expression of CD23[24]. The antigen receptor and CD40 activate small B cells by distinct intracellular signaling pathways. Drugs that block activation by aggregation of membrane Ig (cyclosporin A, acute treatment with phorbol esters or depletion of protein kinase C (PKC) by chronic treatment with phorbol esters, and agents that raise intracellular cAMP concentrations) all are much less effective against or fail to block activation through CD40[24–27]. Ligation of the antigen receptor induces expression of the transcription factors, egr-1 and c-myc, while T-cell help induces comparable levels of c-myc message with little induction of egr-1[28].

## HELPER CYTOKINES

Once activated by antigen, either directly through the antigen receptor or indirectly through presentation of processed antigen to a helper T cell or both, clonal expansion and maturation to antibody secretion are driven largely by soluble cytokines in combination with continuing signals through CD40 and/or the antigen receptor. The original names of the helper cytokines reflected our hope that particular cytokines would produce unique effects on particular cell types: 'B-cell growth factor' to induce B-cell proliferation, and 'B-cell differentiation factor' to induce maturation to antibody synthesis. Now we know that individual cytokines affect many cell types, and have different effects depending on the type and state of activation and differentiation of the target cell. Moreover, different cytokines can have similar effects on the same target cell. CD4 T cells tend towards polarized differentiation states in which they secrete distinct sets of cytokines. These T-cell subsets have done much to rationalize cytokine effects in T-cell effector functions, in that the Th1 subset promotes inflammatory and cytotoxic reactions to viruses and intracellular bacteria, while the Th2 subset promotes antibody formation and immediate hypersensitivity reactions[29].

The Th2 cytokines (IL-4, IL-5, IL-6, IL-10) are generally more effective growth and differentiation factors for B cells than the Th1 cytokines (IL-2, interferon gamma (IFN-γ), TNF-α and lymphotoxin). However, Th1 cell lines express CD40L[30] and can be converted into effective helpers *in vitro* by the addition of IL-4 and neutralizing antibodies to IFN-γ[31]. Th1 lines are effective helpers *in vivo*[32], and the knockout mice show that IL-4 is not required for effective antibody responses *in vivo*. Because of their ability to selectively activate transcription of unswitched heavy chain constant region loci[33], cytokines direct switch recombination and so determine the amounts of various classes of antibodies made during an antibody response. If the response is tilted towards Th2 cytokines, then IgE and the less cytotoxic subclasses of IgG antibody (IgG1 in the mouse) predominate. If the response is tilted towards Th1 cytokines, then IgE is not made and other IgG subclasses predominate. The effects of individual cytokines on Ig synthesis and class switching are examined comprehensively in Part II of this book.

## POSITIVE AND NEGATIVE B-CELL RESPONSES TO ACTIVATING SIGNALS

As mentioned in the introduction, production of a clone of antibody-secreting cells is only one possible outcome of the activating signals described above. The nature of the response depends not only on the signals but on the state of differentiation and the microenvironment of the B cells. It is frequently difficult to determine whether various responses of a population of cells to various signals reflect shaping of the response by the signals or selection by the signals of subpopulations committed to particular responses. The different B-cell subpopulations and the microenvironments in which they respond to antigen are the subjects of Chapters 2 and 3.

### PRIMARY ANTIBODY RESPONSE

The primary antibody response is the response most closely mimicked by polyclonal B-cell activation *in vitro*. The T-cell-dependent primary response occurs in the periarteriolar areas of the spleen, rather than in the follicles[34,35], and results mostly in IgM antibody. The T-cell-independent response to type 2 antigens may involve a specialized B-cell subset, the marginal zone B cell, and includes limited switching favoring a particular IgG isotype (IgG3 in the mouse). *In vitro*, both T-cell-dependent and T-cell-independent responses can be driven with cytokines to undergo extensive Ig class switching. Like the *in vitro* responses, primary antibody responses are short-lived and limited; the generation of long-lived memory cells requires the specialized microenvironment of the germinal center[36]. It has been suggested that the precursors of the primary antibody response are a distinct B-cell subpopulation from those that can enter germinal centers[37], but this conclusion has been challenged[34]. The mucosal antibody response has its own specialized lymphocyte subpopulations, lymphoid tissues, and micro-environments (see Chapter 16).

## GERMINAL CENTER REACTION

Following T-cell-dependent activation, a few B cells enter the primary lymphoid follicles, where they proliferate extensively to create a germinal center composed of rapidly dividing cells with a unique cell surface phenotype, together with a few antigen-specific T cells[35]. Within the oligoclonal germinal centers, the as yet undefined somatic mutation machinery is turned on, and mutations are deliberately introduced into the variable regions of the antibody genes of the proliferating cells[38,39]. Survival of the germinal center cells depends on their ability to bind antigen with their mutated receptors, and when antigen is limiting, competition between circulating antibody and newly mutated antigen receptors on germinal center B cells is thought to drive affinity maturation by preferential survival of rare cells bearing mutated receptors with increased affinity for antigen. Most cells generated in germinal centers are thought to die there. The surviving cells can contribute to the late primary antibody response, which includes higher affinity, mutated antibodies of IgM and other classes. Others revert to long-lived, recirculating memory B cells, which form the basis for the more vigorous secondary antibody response upon re-exposure to antigen. The memory B cells have frequently undergone genomic switch rearrangements, and these memory cells express membrane Ig receptors of IgG, IgA or, more rarely, IgE isotypes. Other changes in surface phenotype of memory cells are associated with adhesion molecules thought to confer new recirculation patterns.

The germinal center reaction and the induction of high-rate somatic mutation has not been replicated *in vitro*, although advances have been made in finding culture conditions which produce extensive, CD40-dependent proliferation without terminal differentiation to antibody formation[40]. Follicular dendritic cells serve as a reservoir for protein antigens in germinal centers and may play other important roles as B-cell activators in the germinal center reaction[41].

## DEATH, ANERGY, EXILE AND SUPPRESSION

Signals through the antigen receptor and soluble and membrane-bound cytokines made by T cells and other cells can also kill, inactivate or shut down B cells and B-cell responses. These mechanisms delete new or somatically mutated B cells which have generated receptors for multivalent self-antigens, and may be important in enabling T cells to negatively regulate antibody formation to foreign antigens and self-antigens.

Newly differentiated B cells in the bone marrow are exquisitely sensitive to activation-induced death by antigen receptor aggregation, and die in the bone marrow if they cannot produce a receptor without antibody activity for multivalent self-antigens[42,43]. Mature B cells of both the B1 and B2 subsets (see Chapter 3) are also killed by receptor ligation without appropriate help[44–47]. Low-level aggregation of antigen receptors by soluble antigens in the absence of help can result in a state of reversible anergy to signals through the antigen receptor, rather than death[6]. These anergic cells are short-lived *in vivo* because they fail to compete effectively with other B cells for migration into lymphoid follicles[48]. Interaction with certain self-antigens or environmental antigens can determine which B cells enter into or selectively survive in the long-lived, self-renewing adult B1 subset, many of whose members are exiled to the peritoneum[45,49–51]. Germinal center B cells are programmed to die unless rescued by antigen and T-cell help[35], and may undergo a phase of heightened susceptibility to tolerance by antigen receptor ligation without help, similar to that of newly differentiated B cells[52].

Several cytokines are very effective at inhibiting B-cell proliferation or blocking activation of resting cells. These inhibitory cytokine effects on lymphocytes and antigen-presenting cells are now the favorite explanation for the mechanism of antigen-specific suppression. Like CD40L, some inhibitory cytokines are membrane-bound members of the TNF family, including membrane TNF-α, lymphotoxin-β, and Fas ligand. Th1 CD4 cells can kill rather than help antigen-presenting B cells through interaction of Fas ligand with Fas, a member of the TNF receptor family on activated B cells and many other cell types that mediates apoptotic cell death[53]. CD40L is very effective at inducing Fas expression and sensitizing B cells for killing by a Th1 cell line, but the B cells can be rescued by antigen receptor aggregation, which uncouples Fas from the death pathway[30] except in anergic B-cells[54]. This is an interesting example of complex interactions among B-cell activation signals that may enable appropriate B-cell responses to foreign antigens while avoiding formation of destructive autoantibodies.

To contribute to an effective antibody response, the B cells must not only receive the appropriate activating signals through its antigen and cytokine receptors, but also avoid these signals and combinations of signals that kill or inactivate it. Ultimately, a satisfactory explanation of the various B-cell responses to activating signals will require an intimate knowledge of how various extracellular signals are integrated through the cytoplasmic signal transduction pathways to regulate the transcriptional, cell cycle progression, and programmed cell death machinery inside the cell.

## REFERENCES

1. Burnett FM. A modification of Jerne's theory of antibody production using the concept of clonal selection. Aust J Sci 1957; 20:67–69.
2. Snapper CM, Yamaguchi H, Moorman MA, Mond JJ. An in vitro model for T

cell-independent induction of humoral immunity. A requirement for NK cells. J Immunol 1994; 152:4884–4892.

3. Coutinho A, Möller G. Immune activation of B cells: evidence for 'one nonspecific triggering signal' not delivered by the Ig receptors. Scand J Immunol 1974; 3:133–146.
4. Parker DC. T cell-dependent B cell activation. Annu Rev Immunol 1993; 11:331–360.
5. Tony H-P, Phillips NE, Parker DC. Role of membrane immunoglobulin (Ig) crosslinking in membrane Ig-mediated, major histocompatibility-restricted T cell–B cell cooperation. J Exp Med 1985; 162:1695–1708.
6. Cooke MP, Heath AW, Shokat KM *et al.* Immunoglobulin signal transduction guides the specificity of B cell–T cell interactions and is blocked in tolerant self-reactive B cells. J Exp Med 1994; 179:425–438.
7. Lenschow DJ, Sperling AI, Cooke MP *et al.* Differential up-regulation of the B7-1 and B7-2 costimulatory molecules after Ig receptor engagement by antigen. J Immunol 1994; 153:1990–1997.
8. Snapper CM, Kehry MR, Castle BE, Mond JJ. Multivalent, but not divalent, antigen receptor cross-linkers synergize with CD40 ligand for induction of Ig synthesis and class switching in normal murine B cells: A redefinition of the TI-2 vs T cell-dependent antigen dichotomy. J Immunol 1995; 154:1177–1187.
9. Armitage RJ, Fanslow WC, Strockbine L *et al.* Molecular and biological characterization of a murine ligand for CD40. Nature 1992; 357:80–82.
10. Noelle RJ, Roy M, Shepherd DM *et al.* A novel ligand on activated helper T cells binds CD40 and transduces the signal for the cognate activation of B cells. Proc Natl Acad Sci USA 1992; 89:6550–6554.
11. Durie FH, Foy TM, Masters SR *et al.* The role of CD40 in the regulation of humoral and cell-mediated immunity. Immunol Today 1994; 15:406–411.
12. Markowitz JS, Rogers PR, Grusby MJ *et al.* B lymphocyte development and activation independent of MHC class II expression. J Immunol 1993; 150:1223–1233.
13. Parker DC. The functions of antigen recognition in T cell-dependent B cell activation. Semin Immunol 1993; 5:413–420.
14. Poudrier J, Owens T. CD54/intercellular adhesion molecule 1 and major histocompatibility complex II signaling induces B cells to express interleukin 2 receptors and complements help provided through CD40 ligation. J Exp Med 1994; 179:1417–1427.
15. Newell MK, VanderWall J, Beard KS, Freed JH. Ligation of major histocompatibility complex class II molecules mediates apoptotic cell death in resting B lymphocytes. Proc Natl Acad Sci USA 1993; 90:10459–10463.
16. Xu J, Foy TM, Laman JD *et al.* Mice deficient for the CD40 ligand. Immunity 1994; 1:423–432.
17. Kawabe T, Naka T, Yoshida K *et al.* The immune response in CD40-deficient mice: impaired immunoglobulin class switching and germinal center formation. Immunity 1994; 1:167–178.
18. Renshaw BR, Fanslow III WC, Armitage RJ et al. Humoral immune responses in CD40 ligand-deficient mice. J Exp Med 1994; 180:1889–1900.
19. Castigli E, Alt FW, Davidson L *et al.* CD40-deficient mice generated by RAG-2 deficient blastocyst complementation. Proc Natl Acad Sci USA 1994; 91:12135–12139.
20. Hill A, Chapel H. The fruits of cooperation. Nature 1993; 361:494.
21. Kündig TM, Schorle H, Bachmann MF *et al.* Immune responses in interleukin-2-deficient mice. Science 1993; 262:1059–1061.

22. Kopf M, Le Gros G, Bachmann M *et al.* Disruption of the murine IL-4 gene blocks Th2 cytokine responses. Nature 1993; 362:245–248.
23. Mond JJ, Lees A, Snapper CM. T cell-independent antigens type 2. Annu Rev Immunol 1995; 13:655–692.
24. Wortis HH, Teutsch M, Higer M *et al.* B-cell activation by crosslinking of surface IgM or ligation of CD40 involves alternative signal pathways and results in different B-cell phenotypes. Proc Natl Acad Sci USA 1995; 92:3348–3352.
25. Kawakami K, Parker DC. Antigen and helper T lymphocytes activate B lymphocytes by distinct signaling pathways. Eur J Immunol 1993; 23:77–84.
26. Lalmanach-Girard A-C, Chiles TC, Parker DC, Rothstein TL. T cell-dependent induction of NF-κ B in B cells. J Exp Med 1993; 177:1215–1219.
27. Kato T, Kokuho T, Tamura T, Nariuchi H. Mechanisms of T cell contact-dependent B cell activation. J Immunol 1994; 152:2130–2138.
28. Klaus SJ, Parker DC. Inducible cell contact signals regulate early activation gene expression during B–T collaboration. J Immunol 1992; 149:1867–1875.
29. Mosmann TR, Coffman RL. Th1 and Th2 cells: different patterns of lymphokine secretion lead to different functional properties. Annu Rev Immunol 1989; 7:145–173.
30. Rothstein TL, Wang JKM, Panka DJ *et al.* Protection against Fas-dependent Th1-mediated apoptosis by antigen receptor engagement in B cells. Nature 1995; 374:163–165.
31. Coffman RL, Seymour BW, Lebman DA *et al.* The role of helper T cell products in mouse B cell differentiation and isotype regulation. Immunol Rev 1988; 102:5–28.
32. Rizzo LV, DeKruyff RH, Umetsu DT. Generation of B cell memory and affinity maturation. Induction with Th1 and Th2 T cell clones. J Immunol 1992; 148:3733–3739.
33. Stavnezer J, Radcliffe G, Lin Y-C *et al.* Immunoglobulin heavy-chain switching may be directed by prior induction of transcripts from constant-region genes. Proc Natl Acad Sci USA 1988; 85:7704–7708.
34. Jacob J, Kelsoe G. In situ studies of the primary immune response to (4-hydroxy-3-nitrophenyl)acetyl. II. A common clonal origin for periarteriolar lymphoid sheath-associated foci and germinal centers. J Exp Med 1992; 176:679–687.
35. MacLennan ICM, Liu Y-J, Johnson GD. Maturation and dispersal of B-cell clones during T cell-dependent antibody responses. Immunol Rev 1992; 126:143–161.
36. Coico RF, Bhogal BS, Thorbecke GJ. Relationship of germinal centers in lymphoid tissue to immunologic memory. VI. Transfer of B cell memory with lymph node cells fractionated according to their receptors for peanut agglutinin. J Immunol 1983; 131:2254–2257.
37. Linton P-J, Decker DJ, Klinman NR. Primary antibody-forming cells and secondary B cells are generated from separate precursor cell subpopulations. Cell 1990; 59:1049–1059.
38. Jacob J, Przylepa J, Miller C, Kelsoe G. In situ studies of the primary immune response to (4-hydroxy-3-nitrophenyl)acetyl. III. The kinetics of V region mutation and selection in germinal center B cells. J Exp Med 1993; 178:1293–1307.
39. Ziegner M, Steinhauser G, Berek C. Development of antibody diversity in single germinal centers: selective expansion of high-affinity variants. Eur J Immunol 1994; 24:2393–2400.
40. Arpin C, Déchanet J, Van Kooten C *et al.* Generation of memory B cells and plasma cells in vitro. Science 1995; 268:720–722.

41. Kosco-Vilbois MH, Gray D, Scheidegger D, Julius M. Follicular dendritic cells help resting B cells to become effective antigen-presenting cells: induction of B7/BB1 and upregulation of major histocompatibility complex class II molecules. J Exp Med 1993; 178:2055–2066.
42. Nemazee DA, Bürki K. Clonal deletion of B lymphocytes in a transgenic mouse bearing anti-MHC class I antibody genes. Nature 1989; 337–562–566.
43. Hartley SB, Crosbie J, Brink R *et al.* Elimination from peripheral tissues of self-reactive B lymphocytes recognizing membrane-bound antigens. Nature 1991; 353:765–769.
44. Russel DM, Dembie Z, Monahan G *et al.* Peripheral deletion of self-reactive B cells. Nature 1991; 354:308.
45. Nisitani S, Tsubata T, Murakami M *et al.* The bcl-2 gene product inhibits clonal deletion of self-reactive B lymphocytes in the periphery but not in the bone marrow. J Exp Med 1993; 178:1247–1254.
46. Parker DC. Induction and suppression of polyclonal antibody responses by anti-lg reagents and antigen-nonspecific helper factors: a comparison of the effects of anti-Fab, anti-IgM, and anti-IgD on murine B cells. Immunol Rev 1980; 52:115–139.
47. Parry SL, Hasbold J, Holman M, Klaus GG. Hypercross-linking surface IgM or IgD receptors on mature B cells induces apoptosis that is reversed by costimulation with IL-4 and anti-CD40. J Immunol 1994; 152:2821–2829.
48. Cyster JG, Hartley SB, Goodnow CC. Competition for follicular niches excludes self-reactive cells from the recirculating B-cell repertoire. Nature 1994; 371:389.
49. Hardy RR, Carmack CE, Li YS, Hayakawa K. Distinctive developmental origins and specificities of murine $CD5^+$ B cells. Immunol Rev 1994; 137:91–118.
50. Arnold LW, Pennell CA, McCray SK, Clarke SH. Development of B-1 cells: segregation of phosphatidyl choline-specific B cells to the B-1 population occurs after immunoglobulin gene expression. J Exp Med 1994; 179:1585–1595.
51. Haughton G, Arnold LW, Whitmore AC, Clarke SH. B-1 cells are made, not born. Immunol Today 1993; 14:84–87.
52. Linton PJ, Rudie A, Klinman NR. Tolerance susceptibility of newly generating memory B cells. J Immunol 1991; 146:4099–4104.
53. Ju ST, Cui H, Panka DJ *et al.* Participation of target Fas protein in apoptosis pathway induced by CD4+ Th1 and CD8+ cytotoxic T cells. Proc Natl Acad Sci USA 1994; 91:4185–4189.
54. Rathmell JC, Cooke MP, Ho WY *et al.* CD95 (Fas)-dependent elimination of self-reactive B cells upon interaction with $CD4^+$ T cells. Nature 1995; 376:181–183.

# 5 Immunoglobulin Class Switching

**MATTHIAS LORENZ and ANDREAS RADBRUCH**
*Institute for Genetics, Cologne, Germany*

## INTRODUCTION

Antibodies (immunoglobulin, Ig) occur in eight (mice) or nine (human) different classes, with respect to the constant region of their heavy chain. The class determines the antibody effector function and thus the kind of humoral immune response towards a particular antigen. Activated B lymphocytes can switch the class of the antibody they express, conserving the antigen-binding part of it. Here we review recent experiments showing that the molecular basis of antibody class switching is a highly specific recombination, which is induced upon activation in B lymphocytes and targeted to distinct classes by cytokines. These cytokines induce switch transcripts of the targeted recombinogenic DNA, and these transcripts or the process of their generation are most probably involved in switch recombination[1] (for reviews see references 2–6).

## INDUCTION AND ROLE OF Ig CLASS SWITCHING

### FUNCTIONAL HETEROGENEITY OF IG CLASSES

Mice have antibodies of the classes IgM, IgD, IgG3, IgG1, IgG2b, IgG2a, IgE and IgA, and humans of the classes IgM, IgD, IgG3, IgG1, IgG2, IgG4, IgE, IgA1 and IgA2. The effector functions attributed to these classes in mice include effective crosslinking by IgM, opsonization, and complement fixation by IgM and murine IgG3, IgG2b and IgG2a. IgA is transported across basal membranes and IgE arms mast cells and granulocytes (for review see reference 7).

### Ig CLASSES IN IMMUNE RESPONSE

The antibody classes expressed in particular immune responses depend on the class switch that is induced in B cells upon antigenic challenge. It has been known for a while that the kind of Ig class switch is dependent on the method of

*Cytokine Regulation of Humoral Immunity: Basic and Clinical Aspects.* Edited by Clifford M. Snapper.

B-cell activation, i.e. the type of antigen, adjuvants, route of immunization, T cells and accessory cells involved, and genetic background of the responding immune system[8–10]. In the mouse, T-cell-dependent humoral immune responses are dominated by IgG1, IgG2a, IgA and IgE, while so-called T-cell-independent responses are dominated by IgM, IgG3 and IgG2b[8, 11–13]. Some examples of typical immune responses are given below, although the topic in general is elaborated in the other chapters of this book. IgG3 is the main class in responses against bacteria, especially in T-cell-'independent' immune responses against carbohydrates[14]. IgG1 is the dominant class in response against soluble proteins and parasites, like the cestode parasite *Mesocestoides corti*. Switching to IgG1 is controlled by cells expressing the cytokine interleukin 4 (IL-4)[15]. IgG2a is the major Ig class in response to viral antigens[16]. Switching to IgG2a is induced by interferon gamma (IFN-$\gamma$)-expressing cells[17]. Extracellular parasites, especially multicellular ones, often provoke a strong IgE response. The class switch to IgE is induced by IL-4 at high concentrations[18–22].

In humans compared to mice, analogous classes of Ig are involved in corresponding antiviral, antibacterial and antiparasite immune responses. Human IgE and IgG4 are analogous to murine IgE and IgG1.

## SEQUENTIAL CLASS SWITCHING

Upon activation, naive B cells, expressing IgM and IgD, can switch to any other class[23,24]. However, sequential switching can also occur, i.e. switching from IgG to IgE or IgA, and from IgE to IgA[25,26]. For murine IgE, sequential switching from IgM to IgG1 and then to IgE sometimes is dominant over direct switching, as shown by the molecular analysis of switched cells[27–30], the existence of expressing Ig of both classes simultaneously[20] and the suppression of switching to IgE by anti-IgG1 antibodies[30,31]. The functional significance of sequential switching to IgE has been controversial: today it seems clear that the sequential switch from IgM to IgG1 to IgE may rather reflect the coincidental induction of switching to IgG1 and IgE by the same cytokine, IL-4. In mice, in which switching to IgG1 is blocked, the frequency of cells switching to IgE is not reduced[32].

## LPS-INDUCED CLASS SWITCHING

*In vitro*, B lymphocytes can be activated by mitogens like lipopolysaccharide (LPS), a component of the outer cell membrane of Gram-negative bacteria. LPS-activated murine, but not human, B cells are induced to switch, even in the absence of added T-cell-derived cytokines. Macrophages and their cytokines have to be present to induce the B cells for proliferation and class switching[33,34]. This system has been used extensively to study class switching *in vitro*[35,36]. After a lag period of about 36 h[37], between 1 in 3 and 1 in 10 splenic B cells, depending on the mouse strain, react for LPS[38], start to divide, and continue to proliferate at generation times of about 10 h[37] until they die, presumably by apoptosis, as has been shown for anti-Ig-activated B cells[39]. LPS activates naive B cells to downregulate IgD expression, become Ig-secreting plasmablasts and undergo Ig class switching at high frequency. Within a few days, 30 per cent of IgG3-expressing[40] and IgG2b-expressing cells are generated, which are the dominant classes induced[23], and nearly all LPS-activated cells generate switched cells in their offspring[23]. Addition of T-cell cytokines like IL-4 to LPS cultures suppresses switching to IgG3 and instead induces switching to IgG1 in up to 30 per cent of lymphoblasts[41].

## THE MOLECULAR BASIS OF Ig CLASS SWITCHING

### STRUCTURE OF THE IgH LOCUS

The Ig heavy chain (IgH) locus spans more than 2000 kb on chromosome 12 of mouse (Figure 5.1) and chromosome 14 of humans. Most of it contains gene segments for the antigen-binding domain of the Ig heavy chain, the variable region ($V_H$). Several hundred kilobases of the 3′ part of the IgH locus carry the gene segments ($C_H$) coding for the constant regions of Ig heavy chains, eight different ones in mouse[42,43] and nine functional genes and two pseudogenes (ψ) in humans. The murine $C_H$ gene segments (black boxes in Figure 5.1) extend over approximately 200 kb and are arranged in the order of 5′ μ–δ–γ3–γ1–γ2b–γ2a–ε–α 3′. The human $C_H$ genes extend over more than 300 kb in the following order: 5′ μ–δ–γ3–γ1–ψε–α1–ψγ–γ2–γ4–ε–α2 3′[44].

$C_H$ gene segments differ not only in sequence but also in structure, i.e. in the number of exons. All $C_H$ gene segments consist of four exons, each coding for one heavy chain domain of the secreted form of Ig, and two additional exons for the membrane form of Ig. The Cα, Cγ and Cδ gene segments in their secreted form[45,46] consist of three exons of about 300 bp in length, and one exon which is reduced in length and codes for the hinge region. The hinge exon contributes to flexibility of the two antigen-binding arms of IgG, IgA and IgD. The Cμ[47] and the Cε gene segments[48,49] have a hinge exon of about 300 bp in length. The Cδ gene segment consists of two exons plus a smaller hinge exon and a membrane-binding exon[45].

In front of each $C_H$ gene segment, repetitive DNA sequences are located, called 'switch regions' ($S_H$) (hatched boxes in Figure 5.1), since they are the apparent substrate of switch recombination.

### SWITCH REGIONS ARE GC-RICH REPETITIVE RECOMBINOGENIC SEQUENCES

The sites of Ig class switch recombination are regions of tandemly repeated DNA sequences, the switch regions, which are located upstream of each $C_H$

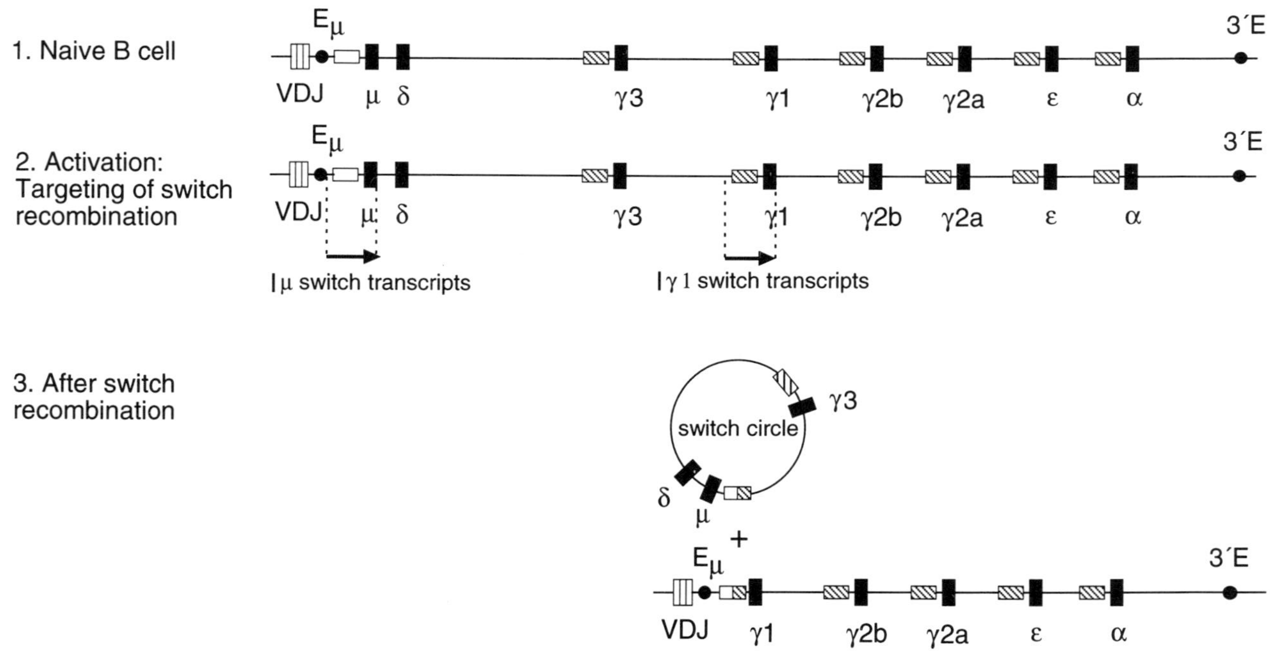


**Figure 5.1** Dynamics of the murine IgH locus during class switching to IgG1. White, hatched and black boxes indicate the μ switch region, other switch regions and the $C_H$ genes, respectively. Eμ, IgH intron enhancer; 3′E, IgH 3′ enhancer

gene, except for Cδ (hatched boxes in Figure 5.1). Switch regions vary in size from 1 kb (sε) to 10 kb (sγ1) and are composed of GC-rich tandem repeats of pentanucleotide sequences like GAGCT and GGGGT[51,52] and stretches of homopurine–homopyrimidine sequences. The tandem repeats vary both in sequence and in length, with 10–40-bp repeats for Sμ, 49-bp repeats for Sγ1, Sγ3 and Sγ2b, 52-bp repeats for Sγ2a, 80-bp repeats for Sα and 40-bp repeats for Sε (for review see reference 53). The degree of homology between the μ, γ, ε and α switch regions is not position-dependent. The sequence of Sμ is more homologous to Sε than to Sα, and least to Sγ[51]. Both human and murine Sγ regions are much less homologous to Sμ than are the respective Sε and Sα regions, but the homology of the various murine Sγs correlates to the distance of a particular Sγ from Sμ (sγ3 > Sγ1 > Sγ2b > Sγ2a)[51].

Switch regions seem to be good substrates for switch recombination as well as for meiotic recombination, since they show considerable length polymorphism, which is probably due to unequal homologous recombination during meiosis[42]. In general bacterial and eukaryotic recombination systems, $S_H$ regions are preferred recombination targets as well[54,55].

The available evidence suggests that switch regions are essential for switch recombination. The molecular basis for this requirement is not yet clear. The recombinogenic property could be due, in part, to the formation of unusual DNA structures promoted by the high GC content of $S_H$ regions. In general, GC-rich regions are found in non-B DNA conformation, and poly(dG)–poly(dC) sequences of supercoiled plasmid DNA induce an altered single-stranded DNA conformation of neighboring DNA sequences[56]. GC-rich regions can also induce triple-stranded D-loops found in contiguous, complementary DNA[57]. The single-stranded DNA of D-loops could serve as a primer for DNA synthesis[57]. It has also been shown that triple helices can be formed by poly(dG)–poly(dC) sequences in supercoiled plasmids[58]. Sen and Gilbert proposed that these oligomeric complexes consist of four DNA strands in parallel orientation, stabilized by Hoogsteen hydrogen-bonded guanine tetrades[59]. If either of these structures exist in activated B cells, they might contribute to pairing or orientation of S regions during switch recombination.

## RECOMBINATION BREAKPOINTS OCCUR IN SWITCH REGIONS

In terms of structure and sequence, switch regions are distinguished targets of switch recombination. So far all attempts have failed to identify particular switch region sequences involved in the switch recombination. However, there is a basic difficulty in studying switch recombination breakpoints and signal sequences associated with them. During amplification and cloning of recombined switch sequences, additional recombination in the bacteria used for cloning could delete parts of those sequences. It has been shown that bacteria or even bacterial extracts can recombine $S_H$ regions efficiently[54].

Switch recombination also may not be a one-hit event by itself. Frequently, intra-switch region recombinations are found in switching cells, especially if particular switch regions are inactivated by targeted mutation[32,60]. The inactive IgH alleles of switched Sγ1 cells nearly always show either recombination between or within switch regions[61]. Successful switch recombination may be a series of recombinations within and between switch regions. More support for this hypothesis comes from comparison of switch recombination products, i.e. the deleted part of the IgH locus, the 'switch circle', and the chromosomal counterproduct. In general, Sμ switch recombination breakpoints are located within the repetitive Sμ sequences of switch circles[62–64], but 5′ thereof on the chromosome[61,65], indicating additional recombinations on the chromosome after the switch. Dunnick *et al.* have compared the sequences of over 150 sites of recombination, mostly compiled from previous publications[66]. No sequences specific for recombinations to distinct classes or recombination as such could be identified at or in close proximity of switch joints, implying that switch recombination is not site specific but region specific[27,61]. Despite the basic homology between the various switch regions, switch recombination seems not to make use of this homology for pairing of DNA strands. Deletions or insertions of one or a few bases are often found at the site of recombination, making switch recombination similar to other types of recombination, like site-directed VDJ recombination or double-strand break repair[67,68].

## CONTROL ELEMENTS FOR TRANSCRIPTION AND RECOMBINATION

Expression of rearranged genes for Ig heavy chains is controlled by $V_H$ promoters and B-cell specific transcriptional enhancers, of which the IgH 'intron' enhancer (for review see reference 69) and the IgH 3′ enhancer have been characterized so far[70–72]. In the mouse, the IgH 'intron' enhancer (Eμ in Figure 5.1) is located between the $J_H$ gene segments and the Cμ gene segments, while the IgH 3′ enhancer (3′ E in Figure 5.1) is located about 16 kb downstream of the Cα gene (Figure 5.1).

As shown by targeted replacement mutation of chimeric mice, the intron enhancer is probably required for rearrangement of V-, D- and J-gene segments early in B-cell differentiation and establishment of a functional Ig heavy chain transcription unit[73,74]. Deletion of the core and 5′ region of the enhancer results in drastic although not complete inhibition of VDJ rearrangement, while deletion of the 3′ region has little effect[74]. Later in B-cell development, the intron enhancer is dispensable for transcription of heavy chain genes[75–77]. For Ig class switching, however, the intron enhancer seems to be required again[60], as will be discussed later in detail.

The 3′ enhancer has been identified as a transcriptional control element of already established Ig heavy chain genes. It is also involved in Ig class switching, since its targeted replacement inhibits switching to IgG2a, IgG2b, IgG3 and IgE *in vitro* and, to a lesser extent, of IgG2b *in vivo*[78]. Since class switching to IgG1 is only marginally effected in the absence of the 3′ enhancer, an additional control element may exist for IgG1 switching.

Apart from the intron and 3′ enhancers, additional control elements are involved in Ig class switching. These specific DNA elements are located upstream of each switch region and control the accessibility of this switch region for switch recombination. The targeted deletion of the murine Sγ1[79] and targeted replacement of the Sγ2b switch control regions[80] abolishes switching to IgG1 and IgG2b, respectively. Apart from controlling switch recombination, these control elements are promoters for transcription, spanning a pseudoexon, the so-called I exon, and the adjacent switch region and constant region gene segments (Figures 5.1 and 5.2). The I exon is spliced to the $C_H$ gene segments to form a stable $I_H$ 'switch' transcript. A similar transcript is also derived from the intron enhancer, which acts as a promoter for a transcript spanning Iμ, Sμ and Cμ[81] (Figure 5.1). The $I_H$ promoters for control of switch recombination and switch transcription are themselves controlled by cytokines, like IFN-γ, IL-4 or transforming growth factor (TGF-β), most of them derived from T lymphocytes. Thus, the old knowledge about control of isotypes in immune responses has finally reached a molecular level. The molecular analysis of signal transduction from cytokine receptors to $I_H$ promoters is currently underway in a variety of research groups, and probably soon will reveal a detailed picture of protein–protein and protein–DNA interactions. Induction of $I_H$ transcription and switch recombination of the adjacent switch regions show a drastic correlation[2]. But only recently a functional connection between the transcription and recombination could be shown, which later will be discussed in detail[1].

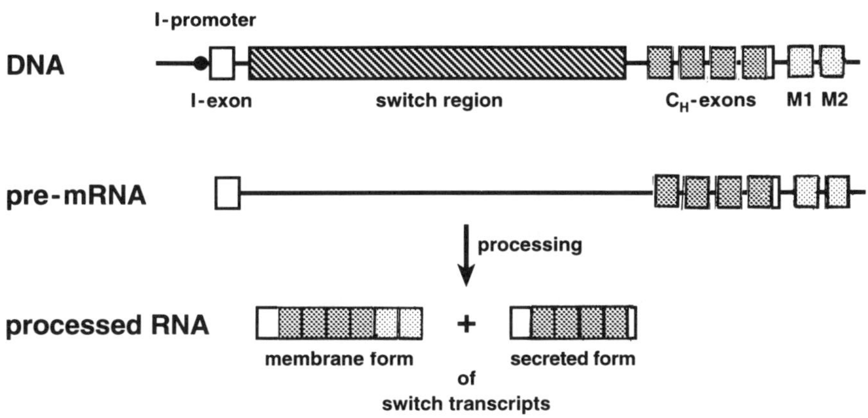


**Figure 5.2** Generalized scheme of processing of switch transcripts. M indicates the membrane exons

### SWITCH TRANSCRIPTS PRECEDE CLASS SWITCHING

In activated B cells, before Ig class switch recombination takes place, specific switch transcripts of the switch donor and the switch acceptor region can be detected (Figure 5.1).

These switch transcripts[81–89] initiate at multiple sites of the I (intervening) regions of DNA, located several hundred base pairs upstream of the corresponding switch region[82,90,91] (Figure 5.2). The initial transcription proceeds through the switch region and $C_H$ gene and terminates at the normal termination site of the corresponding $C_H$ gene. The transcript is processed and stabilized by splicing out of the switch region sequence and the $C_H$ introns, so that the processed switch transcript consists of an I exon spliced to the $C_H$ exons. Analogous to VDJ transcripts, switch transcripts can have the membrane (M1, M2) or secretory exons of the $C_H$ gene (for review see reference 4) (Figure 5.2). Since the transcripts start 5′ of the switch region, they can no longer be produced after switch recombination, and thus have also been termed 'germline' transcripts. The Iμ exon is preserved upon switching from IgM to any other class, and, not surprisingly, switch transcripts containing the Iμ exon spliced to a Cγ2b gene have been identified in cells that have switched to γ2b[92]. Such transcripts could play a role in sequential switching from IgG2b to downstream classes. In general, the 5′ exons of different $I_H$ transcripts do not express significant sequence homology and nor are their sequences conserved between, for example, humans and mice. Between evolutionarily related classes, however, distinct homologies have been described. Nearly all of the switch transcripts contain stop codons in all reading frames and therefore cannot encode peptides of significant length; this is why they also have been termed 'sterile' transcripts.[81,93] The role of switch transcripts in switch recombination is discussed later.

## THE MOLECULAR MECHANISM OF CLASS SWITCHING

### SWITCH TRANSCRIPTION VERSUS SWITCH RECOMBINATION

In the life of B lymphocytes, Ig class switching occurs at high frequency at two stages of differentiation. Fresh B cells, after having assembled their $V_H$- and $V_L$-gene segments in the bone marrow and expressing IgM, are induced by unknown signals to switch to coexpression of IgM and IgD, before antigenic stimulation. Upon activation by antigen, B cells downregulate expression of IgD, and then switch at high frequency from expression of IgM and IgD to expression of any of the IgG, IgA or IgE classes[3]. Coexpression of IgM and IgG, IgA or IgE has been reported, in B lymphocytes from human peripheral blood[94], or murine blood[95], as in murine B-cell blasts activated by mitogens[40] or in certain B lymphoma lines[96]. However, recent results have not confirmed coexpression of IgM together with IgA or IgE in human or murine

B cells, apart from expression of endogenous IgM with passively adsorbed IgG, IgA or IgE[97,98]. For mitogen-activated B-cell blasts, it has been speculated that various Ig classes are expressed together transiently in the process of switching[40]. Today, coexpression of various Ig classes other than IgM and IgD has not been demonstrated beyond doubt for any B cell[99]. This discussion is of basic importance for the understanding of class switching, since stable coexpression of several Ig classes ($C_H$ genes) would rule out recombinatorial mechanisms as the only molecular basis of class switching and would invoke differential control of transcription and RNA processing[100,101].

## LONG TRANSCRIPTS

The coexpression of IgM and IgD, i.e. Cμ- and Cδ-gene segments with the same VDJ gene segment in different Ig heavy chains, by individual cells, is indeed based on a combination of differential use of polyadenylation sites and differential processing of the primary VDJ–Cμ–Cδ transcript[50, 102–104]. This resembles the switch from expression of the membrane form of Ig to the secreted form in activated B-cell blasts. The mRNA encoding the membrane or secreted forms of Ig is produced by differential splicing of RNA and involves the use of alternative polyadenylation sites[105].

Expression of IgM together with IgG, IgA or IgE by individual cells, which would require differential processing of long transcripts encoding VDJ, Cμ and Cγ, Cα and Cϵ, or trans-splicing, as discussed below, has been reported in both normal and transformed B cells. In these cells, despite apparent coexpression of two isotypes, the $C_H$ genes are in 'germline' configuration. Switch recombination is not detectable. However, in all these reports coexpression of various classes of Ig, which is the critical parameter for classifying these cells as switched cells, has been determined by immunofluorescent staining of Ig on the cell surface. Unfortunately, in those experiments it has never been ruled out that Ig of one of the classes had been adsorbed to the cell surface passively, e.g. by class-specific Fc receptors. This has been explicitly discussed for IgM and IgE coexpressing murine splenic B cells[95,97]. B cells from spleens of SJA/9 mice infected with *Nippostrongylus brasiliensis* had been sorted for expression of surface IgM and surface IgE. DNA from these cells did not show switch recombination as detectable by restriction analysis of the bulk population. Based on these results, Yaoita *et al.* proposed a two-step model for class switching. First, differential processing of RNA would result in cells coexpressing IgM and IgE on the cell surface. Second, switch recombination would generate IgE-secreting plasma cells. A critical argument in this work was that SJA/9 mice would not express secreted IgE for passive adsorption, because IgE-secreting plasma cells could not be detected in these mice. However, Katona *et al.* later showed that this might have been a problem of sensitivity. They could demonstrate the existence of IgE-secreting cells and passive uptake of secreted IgE by most of the IgM-expressing B cells of SJA/9 mice.

Transformed B cells from a number of cell lines have been reported to produce IgM and another isotype simultaneously[106,107]. Even in cloned BCL1.2.58 lymphoma cells, expressing IgM and IgG1 of the same idiotype, i.e. specificity[96], and having only one IgH locus left in the genome, the existence of rare switch variants providing IgG1 for passive adsorption to all cells has not been ruled out conclusively[99]. We had observed such a phenomenon while isolating switch variants from a murine hybridoma cell line (Radbruch, unpublished results). More recently, Nolan-Willard *et al.* have failed to demonstrate long transcripts in BCL1 cells by nuclear run-on assays[108].

In an attempt to demonstrate long transcripts containing VDJ and $C\mu$ together with $C\gamma$ or $C\alpha$ directly. Perlmutter and Gilbert[109] have sorted cells expressing IgM and IgA or IgM and IgG on the cell surface, stripped them of surface Ig, incubated them overnight to enable endogenous Ig expression, sorted them again for IgA or IgG expression, and analyzed their RNA for the presence of long transcripts in a sandwich hybridization assay. The RNA was hybridized to membrane-bound $C\gamma$ or $C\alpha$ probes and bound RNA containing also $C\mu$ was then detected with a $C\mu$ probe. Only in sorted IgM and IgG or IgM- and IgA-expressing cells could they detect RNA containing $C\gamma$ or $C\alpha$ and $C\mu$ sequences. However, elegant as it was, this analysis suffered from two basic flaws: first, passive adsorption was not completely ruled out, since it also may have taken place during the overnight incubation; and second, the RNA analysis may not have detected long transcripts, but aggregates of short transcripts with different $C_H$ genes, and derived from different cells.

## TRANS-SPLICING

The attempts to demonstrate long transcripts containing several $C_H$ genes became somewhat outdated when it became clear that class switching is directed to distinct classes by specific cytokines and that these cytokines induce short transcripts of the respective $C_H$ gene and its switch region, the $I_H$ switch transcripts[110–113]. In a modern view, if differential processing of RNA were a mechanism of class switching, it would be trans-splicing of the VDJ-$C\mu$ and $I\gamma$, $I\alpha$ or $I\epsilon$ switch transcripts rather than differential splicing of long transcripts[100,114]. Trans-splicing involves the splicing of two separate RNA precursors into one mRNA (for review see reference 115). Although trans-splicing cannot be a general way of processing of eukaryotic RNA, it has been detected in specialized systems, like certain nematodes. Mammalian cells can trans-splice when transfected with nematode RNA substrates for trans-splicing[116]. For Ig class switching, trans-splicing has been suggested to occur in a transgenic mouse model situation[100] and in the murine BCL1 lymphoma cells described above. Cloned BCL1 cell lines expressing both IgM and IgG1 from one IgH locus contain both mature VDJ-Cγ1 and Iγ1 switch transcripts[108]. If this occurred in individual cells of such a cell line, IgG1 could only be expressed by trans-splicing. However, it was not ruled out in this analysis that a few cells switched to expression of IgG1 by recombination and that expression of endogenous IgG1 and expression of Iγ1 switch transcripts occurred in different cells of the same clone, Iγ1 switch transcript-expressing cells expressing IgG1 by passive adsorption, but not from the endogenous gene, as discussed above.

The same argument holds true for B cells from a transgenic mouse carrying a human VDJ-Cμ transgene. Switching to expression of the human VDJ together with murine Cγ genes occurs in some B cells[114,117]. Again, the bulk of B cells shows no interchromosomal recombination between transgene and endogenous IgH locus, and detection of the switched transgenic VDJ correlates with the induction, by cytokines, of the corresponding Iγ switch transcripts[101]. Again, if expression of the switched Ig and of Iγ switch transcripts occurred in the same cell, one possible explanation of this result would be trans-splicing of VDJ-Cμ to Iγ switch transcripts, although an alternative possible explanation would be expression of the switched Ig, generated by trans-recombination, and of Iγ from the second IgH locus of that cell. More recently, Shimizu and Honjo have described human-VDJ–murine-Cε transcripts in B cells from these mice, generated upon stimulation with IL-4 and lipopolysaccharide (LPS), with IL-4 alone generating only Iε switch transcripts[100]. Again, as well as with trans-splicing, this result would be compatible with induction of trans-switch recombination by LPS, since the human transgene contains the Sμ switch region[117]. Today, we are still waiting for clear evidence for trans-splicing showing that it is a biologically relevant molecular mechanism for class switching.

## SWITCH RECOMBINATON BY LOOP-OUT AND DELETION

Switch recombination was the first molecular mechanism described for class switching. It has been demonstrated in murine myelomas and hybridomas producing IgG, IgA or IgE[118–124], in switch variants from myeloma and hybridoma cell lines[125–128], in human lymphomas[129–132], in murine LPS blasts, i.e. activated normal B cells[36,41,133,134], and in human IgA1$^+$ B cells from peripheral blood[98]. In those cells, Ig class switching had involved an intrachromosomal recombination of the Sμ switch region or adjacent sequences with any of the other switch regions, bringing the VDJ gene into proximity with a Cγ, Cα or Cε gene and deleting the Cμ, Cδ and other intervening $C_H$ genes (Figure 5.1). In most cells, switch recombination had occurred not only on the expressed IgH allele, but also on the allelically excluded one.

Although switch recombination by sister chromatid exchange was discussed earlier[5], it is now clear that switch recombination normally occurs by looping out and deletion of DNA from one strand. The intervening DNA between switch donor and switch acceptor regions is deleted as circular DNA and can be retrieved from switched cells[62–64]. Occasionally, the looped-out DNA is not deleted but inverted, leading to a non-functional IgH locus[30,135]. Recombinations between oncogenes and switch regions[136], as well as recombinations between switch regions in trans[137–140], demonstrate that switch recombination can act in trans, although perhaps only at low frequency.

## SWITCH RECOMBINATION MAY REQUIRE DNA SYNTHESIS

As will be discussed later in detail, switch recombination can be induced *in vitro* by activation of B cells. Although all of the known activation stimuli also induce proliferation of the B cells, it is not clear whether class switching depends on proliferation. It is probably dependent on DNA synthesis, since inhibition of DNA synthesis in LPS-activated murine spleen cells with thymidine or hydroxyurea reduces the frequency of class switching[141]. Comparison of recombined S$\mu$–S$\alpha$ regions from clonally related 129 lymphoma cells with the germline sequence of S$\mu$ and S$\alpha$ reveals that some progeny of a single-switch recombination event have mutations, whereas other progeny do not. Based on these findings Dunnick and Stavnezer have proposed that class switch recombination is mediated by error-prone DNA synthesis of one DNA strand and ligation of the other strand from pre-existing DNA[142,143]. Mutations had been found at the sites of switch recombination earlier, including small deletions or insertions, as has been described for error-prone DNA double-strand break repair[61,67,68].

## PROTEINS INVOLVED IN SWITCH RECOMBINATION

Protein components of the switch recombinase have not yet been identified unambiguously. Several groups have reported identification by mobility shift analysis of proteins from nuclear extracts of activated B lymphocytes binding to switch regions more or less specifically. Such proteins could be part of the switch recombinase or be involved in control of switch recombination. LR1 (LPS-responsive factor 1)[144] binds to sequences of the S$\gamma$1, S$\gamma$3 and S$\mu$ regions, but also to the Ig heavy chain intron enhancer[144], and to the *c-myc* P1 promoter[145], suggesting that LR1 could act as a transcription factor. The LR1–DNA complex is induced by LPS, requires phosphorylation and is present in pre-B cell lines and mitogen-activated primary B cells, but not in unstimulated primary B cells[144]. Recently, this factor has been cloned[146].

BSAP (B-cell specific activator protein)[147], also referred to as S$\alpha$-BP[148] or NF-S$\mu$-B1[149], binds to two distinct sites 5′ of the S$\alpha$ switch region[148] and to repetitive sequence motifs of the S$\mu$ region[149]. BSAP appears to be induced during pro-B cell development, is abundant at the pre-B-cell and mature B-cell stage, but is absent in terminally differentiated plasma cells[148]. Its function is not clear.

The three DNA-binding proteins SNUP, SNAP and SNIP, the last in its complexed form with NFκB, are expressed in mitogen-activated murine splenic B cells and bind to tandem repeats of switch regions. While SNUP specifically interacts with the Sμ region[150], SNAP and SNIP bind to Sγ3, Sγ1 and Sγ2b switch regions[151,152]. Many of the Sγ3 recombination breakpoints occur within the SNAP- and the SNIP/NFκB-binding site[152]. The sequence of the transcription factor NFκB contains a reldomain that can promote dimerization, and the factors might therefore be involved in the alignment of switch regions for switch recombination, which at present is still a speculation.

Recently a murine and human cDNA encoding for a Sμ region binding protein, called Sμ bp-2, was cloned[153,154]. Sμ bp-2 binds to single-stranded DNA containing GGGG stretches, and the deduced amino acid sequence carries motifs shared by the helicase family. Expression of Sμ bp-2 mRNA is ubiquitous and augmented in spleen cells stimulated with LPS plus IL-4.

Summarizing the present information, one could state that the only molecular mechanism for Ig class switching identified so far is class switch recombination. Although this recombination occurs at high frequency *in vitro*, its molecular mechanism and components remain obscure.

## CONTROL OF CLASS SWITCH RECOMBINATION

### INDUCTION OF SWITCH RECOMBINATION

Switch recombination is induced upon activation in naive, IgM- and IgD-expressing B lymphocytes[155] and in memory B cells[156]. *In vitro*, mitogens like bacterial LPS for murine B cells[36] or antigen/mitogen plus CD40 stimulation for murine and human B cells[12,157] switch on high-frequency recombination. Frequencies of class switching can be as high as 10 per cent/cell per generation[61], leading to more than 30 per cent of switched cells within a few days. It remains unclear whether switch recombination is induced in all activated cells or just in distinct subsets. Cells activated *in vitro* by mitogen can be divided into switching cells, showing switch recombination not only on the expressed IgH allele, but frequently also on the allelically excluded IgH[36], and nearly always showing recombination within the Sμ switch region[61], and non-switching cells, expressing IgM until they 'escape' the *in vitro* stimulation by apoptosis. These cells show no signs of switch recombination or intra-Sμ recombination on either IgH allele[61].

Although the switch-inducing stimuli activate not only switch recombination but also proliferation of naive B cells, the functional relation between the two events is not clear. In any case, the reverse correlation does not hold true, i.e. in rapidly proliferating, transformed plasma cells, like myelomas or hybridomas, class switching occurs only at frequencies of less than $10^{-5}$/cell per generation. It has been questioned whether this switching occurs by the physiological switch mechanism at all, rather than being a rare genetic variation[137]. Ig-secreting plasmablasts may even have an inhibitor of switch recombination, as is suggested by fusion of PC140 hybridoma cells, switching at low frequency ($10^{-4}$) from IgM to IgG1[125], with LPS-activated B cells switching at high frequency. Analysis of the hybrid hybridomas shows that switch recombination of the LPS blasts had stopped upon fusion, and switch recombination of the IgH loci of the PC140 myeloma cells is not induced[158]. An inhibitor of switch recombination in plasma cells would make sense in an immune response, to prevent continued switching in Ig-secreting plasma cells, which have left the site of activation by antigen and accessory cells, and are thus no longer under appropriate switch control.

Whether switch recombination occurs during early stages of B-cell development is controversial. Pre-B cells from bone marrow, which lack Ig light chain expression, express cytoplasmic $\mu$ heavy chains[159], but no cytoplasmic $\gamma$ or $\alpha$ heavy chains[160]. Thus, the frequency of Ig class switching seems to be below the level of detection, up to the stage of naive B cells, despite their strong proliferation. On the other hand, the Abelson murine lymphoma cell line 18.81, representing murine pre-B cells and expressing only $\mu$ Ig heavy chains but no light chains, performs switch recombination to IgG2b at frequencies of 0.5–10 per cent[127,128]. Switching to other classes has not been reported for 18.81 cells so far. It remains to be shown whether, with regard to class switching, 18.81 cells really represent pre-B cells. So far, convincing evidence for high-frequency class switching in normal pro- or pre-B cells is not available. Class switching in pre-B cells, if it occurs at all, would be of little physiological relevance anyway, according to current concepts of how immune responses develop by affinity maturation, with preference for decavalent IgM in the initial phase of the response, which is later replaced by affinity-matured, bivalent IgG, IgA or IgE.

## TARGETING RECOMBINATION TO DISTINCT SWITCH REGIONS

In the past few years, it has been shown that class switch recombination does not involve switch regions at random, but is specifically targeted to distinct switch regions by external signals to B cells. Several lines of evidence support this view, which makes switch recombination one of the most spectacular eukaryotic recombination systems, in terms of frequency, specificity and control. First, it was shown for B cells activated *in vitro* under limiting dilution conditions that certain T-cell-derived cytokines can change the frequency of cells switching to distinct classes[15]. At the time, the mechanism of this control remained obscure. This became clearer when switch recombination was identified as the molecular mechanism of class switching in B cells activated *in vitro* by mitogen. Switch recombination in such cells had occurred on both the expressed and the excluded IgH alleles[36]. The IgH allele excluded from expression provided an excellent endogenous substrate to test specific targeting of recombination. In addition, since the cells could not have been selected for expression of this allele, as they could have been for the expressed one, the analysis distinguishes clearly between instruction and selection of cells. For murine B cells activated by a mitogen and the T-cell cytokine, it was shown by restriction analysis of cells switched to IgG1 and sorted for expression of one allele, that both alleles had switched to IgG1[41,134]. Analysis of hybridomas derived from such cultures confirmed this result on a clonal level[61].

For human B cells, targeting of switch recombination has been doubted for a long time, since switch recombination could not be analyzed *in vitro* and analysis of a number of transformed B cells had shown no correlation between switch recombination of the expressed and excluded IgH alleles[161,162]. These cells had been induced to switch *in vivo*, before transformation, and could well have been subjected to coincident induction by several different stimuli, resulting in switch recombination to different Ig classes on both IgH alleles. Recently, clear evidence for targeting of switch recombination in human B cells has been obtained from analysis of a panel of nine clonally unrelated, Epstein–Barr virus (EBV)-transformed B cells from one donor, seven of which have switched to IgG1 on both of their IgH alleles, with the remaining two having only recombined their expressed IgH allele[163]. Even more compelling evidence was obtained for human B cells from peripheral blood, sorted for expression of IgA1 on their cell surface. Restriction analysis of these cells shows that the vast majority of them had performed switch recombination to IgA1 on both IgH alleles[98]. Apart from showing that switch recombination is targeted in human as well as in murine B cells, this result also shows that cells expressing switched Ig on their surface and circulating in the periphery of the immune system have already performed switch recombination, establishing recombination as the molecular basis of class switching in these cells, which are most likely B memory cells.

Targeted switch recombination, if led astray, may also be involved in the transformation of B plasmablasts by c-*myc*. In murine and in rat myelomas c-*myc* is frequently found recombined to that switch region of the excluded IgH allele which corresponds to the one involved in switch recombination of the expressed allele[136]. This is consistent with the idea that c-*myc* translocation can occur as an accident of normal, directed switch recombination[41,61,136].

The third line of evidence for switch recombination being targeted to distinct switch regions comes from the observation that in cell lines which switch to particular Ig classes, as well as in activated B cells induced to switch to particular Ig classes *in vitro*, switch recombination is preceded by transcription of the respective switch regions and $C_H$ genes, resulting in $I_H$

switch transcripts[90,110,111,112,164,165]. This transcription, the transcripts generated or the molecular 'opening' of the respective DNA have been key candidates for the molecular mechanism for targeting of switch recombination to distinct switch regions.

## CONTROL OF SWITCH TRANSCRIPTION

Transcription from the switch promoters (switch transcription) is strictly controlled in B cells (Figure 5.1). This is reflected not only by the presence of detectable transcripts but also by methylation of the respective DNA regions, which are methylated to a larger extent in resting B cells than in other somatic cells, as has been shown for the murine Sγ1 region[166]. Also, protection of the respective DNA is reflected by the lack of DNase I hypersensitive sites[167,168]. Upon induction of switch transcription, DNase I hypersensitive sites are generated around the sites of transcriptional initiation and this area becomes demethylated. Within a few hours, $I_H$ switch transcripts become detectable[90,164,169]. In normal B cells, the induction of switch transcripts is transient and will last for a few days[84,170].

This seems to be different for 18.81 lymphoma cells, which are transformed, cloned pre-B cells, and which express Iγ2b and Iγ3 switch transcripts in the absence of signals from other cell types, and also switch to IgG2b, as has been discussed above[82,84,111,169]. A similar situation is found for I.29 lymphoma cells, some of which switch upon LPS treatment to IgA, IgE and IgG2a *in vitro*[110,112]. These I.29 cells apparently express Iα, Iγ2a and Iε, but no Iγ1 and Iγ2b transcripts[112].

The molecular signals controlling induction of switch transcripts are discussed in detail elsewhere in this book. So far, the signals detected have been cytokines which are secreted mainly by activated $T_H$ lymphocytes, but also by other cell types. The situation is somewhat complex in that the same cytokine can target switch recombination to several Ig classes, e.g. IL-4 to murine IgG1, human IgG4 and both human and murine IgE[90,110,164,170–172], but also inhibit targeting to other Ig classes, like IFN-γ, which acts as an antagonist of IL-4. At present it is not clear how one cytokine can target switching to different classes with different frequencies. The frequencies of B cells expressing Iγ1 switch transcripts upon IL-4 induction is similar to the frequency of IgG1-expressing plasma cells detectable later in culture by *in situ* hybridization[173] or polymerase chain reaction (PCR) analysis[174].

Apart from IL-4, other switch cytokines, like TGF-β and IFN-γ, have been identified. TGF-β induces Iα and Iγ2b transcripts[175] and class switching to IgA and IgG2b. IFN-γ induces Iγ2a and Iγ3 switch transcripts[176] and suppresses the expression of Iγ1[90,165] and Iε switch transcripts in murine B cells stimulated with LPS and IL-4[165,177], but not in IL-4-stimulated human B cells[86].

## ARE SWITCH TRANSCRIPTS INVOLVED IN RECOMBINATION?

In several prokaryotic and eukaryotic recombination systems, transcription as such may play an essential role in the process of recombination. Transcription is a prerequisite for RNA polymerase-mediated recombination of phage lambda in *E. coli*[178] and it enhances mating-type switch recombination in yeast[179]. Homologous recombination between two adjacent genes in yeast is increased when they are being actively transcribed[179,180,181]. It is not yet known how transcription might stimulate recombination. It has been proposed that RNA polymerase-associated topoisomerase might be involved in recombination, or that recombination might be promoted by supercoiling of transcriptionally active DNA[182].

For Ig class switching, transcription of switch regions (Figures 5.1 and 5.2) as such seems to be insufficient to target particular switch regions for recombination[1,183]. Important evidence has been provided recently by targeted genetic modification of the murine germline. Bottaro *et al.* have replaced the IL-4-inducible I$\epsilon$ promoter and the entire I$\epsilon$ exon of the I$\epsilon$ switch transcripts by sequences of the IgH intron enhancer and the $V_H$ promoter. Although from this promoter substantial transcription through the S$\epsilon$ switch region could be induced by LPS, only marginal class switching to IgE was obtained, at frequencies 100-fold less than in wild-type cells, stimulated with LPS and IL-4[183]. Even more drastically, replacement of the I$\gamma$1$^-$ region by the completely heterologous human metallothionein promoter completely abolishes class switching in the presence of switch transcription[1]. In a parallel experiment, however, Lorenz *et al.* have replaced the I$\gamma$1 promoter and the 5′ part of the I$\gamma$1 exon by the metallothionein promoter, now leaving the splice donor site for processing of the I$\gamma$1 transcripts intact. In contrast to the complete replacement, which does not allow processing of switch transcripts or switch recombination, the partial replacement leading to processed artificial switch transcripts allows switch recombination at high frequencies. Thus, processing of switch transcripts or the processed transcripts (Figure 5.1), but not switch transcription as such, seems to be responsible for targeting of switch recombination to distinct switch regions. Switch transcripts could emerge as the first identified component of the switch recombinase, targeting it to specific DNA regions.

## REFERENCES

1. Lorenz M, Jung S, Radbruch A. Switch transcripts in immunoglobulin class switching. Science 1995; 267:1825–1828.
2. Illges H, Mueller W, Radbruch A. Induction of directed switch recombination by cytokines. In: Sorg C (ed.) Molecular Biology of B Cell Developments, vol. 3. Basel: S. Karger 1990, pp. 109–125.
3. Esser C, Radbruch A. Immunoglobulin class switching: molecular and cellular analysis. Annu Rev Immunol 1990; 8:717–735.

4. Vercelli D, Geha RS. Regulation of isotype switching. Curr Opin Immunol 1992; 4:794–797.
5. Harriman W, Volk H, Defranoux N, Wabl M. Immunoglobulin class switch recombination. Annu Rev Immunol 1993; 11:361–384.
6. Coffman RL, Lebman DA, Rothman P. Mechanism and regulation of immunoglobulin isotype switching. Adv Immunol 1993; 54:229–270.
7. Burton DR. Immunoglobulin, functions. In: Roitt IM, Delves PJ (eds) Encyclopedia of Immunology, vol. 2. San Diego: Academic Press 1992, pp. 828–830.
8. Cebra JJ, Komisar JL, Schweitzer PA. CH isotype 'switching' during normal B-lymphocyte development. Annu Rev Immunol 1984; 2:493–548.
9. Slack JH. Genetic control of immunoglobulin isotype restriction. Curr Top Microbiol Immunol 1985; 122:205–209.
10. Long EO, Jacobson S. Pathways of viral antigen processing and presentation to CTL: defined by the mode of virus entry? Immunol Today 1989; 10:45–48.
11. Rosenberg YJ. Isotype-specific T cell regulation of immunoglobulin expression. Immunol Rev 1982; 67:33–58.
12. Severinson E, Bergstedt-Lindqvist S, van-der-Loo W, Fernandez C. Characterization of the IgG response induced by polyclonal B cell activators. Immunol Rev 1982; 67:73–85.
13. Tesch H, Smith FI, Muller-Hermes WJ, Rajewsky K. Heterogeneous and monoclonal helper T cells induce similar anti-(4-hydroxy-3-nitrophenyl)acetyl (NP) antibody populations in the primary adoptive response. I. Isotype distribution. Eur J Immunol 1984; 14:188–194.
14. Perlmutter RM, Hansburg D, Briles DE *et al.* Subclass restriction of murine anti-carbohydrate antibodies. J Immunol 1978; 121:566–572.
15. Layton JE, Vitetta ES, Uhr JW, Krammer PH. Clonal analysis of B cells induced to secrete IgG by T cell-derived lymphokine(s). J Exp Med 1984; 160:1850–1863.
16. Coutelier JP, van-der-Logt JT, Heessen FW *et al.* IgG2a restriction of murine antibodies elicited by viral infections. J Exp Med 1987; 165:64–69.
17. Snapper CM, Paul WE. Interferon-gamma and B cell stimulatory factor-1 reciprocally regulate Ig isotype production. Science 1987; 236:944–947.
18. Finkelman FD, Katona IM, Urban J Jr *et al.* Suppression of in vivo polyclonal IgE responses by monoclonal antibody to the lymphokine B-cell stimulatory factor 1. Proc Natl Acad Sci USA 1986; 83:9675–9678.
19. Savelkoul HF, Lebman DA, Benner R, Coffman RL. Increase of precursor frequency and clonal size of murine IgE-secreting cells by IL-4. J Immunol 1988; 141:749–755.
20. Snapper CM, Finkelman FD, Stefany D *et al.* IL-4 induces co-expression of intrinsic membrane IgG1 and IgE by murine B cells stimulated with lipopolysaccharide. J Immunol 1988; 141:489–898.
21. Bergstedt-Lindqvist S, Moon HB, Persson U *et al.* Interleukin 4 instructs uncommitted B lymphocytes to switch to IgG1 and IgE. Eur J Immunol 1988; 18:1073–1077.
22. Kühn R, Rajewsky K, Muller W. Generation and analysis of interleukin-4-deficient mice. Science 1991; 254:707–710.
23. Coutinho A, Forni L. Intraclonal diversification in immunoglobulin isotype secretion: an analysis of switch probabilities. EMBO J 1982; 1:1251–1257.
24. Finkelman FD, Vitetta ES. Role of surface immunoglobulin in B lymphocyte activation. Fed Proc 1984; 43:2624–2632.
25. Webb CF, Gathings WE, Cooper MD. Effect of anti-gamma 3 antibodies on immunoglobulin isotype expression in lipopolysaccharide-stimulated cultures of mouse spleen cells. Eur J Immunol 1983; 13:556–559.

26. Iwasato T, Arakawa H, Shimizu A *et al.* Biased distribution of recombination sites within S regions upon immunoglobulin class switch recombination induced by transforming growth factor beta and lipopolysaccharide. J Exp Med 1992; 175:1539–1546.
27. Petrini J, Shell B, Hummel M, Dunnick W. The immunoglobulin heavy chain switch: structural features of gamma 1 recombinant switch regions. J Immunol 1987; 138:1940–1946.
28. Katzenberg DR, Birshtein BK. Sites of switch recombination in IgG2b- and IgG2a-producing hybridomas. J Immunol 1988; 140:3219–3127.
29. Yoshida K, Matsuoka M, Usuda S *et al.* Immunoglobulin switch circular DNA in the mouse infected with Nippostrongylus brasiliensis: evidence for successive class switching from mu to epsilon via gamma 1. Proc Natl Acad Sci USA 1990; 87:7829–7833.
30. Siebenkotten G, Esser C, Wabl M, Radbruch A. The murine IgG1/IgE class switch program. Eur J Immunol 1992; 22:1827–1834.
31. Mandler R, Finkelman FD, Levine AD, Snapper CM. IL-4 induction of IgE class switching by lipopolysaccharide-activated murine B cells occurs predominantly through sequential switching. J Immunol 1993; 150:407–418.
32. Jung S, Siebenkotten G, Radbruch A. Frequency of immunoglobulin E class switching is autonomously determined and independent of prior switching to other classes. J Exp Med 1994; 179:2023–2026.
33. Corbel C, Melchers F. Requirement for macrophages or for macrophage- or T cell-derived factors in the mitogenic stimulation of murine B lymphocytes by lipopolysaccharides. Eur J Immunol 1983; 13:528–533.
34. Melchers F, Corbel C, Leptin M, Lemhardt W. Activation and cell cycle control of murine B lymphocytes. J Cell Sci Suppl 1985; 3:77–82.
35. Kearney JF, Lawton AR. B lymphocyte differentiation induced by lipopolysaccharide. I. Generation of cells synthesizing four major immunoglobulin classes. J Immunol 1975; 115:671–676.
36. Radbruch A, Sablitzky F. Deletion of Cmu genes in mouse B lymphocytes upon stimulation with LPS. EMBO J 1983; 2:1929–1935.
37. Seyschab H, Friedl R, Schindler D *et al.* The effects of bacterial lipopolysaccharide, anti-receptor antibodies and recombinant interferon on mouse B cell cycle progression using 5-bromo-2′-deoxyuridine/Hoechst 33258 dye flow cytometry. Eur J Immunol 1989; 19:1605–1612.
38. Andersson J, Coutinho A, Melchers F. Frequencies of mitogen-reactive B cells in the mouse. I. Distribution in different lymphoid organs from different inbred strains of mice at different ages. J Exp Med 1977; 145:1511–1519.
39. Tsubata T, Murakami M, Honjo T. Antigen-receptor cross-linking induces peritoneal B-cell apoptosis in normal but not autoimmunity-prone mice. Curr Biol 1994; 4:8–17.
40. Kearney JF, Cooper MD, Lawton AR. B cell differentiation induced by lipopolysaccharide. IV. Development of immunoglobulin class restriction in precursors of IgG-synthesizing cells. J Immunol 1976; 117:1567–1572.
41. Radbruch A, Muller W, Rajewsky K. Class switch recombination is IgG1 specific on active and inactive IgH loci of IgG1-secreting B-cell blasts. Proc Natl Acad Sci USA 1986; 83:3954–3957.
42. Shimizu A, Takahashi N, Yaoita Y, Honjo T. Organization of the constant-region gene family of the mouse immunoglobulin heavy chain. Cell 1982; 28:499–506.
43. Honjo T, Kataoka T. Organization of immunoglobulin heavy chain genes and allelic deletion model. Proc Natl Acad Sci USA 1978; 75:2140–2144.
44. Hofker MH, Walter MA, Cox DW. Complete physical map of the human

immunoglobulin heavy chain constant region gene complex. Proc Natl Acad Sci USA 1989; 86:5567–5571.

45. Tucker PW, Liu CP, Mushinski JF, Blattner FR. Mouse immunoglobulin D: messenger RNA and genomic DNA sequences. Science 1980; 209:1353–1360.
46. Sakano H, Maki R, Kurosawa Y *et al.* Two types of somatic recombination are necessary for the generation of complete immunoglobulin heavy chain genes. Nature 1980; 286:676–683.
47. Kawakami T, Takahashi N, Honjo T. Complete nucleotide sequence of mouse immunoglobulin mu gene and comparison with other immunoglobulin heavy chain genes. Nucleic Acids Res 1980; 8:3933–3945.
48. Ishida N, Ueda S, Hayashida H *et al.* The nucleotide sequence of the mouse immunoglobulin epsilon gene: comparison with the human epsilon gene sequence. Embo J 1982; 1:1117–1123.
49. Liu FT, Albrandt K, Sutcliffe JG, Katz DH. Cloning and nucleotide sequence of mouse immunoglobulin epsilon chain cDNA. Proc Natl Acad Sci USA 1982; 79:7852–7856.
50. Tucker P. Transcriptional regulation of IgM and IgD. Immunol Today 1985; 6:181–182.
51. Nikaido T, Yamawaki-Kataoka Y, Honjo T. Nucleotide sequences of switch regions of immunoglobulin C epsilon and C gamma genes and their comparison. J Biol Chem 1982; 257:7322–7329.
52. Stanton LW, Marcu KB. Nucleotide sequence and properties of the murine gamma 3 immunoglobulin heavy chain gene switch region: implications for successive C gamma gene switching. Nucleic Acids Res 1982; 10:5993–6006.
53. Gritzmacher CA. Molecular aspects of heavy-chain class switching. Crit Rev Immunol 1989; 9:173–200.
54. Kataoka T, Takeda S, Honjo T. Escherichia coli extract-catalyzed recombination in switch regions of mouse immunoglobulin genes. Proc Natl Acad Sci USA 1983; 80:2666–2670.
55. Katz A, Kahana C. Rearrangement between ornithine decarboxylase and the switch region of the gamma 1 immunoglobulin gene in alpha-difluoromethylornithine resistant mouse myeloma cells. EMBO J 1989; 8:1163–1167.
56. Kohwi-Shigematsu T, Kohwi Y. Poly(dG)-poly(dC) sequences, under torsional stress, induce an altered DNA conformation upon neighboring DNA sequences. Cell 1985; 43:199–206.
57. Usdin K, Furano AV. Rat L (long interspersed repeated DNA) elements contain guanine-rich homopurine sequences that induce unpairing of contiguous duplex DNA. Proc Natl Acad Sci USA 1988; 85:4416–4420.
58. Kohwi Y, Kohwi-Shigematsu T. Magnesium ion-dependent triple-helix structure formed by homopurine-homopyrimidine sequences in supercoiled plasmid DNA. Proc Natl Acad Sci USA 1988; 85:3781–3785.
59. Sen D, Gilbert W. Formation of parallel four-stranded complexes by guanine-rich motifs in DNA and its implications for meiosis. Nature 1988; 334:364–366.
60. Gu H, Zou YR, Rajewsky K. Independent control of immunoglobulin switch recombination at individual switch regions evidenced through Cre-IoxP-mediated gene targeting. Cell 1993; 73:1155–1164.
61. Winter E, Krawinkel U, Radbruch A. Directed Ig class switch recombination in activated murine B cells. EMBO J 1987; 6:1663–1671.
62. von-Schwedler U, Jack HM, Wabl M. Circular DNA is a product of the immunoglobulin class switch rearrangement. Nature 1990; 345:452–456.
63. Iwasato T, Shimizu A, Honjo T, Yamagishi H. Circular DNA is excised by immunoglobulin class switch recombination. Cell 1990; 62:143–149.
64. Matsuoka M, Yoshida K, Maeda T *et al.* Switch circular DNA formed in

cytokine-treated mouse splenocytes: evidence for intramolecular DNA deletion in immunoglobulin class switching. Cell 1990; 62:135–142.

65. Szurek P, Petrini J, Dunnick W. Complete nucleotide sequence of the murine gamma 3 switch region and analysis of switch recombination sites in two gamma 3-expressing hybridomas. J Immunol 1985; 135:620–626.
66. Dunnick W, Hertz GZ, Scappino L, Gritzmacher C. DNA sequences at immunoglobulin switch region recombination sites. Nucleic Acids Res 1993; 21:365–372.
67. Roth DB, Wilson JH. Nonhomologous recombination in mammalian cells: role for short sequence homologies in the joining reaction. Mol Cell Biol 1986; 6:4295–4304.
68. Roth DB, Chang XB, Wilson JH. Comparison of filler DNA at immune, nonimmune, and oncogenic rearrangements suggests multiple mechanisms of formation. Mol Cell Biol 1989; 9:3049–3057.
69. Sen R, Baltimore D. Factors regulating gene transcription. In: Honjo T, Alt FW, Rabbits TH (eds) Immunoglobulin Genes. Boston: Academic Press 1989, pp. 327–342.
70. Pettersson S, Cook GP, Bruggemann M *et al.* A second B cell-specific enhancer 3′ of the immunoglobulin heavy-chain locus. Nature 1990; 344:165–168.
71. Lieberson R, Giannini SL, Birshtein BK, Eckhardt LA. An enhancer at the 3′ end of the mouse immunoglobulin heavy chain locus. Nucleic Acids Res 1991; 19:933–937.
72. Dariavach P, Williams GT, Campbell K *et al.* The mouse IgH 3′-enhancer. Eur J Immunol 1991; 21:1499–1504.
73. Serwe M, Sablitzky F. V(D)J recombination in B cells is impaired but not blocked by targeted deletion of the immunoglobulin heavy chain intron enhancer. EMBO J 1993; 12:2321–2327.
74. Chen J, Trounstine M, Alt FW *et al.* Immunoglobulin gene rearrangement in B cell deficient mice generated by targeted deletion of the JH locus. Int Immunol 1993; 5:647–656.
75. Wabl MR, Burrows PD. Expression of immunoglobulin heavy chain at a high level in the absence of a proposed immunoglobulin enhancer element in cis. Proc Natl Acad Sci USA 1984; 81:2452–2455.
76. Klein S, Sablitzky F, Radbruch A. Deletion of the IgH enhancer does not reduce immunoglobulin heavy chain production of a hybridoma IgD class switch variant. EMBO J 1984; 3:2473–2476.
77. Klein S, Gerster T, Picard D *et al.* Evidence for transient requirement of the IgH enhancer. Nucleic Acids Res 1985; 13:8901–8912.
78. Cogne M, Lansford R, Bottaro A *et al.* A class switch control region at the 3′ end of the immunoglobulin heavy chain locus. Cell 1994; 77:737–747.
79. Jung S, Rajewsky K, Radbruch A. Shutdown of class switch recombination by deletion of a switch region control element. Science 1993; 259:984–987.
80. Zhang J, Bottaro A, Li S *et al.* A selective defect in IgG2b switching as a result of targeted mutation of the I gamma 2b promoter and exon. EMBO J 1993; 12:3529–3537.
81. Lennon GG, Perry RP. C mu-containing transcripts initiate heterogeneously within the IgH enhancer region and contain a novel 5′-nontranslatable exon. Nature 1985; 318:475–478.
82. Lutzker S, Alt FW. Structure and expression of germ line immunoglobulin gamma 2b transcripts. Mol Cell Biol 1988; 8:1849–1852.
83. Xu M, Stavnezer J. Structure of germline immunoglobulin heavy-chain gamma 1 transcripts in interleukin 4 treated mouse spleen cells. Dev Immunol 1990; 1:11–17.

84. Rothman P, Chen YY, Lutzker S *et al.* Structure and expression of germ line immunoglobulin heavy-chain epsilon transcripts: interleukin-4 plus lipopolysaccharide-directed switching to C epsilon. Mol Cell Biol 1990; 10:1672–1679.
85. Gaff C, Gerondakis S. RNA splicing generates alternate forms of germline immunoglobulin alpha heavy chain transcripts. Int Immunol 1990; 2:1143–1148.
86. Gauchat JF, Lebman DA, Coffman RL *et al.* Structure and expression of germline epsilon transcripts in human B cells induced by interleukin 4 to switch to IgE production. J Exp Med 1990; 172:463–473.
87. Neale GA, Kitchingman GR. mRNA transcripts initiating within the human immunoglobulin mu heavy chain enhancer region contain a non-translatable exon and are extremely heterogeneous at the 5′ end. Nucleic Acids Res 1991; 19:2427–2433.
88. Nilsson L, Islam KB, Olafsson O *et al.* Structure of TGF-beta 1-induced human immunoglobulin C alpha 1 and C alpha 2 germ-line transcripts. Int Immunol 1991; 3:1107–1115.
89. Sideras P, Nilsson L, Islam KB *et al.* Transcription of unrearranged Ig H chain genes in human B cell malignancies. Biased expression of genes encoded within the first duplication unit of the Ig H chain locus. J Immunol 1992; 149:244–252.
90. Berton MT, Uhr JW, Vitetta ES. Synthesis of germ-line gamma 1 immunoglobulin heavy-chain transcripts in resting B cells: induction by interleukin 4 and inhibition by interferon gamma. Proc Natl Acad Sci USA 1989; 86:2829–2833.
91. Sideras P, Mizuta TR, Kanamori H *et al.* Production of sterile transcripts of C gamma genes in an IgM-producing human neoplastic B cell line that switches to IgG-producing cells. Int Immunol 1989; 1:631–642.
92. Li SC, Rothman PB, Zhang J *et al.* Expression of I mu-C gamma hybrid germline transcripts subsequent to immunoglobulin heavy chain class switching. Int Immunol 1994; 6:491–497.
93. Alt FW, Rosenberg N, Enea V *et al.* Multiple immunoglobulin heavy-chain gene transcripts in Abelson murine leukemia virus-transformed lymphoid cell lines. Mol Cell Biol 1982; 2:386–400.
94. Miyawaki T, Butler JL, Radbruch A *et al.* Isotype commitment of human B cells that are transformed by Epstein-Barr virus. Eur J Immunol 1991; 21:215–220.
95. Yaoita Y, Kumagai Y, Okumura K, Honjo T. Expression of lymphocyte surface IgE does not require switch recombination. Nature 1982; 297:697–699.
96. Chen YW, Word C, Dev V *et al.* Double isotype production by a neoplastic B cell line. II. Allelically excluded production of mu and gamma 1 heavy chains without CH gene rearrangement. J Exp Med 1986; 164:562–579.
97. Katona IM, Urban J Jr, Finkelman FD. B cells that simultaneously express surface IgM and IgE in Nippostrongylus brasiliensis-infected SJA/9 mice do not provide evidence for isotype switching without gene deletion. Proc Natl Acad Sci USA 1985; 82:511–515.
98. Irsch J, Irlenbusch S, Radl J *et al.* Switch recombination in normal IgA1 + B lymphocytes. Proc Natl Acad Sci USA 1994; 91:1323–1327.
99. Radbruch A, Irlenbusch S. Directed Ig class switch recombination. Monogr Allergy 1988; 24:191–196.
100. Shimizu A, Honjo T. Synthesis and regulation of trans-mRNA encoding the immunoglobulin epsilon heavy chain. Faseb J 1993; 7:149–154.
101. Han H, Okamoto M, Honjo T, Shimizu A. Regulated expression of immunoglobulin trans-mRNA consisting of the variable region of a transgenic mu chain and constant regions of endogenous isotypes. Int Immunol 1991; 3:1197–1206.

102. Moore KW, Rogers J, Hunkapiller T *et al.* Expression of IgD may use both DNA rearrangement and RNA splicing mechanisms. Proc Natl Acad Sci USA 1981; 78:1800–1804.
103. Maki R, Roeder W, Traunecker A *et al.* The role of DNA rearrangement and alternative RNA processing in the expression of immunoglobulin delta genes. Cell 1981; 24:353–365.
104. Knapp MR, Liu CP, Newell N *et al.* Simultaneous expression of immunoglobulin mu and delta heavy chains by a cloned B-cell lymphoma: a single copy of the VH gene is shared by two adjacent CH genes. Proc Natl Acad Sci USA 1982; 79:2996–3000.
105. Kemp DJ, Morahan G, Cowman AF, Harris AW. Production of RNA for secreted immunoglobulin mu chains does not require transcriptional termination 5′ to the microM exons. Nature 1983; 301:84–86.
106. Morse H, Pumphrey JG, Potter M, Asofsky R. Murine plasma cells secreting more than one class of immunoglobulin heavy chain. I. Frequency of two or more M-components in ascitic fluids from 788 primary plasmacytomas. J Immunol 1976; 117:541–547.
107. Mackenzie T, Dosch HM. Clonal and molecular characteristics of the human IgE-committed B cell subset. J Exp Med 1989; 169:407–430.
108. Nolan-Willard M, Berton MT, Tucker P. Coexpression of mu and gamma 1 heavy chains can occur by a discontinuous transcription mechanism from the same unrearranged chromosome. Proc Natl Acad Sci USA 1992; 89:1234–1238.
109. Perlmutter AP, Gilbert W. Antibodies of the secondary response can be expressed without switch recombination in normal mouse B cells. Proc Natl Acad Sci USA 1984; 81:7189–7193.
110. Stavnezer J, Radcliffe G, Lin YC *et al.* Immunoglobulin heavy-chain switching may be directed by prior induction of transcripts from constant-region genes. Proc Natl Acad Sci USA 1988; 85:7704–7708.
111. Yancopoulos GD, DePinho RA, Zimmerman KA *et al.* Secondary genomic rearrangement events in pre-B cells: VHDJH replacement by a LINE-1 sequence and directed class switching. EMBO J 1986; 5:3259–3266.
112. Stavnezer-Nordgren J, Sirlin S. Specificity of immunoglobulin heavy chain switch correlates with activity of germline heavy chain genes prior to switching. EMBO J 1986; 5:95–102.
113. Alt FW, Blackwell TK, DePinho RA *et al.* Regulation of genome rearrangement events during lymphocyte differentiation. Immunol Rev 1986; 89:5–30.
114. Shimizu A, Nussenzweig MC, Han H *et al.* Trans-splicing as a possible molecular mechanism for the multiple isotype expression of the immunoglobulin gene. J Exp Med 1991; 173:1385–1393.
115. Agabian N. Trans splicing of nuclear pre-mRNAs. Cell 1990; 61:1157–1160.
116. Bruzik JP, Maniatis T. Spliced leader RNAs from lower eukaryotes are trans-spliced in mammalian cells. Nature 1992; 360:692–695.
117. Shimizu A, Nussenzweig MC, Mizuta TR *et al.* Immunoglobulin double-isotype expression by trans-mRNA in a human immunoglobulin transgenic mouse. Proc Natl Acad Sci USA 1989; 86:8020–8023.
118. Davis MM, Kim SK, Hood LE. DNA sequences mediating class switching in alpha-immunoglobulins. Science 1980; 209:1360–1365.
119. Kataoka T, Kawakami T, Takahashi N, Honjo T. Rearrangement of immunoglobulin gamma 1-chain gene and mechanism for heavy-chain class switch. Proc Natl Acad Sci USA 1980; 77:919–923.
120. Rabbitts TH, Forster A, Dunnick W, Bentley DL. The role of gene deletion in the immunoglobulin heavy chain switch. Nature 1980; 283:351–356.
121. Hurwitz JL, Coleclough C, Cebra JJ. CH gene rearrangements in IgM-bearing B

cells and in the normal splenic DNA component of hybridomas making different isotypes of antibody. Cell 1980; 22:349–359.

122. Eckhardt LA, Tilley SA, Lang RB *et al.* DNA rearrangements in MPC-11 immunoglobulin heavy chain class-switch variants. Proc Natl Acad Sci USA 1982; 79:3006–3010.
123. Stavnezer J, Marcu KB, Sirlin S *et al.* Rearrangements and deletions of immunoglobulin heavy chain genes in the double-producing B cell lymphoma. I.29. Mol Cell Biol 1982; 2:1002–1013.
124. Cory S. Activation of cellular oncogenes in hemopoietic cells by chromosome translocation. Adv Cancer Res 1986; 47:189–234.
125. Preud'homme J-L, Birshtein BK, Scharff MD. Variants of a mouse myeloma cell line that synthesize immunoglobulin heavy chains having an altered serotype. Proc Natl Acad Sci USA 1975; 72:1427–1430.
126. Radbruch A, Liesegang B, Rajewsky K. Isolation of variants of mouse myeloma X63 that express changed immunoglobulin class. Proc Natl Acad Sci USA 1980; 77:2909–2913.
127. Burrows PD, Beck GB, Wabl MR. Expression of mu and gamma immunoglobulin heavy chains in different cells of a cloned mouse lymphoid line. Proc Natl Acad Sci USA 1981; 78:564–568.
128. Burrows PD, Beck-Engeser GB, Wabl MR. Immunoglobulin heavy-chain class switching in a pre-B cell line is accomplished by DNA rearrangment. Nature 1983; 306:243–246.
129. Vogler LB, Preud'homme JL, Seligmann M *et al.* Diversity of immunoglobulin expression in leukaemic cells resembling B-lymphocyte precursors. Nature 1981; 290:339–341.
130. Foroni L, Catovsky D, Rabbitts TH, Luzzatto L. DNA rearrangements of immunoglobulin genes correlate with phenotypic markers in B-cell malignancies. Mol Biol Med 1984; 2:63–79.
131. Brown NA, Liu C, Berenson JR *et al.* Immunoglobulin JH, C mu, and C gamma gene rearrangements in human B lymphocytes clonally transformed by Epstein-Barr virus. Proc Natl Acad Sci USA 1985; 82:556–560.
132. Borzillo GV, Cooper MD, Bertoli LF *et al.* Lineage and stage specificity of isotype switching in humans. J Immunol 1988; 141:3625–3633.
133. Hurwitz JL, Cebra JJ. Rearrangements between the immunoglobulin heavy chain gene JH and C mu regions accompany normal B lymphocyte differentiation in vitro. Nature 1982; 299:742–744.
134. Kepron MR, Chen YW, Uhr JW, Vitetta ES. IL-4 induces the specific rearrangement of gamma 1 genes on the expressed and unexpressed chromosomes of lipopolysaccharide-activated normal murine B cells. J Immunol 1989; 143:334–339.
135. Jack HM, McDowell M, Steinberg CM, Wabl M. Looping out and deletion mechanism for the immunoglobulin heavy-chain class switch. Proc Natl Acad Sci USA 1988; 85:1581–1585.
136. Tian SS, Faust C. Rearrangement of rat immunoglobulin E heavy-chain and c-myc genes in the B-cell immunocytoma IR162. Mol Cell Biol 1987; 7:2614–2619.
137. Sablitzky F, Radbruch A, Rajewsky K. Spontaneous immunoglobulin class switching in myeloma and hybridoma cell lines differs from physiological class switching. Immunol Rev 1982; 67:59–72.
138. Kipps TJ, Herzenberg LA. Homologous chromosomes recombination generating immunoglobulin allotype and isotype switch variants. EMBO J 1986; 5:263–268.
139. Beck-Engeser G, Jack HM, Wabl M. Allelic inclusion in a pre-B-cell line that generates immunoglobulin heavy chain genes in vitro. Proc Natl Acad Sci USA 1987; 84:1060–1064.

140. Gerstein RM, Frankel WN, Hsieh CL *et al.* Isotype switching of an immunoglobulin heavy chain transgene occurs by DNA recombination between different chromosomes. Cell 1990; 63:537–548.
141. Severinson Gronowics E, Doss C, Scröder J. Activation to IgG secretion by lipopolysaccharide requires several proliferation cycles. J Immunol 1979; 123:2057–2062.
142. Dunnick W, Wilson M, Stavnezer J. Mutations, duplication, and deletion of recombined switch regions suggest a role for DNA replication in the immunoglobulin heavy-chain switch. Mol Cell Biol 1989; 9:1850–1856.
143. Dunnick W, Stavnezer J. Copy choice mechanism of immunoglobulin heavy-chain switch recombination. Mol Cell Biol 1990; 10:397–400.
144. Williams M, Maizels N. LR1, a lipopolysaccharide-responsive factor with binding sites in the immunoglobulin switch regions and heavy-chain enhancer. Genes Dev 1991; 5:2353–2361.
145. Brys A, Maizels N. LR1 regulates c-myc transcription in B-cell lymphomas. Proc Natl Acad Sci USA 1994; 91:4915–4919.
146. Williams M, Hanakahi LA, Maizels N. Purification and properties of LR1, an inducible DNA binding protein from mammalian B lymphocytes. J Biol Chem 1993; 268:13731–13737.
147. Barberis A, Widenhom K, Vitelli L, Busslinger M. A novel B-cell lineage-specific transcription factor present at early but not late stages of differentiation. Genes Dev 1990; 4:849–859.
148. Waters SH, Saikh KU, Stavnezer J. A B-cell-specific nuclear protein that binds to DNA sites 5′ to immunoglobulin S alpha tandem repeats is regulated during differentiation. Mol Cell Biol 1989; 9:5594–5601.
149. Xu L, Kim MG, Marcu KB. Properties of B cell stage specific and ubiquitous nuclear factors binding to immunoglobulin heavy chain gene switch regions. Int Immunol 1992; 4:875–887.
150. Wuerffel RA, Nathan AT, Kenter AL. Defection of an immunoglobulin switch region-specific DNA-binding protein in mitogen-stimulated mouse splenic B cells. Mol Cell Biol 1990; 10:1714–1718.
151. Kenter AL, Wuerffel R, Sen R *et al.* Switch recombination breakpoints occur at nonrandom positions in the S gamma tandem repeat. J Immunol 1993; 151:4718–4731.
152. Wuerffel R, Jamieson CE, Morgan L *et al.* Switch recombination breakpoints are strictly correlated with DNA recognition motifs for immunoglobulin S gamma 3 DNA-binding proteins. J Exp Med 1992; 176:339–349.
153. Mizuta TR, Fukita Y, Miyoshi T *et al.* Isolation of cDNA encoding a binding protein specific to 5′-phosphorylated single-stranded DNA with G-rich sequences. Nucleic Acids Res 1993; 21:1761–1766.
154. Fukita Y, Mizuta TR, Shirozu M *et al.* The human S my bp-2, a DNA-binding protein specific to the single-stranded guanine-rich sequence related to the immunoglobulin mu chain switch region. J Biol Chem 1993; 268:17463–17470.
155. Nossal GJV, Szenberg A, Ada GL, Austin CM. Single cell studies on 19S antibody production. J Exp Med 1964; 119:485–502.
156. Siekevitz M, Kocks C, Rajewsky K, Dildrop R. Analysis of somatic mutation and class switching in naive and memory B cells generating adoptive primary and secondary responses. Cell 1987; 48:757–770.
157. Banchereau J, Bazan F, Blanchard D *et al.* The CD40 antigen and its ligand. Annu Rev Immunol 1994; 12:881–922.
158. Klein S, Radbruch A. Inhibition of class switch recombination in plasma cells. Cell Immunol 1994; 157:106–117.

159. Burrows P, Lejeune M, Kearney JF. Evidence that murine pre-B cells synthesise mu heavy chains but no light chains. Nature 1979; 280:838–840.
160. Kubagawa H, Gathings WE, Levitt D *et al.* Immunoglobulin isotype expression of normal pre-B cells as determined by immunofluorescence. J Clin Immunol 1982; 2:264–269.
161. Borzillo GV, Cooper MD, Kubagawa H *et al.* Isotype switching in human B lymphocyte malignancies occurs by DNA deletion: evidence for nonspecific switch recombination. J Immunol 1987; 139:1326–1335.
162. Webb CF, Cooper MD, Burrows PD, Griffin JA. Immunoglobulin gene arrangements and deletions in human Epstein-Barr virus-transformed cell lines producing different IgG and IgA subclasses. Proc Natl Acad Sci USA 1985; 82:5495–5499.
163. Irsch J, Hendriks R, Tesch H *et al.* Evidence for a human IgG1 class switch program. Eur J Immunol 1993; 23:481–486.
164. Esser C, Radbruch A. Rapid induction of transcription of unrearranged S gamma 1 switch regions in activated murine B cells by interleukin 4. EMBO J 1989; 8:483–488.
165. Severinson E, Fernandez C, Stavnezer J. Induction of germ-line immunoglobulin heavy chain transcripts by mitogens and interleukins prior to switch recombination. Eur J Immunol 1990; 20:1079–1084.
166. Burger C, Radbruch A. Protective methylation of immunoglobulin and T cell receptor (TcR) gene loci prior to induction of class switch and TcR recombination. Eur J Immunol 1990; 20:2285–2291.
167. Schmitz J, Radbruch A. An interleukin 4-induced DNase I hypersensitive site indicates opening of the gamma 1 switch region prior to switch recombination. Int Immunol 1989; 1:570–575.
168. Berton MT, Vitetta ES. Interleukin 4 induces changes in the chromatin structure of the gamma 1 switch region in resting B cells before switch recombination. J Exp Med 1990; 172:375–378.
169. Lutzker S, Rothman P, Pollock R *et al.* Mitogen- and IL-4-regulated expression of germ-line Ig gamma 2b transcripts: evidence for directed heavy chain class switching. Cell 1988; 53:177–184.
170. Rothman P, Lutzker S, Cook W *et al.* Mitogen plus interleukin 4 induction of C epsilon transcripts in B lymphoid cells. J Exp Med 1988; 168:2385–2389.
171. Kitani A, Strober W. Regulation of C gamma subclass germ-line transcripts in human peripheral blood B cells. J Immunol 1993; 151:3478–3488.
172. Kunimoto DY, Sneller MC, Claflin L *et al.* Molecular analysis of double isotype expression in IgA switching. J Immunol 1993; 150:1338–1347.
173. Turaga PS, Berton MT, Teale JM. Frequency of B cells expressing germ-line gamma 1 transcripts upon IL-4 induction. J Immunol 1993; 151:1383–1390.
174. Goodman DJ, Gaff C, Gerondakis S. The IL-4 induced increase in the frequency of resting murine splenic B cells expressing germline Ig heavy chain gamma 1 transcripts correlates with subsequent switching to IgG1. Int Immunol 1993; 5:199–208.
175. McIntyre TM, Klinman DR, Rothman P *et al.* Transforming growth factor β1 selectivity stimulates immunoglobulin G2b secretion by lipopolysaccharide-activated murine B cells. J Exp Med 1993; 177:1031–1037.
176. Snapper CM, McIntyre TM, Mandler R *et al.* Induction of IgG3 secretion by interferon γ. A model for T cell-independent class switching in response to T cell-independent type 2 antigens. J Exp Med 1992; 175:1367–1371.
177. Xu L, Rothman P. IFN-gamma represses epsilon germline transcription and subsequently down-regulates switch recombination to epsilon. Int Immunol 1994; 6:515–521.

178. Ikeda H, Matsumoto T. Transcription promotes recA-independent recombination mediated by DNA-dependent RNA polymerase in Escherichia coli. Proc Natl Acad Sci USA 1979; 76:4571–4575.
179. Voelkel-Meiman K, Keil RL, Roeder GS. Recombination-stimulating sequences in yeast ribosomal DNA correspond to sequences regulating transcription by RNA polymerase I. Cell 1987; 48:1071–1079.
180. Keil RL, Roeder GS. Cis-acting, recombination-stimulating activity in a fragment of the ribosomal DNA of S. cerevisiae. Cell 1984; 39:377–386.
181. Thomas BJ, Rothstein R. Elevated recombination rates in transcriptionally active DNA. Cell 1989; 56:619–630.
182. Thomas BJ, Rothstein R. Sex, maps, and imprinting. Cell 1991; 64:1–3.
183. Bottaro A, Lansford R, Xu L *et al.* S region transcription per se promotes basal IgE class switch recombination but additional factors regulate the efficiency of the process. EMBO J 1994; 13:665–674.

# Part II

# CYTOKINES

# 6 Cellular Sources and Regulation of Cytokine Production

**WILLIAM C. GAUSE and PIN LU**
*Uniformed Services University of the Health Sciences, Bethesda, Maryland, USA*

*Victory in war is not repetitious,*
*but adapts itself endlessly.*
Sun Tzu, The Art of War, ≈2000 B.P.

## INTRODUCTION

Many of the basic tenets that have laid the foundation for modern immunology were originally derived from experiments with a variety of easily obtainable haptens and antigens such as TNP (trinitrophenyl), bovine serum albumin, or sheep red blood cells (SRBCs). Although findings obtained with these antigens were of great significance and continue to contribute fundamental insights in immunology, they can also be misleading, since the foreign antigens, namely pathogens, that the host immune system has co-evolved with over millions of years are quite different. Most importantly, they are complex living organisms with rapid generation times that can rapidly adapt to inhospitable environments. Consequently, certain pathogens have developed ways of manipulating the host immune system to avoid destruction and optimize propagation, and the host has responded with countermeasures and also with mechanisms for rapidly recognizing these antigens and directing a distinct response that is effective against them. As a result, responses that are effective against one pathogen may be ineffective or even promote disease against others. This ongoing co-evolutionary process makes it difficult at times to identify which components of the immune response are actually host protective against a particular pathogen and underscores the importance of studying the immune response to a variety of pathogens to gain an understanding of the host response to infectious disease. In this chapter we will emphasize the cell populations and factors involved in the initiation and progression of immune responses to pathogens with a particular emphasis on the differentiation of naive $CD4^+$ T cells into effector T-helper cells that can provide help for B-cell activation and immunoglobulin (Ig) secretion (Table

*Cytokine Regulation of Humoral Immunity: Basic and Clinical Aspects.* Edited by Clifford M. Snapper.

6.1). We will not discuss the chemokines in detail and will only discuss the inflammatory cytokines with respect to their role in influencing T-helper cell differentiation. Also, although superantigens are important in a number of infectious diseases, they have been well covered in several other reviews[1–3] and will not be discussed in detail here.

The immune response to a pathogen is initiated when certain cell populations, such as macrophages or natural killer (NK) cells, are activated through antigen-non-specific mechanisms to become effector cells that can directly target the pathogen or cells infected by the pathogen. Many of these effector cell populations of the nonadaptive or innate immune response can

**Table 6.1** Cytokines secreted by cells associated with the immune response

| Cell type | Cytokines produced |
|---|---|
| CD4$^+$ T cell | GM-CSF[67], IFN-α/β[68,69], IFN-γ[70], TNF-α/β[70,71], TGF-β[72], IL-2[67,73], IL-3[67,70], IL-4[67,70], IL-5[70], IL-6[74], IL-9[75], IL-1[29], IL-13[70,76] |
| CD8$^+$ T cell | GM-CSF[77], TNF-α/β[71,78], IFN-γ[79,80], TGF-β[81], IL-2[82], IL-3[79], IL-4[64,66], IL-5[66], IL-6[83,84], IL-10[29,85] |
| TCR-γ/δ$^+$ T cell | GM-CSF[86], IFN-γ[87], TNF-α[88], IL-2[89], IL-4[88,90], IL-5[91] |
| B cell | GM-CSF[92], IFN-α[68,93], TNF-α[94], IL-1α/β[95,96], IL-2[97], IL-6[98], IL-7[99], IL-8[100], IL-10[29,101] |
| Macrophage | IFN-α/β[68,102], IFN-γ[26], TNF-α[103,104], TGF-β[105], IL-1α/β[106,107], IL-6[30,31], IL-10[29,108], IL-12[109], IL-15[110] |
| Monocyte | IFN-α[102], TGF-β[111], TNF-α[103,104], IL-1β[106,107], IL-6[112], IL-8[113], IL-10[29], IL-15[110] |
| NK cell | GM-CSF[114], TNF-α[115], IFN-γ[115], IL-4[116], IL-8[117] |
| Mast cell | GM-CSF[118], TNF-α[118,119], TGF-β[118], IL-1β[119,120], IL-3[121], IL-4[122], IL-5[123], IL-6[118,119,123], IL-8[119], IL-12[124] |
| Eosinophil | GM-CSF[125], TNF-α[125], TGF-α/β[126], IL-3[127], IL-5[40], IL-8[125,128] |
| Basophil | IL-4[129] |
| Neutrophil | IFN-α[32], TNF-α[32], IL-1β[32,107], IL-3[32], IL-8[113,130], IL-12[32] |
| Langerhans cell | GM-CSF[131], TNF-β[131], IFN-γ[131], IL-1α[131], IL-6[131], IL-8[131], IL-10[131] |
| Thymocyte | IFN-γ[132,133], IL-2[132,134], IL-3[135], IL-4[132–134], IL-6[134], IL-10[132,136] |
| Epithelial cell | GM-CSF[137], IFN-β[68,138], TNF-α[139], TGF-β[140], IL-1α/β[107], IL-3[139], IL-6[39,141], IL-7[139], IL-8[39,141], IL-10[139], IL-11[142] |
| Endothelial cell | GM-CSF[143], IFN-α/β[68], IL-1α/β[107,144], IL-6[145], IL-8[130,146], IL-11[147] |
| Fibroblast | IFN-β[68,148], TNF-α[149], TGF-β[150,151], IL-1α[149], IL-6[152], IL-8[130,153], IL-11[154] |
| Keratinocyte | TGF-β[155], IL-1α/β[107,156,157], IL-3[158], IL-7[159], IL-8[130,160], IL-10[29,161] |
| Bone marrow stromal cell | TGF-β[162], IL-1α[163], IL-6[164], IL-7[165], IL-11[154] |
| Thymic stromal cell | IL-7[166] |
| Astrocyte | TNF-α[167], IL-1β[107,168], IL-5[169], IL-6[168,170] |

GM-CSF, granulocyte/macrophage colony-stimulating factor.

also secrete restricted sets of cytokines and/or express certain cell surface molecules that together can produce a milieu that influences the development of the antigen-specific T and B lymphocytes, which mediate the adaptive response. Following antigen presentation by professional antigen-presenting cells (APCs) in this milieu, naive antigen-specific $CD4^+$ T cells are activated and go on to differentiate to cytokine-producing effector T cells, which can provide help for B cells. In addition, cytokine production by these T-helper effector cells further amplifies the response, supporting the activation and further proliferation of a variety of effector cells, including NK cells and $CD8^+$ T cells in the case of an interferon gamma (IFN-γ)-dominant (type 1) response, and eosinophils and mast cells in the case of an IL-4-dominant (type 2) response. Although the type 1 and the type 2 responses have previously been referred to as Th1 or Th2 responses respectively, this terminology is misleading, since many of the Th1/Th2 cytokines, including IFN-γ and interleukin-4 (IL-4), originally identified as being produced by Th cells are also made by a variety of other cell types. In both type 1 and type 2 responses, antibodies play an important role, with IgG2a being elevated in the former and IgG1 and IgE being increased in the latter.

## INITIATION OF THE IMMUNE RESPONSE

### TYPE 1 OR IFN-γ-DOMINANT RESPONSE

Within hours after immunization with a pathogen, a pronounced and highly restricted cytokine pattern is detectable in lymphoid organs. These cytokines are derived from cells that have been activated by conserved microbial structures expressed by the pathogen. These structures are not necessarily antigenic but rather are molecules characteristic of particular groups of pathogens that host cells mediating an immune response have evolved to recognize. Receptors exist on the surface of host immune cell populations that can directly recognize the microbial structures and be activated by them to produce specific cytokines. The lipopolysaccharide (LPS) component of Gram-negative bacteria is one of the best understood of these structures. LPS is an integral component of the bacterial cell wall and as such is highly conserved among a large group of bacteria and cannot easily be altered by these pathogens[4]. LPS is thus well suited to be selected during the evolutionary process as a recognition structure by the immune system to rapidly recognize and target invading Gram-negative bacteria. Macrophages[4], and also several other cell types[5,6], can be activated by LPS. Macrophages activated by LPS rapidly produce a variety of mediators that have bactericidal activities (e.g. nitrous oxide intermediates) and they also secrete cytokines, including IL-12, IFN-α, IL-1, IL-6, transforming growth factor beta (TGF-β), tumor necrosis factor alpha (TNF-α) and IL-10[4,7]. These cytokines can have both local and systemic effects that mediate host defense during the innate response or at higher concentrations of LPS can be associated with septic shock. Several of these cytokines are particularly important in triggering the production of other cytokines and also influencing the development of the adaptive response. For example, IL-12, which can be produced by monocytes and macrophages, can cause a cascade of effects, including spleen cell IFN-γ and IL-10 induction[8] and $CD4^+$ T-cell activation, resulting in enhanced priming for IFN-γ production[9]. Thus LPS, a single highly conserved constituent of gram-negative bacteria, can quickly cause cells of the innate immune system to secrete a restricted set of cytokines.

As might be expected, a similar cytokine pattern is observed following immunization with various Gram-negative bacteria, including *Salmonella typhimurium* (IL-6, IFN-γ and IL-10)[10–12] (Gause, unpublished) and *Brucella abortus* (IL-12, IL-6, IL-10 and IFN-γ)[13]. In many cases, the route of immunization and the particular tissue analyzed does not seem to affect the induction of this pattern, since it is observed with live *Salmonella* either orally or i.v. in the Peyer's patches or spleen respectively or with killed *Brucella abortus* following i.v. injection or injection in the footpad and analysis of the spleen or popliteal lymph node respectively[10–13]. In contrast, injection with peptide Ags (antigens) or other artificial Ags such as SRBCs results in considerable variation in the cytokine pattern, depending on the route of immunization or the concentration of Ag[14,15]. Presumably the LPS component is initiating this conserved and restricted cytokine pattern observed in response to Gram-negative bacteria. However, apparently other constituents can also elicit this particular pattern, since elevations in IFN-γ, IL-10 and IL-6 gene expression are observed within 6 h after infection with the Gram-positive bacterium *Listeria monocytogenes*[16], which of course does not express LPS. Furthermore, infection with Venezuelan equine encephalitis virus (VEE)[18] also induces a similar cytokine pattern, again characterized by elevations in IFN-γ, IL-10 and IL-6, suggesting that conserved structures characteristic of viruses can also elicit production of this restricted set of cytokines. Recently, elevations in IL-12 gene expression have also been observed in mice infected with VEE[18], mouse hepatitis virus, mouse adenovirus, and predominantly in macrophages of mice infected with lactate dehydrogenase-elevating virus[19]. Thus, as in bacteria, IL-12 may regulate subsequent cytokine production following viral infection. IFN-α/β may also be important in upregulating IL-10 and IFN-γ production in viruses, as we have recently observed that administration of anti-IFN-α/β antibody (provided by Dr Ion Gresser, CNRS) can downregulate elevations in IFN-γ and IL-10 gene expression induced by VEE infection[18].

At this early stage of the immune response to both viruses and whole bacteria the primary source of the elevated IFN-γ is probably from NK cells, which can be activated by cytokines, in particular IL-12 and IL-2, but which may also be activated following recognition of specific conserved structures on the pathogen[20–22]. NK cells, through the production of IFN-γ, can also induce B-cell Ig isotype switching to IgG2a and IgG3[23–25] (Snapper, personal communication). Some reports suggest that macrophages may also produce IFN-γ[26], but whether macrophages are an important source of this cytokine *in vivo* is uncertain. Recently, γ/δ T cells from *L. monocytogenes*-infected mice were shown to express markedly increased levels of cytoplasmic IFN-γ as early as 24 h after immunization, suggesting the possibility that this population may also be an important source of IFN-γ at initial stages of the immune response[27]. Several other pathogens have also been shown to stimulate γ/δ T cells to produce IFN-γ[28].

Elevated IL-10 may be derived from B cells, in particular B1 B cells, monocytes and macrophages, since all three populations produce IL-10 upon activation[4,29]. The source of elevated IL-6 during the *in vivo* immune response is also uncertain but may include monocytes and macrophages[30,31]. Neutrophils have also been found to produce a number of cytokines, including IL-6, IL-3, TNF-α and TGF-β[32]. Because they are activated early in the response to a pathogen, they could potentially be important in influencing the course of the immune response; however, this cell population has yet to be shown to be an important cytokine source *in vivo*. More typically, TNF-α, TGF-β and also IL-12 and IL-1 are derived from macrophages[4,33].

Thus a conserved pattern of cytokine expression, including elevations in IL-12, IFN-γ, IL-6 and IL-10, is elicited within 24 h after immunization with any one of several different types of pathogens, including both bacteria and viruses. With the exception of LPS[4,7], and perhaps double-stranded RNA[34], few microbial structures have been identified that can elicit this cytokine pattern. However, as we shall see, the early induction of these cytokines by antigen-non-specific effector cells of the innate immune response is predictive of the appearance of an adaptive IFN-γ-dominant (type 1-like) T-cell response that favors cell-mediated immunity, and several of these cytokines, including IL-12, IFN-γ and perhaps IFN-α, appear critical in influencing its development.

## TYPE 2 OR IL-4-DOMINANT RESPONSE

Nematode parasites, on the other hand, elicit a quite different set of cytokines than bacterial and viral pathogens. Unlike bacteria and viruses, nematode parasites are larger than individual cells of the host and consequently must invade the host by digestion of epithelial cell barriers and penetration into the intercellular spaces. This different route of entry may trigger other cell populations, in particular mast cells or epithelial cells, to intially respond. Within 24 h after oral inoculation with the nematode parasite *Heligmosomoides polygyrus*, pronounced elevations in IL-3, IL-5 and IL-9 mRNA are detected by quantitative reverse transcriptase polymerase chain reaction (RT-PCR) in the Peyer's patches and the gut mucosa of the small intestine[35]. In contrast, within 6 h after inoculation no elevations were detected in IL-4, IL-12, TNF-α, TGF-β, IL-1, IFN-γ, IL-10 or IL-6[35] (Gause, unpublished). This response to oral infection is specific to the pathogen and not the route of immunization, since oral inoculation with *Salmonella typhimurium* induces elevations in IFN-γ, IL-6 and IL-10, with elevations in IL-5 or IL-9 not detected in the Peyer's patch[12]. These findings are particularly relevant to the development of oral vaccines, since they suggest that one can influence the mucosal response by employing different vaccine delivery systems[36].

The cellular source of the elevated IL-5 and IL-9 in response to nematode parasites is uncertain, although elevations are maintained in the gut mucosa of nude and SCID mice, suggesting a non-B/non-T cell, perhaps of the mast cell lineage[35]. If this is the case, it is somewhat surprising that they do not express IL-4, since mast cells/basophils have been shown to produce IL-4 upon activation[37]. IL-4 mRNA is not actually elevated until day 4 after *H. polygyrus* inoculation, and the TCR-$\alpha\beta^+$, $CD4^+$ T cells are the only source detectable by cell sorting[35]. Recently, mucosal epithelial cells have been shown to produce a variety of cytokines, including TNF-α, IL-6 and IL-8[38,39], and although they have not been shown to produce IL-5 or IL-9, stimulation of these cells with agents that can evoke an IL-4-dominant response has not yet been reported. Another possible source of elevated cytokines at early stages of an IL-4-dominant response is the eosinophil, which has been shown to produce IL-5[40]. Similar studies with *Nippostrongylus brasiliensis* have also shown IL-5 and IL-9 but not IL-4 to be elevated in the gut shortly after immunization (Madden and Gause, unpublished data). The conserved constituent of nematode parasites that stimulates the rapid gut cytokine response has not been identified. One possible candidate may comprise proteolytic enzymes which are used by the nematode to penetrate the host intestinal epithelial cells[41]. Recent findings suggest that γδ T cells in the peritoneal cavity and the spleen produce elevated IL-4 by several days after i.p. injection of *N. brasiliensis*[27], implicating this cell population as capable of producing either type 1 (in the case of *Listeria* infection) or type 2 cytokines, depending on the pathogen involved.

These findings suggest that pathogens can induce distinct cytokine responses within hours after infection. The subsequent cytokine milieu may produce conditions that favor the development of an adaptive immune response tailored to be protective against the specific pathogen involved. This is well documented in the IFN-γ-dominant response but as yet the cytokine elevations associated with the initiation of an IL-4-dominant response have not been shown to influence T-cell differentiation to IL-4 production. From an evolutionary viewpoint, this rapid and restricted host response maximizes an effective counteraction against the pathogen by both quickly providing protection via activation of the nonadaptive immune elements and by influencing the development of the antigen-specific T and B cells.

## THE ADAPTIVE RESPONSE

### TYPE 2 OR IL-4-DOMINANT RESPONSE

Proliferation of naive TCR-α/β⁺, CD4⁺ T cells followed by their differentiation into cytokine-producing effector T-helper cells requires both signaling through the antigen-specific T-cell receptor (TCR) and a costimulatory signal. Signaling through the TCR in the absence of the appropriate costimulatory signal renders the T cell anergic or in some cases triggers programmed cell death[42,43]. Additional signals are important in shaping the T-cell response toward production of particular sets of cytokines. The professional APCs, including the dendritic cells, macrophages and activated B cells, provide the costimulatory activity for T cells, and these APCs and several other cell types, including NK cells and perhaps also γδ T cells, neutrophils and cells of the mast cell/basophil lineage, provide additional signaling that influences T-cell differentiation. We have recently demonstrated the requirement of the costimulatory signal provided by B7 interactions with T-cell CD28/CTLA4 for T cells to differentiate to cytokine-producing cells during a mucosal immune response. Blocking B7 ligand interactions by *in vivo* administration of the fusion protein CTLA4-Ig inhibited mesenteric lymph node (MLN) TCR-α/β⁺, CD4⁺ T-cell IL-4 production following *H. polygyrus* oral inoculation[44]. Naive T cells were probably the source of elevated IL-4 in this primary response since administration of CTLA4-Ig 3–4 days after inoculation or during a challenge response did not suppress subsequent elevations in T-cell cytokine production, further suggesting that both effector and memory T cells do not require CD28/CTLA4 costimulatory signals for IL-4 production *in vivo*[45]. These findings suggest that in this response naive T-helper cells, provided they have CD28/CTLA4 costimulation, can rapidly differentiate within about 4–5 days to IL-4-secreting cells that can provide helper function for B cells which differentiate to secrete IgE and IgG1. Once stimulated, the T-helper cells also secrete IL-5 and show elevations in IL-3 and IL-9 gene expression but do not express elevated IL-2, IFN-γ or IL-10 mRNA[35]. By 8–10 days after inoculation the primary source of elevated IL-5 and IL-9 is CD4⁺ T cells, with non-T cells being a minor source of cytokines at this later stage of the response. T-cell differentiation in the presence of a potent antigen, such as a nematode parasite, with its many associated constituents, can thus proceed directly to a restricted type 2-like pattern without initially exhibiting a Th0 cell phenotype. Differentiation to IL-4 production also appears to be IL-2 independent, since elevations in IL-2 gene expression are not detected during the response, and *in vivo* administration of anti-IL-2/anti-IL-2R antibodies does not effect elevations in serum IgE levels in nematode-infected mice (Finkelman, personal communication). Recently, a novel NK.1.1$^+$, CD4$^+$ T-cell population has been identified in the spleen that is induced to produce IL-4 within several hours after *in vivo* anti-CD3 monoclonal antibody (mAb)administration[46]. It is possible that this population may be a source of the initial elevations in IL-4 production detected by 4–6 days after oral *H. polygyrus* inoculation. The lack of a requirement of IL-2 for IL-4 production is also consistent with detection of elevated serum IgG1 levels and IL-4 in IL-2 null mice[47] (Sedar, personal communication), although the definitive experiment examining whether IL-4 production is elevated in T cells from IL-2 gene knockout mice inoculated with *H. polygyrus* has not yet been performed.

The early signals that trigger these MLN T cells to rapidly differentiate into IL-4-producing cells following *H. polygyrus* inoculation are unknown, although the initial increases in IL-3, IL-5 and IL-9 by non-T cells may contribute to the required milieu. Once IL-4 is produced by these T cells, it apparently functions in an autocrine manner, since anti-IL-4 mAb administration as late as 3–4 days after *H. polygyrus* inoculation can markedly inhibit IL-4 secretion at day 8 after inoculation (Gause and Finkelman, unpublished). Other T-cell responses to nematode parasites, in particular *Trichuris*, show similar cytokine patterns[48]. Following immunization with the filarial nematode *Brugia pahangi*[49], elevations in IL-5, IL-9 and IL-4, in the absence of elevations in IFN-γ, are observed in splenic lymphocytes. The pattern of similar cytokines being elicited from different tissues and often different cell types appears to be a common motif characteristic of the immune response to pathogens.

In the very different granulomatous response in the lung to eggs of *Schistosoma mansoni*, elevations in IL-4 gene expression by T cells are preceded by IL-2 elevations, and *in vivo* administration of anti-IL-2/IL-2R antibodies blocks IL-4 mRNA elevations[50], suggesting that under different conditions T cells may require IL-2 signaling for their differentiation to IL-4 production *in vivo*, as has been suggested from *in vitro* studies[51,52]. Following immunization of genetically susceptible Balb/c mice with *Leishmania major* promastigotes, CD4$^+$ T cells develop yet another cytokine pattern, characterized by IL-4 and IL-10 elevations, which is more consistent with the classical Th2 paradigm, but in the context of the responses to the other pathogens already discussed it is clear that the cytokine patterns produced in response to different pathogens are considerably more complex than the original Th1/Th2 model predicted, and that expression of type 2 cytokines by CD4$^+$ T cells is independently regulated, particularly in the case of IL-10.

## TYPE 1 OR IFN-γ-DOMINANT RESPONSE

The role of CD28 costimulatory molecules in the development of type 1 $CD4^+$ T cells producing IFN-γ and other type 1 cytokines *in vivo* has not yet been directly examined. However, the immune response to *Leishmania major* infection, as measured by footpad size and serum Ig levels, is inhibitable by blocking B7-dependent costimulation in Balb/c but not C57BL/6 mice, suggesting that priming for type 1 cytokine production is less dependent on B7 costimulation than priming for type 2 cytokine production[53]. However, since the type 1 response in BL/6 mice is initially non-T-cell mediated, T cells have to be directly examined in *Leishmania*-infected BL/6 mice to confirm whether they require B7 signals for cytokine production. Also, the cell-mediated immune response associated with graft rejection is blocked by CTLA4 Ig administration[54,55], and if this response is, as would be expected, mediated by IFN-γ, then this variation of a type 1 response is B7/dependent.

The cytokines made by $CD4^+$ T cells in a type 1 or IFN-γ-dominant response to pathogens are frequently not the same cytokines as those originally identified in long-term Th1 cell clones derived from mice immunized with artificial Ags. Perhaps surprisingly, most immune responses to whole pathogens, killed or viable, that elicit IFN-γ production are associated with a distinct cytokine pattern that includes the production of both IL-10 and IFN-γ by $CD4^+$ T cells. This cytokine pattern has been observed in $CD4^+$ T cells associated with the immune response to a number of pathogens, including killed *Brucella abortus*[13], *Influenza pneumonia*[17,56] and Borna disease virus[57], and, based on depletion studies, probably also occurs in T cells during the immune response to *Listeria monocytogenes*[16]. Except for *Brucella abortus*, in which the cellular source for IL-6 has not been identified, IL-6 elevations are also derived from T cells following immunization with the aforementioned pathogens. As mentioned previously, IL-10, IFN-γ and also IL-6 are also made by cells during the initial innate immune response to many bacteria and viruses. Thus many of the same cytokines are produced both by cells characteristic of the nonadaptive type 1 immune response and by antigen-specific T cells contributing to the adaptive type 2 response. Production of both IFN-γ and IL-6 have been well documented as promoting host-protective cell-mediated responses to both bacteria and viruses, but the role of elevations in IL-10 during the IFN-γ-dominant response is uncertain. One possibility is that IL-10, which can suppress IL-12 secretion by macrophages and IFN-γ production by NK cells[58], may function to downregulate a cell-mediated response, which under some circumstances may be associated with host-damaging inflammatory reactions. Exogenous IL-12 administration during LCMV (lymphocytic choriomeningitis virus) infection is associated with increased TNF-α production, which causes toxicity and decreased resistance to disease[59,60]. This disruption of the response by the presence of additional IL-12 suggests that the potential for such toxicity exists physiologically and that regulatory controls, perhaps including IL-10, may normally prevent such harmful responses. This possibility is of course, testable now that IL-10 gene knockout mice are available.

Several cytokines produced at early stages of the IFN-γ-dominant immune response may influence the development of the subsequent adaptive immune response. IL-12, in particular, can act directly on $CD4^+$ T cells to enhance priming for IFN-γ production and inhibit the development of IL-4-producing T-helper cells[9]. IL-12-mediated induction of IFN-γ production by NK cells may also favor T-cell differentiation toward IFN-γ production. Some studies suggest that TNF-α[58] and IFN-α/β[34] may also influence T cells toward IFN-γ production.

TCR-α/$\beta^+$, $CD8^+$ cells are usually considered as precursor cytotoxic T cells which differentiate to effector cells during the IFN-γ-dominant response. However, there is also a considerable literature dealing with $CD8^+$ T cells functioning as suppressor cells. A number of investigators have suggested that this suppressor function may result from the secretion of immunoregulatory cytokines, including IL-4 and IFN-γ[61]. Immune deviation may then result, with the nature (e.g. type 1 versus type 2) rather than the strength of the response being altered. Generally, $CD8^+$ T cells have been found to produce the type 1 cytokines, including IFN-γ and TNF-β[62,63]. However, $CD8^+$ T cells have now also been demonstrated to produce type 2 cytokines, including IL-4 and IL-5 when cultured *in vitro* with T-cell mitogens and IL-4[64–66]. Similar to the effects observed with $CD4^+$ T-helper cells, culture of $CD8^+$ T-cell effectors with IL-12 and IL-2 favored IFN-γ production while culture with IL-4 favored IL-4 and IL-5 production[66]. Furthermore, separate $CD8^+$ T-cell clones have been isolated that secrete either IFN-γ or IL-4 from patients with leprosy[61]. Whether cytokine production by this cell population is an important component of the *in vivo* immune response has yet to be determined, and it is clear that this population should be carefully examined for cytokine production in future studies.

## SUMMARY

In summary, the advent and further development of several techniques, including RT-PCR, ELISPOT and immunohistology, have permitted cytokine production by specific cell populations following immunization with whole pathogens to be examined. The complexity of the immune response that has been observed is necessary and expected, given that it has coevolved with a large variety of pathogens which are continuously attempting to circumvent its effectiveness. Since these organisms often have short generation times, it is advantageous for the host to rapidly respond to the particular invading pathogen with a specific immune response. When *in vivo* cytokine expression is measured either by mRNA or protein levels, it is apparent that a specific pattern is indeed elicited and that this highly reproducible pattern is detected within hours after infection. The specific response is not antigen specific but is instead triggered by general constituents characteristic of certain groups of pathogens that are often vulnerable to a particular kind of attack by effector cells of the innate immune response. Cytokines secreted by these activated effector cells result in a cytokine milieu favoring the rapid development of Ag-specific effector T-helper cells, which also require TCR and costimulatory molecule signaling. These effector T-helper cells in turn produce specific cytokines that amplify the pathogen-specific response initiated by the antigen-non-specific cells. Understanding which cytokines cells of the innate immune response secrete following infection and how these cells are triggered to undergo activation is thus of considerable importance, since it is these cells that are probably the primary players in influencing whether a type 1 or a type 2 response will develop.

## REFERENCES


1. Janeway CA. Are there cellular superantigens? Immunol Rev 1993; 131:189–200.
2. Held W, Acha-Orbea H, MacDonald HR, Waanders GA. Superantigens and retroviral infection: insights from mouse mammary tumor virus. Immunol Today 1994; 15:184–190.
3. Marrack P, Hugo P, McCormack J, Kappler J. Death and T cells. Immunol Rev 1993; 133:119–129.
4. Manthey C, Vogel SN. Interactions of lipopolysaccharide with macrophages. In: Zwilling BS, Eisenstein TK (eds) Macrophage–Pathogen Interactions. New York: Marcel Dekker, Inc. 1994, pp. 63–81.
5. Takanaski S, Nonaka R, Xing Z *et al.* Interleukin 10 inhibits lipopolysaccharide-induced survival and cytokine production by human peripheral blood eosinophils. J Exp Med 1994; 180 (2):711–715.
6. Leal-Berumen I, Conlon P, Marshall JS. IL-6 production by rat peritoneal mast cells is not necessarily preceded by histamine release and can be induced by bacterial lipopolysaccharide. J Immunol 1994; 152 (11):5468–5476.
7. Heinzel FP, Rerko RM, Ling P *et al.* Interleukin 12 is produced in vivo during endotoxemia and stimulates synthesis of gamma interferon. Infect Immun 1994; 62:4244–4249.
8. Morris SC, Madden KB, Adamovicz JJ *et al.* Effects of IL-12 on in vivo cytokine gene expression and Ig isotype selection. J Immunol 1994; 152:1047–1056.
9. Seder RA, Gazzinelli R, Sher A, Paul WE. Interleukin 12 acts directly on $CD4^+$ T cells to enhance priming for interferon gamma production and diminishes interleukin 4 inhibition of such priming. Proc Natl Acad Sci USA 1993; 90 (21):10188–10192.
10. Ramarathinam L, Niesel DW, Klimpel GR. Ity influences the production of IFN-gamma by murine splenocytes stimulated in vitro with Salmonella typhimurium. J Immunol 1993; 150:3965–3972.

11. Ramarathinam L, Niesel DW, Klimpel GR. Salmonella typhimurium induces IFN-gamma production in murine splenocytes. J Immunol 1993; 150:3973–3981.
12. Svetic A, Urban JF, Finkelman FD *et al.* Elevations in IL-5 and IL-9 gene expression precede a Th2-like response. J Immunol 1993; 150:93a(abstract).
13. Svetic A, Jian YC, Lu P *et al.* Brucella abortus induces a novel cytokine gene expression characterized by elevated IL-10 and IFN-gamma in CD4+ T cells. Int Immunol 1993; 5:877–884.
14. Pfeffer C, Sette A, Bottomly K. Priming of Th1 or Th2 in vivo is a function of TCR-ligand density. J Cell Biochem 1995; 21a:127(abstract).
15. Xu-Amano J, Beagley KW, Mega J *et al.* Induction of T helper cells and cytokines for mucosal IgA responses. Adv Exp Med Biol 1992; 327:107–117.
16. Ehlers S, Mielke MEA, Blankenstein T, Hahn H. Kinetic analysis of cytokine gene expression in the livers of naive and immune mice infected with *Listeria monocytogenes*: the intermediate early phase in innate resistance and acquired immunity. J Immunol 1992; 149:3016.
17. Sarawar SR, Doherty PC. Concurrent production of interleukin-2, interleukin-10, and gamma interferon in the regional lymph nodes of mice with influenza pneumonia. J Virol 1994; 68(5):3112–3119.
18. Grieder FB, Nguyen H, Zhou X *et al.* A specific Th1/Th2 cytokine pattern is rapidly elicited following infection with Venezuelan Equine Encephalitis Virus. J Cell Biochem 1995; 19a:285(abstract).
19. Coutelier JP, Broeck J, Wolf SF. Interleukin-12 gene expression after viral infection in the mouse. J Virol 1995; 69:1955–1958.
20. Brunda MJ. Interleukin-12. J Leukocyte Biol 1994; 55:280–288.
21. Aste-Amezaga M, D'Andrea A, Kubin M, Trinchieri G. Cooperation of natural killer cell stimulatory factor/interleukin-12 with other stimuli in the induction of cytokines and cytotoxic cell-associated molecules in human T and NK cells. Cell Immunol 1994; 156:480–492.
22. Bonnema JD, Rivlin KA, Ting AT *et al.* Cytokine-enhanced NK cell-mediated cytotoxicity. Positive modulatory effects of IL-2 and IL-12 on stimulus-dependent granule exocytosis. J Immunol 1994; 152:2098–2104.
23. Snapper CM, Yamaguchi H, Moorman MA, Mond JJ. An in vitro model for T cell-independent induction of humoral immunity. A requirement for NK cells. J Immunol 1994; 152:4884–4892.
24. Snapper CM, Yamaguchi H, Moorman MA, Mond J. An in vitro model for T cell-independent induction of humoral immunity. J Immunol 1994; 151:5251–5260.
25. Snapper CM, McIntyre TM, Mandler R *et al.* Induction of IgG3 secretion by interferon gamma: a model for T cell-independent class switching in response to T cell-independent type 2 antigens. J Exp Med 1992; 175:1367–1371.
26. Fultz MJ, Barber BA, Dieffenbach CW, Voegl SN. Induction of IFN-gamma in macrophages by lipopolysaccharide. Int Immunol 1993; 5:1383–1392.
27. Ferrick DA, Schrenzel MD, Mulvania T *et al.* Differential production of interferon-gamma and interleukin-4 in response to Th1 and Th2-stimulating pathogens by gamma/delta T cells in vivo. Nature 1995; 373:255–256.
28. Kaufman SHE. Immunity to intracellular bacteria. Annu Rev Immunol 1994; 153:2302–2312.
29. Moore KW, O'Garra A, De Waal MR *et al.* Interleukin-10. Annu Rev Immunol 1993; 11:165–190.
30. Van Heeckeren AM, Rikihisa Y, Park J, Fertel R. Tumor necrosis factor alpha, interleukin-1 alpha, interleukin-6, and prostaglandin E2 production in murine peritoneal macrophage infected with Ehrlichia risticii. Infect Immun 1993; 61:4333–4337.

31. Temeles DS, McGrath HE, Kittler EL *et al.* Cytokine expression from bone marrow derived macrophages. Exp Hematol 1993; 21:388–393.
32. Cassatella MA. The production of cytokines by polymorphonuclear neutrophils. Immunol Today 1995; 16:21–26.
33. Salkowski CA, Neta R, van Rooijen N, Vogel SN. In vivo analysis of cytokine mRNA expression after endotoxin challenge of macrophage-depleted mice. J Immunol 1995; 155:3168.
34. Finkelman FD, Svetic A, Gresser I *et al.* Regulation by IFN-α of immunoglobulin isotype selection and lymphokine production in mice. J Exp Med 1991; 174:1179–1188.
35. Svetic A, Madden KB, Zhou XD *et al.* A primary intestinal helminthic infection rapidly induces a gut-associated elevation of Th2-associated cytokines and IL-3. J Immunol 1993; 150:3434–3441 (abstract).
36. Jackson RJ, Staats HF, Xu-Amano J *et al.* Oral vaccine models: multiple delivery systems employing tetanus toxoid. Ann N Y Acad Sci 1994; 730:217–234.
37. Ben-Sasson SZ, Le-Gros G, Conrad DH *et al.* Cross-linking Fc receptors stimulates splenic non-B, non-T cells to secrete IL-4 and other lymphokines. Proc Natl Acad Sci USA 1990; 87:1421.
38. Eckmann L, Jung H, Yang S-K *et al.* A distinct array of proinflammatory cytokines is expressed in human colon epithelial cells in response to bacterial invasion. J Cell Biochem 1995; 19A:245(abstract).
39. Hedges S, Agace W, Svensson M *et al.* Uroepithelial cells are part of a mucosal cytokine network. Infect Immun 1994; 62:3215–3221.
40. Dubucquoi S, Desreumaux P, Janin A *et al.* Interleukin 5 synthesis by eosinophils: association with granules and immunoglobulin-dependent secretion. J Exp Med 1994; 179:703–708.
41. Urban JF, Madden KB, Svetic A *et al.* The importance of Th2 cytokines in protective immunity to nematodes. Immunol Rev 1992; 127:205–220.
42. Schwartz RH. Costimulation of T lymphocytes: the role of CD28, CTLA-4, and B7/BB1 in interleukin-2 production and immunotherapy. Cell 1993; 71:1065–1068.
43. Jenkins MK, Pardoll DM, Mizuguchi J *et al.* Molecular events in the induction of a nonresponsive state in IL-2 producing helper T lymphocyte clones. Proc Natl Acad Sci USA 1987; 84:5409–5414.
44. Lu P, Zhou X, Chen SJ *et al.* CTLA-4 ligands are required in an in vivo interleukin 4 response to a gastrointestinal nematode parasite. J Exp Med 1994; 180:693–698.
45. Gause WC, Zhou X-D, Chen S-J *et al.* The CTLA-4 counter-receptor is required for T cell IL-4 production during the primary but not challenge mucosal immune response to a gastrointestinal nematode. J Cell Biochem 1995; 21A:165(abstract).
46. Yoshimoto T, Paul WE. $CD4^+$, $NK1.1^+$ T cells promptly produce interleukin 4 in response to in vivo challenge with anti-CD3. J Exp Med 1994; 179:1285–1295.
47. Kundig TM, Schorle H, Bachman MF *et al.* Immune responses in interleukin-2-deficient mice. Science 1993; 262:1059–1061.
48. Else KJ, Finkelman FD, Maliszewski CR, Grencis RK. Cytokine-mediated regulation of chronic intestinal helminth infections. J Exp Med 1994; 179:347–351.
49. Bancroft AJ, Grencis RK, Else KJ, Devaney E. The role of CD4 cells in protective immunity to *Brugia pahangi*. Parasite Immunol 1994; 16:385–387.
50. Wynn TA, Eltoum I, Cheever AW *et al.* Analysis of cytokine gene mRNA

expression during primary granuloma formation induced by eggs of *Schistosoma mansoni*. J Immunol 1993; 151:1430–1440.

51. Ben-Sasson SZ, Le-Gros G, Conrad DH *et al.* IL-4 production by T cells from naive donors: IL-2 is required for IL-4 production. J Immunol 1990; 145:1127–1136.
52. Le Gros G, Ben-Sasson SZ, Sedar R *et al.* Generation of interleukin 4 (IL-4)-producing cells in vivo and in vitro. IL-2 and IL-4 are required for in vitro generation of IL-4 production. J Exp Med 1990; 172:921–929.
53. Corry DB, Reiner SL, Linsley PS, Locksley RM. Differential effects of blockade of CD28-B7 on the development of Th1 or Th2 receptor cells in experimental Leishmaniasis. J Immunol 1994; 153:4142–4148.
54. Lenschow DJ, Zeng Y, Thistlethwaite JR *et al.* Long-term survival of xenogeneic islet grafts induced by CTLA4-Ig. Science 1992; 257:789–792.
55. Turka LA, Linsley PS, Lin H *et al.* T cell activation by the CD28 ligand B7 is required for cardiac allograft rejection in vivo. Proc Natl Acad Sci USA 1992; 89:11102–11105.
56. Sarawar SR, Sangster M, Coffman RL, Doherty DC. Administration of anti-IFN-gamma antibody to beta 2-microglobulin-deficient mice delays influenza virus clearance but does not switch the response to T helper cell 2 phenotype. J Immunol 1994; 153 (3):1246–1253.
57. Planz O, Bilzer T, Stitz L. Immunopathogenic role of T-cell subsets in Borna disease virus-induced progressive encephalitis. J Virol 1995; 69 (2):896–903.
58. Tripp CS, Wolf SF, Unanue ER. Interleukin 12 and tumor necrosis factor alpha are costimulators of interferon gamma production by natural killer cells in severe combined immunodeficiency mice with listeriosis, and interleukin 10 is a physiologic antagonist. Proc Natl Acad Sci USA 1994; 90:3725–3829.
59. Bruserd O, Ehninger G, Hamann W, Pawelec G. Secretion of IL-2, IL-3, IL-4, IL-6 and GM-CSF by $CD4^+$ and $CD8^+$ TCR alpha beta+ T-cell clones derived early after allogeneic bone marrow transplantation. Scand J Immunol 1993; 38:65–74.
60. Biron CA, Cousens LP, Orange JS *et al.* Cytokine regulation of NK and T cell responses to viral infection. J Cell Biochem 1995; 19A:271(abstract).
61. Salgame PR, Abrams JS, Clayberger C *et al.* Differing lymphokine profiles of functional subsets of human CD4 and CD8 T cell clones. Science 1991; 254:279–282.
62. Klein JR, Raulet DH, Pasternack MC, Bevan MJ. Cytotoxic T lymphocytes produce immune interferon in response to antigen or mitogen. J Exp Med 1982; 155:1198.
63. Morris AG, Lin Y-L, Askonas BA. Immune interferon release when a cloned cytotoxic T-cell line meets its correct influenza-infected target cell. Nature 1982; 295:150–152.
64. Seder RA, Boulay JL, Finkelman FD *et al.* CD8 T cells can be primed in vitro to produce IL-4. J Immunol 1992; 148:1652–1656.
65. Erard F, Wild M-T, Garcia-Sanz JA, Le Gros G. Switch of CD8 T cell to noncytolytic CD8−, CD4− cells that make Th2 cytokines and help B cells. Science 1993; 260:1802–1805.
66. Croft M, Carter L, Swain SL, Dutton RW. Generation of polarized antigen-specific CD8 effector populations: reciprocal action of interleukin (IL)-4 and IL-12 in promoting type 2 versus type 1 cytokine profiles. J Exp Med 1994; 180 (5):1715–1728.
67. Mosmann TR, Cherwinski H, Bond MW *et al.* Two types of murine helper T cell clone I. Definition according to profiles of lymphokine activities and secreted proteins. J Immunol 1986; 136:2345–2356.

68. Friedman RM. Interferons. In: Oppenheim JJ, Shevach EM (eds) Textbook of immunophysiology. New York: Oxford Pub. 1988, p. 194.
69. Klimpel GR, Infante AJ, Patterson J *et al.* Virus-induced interferon alpha/beta (IFN-alpha/beta) production by T cells and by Th1 and Th2 helper T cell clones: a study of the immunoregulatory actions of IFN-gamma versus IFN-alpha/beta on functions of different T cell populations. Cell Immunol 1990; 128:603–618.
70. Mosmann TR, Coffman RL. Th1 and Th2 cells: different patterns of lymphokine secretion lead to different functional properties. Annu Rev Immunol 1989; 7:145.
71. Bruserud O, Hamann W, Patel S *et al.* IFN-gamma and TNF-alpha secretion by CD4+ and CD8+ TCR alpha beta + T cell clones derived early after allogeneic bone marrow transplantation. Eur J Haematol 1993; 51:73–79.
72. Gold KN, Weyand CM, Goronzy JJ. Modulation of helper T cell function by prostaglandins. Arthritis Rheum 1994; 37:925–933.
73. Altman A, Katz DH. The biology of monoclonal lymphokines secreted by T cell lines and hybridomas. Adv Immunol 1982; 33:73–166.
74. Hirano T, Yaga T, Nakano N. Purificaiton to homogeneity and characterization of human B cell differentiation factor (BCDF or BSFp-2). Proc Natl Acad Sci USA 1985; 82:5490–5494.
75. Renauld JC, Goethals A, Houssiau F *et al.* Human P40/IL-9. Expression in activated CD4+ T cells, genomic organization, and comparison with the mouse gene. J Immunol 1990; 144:4235–4241.
76. Reiner SL, Zheng S, Wang ZE *et al.* Leishmania promastigotes evade interleukin 12 (IL-12) induction by macrophages and stimulate a broad range of cytokines from CD4+ T cells during initiation of infection. J Exp Med 1994; 179:447–456.
77. Bruserud O, Ehninger G, Hamann W, Pawelec G. Secretion of IL-2, IL-3, IL-4, IL-6, and GM-CSF by CD4+ and CD8+ TCR alpha beta+ T-cell clones derived early after allogeneic bone marrow transplantation. Scand J Immunol 1993; 38:65–74.
78. Adamthwaite D, Cooley MA. CD8+ T-cell subsets defined by expression of CD45 isoform differ in their capacity to produce IL-2, IFN-gamma and TNF-beta. Immunology 1994; 81:253–260.
79. Koyasu S, Nakauchi H, Kitamura K *et al.* Production of interleukin 3 and gamma-interferon by an antigen-specific mouse suppressor T cell clone. J Immunol 1985; 134:3130–3136.
80. Matsuyama M, Sugamua K, Kawade Y, Hinuma Y. Production of immune interferon by human cytotoxic T cell clones. J Immunol 1982; 129:450.
81. Chen Y, Mohapatra S, Mohapatra SS, Sehon AH. Cytokine gene expression of CD8+ suppressor T cells induced by tolerogenic conjugates of antigen and mPEG. Cell Immunol 1993; 149:409–421.
82. Fong TA, Mosmann TR. Alloreactive murine CD8+ T cell clones secrete the Th1 pattern of cytokines. J Immunol 1990; 144:1744–1752.
83. Lorre K, Kasran A, Van Vaeck F *et al.* Interleukin-1 and B7/CD28 interaction regulate interleukin-6 production by human T cells. Clin Immunol Immunopathol 1994; 70:81–90.
84. Bruserud O, Ehninger G, Hamann W, Pawelec G. Secretion of IL-2, IL-3, IL-4, IL-6 and GM-CSF by $CD4^+$ and CD8+ TCR alpha beta+ T-cell clones derived early after allogeneic bone marrow transplantation. Scand J Immunol 1994; 38:65–74.
85. Hisatsune T, Nishijima K, Minai Y *et al.* Autoreactive CD8+ T cell clones producing immune suppressive lymphokines IL-10 and interferon-gamma. Cell Immunol 1994; 154:181–192.

86. Spites H, Paliard X, Vandekerckhove Y, de Vries JE. Functional and phenotypic differences between CD4+ and CD4− T cell receptor-gamma delta clones from peripheral blood. J Immunol 1991; 147:1180–1188.
87. Follows GA, Munk ME, Gatrill AJ *et al.* Interferon-gamma and IL-2 but no detectable interleukin 4 in gamma/delta T cell cultures after activation with bacteria. Infect Immun 1992; 60:1231.
88. Schlaak JF, Herman E, Gallati H *et al.* Differential effects of IL-10 on proliferation and cytokine production of human gamma/delta and alpha/beta T cells. Scand J Immunol 1994; 39:209–215.
89. Munk ME, Gatrill A, Kaufmann SHE. Antigen-specific target cell lysis and interleukin-2 secretion by Mycobacterium tuberculosis-activated gamma delta T cells. J Immunol 1990; 145:2434–2439.
90. Chomarat P, Kjeldsen-Kragh J, Quayle AJ *et al.* Different cytokine production profiles of gamma delta T cell clones: relation to inflammatory arthritis. Eur J Immunol 1994; 24:2087–2091.
91. Taguchi T, Aicher WK, Fujihashi K *et al.* Novel function for intestinal intraepithelial lymphocytes. Murine CD3+ gamma/delta TCR+ T cells produce IFN-gamma and IL-5. J Immunol 1995; 147:3736–3744.
92. Corcione A, Baldi L, Zupo S *et al.* Spontaneous production of granulocyte colony-stimulating factor in vitro by human B-lineage lymphocytes is a distinctive marker of germinal center cells. J Immunol 1994; 153:2868–2877.
93. Capobianchi MR, Malavasi F, Mattana P *et al.* Membrane interactions involved in the induction of acid labile interferon alpha. J Biol Regul Homeost Agents 1990; 4:19–24.
94. Xia HZ, Kammapell CC, Fu SM, Sung SS. Differential regulation of human B-lymphocyte tumor necrosis factor-alpha (TNF-alpha) and lymphotoxin (TNF-beta) production by protein phosphatase 1 and 2A inhibitor. Blood 1993; 82:2806–2812.
95. Abken H, Fluck J, Willecks K. Four cell-secreted cytokines act synergistically to maintain long term proliferation of human B cell lines in vitro. J Immunol 1992; 149:2785–2794.
96. Schena M, Gaidano G, Gottardi D *et al.* Molecular investigation of the cytokines produced by normal and malignant B lymphocytes. Leukemia 1992; 6:120–125.
97. Lagoo A, Tseng CK, Sell S. Molecular signals in B cell activation. I. Differential refractory effects of incomplete signaling by ionomycin or PMA relate to autocrine IL-2 production and IL-2R expression. Cell Immunol 1990; 127:483–496.
98. Blomhoff HK, Smeland EB, Erikstein B *et al.* Vitamin A is a key regulator for cell growth, cytokine production, and differentiation in normal B cells. J Biol Chem 1992; 267:23988–23992.
99. Benjamin D, Sharma V, Knobloch TJ *et al.* B cell IL-7. Human B cell lines constitutively secrete IL-7 and express IL-7 receptors. J Immunol 1994; 152:4749–4757.
100. Srivastava MD, Srivastava R, Srivastava BI. Constitutive production of interleukin-8 (IL-8) by normal and malignant human B-cells and other cell types. Leukocyte Res 1993; 17:1063–1069.
101. Song F, Matsuzaki G, Mitsuyama M, Nomoto K. The role of B cells in in vitro induction of IFN-gamma-producing CD4+ T cells specific to Listeria monocytogenes: positive and IL-10-mediated negative regulation. Cell Immunol 1994; 157:403–414.
102. Hayes MP, Enterline JC, Gerrard TL, Zoon KC. Regulation of interferon production by human monocytes: requirements for priming for lipopolysaccharide-induced production. J Leukocyte Biol 1991; 50:176–181.

103. Carswell EA, Old LJ, Kassel RL *et al.* An endotoxin-induced serum factor that causes necrosis of tumors. Proc Natl Acad Sci USA 1975; 72:3666–3670.
104. Fisch H, Gifford GE. In vitro production of rabbit macrophage tumor cell cytotoxin. Int J Cancer 1983; 32:105–112.
105. Khalil N, Whitman C, Zuo L *et al.* Regulation of alveolar macrophage transforming growth factor-beta secretion by corticosteroids in bleomycin-induced pulmonary inflammation in the rat. J Clin Invest 1993; 92:1812–1818.
106. Beuscher HU, Rausch UP, Otterness IG, Tollinghoff M. Transition from interleukin 1 beta (IL1 beta) to IL1 alpha production during maturation of inflammatory macrophages in vivo. J Exp Med 1992; 175:1793–1797.
107. Durum SK, Schmidt JA, Oppenheim JJ. IL-1: an immunological perspective. Annu Rev Immunol 1985; 3:263.
108. Benjamin D, Park CD, Sharma V. Human B cell interleukin 10. Leuk Lymphoma 1994; 12:205–210.
109. Wolf SF, Temple PA, Kobayashi M *et al.* Cloning of cDNA for natural killer cell stimulatory factor. J Immunol 1991; 146:3074–3081.
110. Grabstein KH, Eisenman J, Shanebeck K *et al.* Cloning of a T cell growth factor that interacts with the beta chain of the interleukin-2 receptor. Science 1994; 264:965–968.
111. Miller-Graziano CL, Zhu D, Kodys K. Differential induction of human monocyte transforming growth factor beta 1 production and its regulation by interleukin 4. J Clin Invest 1994; 14:61–72.
112. May LT, Ghrayeb J, Santhanan U *et al.* Synthesis and secretion of multiple forms of beta2-interferon/B-cell differentiation factor 2/hepatocyte-stimulating factor by human fibroblast and monocytes. J Biol Chem 1995; 263:7760–7766.
113. Takahashi GW, Andrews DF, Lilly MB *et al.* Effect of granulocyte-macrophage colony-stimulating factor and interleukin-3 on interleukin-8 production by human neutrophils and monocytes. Blood 1993; 81:357–364.
114. Saito S, Nishikawa K, Morii T *et al.* Cytokine production by CD16-CD56 bright natural killer cells in the human early pregnancy decidua. Int Immunol 1993; 5:559–563.
115. Christmas SE, Meager A, Moore M. Production of interferon and tumor necrosis factor by cloned human natural cytotoxic lymphocyte and T cells. Clin Exp Immunol 1987; 69:441–450.
116. Lorenzen J, Lewis CE, McCracken D *et al.* Human tumor-associated NK cells secrete increased amounts of interferon gamma and interleukin-4. Br J Cancer 1991; 64:457–462.
117. Saito S, Kasahara T, Sakakura S *et al.* Interleukin-8 production by CD16-CD56 bright natural killer cells in the human early pregnancy decidua. Biochem Biophys Res Commun 1994; 200:378–383.
118. Gordon JR, Burd PR, Galli SJ. Mast cells as a source of multifunctional cytokines. Immunol Today 1990; 11:458–464.
119. Grabbe J, Welker P, Moller A *et al.* Comparative cytokine release from human monocytes, monocyte-derived immature mast cells, and a human mast cell line (HMC-1). J Invest Dermatol 1994; 103:504–508.
120. Gordon JR, Galli SJ. Mast cells as a source of both preformed and immunological inducible TNF-alpha/cachectin. Nature 1990; 346:274–276.
121. Wodnar-Filipowicz A, Heusser CH, Moroni C. Production of the haemopoietic growth factors GM-CSF and interleukin-3 by mast cells in response to IgE receptor-mediated activation. Nature 1989; 339:150–152.
122. Plaut M, Pierce JH, Watson CJ *et al.* Mast cell lines produce lymphokines in response to cross-linkage of FceRI or to calcium ionophores. Nature 1989; 339:64–67.

123. Bradding P, Roberts JA, Britten KM *et al.* Interleukin-4, -5, and -6 and tumor necrosis factor-alpha in normal and asthmatic airways: evidence for the human mast cell as a source of these cytokines. Am J Respir Cell Mol Biol 1994; 10:471–480.
124. Smith TJ, Ducharme LA, Weis JH. Preferential expression of interleukin-12 or interleukin-4 by murine bone marrow mast cells derived in mast cell growth factor or interleukin-3. Eur J Immunol 1994; 24:822–826.
125. Takanaski S, Nonaka R, Xing Z *et al.* Interleukin 10 inhibits lipopolysaccharide-induced survival and cytokine production by human peripheral blood eosinophils. J Exp Med 1994; 180:711–715.
126. Elovic A, Wong DT, Weller PF *et al.* Expression of transforming growth factors-alpha and beta 1 messenger RNA and product by eosinophils in nasal polyps. J Allergy Clin Immunol 1995; 93:864–869.
127. Hom JT, Estridge T. FK506 and rapamycin modulate the functional activities of human peripheral blood eosinophils. Clin Immunol Immunopathol 1993; 68:293–300.
128. Braun RK, Franchini M, Erard F *et al.* Human peripheral blood eosinophils produce and release interleukin-8 on stimulation with calcium ionophore. Eur J Immunol 1993; 23:956–960.
129. Paul WE. Interleukin-4 production by Fc epsilon R+ cells. Skin Pharmacol 1991; 4:8–14.
130. Schall TJ. Biology of the Rantes/SIS cytokine family. Cytokine 1991; 3:165–183.
131. Srivastava BI, Srivastava A, Srivastava MD. Phenotype, genotype and cytokine production in acute leukemia involving progenitors of dendritic Langerhans cells. Leukocyte Res 1994; 18:499–511.
132. Bendelac A, Matzinger P, Seder RA *et al.* Activation events during thymic selection. J Exp Med 1992; 175:731–742.
133. Arase H, Arase N, Nakagawa K *et al.* NK1.1+, CD4+, CD8− thymocytes with specific lymphokine secretion. Eur J Immunol 1993; 23:307–310.
134. Wang Y, Watson RR. Vitamin E supplementation at various levels alters cytokine production by thymocytes during retrovirus infection causing murine AIDS. Thymus 1994; 22:153–156.
135. Leclercq G, De Smedt M, Plum J. Cytokine production and responsiveness of fetal T-cell receptor V gamma 3 thymocytes. Scand J Immunol 1992; 36:833–841
136. leite de Moraes MD, Minoprio P, Dy M *et al.* Endogenous IL-10 and IFN-gamma production controls thymic cell proliferation in mice acutely infected by Trypanosoma cruzi. Scand J Immunol 1994; 39:51–58.
137. Pedersen H, Andersen A, Ropke C. Human thymic epithelial cells in serum-free culture: changes in cytokine production in primary and successive culture periods. Immunol Lett 1994; 41:43–48.
138. Kirnbauer R, Kock A, Schwarz T *et al.* IFN-beta 2, B cell differentiation factor 2, or hybridoma growth factor (IL-6) is expressed and released by human epidermal cells and epidermoid carcinoma cell lines. J Immunol 1989; 142:1922–1928.
139. Stadnyk AW. Cytokine production by epithelial cells. FASEB J 1994; 8:1041–1047.
140. Campochiaro PA. Cytokine production by retinal pigmented epithelial cells. Int Rev Cytol 1993; 146:75–82.
141. Savnborg C, Agace W, Hedges S *et al.* Bacterial adherence and mucosal cytokine production. Ann N Y Acad Sci 1994; 730:162–181.
142. Elias JA, Zheng T, Einarsson O *et al.* Epithelial interleukin-11. Regulation by cytokines, respiratory syncytial virus, and retinoic acid. J Biol Chem 1994; 269:22261–22268.

143. Maruyama H, Toda K, Uno K *et al.* Murine endothelial cell line cells, F-2: interactions with leukocyte and cytokine production. Microbiol Immunol 1993; 37:895–903.
144. Delomenie C, Wautier-Pepin MP, Chappey O, Wautier JL. Modulation of human endothelial cell activation by antiproliferative cytokines: exploration of arachidonic acid and intracellular cytokine pathways as possible mechanisms of action. Exp Cell Res 1993; 207:122–130.
145. Feder LS, Todaro JA, Laskin DL. Characterization of interleukin-1 and interleukin-6 production by hepatic endothelial cells and macrophages. J Leukocyte Biol 1993; 53:126–132.
146. Jeannin P, Delneste Y, Gosset P *et al.* Histamine induces interleukin-8 secretion by endothelial cells. Blood 1994; 84:2229–2233.
147. Suen Y, Chang M, Lee SM *et al.* Regulation of interleukin-11 protein and mRNA expression in neonatal and adult fibroblasts and endothelial cells. Blood 1994; 84:4125–4134.
148. Sano E, Iizuka M, Kobayashi S. Effect of glucocorticoid hormones on growth of human fibroblast cells and interferon production in a microcarrier culture system. Cell Struct Funct 1987; 12:509–517.
149. Rossano F, Rizzo A, Sanges MR *et al.* Human monocytes and gingival fibroblasts release tumor necrosis factor-alpha, interleukin-1 alpha and interleukin-6 in response to particulate and soluble fractions of Prevotella meloaninogenica and Fusobacterum nucleatum. Int J Clin Lab Res 1993; 23:165–168.
150. DeLarco J, Todaro G. Growth factors from sarcoma virus-transformed cells. Proc Natl Acad Sci USA 1978, 75: 4001–4008.
151. Kelly J, Fabisiak JP, Hawes K, Absher M. Cytokine signaling in lung: transforming growth factor-beta secretion by lung fibroblasts. Am J Physiol 1991; 260:pL123–pL128.
152. Zilberstein A, Ruggieri R, Korn JH, Revel M. Structure and expression of cDNA and genes for human interferon-beta-2, a distinct species inducible by growth-stimulatory cytokines. EMBO J 1986; 5:2529–2537.
153. Rathanaswami P, Hachicha M, Wong WL *et al.* Synergistic effect of interleukin-1 beta and tumor necrosis factor alpha on interleukin-8 gene expression in synovial fibroblasts. Evidence that interleukin-8 is the major neutrophil-activating chemokine released in response to monokine activation. Arthritis Rheum 1993; 36:1295–1304.
154. Du XX, Williams DA. Interleukin-11: a multifunctional growth factor derived from the hematopoietic microenvironment. Blood 1994; 83:2023–2030.
155. Batova A, Danielpour D, Pirisi L, Creek KE. Retinoic acid induces secretion of latent transforming growth factor beta 1 and beta 2 in normal and human papillomavirus type 16-immortalized human keratinocytes. Cell Growth Differ 1992; 3:763–772.
156. Kutsch CL, Norris DA, Arend WP. Tumor necrosis factor-alpha induces interleukin-1 alpha and interleukin-1 receptor antagonist production by cultured human keratinocytes. J Invest Dermatol 1993; 101:79–85.
157. Gueniche A, Viac Charveron M, Schmitt D. Effect of gamma-interferon on IL-1 alpha, beta and receptor antagonist production by normal human keratinocytes. Exp Dermatol 1994; 3:113–118.
158. Peterseim UM, Sarkar SN, Kupper TS. Production of IL-3 by non-transformed primary neonatal murine keratinocytes: evidence for constitutive IL-3 gene expression in neonatal epidermis. Cytokine 1993; 5:240–249.
159. Heufler C, Topar G, Grasseger A *et al.* Interleukin 7 is produced by murine and human keratinocytes. J Exp Med 1993; 178:1109–1114.

160. Takematsu H, Tagami H. Mode of release of interleukin-8 from proliferating human epidermal keratinocytes in vitro. Exp Dermatol 1993; 2:121–124.
161. Nickoloff BJ, Fivenson DP, Kunkel SL *et al.* Keratinocyte interleukin-10 expression is upregulated in tape-stripped skin, poison ivy dermatitis, and Sezary syndrome, but not in psoriatic plaques. Clin Immunol Immunopathol 1994; 73:63–68.
162. Lagneaux L, Delforgr A, Doval C *et al.* Excessive production of transforming growth factor-beta by bone marrow stromal cells in B-cell chronic lymphocytic leukemia inhibits growth of hematopoietic precursors and interleukin-6 production. Blood 1993; 82:2379–2385.
163. Tasaka K, Mio M, Shimazawa M, Nakaya N. Histamine-induced production of interleukin-1 alpha from murine bone marrow stromal cells and its inhibition by H2 blockers. Mol Pharmacol 1993; 43:365–371.
164. Agui T, Xin X, Cai Y *et al.* Stimulation of interleukin-6 production by endothelin in rat bone marrow-derived stomal cells. Blood 1994; 84:2531–2538.
165. Anthony EN, Schmierer AE, March CJ *et al.* B cell precursor growth-promoting activity: purification and characterization of a growth factor active on lymphocyte precursors. J Exp Med 1988; 167:988–1002.
166. Sakata T, Iwagami S, Tsuruta Y *et al.* Constitutive expression of interleukin-7 mRNA and production of IL-7 by a cloned murine thymic stromal cell line. J Leukocyte Biol 1990; 48:205–212.
167. Brenner T, Yamin A, Abramsky O, Gallily R. Stimulation of tumor necrosis factor-alpha production by mycoplasmas and inhibition by dexamethasone in cultured astrocytes. Brain Res 1993; 608:273–279.
168. Sharif SF, Hariri RJ, Chang VA *et al.* Human astrocyte production of tumour necrosis factor-alpha, interleukin-1 beta, and interleukin-6 following exposure to lipopolysaccharide endotoxin. Neurol Res 1993; 15:109–112.
169. Sawada M, Suzumura A, Itoh Y, Marunouchi T. Production of interleukin-5 by mouse astrocytes and microglia in culture. Neurosci Lett 1993; 155:175–178.
170. Maimone D, Cioni C, Rosa S *et al.* Norepinephrine and vasoactive intestinal peptide induce IL-6 secretion by astrocytes: synergism with IL-1 beta and TNF alpha. J Neuroimmunol 1993; 47:73–81.

# 7 Interleukin-2

**MELISSA J. McILRAITH and PETER E. LIPSKY**
*The University of Texas Southwestern Medical Center at Dallas, Dallas, Texas, USA*

## INTRODUCTION

Interleukin-2 (IL-2) is a 17-kDa glycoprotein that was initially identified as a component of an activated T-cell supernatant that was capable of stimulating proliferation of T cells, and was, therefore, originally designated a T-cell growth factor[1,2]. Molecular cloning of the IL-2 gene from T cells and subsequent production of recombinant IL-2[3] has allowed investigation of the role this cytokine plays in other aspects of immunologic responses. These studies have revealed the important role of IL-2 in regulation of B-cell function in both murine and human systems. IL-2 has been characterized as a non-specific B-cell growth factor and as a stimulatory molecule for B-cell differentiation and subsequent immunoglobulin (Ig) production and secretion. Recent studies have begun to characterize the intracellular pathways by which IL-2 exerts its effects on B cells, focusing on those aspects that may be convergent or divergent from pathways delineated for other cytokines.

IL-2 can be placed in the hematopoietin family, based upon structural similarities of the receptors for these cytokines, as well as common structural motifs among the cytokines themselves[4,5]. The extracellular domains of these receptors consist of two fibronectin type III domains. The membrane-distal domain contains a set of four spaced cysteines, whereas the membrane-proximal domain contains a WSXWS motif. The cytokine members of the group whose structures have been characterized (IL-2, growth hormone, IL-4, IL-5 and granulocyte/macrophage colony-stimulating factor (GM-CSF)[6] share a similar tertiary structure that has been described as a 'four-helix bundle with long overhand loops' (reviewed in reference 7). Although some members of this family have been characterized as closely related molecules by chromosomal association of the genes encoding the cytokines[8–10], IL-2 is not included in this group, because its regulation and functions are distinct from those of the other hematopoietins.

*Cytokine Regulation of Humoral Immunity: Basic and Clinical Aspects.* Edited by Clifford M. Snapper.

## SOURCE

IL-2 is mainly produced by activated T cells. In the mouse, IL-2 is produced by the Th1 subset, although Th0 cells are also capable of IL-2 production[11–13]. This differential IL-2 production partially correlates with Th1 support of cell-mediated immune responses versus Th2 support of humoral responses[14]. It has become clear, however, that Th1 cells are able to support the differentiation of antibody-secreting cells, although the isotypes of Ig differ from that supported by Th2 cells[15,16]. This and more direct results have clearly indicated that IL-2 has direct effects on B cells, including support of growth, maturation, and differentiation to antibody-secreting cells. In addition, there is some evidence that activated B cells may themselves be able to secrete small amounts of IL-2, indicating that an autocrine pathway may exist for this cytokine in B cells.[17]

## RECEPTOR

The IL-2 receptor complex has been studied in both T and B cells. The overall structure appears to be essentially the same in both cell types and includes three polypeptide chains denoted alpha ($\alpha$), beta ($\beta$) and gamma ($\gamma$). These chains combine to form receptors with different affinities for IL-2 (reviewed in references 18 and 19).

The $\alpha$ chain (also termed the Tac antigen, CD25) has an apparent molecular mass of 55 kDa and by itself binds IL-2 with low affinity ($k_D \sim 10^{-8}$ M)[20–22]. The cytoplasmic domain of the $\alpha$ chain contains only 13 amino acids (AA) and is not thought to be involved in cytoplasmic signaling.

The heterodimerization of the $\beta$ and $\gamma$ chains creates an IL-2 receptor of intermediate affinity ($k_D \sim 10^{-9}$ M). The $\beta$ chain, with apparent molecular mass of 75 kDa, has a cytoplasmic domain of 286 AA[23], whereas the $\gamma$ chain (64 kDa) possesses a cytoplasmic region of 86 AA[24]. The importance of these chains of the IL-2 receptor in responses has been investigated in experiments utilizing chimeric constructs consisting of the extracellular portion of the IL-2R $\alpha$ chain in combination with the cytoplasmic domains of the $\beta$ or $\gamma$ chains[25]. Anti-IL-2R $\alpha$ chain antibodies triggered proliferation of cells transfected with these constructs, but not those expressing the intact $\alpha$ chain, indicating that the essential signaling properties of the IL-2R are contained in these two cytoplasmic regions.

Extensive characterization of the $\beta$ chain cytoplasmic domain by mutational analysis has allowed some assignment of functional regions to this portion of the molecule[26]. Cells expressing a truncated cytoplasmic region, in which the 'serine-rich' (AA 267–322) subregion was deleted, did not proliferate in response to IL-2, whereas cells expressing a construct lacking the 'acidic' (AA 313–382) subregion were able to respond to IL-2, although less well than wild-type receptor-expressing cells. Similar experiments have demonstrated that both the 'acidic' and 'serine-rich' regions are necessary for induction of $p21^{ras}$ and c-jun and c-fos expression in response to IL-2, and that each region appears to contain motifs important for interactions with specific protein tyrosine kinases (PTK)[26–29]. These findings indicate that although the β chain itself lacks a catalytic domain, the cytoplasmic portion of this molecule contains regions that have distinct roles in the transduction of IL-2-initiated signals. The importance of characterization of the β chain is further underlined by the recent evidence that has linked the β chain to activities of other IL receptor complexes. Preliminary data have indicated involvement of the β chain in responsiveness to IL-15 (IL-T), a cytokine produced by a variety of non-lymphoid cell lines as well as some leukemia cell lines, that largely mimics the biological activities of IL-2[30,31].

The γ chain of IL-2R is less well characterized but appears to be required for the internalization of IL-2R[24,32] and has been implicated in multiple cytokine response pathways. The documented involvement of the γ chain in the IL-2[24], IL-4[33], IL-7[34], IL-9[27], IL-15[30] and possibly IL-13[35] receptor complexes has led to the proposal that this polypeptide be donated the common cytokine gamma chain (γc)[34]. The essential nature of the γ chain has been demonstrated by the mapping of this gene to the same genetic locus as that responsible for X-linked severe combined immunodeficiency[36,37]. The absence of a functional γ chain in this disease state leads to a block in T-cell and natural killer (NK) cell differentiation, and while B cells are present, they appear to manifest altered responsiveness to cytokines. Studies utilizing anti-Ig or sCD40L in combination with cytokines to activate B cells from X-SCID patients revealed abrogation of responses to IL-2 and IL-15, but not to IL-4 or IL-13[38]. In contrast, analysis of B cells from mice in which expression of the γc chain has been deleted revealed defective responses to mitogen plus IL-2, IL-7 or IL-4[39]. These findings emphasize the importance of IL-2Rγ in T- and NK-cell generation and in B-cell function; however, the exact nature of the immune defect in X-SCID has not been delineated[40,41]. Whether this condition reflects a requirement for IL-2, IL-4, IL-7, IL-9, IL-13 or IL-15 in maturation of T and NK cells remains to be determined, and is indeed currently under examination in the mouse with the use of cytokine gene deletion transgenic animals[42–45].

The combination of the α, β and γ chains forms the high-affinity IL-2 receptor ($K_d \sim 10^{-11}$ M). This receptor utilizes both the rapid on-rate of the α chain and the slow off-rate of the β chain to increase the binding affinity over that of the intermediate-affinity receptor, while engaging the same signaling mechanisms (reviewed in references 18 and 46). Expression of high-affinity receptors is thought to be the hallmark of fully IL-2-responsive cells.

Although data are limited, there is no evidence that the structure or signaling potential of the IL-2 receptor differs in T and B cells. Therefore, it can be assumed, but requires rigorous verification, that the functional outcome of signaling B cells through the IL-2 receptor results from the induction of related biochemical events to those by which T cells are stimulated. The specific biochemical pathways involved in unique aspects of B-cell function have not been delineated, however.

## IL-2-INITIATED INTRACELLULAR SIGNALING

The mechanisms by which IL-2 exerts its effects on cellular activation and proliferation have begun to be characterized. Analyses of the IL-2-induced intracellular signaling pathways as well as examination of specific gene transcription stimulated in response to IL-2 have been carried out using cell lines of different lymphoid lineages, and give similar results.

Phosphorylations of intracellular proteins in response to extracellular stimuli appear to be pivotal events in transduction of signals to the nucleus. Analysis of protein phosphorylation in response to IL-2 has revealed rapid tyrosine phosphorylation of several cellular proteins, including the β chain of the IL-2 receptor (reviewed in references 18, 19 and 46). Serine/threonine kinases appear to be activated by IL-2 as analyzed in the human B-cell line SKW6.4[47]. Isolation of serine/threonine phosphorylated proteins from membrane preparations of these cells stimulated with IL-2 identified labeled proteins of 47, 49 and 91 kDa. Interestingly, stimulation of these membranes with other cytokines, such as IL-4 or IL-6, also induced phosphorylation of these same proteins, indicating that there was activation either of the same kinases by these cytokines, or different kinases with the same targets. Stimulation of whole cells with these cytokines led to phosphorylation of additional proteins of molecular mass 45–50 kDa and 85–90 kDa. Activation of both tyrosine and serine/threonine protein kinases appears to be necessary for signal transduction in this cell line, as inhibition of either abrogates cytokine-induced IgM secretion.

Tyrosine kinase activation appears to be linked to the β chain of the IL-2 receptor, as this molecule in T cells is itself phosphorylated in response to IL-2[48] and associated with multiple non-receptor-type PTKs, including the src-like kinase $p56^{lck}$[49–51]. IL-2 stimulation of B cells induces activation of another src-like kinase, $p56^{lyn}$[52]. Other substrates for the activated tyrosine kinase include phosphatidylinositol kinase (PI-3 kinase)[53–55], GTPase activating protein (GAP)[56], the serine/threonine kinase Raf-1[57,58], Jak1 and Jak3[27–29], and also an 85-kDa protein distinct from PI-3 kinase[59].

Among the proteins phosphorylated by IL-2 stimulation are included two members of the Janus family of kinases, Jak1 and Jak3[27–29]. After tyrosine phosphorylation and activation, these kinases associate selectively with the serine-rich domain of IL-2Rβ and the C-terminal region of IL-2Rγ respectively. Activation of these kinases and their association with the β and γ chains of the IL-2R appear to be necessary events in IL-2 signaling.

Tyrosine kinases appear to be responsible for the activation of p21$^{ras}$, as the accumulation of the active p21$^{ras}$–GTP complex is abrogated by a specific inhibitor of tyrosine kinases[60,61]. Functional characterization of the proteins phosphorylated in response to IL-2 as well as analysis of downstream signaling events initiated as a consequence of Raf-1 and p21$^{ras}$ activation may clarify the mechanisms of IL-2 stimulation of cell cycle entry and differentiation[58]. Events induced in this pathway of activation include stimulation of transcription of a number of genes thought to be active in control of cell cycle regulation, including *src* family PTK induction of the nuclear protooncogenes c-*fos* and c-*jun*[62], as well as other members of this gene family. These gene products, as well as c-myc induced by β-chain-associated Syk PTK[51], may be important regulators of cellular proliferation stimulated by IL-2. Recent evidence has also delineated a role for the proto-oncogene *bcl*-2 in stimulation of hematopoietic cell proliferation. Expression of any two of activated p56$^{lck}$, Bcl-2 or c-myc promoted cell cycle progression in the BAF-B03 cell line[63]. Analysis of other possible transmembrane signaling mechanisms such as those that occur in response to ligation of antigen receptors revealed no requirement for phosphatidylinositol hydrolysis[64,65], inositol triphosphate (InsP3)-induced $Cd^{2+}$ release[66], or protein kinase C activation[67,68] in IL-2-mediated signaling. Large and sustained $Ca^{2+}$ influx, as induced by the calcium ionophore ionomycin, inhibits IL-2-induced proliferation[69], as does accumulation of cAMP[69–71]. These events are distinct from those which result from stimulation of the IL-4 receptor with its cognate ligand, in which case cAMP accumulation, phospholipase C activation, and InsP3-induced $Ca^{2+}$ release are obligatory signaling events[72].

Examination of IL-2-induced signals as a whole has enabled classification of these events into two general groups (reviewed in reference 46). These events include those that occur within minutes of IL-2 binding, termed the immediate early events, and those that arise after longer exposure to IL-2, the late events. The former group includes association of p56$^{lyn}$ with the IL-2R β chain, phosphorylation of cellular proteins, and induction of a number of genes, including those for several cellular proto-oncogenes, multiple cytokines, and a novel protein tyrosine kinase (ITK). The late gene products appear to be involved in metabolism and growth, and include glycolytic enzymes, cyclins, cytolytic enzymes and the J chain of IgM, as well as some novel genes that have not yet been characterized.

## IL-2 EFFECTS ON B CELLS

IL-2 was initially characterized as a factor with growth- and differentiation-promoting properties for T cells. When additional effects were observed, such as an increase in Ig synthesis by mixed populations of lymphocytes or anti-IL-2 abrogation of Ig synthesis in Th-cell-supported Ig production[73,74], this was ascribed to an indirect effect related to expansion of helper T cells[75]. With the advent of cloned cell lines and techniques capable of separating different populations of freshly isolated lymphocytes obtained from blood or lymphoid organs, it became feasible to characterize the effects of lymphokines such as IL-2 on individual cell types directly.

Initial experiments that examined the effects of IL-2 on B cells in the absence of T-cell help demonstrated no effect on functional responses of resting normal B cells and some B-cell lines[76–79]. However, when the effect of IL-2 was examined in combination with other co-stimuli, IL-2 was found to amplify B-cell responses dramatically. Both enhancement of proliferation and antibody production were noted in a variety of model systems[80,81]. For example, IL-2 was found to support the generation of antibody-secreting cells in response to sheep red blood cells (SRBC)[82,83]. Further support for a role of IL-2 in B-cell responses was provided by results indicating that IL-2 was able to replace accessory cells in supporting the generation of antigen-specific-antibody-forming cells from lipopolysaccharide (LPS)-stimulated murine spleen cells[84]. IL-2 was also found to enhance IgM production by murine B cells in response to both T-cell-dependent antigens and types 1 and 2 T-cell-independent antigens[85]. In addition, IL-2 was found to provide the 'second signal' necessary to induce the sustained proliferation of normal or malignant murine B cells or human B cells stimulated by crosslinking surface Ig[86–88].

These results clearly indicated that IL-2 directly influenced B-cell responses and led to studies examining the mechanism by which IL-2 affected B-cell function. If the IL-2-mediated effects on B cells were not mediated by T cells or other accessory cells, it was surmised that B cells must be able to interact directly with IL-2 and, therefore, must express IL-2 receptors. The development of IL-2 receptor-specific monoclonal antibodies[89,90] allowed characterization of IL-2 receptor expression on both T and B cells, and these reagents were used to examine whether B cells constitutively or in an activation-dependent manner express IL-2 receptors or upregulate expression of IL-2 receptors in response to specific activation signals.

## IL-2 RECEPTOR EXPRESSION

Purified B-cell preparations, including both murine and human malignant B-cell lines as well as freshly isolated cells from murine spleen and human spleen, peripheral blood and lymph node, were used in combination with polyclonal activators in order to examine the expression of IL-2 receptors, and the effects of IL-2 on these activated cell populations[25,91]. A lymphokine-responsive clone (3B3) of the murine *in vitro* derived Ly-1$^+$ (CD5) B-cell leukemia line, BCL1, responded directly to IL-2 by proliferating and secreting IgM[92]. This clone was found to express IL-2 receptors constitutively. By contrast, a Ly-1$^-$ *in vivo* derived BCL1 clone that did not express IL-2 receptors did not respond to IL-2. Constitutive IL-2 receptor expression by an immortalized B-cell line was also observed in human B cells that had undergone a loss of growth regulation[93].

Extensive characterization of freshly isolated B cells and cloned B cell lines from B-cell chronic lymphocytic leukemias (BCLL) and B-cell lymphomas has documented constitutive IL-2 receptor expression on a portion of these cells, as defined by monoclonal antibody (mAb) to the α chain of the IL-2R and resultant responsiveness to IL-2[94–101]. IL-2 alone could upregulate expression of IL-2 receptor, cause an increase in cell size consistent with activation, promote DNA synthesis, and induce Ig secretion by some of the IL-2R α-chain-expressing cells, indicating that high-affinity IL-2 receptors were also likely to be present or inducible[98]. In a variety of immortalized human B-cell lines, including a pre-B-cell acute lymphoblastic leukemia (BALL)[101], a prolymphocytic leukemia[102], an HTLV-transformed B-cell line[103,104], and hairy cell leukemia lines[105], expression of the α chain of the IL-2R was also detected without *in vitro* activation. In BCLL cells that did not constitutively express the IL-2R α chain, it could be induced by activation with protein kinase C activating phorbol esters (12-O-tetradecanoylphorbol 13-acetate(TPA)) alone or in combination with a calcium ionophore, B-cell differentiation factors, and presumably by IL-2 along with TPA or phytohemagglutinin (PHA), anti-Ig, or *Staphylococcus aureus* Cowan strain 1 (SAC), as these latter stimuli induced IL-2 responsiveness[106–112]. Other leukemic cell lines could be induced to express the α chain of the IL-2R (some BALL[113], CML-BC[114]) in response to PHA or TPA, or in the case of an immature leukemic cell line expressing B-cell-specific antigens, high-affinity IL-2 receptor expression could be induced in response to PMA[115].

Binding experiments have revealed the presence of high-affinity IL-2 receptors on some BALL cells[101]. Direct responsiveness of some of these cell lines to IL-2 is consistent with high- or intermediate-affinity receptor expression. Whereas the majority of B leukemic cells that expressed the α chain of the IL-2R or high-affinity receptors either constitutively or in response to activation stimuli were IL-2 responsive as measured by IL-2-induced proliferation or Ig secretion, expression of IL-2 receptors on these cells did not correlate absolutely with the ability of IL-2 to affect cell function directly[105,116]. Thus, other features of these cells, independent of IL-2 receptor expression, influenced responsiveness to this cytokine.

The data clearly show that many murine and human transformed B-cell lines constitutively express IL-2 receptors and can be functionally stimulated by IL-2. This evaluation has clearly established that B-lineage cells respond directly to this cytokine. The capacity of normal B cells to express IL-2 receptors and the ability of these cells to respond to IL-2 is more complex. Moreover, the exact role of IL-2 in modifying B-cell responsiveness directly *in vivo* during normal immune responses is problematic and not fully resolved.

Analysis of normal murine and human B cells yielded different results than observed for transformed B-cell lines when expression of IL-2 receptor and responsiveness were characterized. Examination of normal murine or human spleen B cells and human lymph node and peripheral blood cells initially indicated that these cells did not express the α chain of the IL-2 receptor in the absence of an *in vitro* activation stimulus and were unresponsive to IL-2[78,117–120]. By contrast, direct stimulation of purified human B cells with IL-2 was noted when large concentrations were employed to stimulate tonsillar B cells[121–125]. Subsequent separation of small, dense B cells (presumably resting cells) and large, less dense cells (thought to be *in vivo* activated) revealed that the IL-2-responsive population resided within the large cell fraction[126,127].

Poor or no direct response to IL-2 was noted with human peripheral blood B cells, a population that would be expected to contain fewer activated B cells[128]. These results and subsequent examination of IL-2 receptor expression by fractionated B cells appear to indicate that truly resting B cells which have not been activated during purification do not express the α chain of the IL-2R.

Analysis of expression of the β chain of the IL-2 receptor on peripheral blood B cells has revealed that this chain may be expressed at low levels by non-activated human B cells and, therefore, may be involved in initial IL-2 signaling[129,130]. Experimental results demonstrating stimulatory properties of IL-2 on B cells and B-cell lines that fail to express the IL-2 receptor α chain support the conclusion that under some circumstances IL-2 may directly stimulate B cells by binding to the β chain that can be constitutively expressed by some B cells[131–133]. In general, these responses are characterized by the requirement for larger concentrations of IL-2, reflecting the diminished affinity of IL-2 receptors that do not include the α chain[134]. The characteristics as well as differentiation and activation status of the B cells that constitutively express the β chain of the IL-2 receptor have not been defined. Moreover, the importance or role of such B cells in immune responses *in vivo* have not been determined.

## IL-2 AS A GROWTH AND DIFFERENTIATION FACTOR FOR B CELLS

In most experimental systems examining B-cell responses to IL-2, an initial activation stimulus is required for B cells to acquire the ability to respond to IL-2. This may reflect *in vivo* immune responses in which initial B-cell stimulation by antigen results in subsequent responsiveness to T-cell-derived factors. This initial contact with antigen presumably involves signaling through the antigen receptor, surface Ig. Therefore, model systems have been developed to mimic this interaction in order to study the acquisition of responsiveness to T-cell-derived cytokines. These model systems involve activation of B cells by stimulation with the mitogens *Staphylococcus aureas* Cowan strain 1 (SAC) or anti-Ig antibodies, both of which engage B-cell surface Ig; LPS or membranes from Gram-negative bacteria; PHA or pokeweed mitogen (PWM); as well as agents designed to stimulate the intracellular second messenger cascade directly, including protein kinase C (PKC) activating phorbol esters alone or in combination with a calcium ionophore. Initial activation of B cells with these polyclonal activators has allowed delineation of the acquisition of IL-2 responsiveness and subsequent details of IL-2 signaling and responsiveness.

## MURINE B CELLS

In studies involving murine spleen cells, LPS has been most frequently used to provide an initial activation stimulus. Incubation of murine spleen cells with LPS induces enlargement of these cells and subsequent responsiveness to other immunomodulatory factors, and, in some cases, directly stimulates proliferation[91]. LPS-stimulated B-cell blasts have been examined for responsiveness to IL-2. Both the influence of this cytokine as a growth factor for B cells, and its function as a differentiation factor, have been examined. In cultures of murine LPS-stimulated spleen B cells, IL-2 alone has been shown to be capable of directly stimulating proliferation of the B-cell blasts or enhancing LPS-stimulated proliferation[135,136]. This result is consistent with the finding that IL-2 promoted proliferation of murine B cells activated by hapten-conjugated Ficoll[137]. Also supporting a direct role for IL-2 as a murine B-cell growth factor are the results obtained using anti-IgM as an inducer of B-cell blastogenesis and the demonstration that IL-2 enhanced proliferation of the resultant B-cell blasts [86,138]. These data provide direct evidence of a role for IL-2 in support of proliferation of activated B cells and document that IL-2 can act as a growth factor for murine B cells.

Additional experiments have addressed the role of IL-2 as a differentiation factor for activated murine B cells. Using murine spleen cells stimulated by LPS, anti-IgM or antigen, direct effects of IL-2 on Ig production by B cells have been examined. In a number of experiments employing these various activation stimuli, IL-2 was able to promote differentiation of activated B-cell precursors into Ig-secreting effector cells[86,139]. Similarly, LPS stimulated spleen B-cell blasts that proliferated but did not differentiate into antibody-forming cells (AFCs) in the absence of another stimulus were induced to generate AFCs by IL-2[91]. When LPS-activated B cells were fractionated into large, low-density and small, high-density cell populations, stimulation of each with IL-2 and antigen induced an antibody response, although the small cells were unable to proliferate in response to IL-2. These results indicate that IL-2 has a distinct role in the differentiation of B cells into Ig-secreting cells that is not necessarily dependent on proliferation[136]. Similarly, when resting and partially *in vivo* activated spleen cells were fractionated by density gradient centrifugation and examined for the ability to mount a polyclonal response upon stimulation with insoluble anti-Ig, IL-2 was noted to enhance the Ig secretion by each population[140]. In other experiments utilizing the activation properties of anti-Ig, IL-2 was noted to synergize with other cytokines in upregulating Ig synthesis by anti-Ig-stimulated B cells[139]. IL-2 was also able to enhance specific antibody responses by resting B cells stimulated with the T-cell-independent antigen TNP-Ficoll[140]. Finally, IL-2 was able to induce Ig production by the malignant B-cell line BCL1 without additional stimulation because these cells express IL-2 receptors constitutively[92]. These results clearly establish that IL-2 is both a growth and differentiation factor for a number of functionally defined murine B-cell subsets. The capacity of IL-2 to induce B-cell differentiation appears to be distinct from its capacity to support the growth of activated B cells. Initial activation signals are required to induce high-affinity IL-2 receptor expression for the B-cell growth and differentiation properties of IL-2 to become apparent.

The data indicating a role for IL-2 in murine B-cell differentiation by cells stimulated to express IL-2 receptors are consistent with results obtained in cultures of murine B cells stimulated by T-helper cell clones (Th). Activated Th can induce blast formation by B cells, and when these blasts are isolated and stimulated with IL-2, Ig of multiple isotypes is secreted[141]. Similarly, in cultures of B cells with Th1 cells, the use of inhibitors of cytokine production has clearly shown that IL-2 alone is sufficient to induce Ig synthesis by the B cells[142]. These activated T cells probably express CD40L which, in combination with IL-2, was shown to be necessary to stimulate antigen-specific Ig production in murine B cells[143]. IL-2 responsiveness in this system is therefore likely to be induced by CD40 ligation that upregulates IL-2R expression.

These results are consistent with findings demonstrating that a variety of Th1 clones that produce IL-2 have the capacity to promote Ig production by murine B cells. Examination of the interaction molecules involved in IL-2-supported and T-cell-dependent B-cell differentiation have revealed the necessity for signals in addition to those induced by CD40–CD40L interactions, as ligation of CD40 alone on murine B cells does not render them responsive to IL-2[144]. However, IL-2 can prepare CD40L-stimulated B cells to manifest enhanced Ig production upon subsequent stimulation with dextran-conjugated anti-IgD and IFN-γ[145].

Taken together, the data clearly show that IL-2 is a non-specific growth and differentiation factor for activated murine B cells. Both B cells responsive to T-cell-independent antigens and those responsive to T-cell-dependent antigens can be induced to grow and differentiate after initial activation in response to IL-2.

Increasing evidence has demonstrated that arrays of specific cytokines may be essential to regulate B-cell responses. Cytokines with broad effects, such as IL-2, may be influenced by the action of other cytokines to produce a more directed response, whereas additional cytokines may render cells more responsive to IL-2. For example, IL-5 has been shown to upregulate IL-2R expression on DNP primed murine B cells[146], BCL1 cells[147], and B cells polyclonally activated either by crosslinking ICAM-1 and MHC II[144], or by LPS[146,148,149]. IL-5 can also synergize with IL-2 to induce Ig secretion from LPS-stimulated B cells[149] and with IL-4/IL-5 to enhance IgG4 secretion from anti-Ig-induced B-cell blasts[139,150]. IL-5 has an almost additive effect on IL-2-induced J chain transcription in BCL1 cells, although the same promoter binding proteins appear to be involved, indicating the possible convergence of two activation pathways[151].

Murine IL-2 appears to synergize with anti-Ig and BCGF-α to stimulate proliferation of LPS-activated B cells[152], and IL-6 upregulates antigen-specific Ig secretion activated by IL-2 stimulation of antigen-primed spleen B cells[153].

Transforming growth factor beta (TGF-β) has been shown to induce isotype switch to IgA preferentially, although IL-2 plays a role in both production and switch to IgA secretion by B cells[154,155].

IL-4 stimulates IL-2Rβ expression in murine splenic B cells and synergizes with interferon gamma (IFN-γ) or anti-IgM for higher levels of expression[156]. However, *in vivo* studies indicate that IL-2 inhibits IL-4-dependent IgE and IgG1 production as examined in a model system utilizing Nb (*Nippostrongylus brasiliensis*) infection to induce IL-4-producing $CD4^+$ T cells. Similarly, IL-2 suppresses IL-4-induced IgE and IgG1 germline transcription and switch recombination by normal B cells activated with LPS[157].

IL-2 also plays a role in B-cell responses to TI-2 antigens. Thus, dextran-conjugated anti-IgD antibodies stimulated resting murine B-cell proliferation, but not differentiation[140,158]. IL-2, in combination with IL-1, was unable to stimulate significant Ig production by these cells, but did render them responsive to induction of Ig production by IL-3 or GM-CSF, the combination of IL-3/GM-CSF being synergistic[159], and by IFN-γ, which could also synergize with IL-3 and GM-CSF[145]. Similarly, activation of resting murine B cells with CD40L and the combination of IL-1 and IL-2 did not induce Ig secretion unless the cells received a further activation signal via surface IgD ligation. This response could be enhanced by IFN[145].

IL-2 appears to be a critical factor in the *in vitro* growth and differentiation of both murine T and B cells, but the essential nature of IL-2 in immune responses *in vivo* is not as clearly defined. The availability of gene targeting techniques has allowed generation of homozygous IL-2-deficient mice in which the requirement for IL-2 could be assessed. In initial experiments examining B-cell maturation in these mice, cross examination surprisingly revealed roughly normal T- and B-cell development[45]. Examination of B-cell subsets, however, revealed a diminution of mature $B220^+$, $Ig^+$ B cells in both bone marrow and lymph nodes of IL-2 knockout mice as compared to wild-type mice. This apparent partial block in maturation occurred in concert with a relative increase in the number of pro- and pre-B cells in the bone marrow of IL-2-deficient mice, indicating that the absence of IL-2 in these animals may lead to dysregulation of B-cell maturation.

Analysis of the activation status and function of B cells in the animals deficient in IL-2 production revealed an increased number of activated B-cell blasts in the lymph node compared to that found in wild-type animals[44]. The presence of increased numbers of activated B cells correlated with an elevated number of IgG- and IgA-secreting cells in these animals. Both of these abnormalities were presumably the result of T-cell-independent stimulation of the B cells owing to the development of inflammatory bowel disease triggered by normal enteric bacterial flora[160]. Abnormalities in T-cell-dependent B-cell responses were suggested by the deficient capacity of IL-2 knockout T cells to support Ig production by anti-IgM-stimulated normal B cells unless exogenous IL-2 was present[45].

As provocative as these results appear to be, they do not provide direct evidence of a role for IL-2 in B-cell responsiveness, as all of the results could be explained by an indirect, but necessary, action of IL-2 in the maturation of helper T cells. It is clear, however, that there is no absolute defect in B-cell function in the IL-2 knockout mice. Thus, they not only respond to T-cell-independent stimulation, but can also produce antibody to viral antigens *in vivo*, although the maturation of this response with switch to IgG antibody is considerably delayed[43]. The possibility that production of cytokines with similar activities to those of IL-2, such as IL-15[31,161], might account for the lack of more significantly delayed T-cell-dependent humoral responses has not been examined.

## HUMAN B-CELL RESPONSES TO IL-2

BCLL cell lines, in keeping with constitutive IL-2 receptor expression, can respond directly to IL-2[162]. Addition of IL-2 to these cells can induce both proliferation[99,163,164] and secretion of IgM[93,165–167], indicating a role for IL-2 in both processes. Unlike immortalized B-cell lines in which a loss of growth regulation has occurred, normal resting human B cells do not constitutively express the IL-2 receptor[78,117,168]. Stimulation with SAC induces normal resting human B cells to express the IL-2 receptor α chain[78,117,120,168–172] and to respond to IL-2 with differentiation[117,118,125,167,173–178] and a level of proliferation greater than that induced by SAC alone[118,179–186]. Most B cells activated for 3 days with SAC were found to express the α chain of the IL-2 receptor[187]. Moreover, IL-2 drove these cells to progress through the cell cycle, as more than 30 per cent of the B cells were found to be in G2 + M in the presence of IL-2[184]. Fractionation of SAC-activated B cells revealed that more than 80 per cent of the large, low-density cells expressed IL-2 receptors, whereas only 45 per cent of the partially activated fraction expressed IL-2 receptors, and few of the high-density resting population expressed the α chain of the IL-2 receptor[171]. These results clearly indicate that IL-2 receptors are expressed by human B-cell blasts, the population that is induced to respond to IL-2.

When SAC-activated B cells were cultured for a further 4 days without stimulation, the cells progressively expressed less of the α chain of the IL-2 receptor and became less responsive to IL-2, whereas IL-2 maintained expression of IL-2 receptors[187]. These results show that once IL-2 receptors are expressed, maintenance of their expression and responsiveness to IL-2 is upregulated by IL-2 signaling. Thus, IL-2 itself appears to be required to facilitate not only proliferation and differentiation, but also maintenance of the IL-2-responsive state. Similarly, cells initially stimulated with SAC and IL-2 and subsequently examined for IL-2 responsiveness were found to proliferate and differentiate to a higher degree than those activated with SAC alone, consistent with a role for IL-2 in the initial induction of B-cell IL-2 responsiveness[118].

IL-2 has been demonstrated to induce or enhance proliferation of SAC-activated human B cells isolated from both peripheral blood and lymphoid organs. SAC-stimulated B cells from blood, spleen and lymph nodes were all documented to respond to IL-2 with enhanced proliferation, although lymph node cells showed a reduced level of IL-2-induced proliferation[117]. In addition, IL-2 alone stimulated Ig secretion from SAC-activated cells. Again, lymph node B cells appeared to be refractory to SAC + IL-2 stimulation and did not secrete antibody in response to these signals. The explanation for the inability of lymph node B cells to secrete Ig in response to SAC and IL-2 is unclear, but the result is consistent with the conclusion that the stage of B-cell activation or differentiation at which IL-2 acts may be limited.

Studies of tonsillar B cells have documented proliferative and differentiative responses to SAC + IL-2 stimulation, but variability between individual donors has been noted. In addition, tonsillar B cells have been noted to produce Ig of various isotypes in response to stimulation with recombinant CD40 ligand and IL-2[188]. These results clearly show that human B cells can proliferate and differentiate into Ig-secreting cells in response to T-cell-independent and T-cell-dependent polyclonal activation signals and IL-2.

Other methods of initial activation have also been used to delineate the effect of IL-2 on human B-cell proliferation and differentiation. Ligation of B-cell surface Ig with anti-Ig stimulates expression of the α chain of the IL-2 receptor[78,189,190] and some B-cell proliferation[131,142,191–193]. IL-2 augments anti-Ig-stimulated cell cycle entry[117] and also induces some Ig production from these activated cells[117,190]. LPS-activated tonsillar B cells also produce Ig in response to IL-2[194]. Activation with a Gram-negative bacterial membrane induces B cells to express the α chain of the IL-2 receptor and responsiveness to IL-2 manifested by proliferation and enhancement of Ig production[195]. Other polyclonal activators, including PWM, also induce IL-2 receptor expression on normal human B cells[196,197].

Peripheral blood B cells from different individuals have been shown to manifest markedly different responses to SAC and IL-2, with high- and low-responder phenotypes noted[198]. These high- and low-response phenotypes revealed by stimulation with SAC and IL-2 were stable over a period of months. Cell cycle analysis revealed that B cells isolated from low responders showed less cell cycle advancement after SAC and IL-2 stimulation, as well as less expression of the α chain of the IL-2 receptor than those of high responders. Examination of Ig secretion demonstrated that the low responders secreted no Ig in response SAC + IL-2, but that Ig-secreting cell (ISC) formation was inducible in the high-responder population. These results may reflect differences in the *in vivo* activation status of B cells, although the explanation of these findings has not been completely delineated. Since SAC has been claimed to stimulate $CD5^+$ B cells primarily[199], the differences could also reflect variability in the appearance of this population in peripheral blood. Of importance is the fact that the basis of the high- and low-responder phenotype does not appear to relate to intrinsic differences in IL-2 responsiveness, but rather to the capacity of SAC to induce IL-2 responsiveness as manifested by expression of the α chain of the IL-2 receptor. To date, little variation in IL-2 responsiveness has been noted in normal individuals.

In studies examining B-cell responses to T-cell-dependent antigen, IL-2 was able to induce Ig production by B cells activated in the presence of T cells and influenza virus[200]. The IL-2-responsive cells were found to be in the low-density activated population, again indicating that activated B cells express IL-2 receptors and become responsive to IL-2. In this system, antigen presentation to specific T cells is likely to lead to T-cell expression of the CD40 ligand and their resultant capacity to induce B-cell IL-2 responsiveness by ligation of B-cell CD40, as has been shown for polyclonally activated T cells and B cells stimulated by recombinant CD40 ligand. The details of the pathway of B-cell activation in this antigen-specific model system have not been analyzed. Studies utilizing membrane-bound CD40L to stimulate B cells showed that IL-2 enhanced CD40L or CD40L and IL-4 stimulated proliferation. Ig secretion by CD40L-stimulated cells was also enhanced by IL-2, whereas IL-2 did not affect CD40/IL-4-induced IgG4 or IgE secretion[188]. Data obtained using anti-CD40 mAb to stimulate normal B cells, including both the $CD5^-$ and $CD5^+$ populations[201], indicated the capacity of immobilized anti-CD40 or soluble CD40L to render B cells directly responsive to IL-2 for Ig secretion[202–204], enhancement of IL-4-induced IgM and IgA production[205], synergy with IL-10 for Ig secretion[201,104,206], and, in contrast to membrane-bound recombinant CD40L stimulation, inhibition of IL-4-induced IgE and IgG4 production[202]. These results indicate that the CD40 signaling pathway may induce B-cell responsiveness to IL-2, perhaps partially via enhancement of IL-2R expression on B cells[206]. However, other studies involving both normal B cells[207] and BCLL cell lines[107] have indicated that signaling via CD40 alone is not sufficient to cause IL-2 responsiveness, as indicated by lack of Ig production in response to anti-CD40 and IL-2 stimulation. These differences may result from the manner in which CD40 ligation is achieved (membrane bound or soluble form), other factors which may be expressed in the cultures, or differences in the *in vivo* activation status of B cells from different sources, such as tonsil versus peripheral blood. Human B cells stimulated with a T-cell-independent antigen, TNP-Ficoll, also became responsive to the growth and differentiative effects of IL-2[208–210]. Similarly, B cells directly stimulated to enter the cell cycle via activation of intracellular signaling pathways by a phorbol ester and ionomycin respond to IL-2 by producing Ig of multiple isotypes[211].

These results clearly indicate a role for IL-2 in proliferation and differentiation of human B cells activated by both T-cell-dependent and T-cell-independent stimuli. Although it appears certain that IL-2 alone is sufficient to induce B cells that have been activated in a variety of ways to proliferate and differentiate, it remains unresolved whether IL-2 is necessary for these responses. A number of cytokines or activation signals appear to be able to promote initial B-cell proliferation as well as their sustained growth. Therefore, IL-2 is not necessary to promote initial clonal expansion of activated B cells. IL-2 appears to play a more essential role in the induction of Ig production. When resting B cells are activated by specific signals such as monoclonal antibodies to CD40, it is clear that IL-4, and perhaps its surrogate IL-13, is sufficient to promote Ig production[207,212–215]. However, in most other circumstances, including those in which B cells are stimulated by SAC or by activated fixed T cells, IL-2 appears to play a necessary role in Ig production. Studies examining the effects of other cytokines on SAC- and IL-2-induced proliferation and Ig production have revealed the presence of cytokine crosstalk *in vitro*. IL-6 was shown to enhance Ig secretion by normal B cells activated by SAC and IL-2[216–218] in the presence[219] or absence[220] of enhanced proliferation, perhaps via upregulation of IL-2R, as has been demonstrated on Epstein–Barr virus (EBV)-transformed B cells[221]. Release of soluble CD23 from SAC-activated B cells was increased by the combination of IL-2 and IL-6, possibly indicating a role for this cytokine interaction in regulation of IgE synthesis and B-cell differentiation[219–223].

It has recently been demonstrated that IL-12 can synergize with IL-2 to stimulate Ig production and proliferation of SAC-activated B cells, and to modestly enhance IL-2Rβ expression on SAC- or SAC + IL-2-stimulated cells[224].

IL-5 has also been shown to stimulate increased Ig production from SAC- and IL-2[184,225] or T-cell-activated B cells[226], consistent with its ability to upregulate IL-2R expression on human [147] and murine[146,148,149] B cells, thereby rendering them more IL-2 responsive.

IL-2R expression on polyclonally activated B cells was also enhanced in the presence of IL-1[227], and this cytokine synergized with IL-2 for increased

Ig production[217] and proliferation[175] by SAC-activated B cells. IL-3 was also shown to increase SAC + IL-2-stimulated Ig secretion[218].

IL-10 appears to stimulate enhanced expression of CD25 on SAC- or SAC + IL-2-activated B cells[228]. However, lack of increased IL-2 responsiveness by the B cells may indicate that the synergy between IL-10 and IL-2 for Ig production in this system may occur during maturation and not the initial activation phase.

Tumor necrosis factor alpha (TNF-α) also appears to render SAC-activated cells more responsive to IL-2 and enhances both proliferation and differentiation[175]. Interestingly, anti-Ig stimulation of tonsil B cells appears to upregulate TNFR-1 expression, particularly on mantle zone B cells[229]. The ability of B cells to produce TNF-α and IL-6 upon SAC + IL-2 stimulation may indicate autocrine pathways for these cytokines in perpetuating or enhancing immune responses[230].

In contrast to these synergistic cytokine relationships, IL-4 and IL-2 appear to be antagonistic in most situations. IL-2 appears to inhibit IL-4-induced IgE and IgG4 production *in vivo*[231]. Similarly, SAC + IL-2[220], SAC + IL-2/IL-6[232], anti-Ig + IL-2[110,191], and antigen + IL-2[233,234] -induced proliferation and differentiation are suppressed by IL0-4. This suppression is dependent upon actions of IL-4 during activation, as addition of IL-4 before IL-2 abrogated IL-2 responsiveness[168], and IL-4 enhances proliferation and differentiation of SAC-preactivated cells[194]. Studies involving examination of IL-2R expression on T cells in response to IL-4 indicate the possibility of IL-2R–IL-4R interactions, possibly via the γc chain, which is thought to be involved in both receptors[33,235,236] IL-4 suppression of SAC and IL-2 responses can be partially abrogated by IFN-γ, IFN-α, IL-1, or low molecular weight B-cell growth factor (LMW/BCGF), indicating a complicated network of cytokine interactions[170].

In contrast to the above results, IL-4 enhances Ig production from LPS + IL-2-stimulated B cells[194], and the combination of IL-2 and IL-4 is necessary to induce Ig secretion in CsA (cyclosporine) blocked neonatal cultures of T and B cells[237], indicating that the mode of activation renders cells differentially responsive to cytokines. Similarly, IFN-γ enhances anti-Ig + IL-2-induced B-cell proliferation[110,191], but inhibits SAC + IL-2/IL-6-induced Ig secretion[216].

Although these results indicate that other cytokines, including IL-6, IL-10 and IL-12, can play a role in enhancing the amount of Ig produced, IL-2 plays an essential role in that all Ig production is inhibited by mAb to the IL-2 receptor. The results are consistent with the conclusion that IL-2 plays a sufficient role in proliferation and differentiation of activated B cells and a necessary role in differentiation of B cells resulting from many, but not all, stimuli.

## ISOTYPE PRODUCTION

A number of cytokines have been shown to influence production of specific Ig heavy chain isotypes. Isotype-specific effects of cytokines can result either from costimulation of B cells to undergo switch recombination to specific downstream heavy chain isotypes or by selectively stimulating production of Ig by post-switch B cells that already express a given downstream isotype. Examples of the former effect include the action of IL-4 on the induction of switch to IgE and that of TGF-β to switch to IgA, whereas IL-5 in the mouse stimulates IgA production by post-switch IgA expressing B cells[154,238–241]. The possibility that IL-2 induces production of specific Ig heavy chain isotypes has been explored in a number of systems.

Experiments examining production of specific heavy chain isotypes by *in vitro* stimulated human B cells that have employed costimulation assays with various polyclonal activators have demonstrated that IL-2 supports production of all Ig isotypes. In one study, for example, examining cytokine effects on IgE production by mononuclear cells, IL-2 was found to increase the secretion of this isotype by six-fold, and the combination of IL-2 and IL-4 induced greater amounts of IgE than either cytokine alone[242]. Upregulation of the secretion of specific Ig isotypes by IL-2 in this mixed cell system could be the result of an effect of IL-2 directly on the B cells, either by promotion of the specific Ig isotype by post-switch B cells previously committed to produce it, or by influencing Ig isotype switch of cells previously producing other isotypes. Alternatively, the effects of IL-2 in this mixed cell culture could be indirect as a result of the impact of IL-2 on other cells, such as T cells, whose activation, growth and differentiation can be dramatically influenced by IL-2. Such IL-2-stimulated T cells could then influence B-cell responses. Similarly, NK cells or monocytes can also be stimulated by IL-2[243] and may produce cytokines which influence B-cell responses, as demonstrated in a murine model of TI-2 antigen B-cell stimulation[244]. Incubation of purified resting spleen B cells with dextran-conjugated anti-IgD and IL-2 failed to induce Ig secretion by these cells. However, addition of NK cells or activated NK cell supernatant supported B-cell maturation to Ig secretion. The factor involved in this NK-cell-induced B-cell differentiation has not yet been characterized. Other experiments have indicated a role for IFN-γ in rIL-2 stimulated NK cell induction of murine B-cell IgG2a production[245].

In order, therefore, to address the direct effect of IL-2 on human B-cell function, a number of studies have been carried out using highly purified B cells from various sources. One such set of experiments examined the effects of IL-2 on isotype production by purified human B cells isolated from tonsil, blood and spleen. In this study, a variety of polyclonal B-cell activators was employed[246]. SAC + IL-2 activation of tonsil B cells caused an upregulation of IgG1 production in relation to the other isotypes. Activation of the same cell population with LPS and IL-2 revealed a different profile of isotype production, with IgM being the predominant isotype, but with a significant induction of IgG2 secretion. Cells stimulated with IL-2 alone secreted some Ig, with IgM and IgG2 appearing as the predominant isotypes. This probably resulted from the presence of some *in vivo* activated B cells in the tonsil population. Stimulation of blood and spleen cells revealed less differential stimulation by SAC and LPS. SAC in combination with IL-2 induced production of all isotypes from these cells, but to a lower extent than in tonsil cells and without the dramatic upregulation of IgG1 production seen with the tonsil-derived cells. LPS stimulation of blood and spleen cells leads to less Ig production of all isotypes than that found in tonsil B cells activated similarly.

Additional studies examined Ig production by tonsillar B cells stimulated to enter the cell cycle by a phorbol ester and ionomycin[211]. These cells responded to IL-2 with production of multiple Ig isotypes, including IgM, IgA, IgG1 and IgG3. Finally, analysis of Ig production by adult human peripheral blood B cells in response to SAC and IL-2 demonstrated secretion of all isotypes, including IgE, with an enhancement of IgG1 synthesis in comparison to other cytokines[196,207,220]. Increased IgG1 production by human B cells in response to IL-2 was also shown in a system utilizing T cells as the B-cell stimulus[247,248]. In a T-cell/B-cell collaboration system involving co-culture of human B cells with an activated T-cell clone which secreted IL-2, synthesis of IgG1 was stimulated[249]. These results are consistent with the conclusion that B cells from different sources have different capacities to produce Ig isotypes, depending on the nature of the stimulus. However, no isotype-specific effect of IL-2 emerged. Rather, IL-2 appeared to promote secretion of a variety of Ig isotypes, the specific nature of which was determined by the source of the B cells and the costimulus. In one situation or the other, IL-2 could promote secretion of IgM as well as each of the IgG isotypes, IgA and IgE. There may be some bias toward production of IgG1 by IL-2 costimulation, but this effect is not absolute and may relate to the nature of the polyclonal activator employed or the differentiation state of the B cell examined.

Unresolved from these studies was whether IL-2 induced Ig production from post-switch B cells committed to a specific isotype or whether IL-2 could induce isotype switching to all downstream isotypes, since the population of B cells employed in most studies is a mixture of naive and pre-switch B cells and post-switch memory B cells. It has become clear from results of a number of investigators that IL-2 can induce Ig production from activated post-switch memory B cells that have previously switched to produce all downstream isotypes. However, the capacity of IL-2 to promote switch recombination has not been as clearly established, nor has the possible isotype specificity of this effect been completely delineated.

A number of approaches have been employed to determine whether IL-2 can induce switch recombination in naive B cells and whether such switching might be isotype specific. The most informative of these have been experiments employing purified populations of naive B cells. One such approach has utilized neonatal cord blood lymphocytes as a responding population[237,250]. When neonatal B cells were cultured with activated T cells that had been stimulated with monoclonal antibodies to the CD3 molecular complex, little Ig secretion was induced. Addition of IL-2, however, induced production of all isotypes of Ig, including IgE. Since neonatal cord blood B cells are entirely composed of naive pre-switch cells, these results are clearly consistent with the conclusion that IL-2 had induced Ig class switching non-specifically. Although other cytokines, including IL-4 and IL-6, enhanced Ig production, the effects of these additional cytokines were not isotype specific and were dependent on the presence of IL-2, as they were completely blocked by a mAb to the IL-2 receptor. In these experiments, however, isotype switch was only observed when B cells were costimulated with IL-2 and activated T cells, leaving open the question of the direct role of IL-2 in this process.

Experiments, utilizing cyclosporin to block cytokine production have also examined the role of T-cell-derived cytokines in switch recombination of naive adult B cells stimulated with activated T cells[251,252]. In these experiments, naive B cells from adult peripheral blood were obtained by sorting B cells expressing surface IgD. These cells have been shown to contain only pre-switch naive B cells. When these cells were cultured with anti-CD3 activated T cells in the presence of cyclosporin, no Ig was produced. However, when cultures were supplemented with IL-2, IgM as well as IgG and IgA were produced, implying that switch recombination had been induced. Similar results have been reported from experiments examining responses of human pre-immune cord blood B cells[250]. These results make it unlikely that T-cell-derived cytokines play a role in this process but do not rule out the possibility that other T-cell influences may play a role in switch recombination. Since, however, expression of CD40 ligand, one of the major T-cell surface molecules involved in T cell–B cell collaboration, is inhibited by cyclosporin[253], it is less likely that this molecule is necessary. Rather a direct role for IL-2 as an inducer of switch recombination to all downstream isotypes is implied.

In order to explore the role of IL-2 in Ig class switching more completely, an analysis of the initial molecular events was undertaken. One of the early molecular events in Ig heavy chain isotype switch is the induction of transcription of unrearranged heavy chain constant region genes[254–257]. The induction of these germline transcripts is followed by deletional DNA recombination of the heavy chain gene to be expressed. These germline transcripts (also called sterile transcripts) begin in a region known as the I region that is 5′ of the switch region for a given constant chain gene, and continue through the constant region gene. These transcripts are spliced and transported to the cytoplasm, but there does not appear to be a protein product, as each transcript contains multiple stop codons. Possible functions of sterile transcription include increasing the access of recombinases to the region being transcribed or facilitation of the action of the recombinase machinery. Although the exact role of sterile transcripts has not yet been elucidated, the process appears to be a prerequisite for switching, as demonstrated by the observations that interference with transcription by targeted disruption of promoter elements[258] or by anti-sense techniques inhibits switch recombination[259].

Analysis of germline transcrption in highly purified adult B cells revealed the capability of IL-2 to induce sterile IgG and IgE transcripts after stimulation with SAC[212]. Similarly, IL-2 induced IgG2 sterile transcripts and increased sterile IgG1 transcripts in SAC-activated $IgM^+$ adult peripheral blood B cells[260]. These results clearly indicate that IL-2 can induce the first step of switch recombination in activated naive B cells, without the influence of T cells. Additional experiments will be required to show whether there is specificity of the transcripts induced and whether IL-2 alone can promote subsequent steps in switch recombination and secretion of some or all downstream Ig isotypes.

## CONCLUSIONS

Although IL-2 was originally characterized as a T-cell growth factor, subsequent investigation has revealed roles for IL-2 in the stimulation of B-cell activation, proliferation and differentiation in both mice and humans. The presence of IL-2 at the time of B-cell activation appears to promote a cytokine-responsive state, and this, as well as the B-cell growth- and differentiation-promoting properties of IL-2, may have significant effects on the magnitude of immune responses. The importance of delineating the role of IL-2 in *in vivo* immune responses is underlined in consideration of clinical uses for IL-2. Intravenous IL-2 has been used in some patients with hypogammaglobulinemia to induce long-term production of protective Ig, indicating that this type of therapy may be useful in rescuing B-cell hyporesponsiveness, although the locus of action of IL-2 in this circumstance remains unclear[261]. Further characterization of possible stimulatory or inhibitory IL-2 effects on multiple cell types will be necessary before the full consequences of administration of this cytokine can be known.

IL-2 appears to exert pleiotropic effects on B-cell functions. Because it affects many interrelated aspects of B-cell biology, it has been difficult to isolate specific and unique effects of this cytokine on B-cell function. Lacking at this point is a clear-cut analysis of the role of specific signaling pathways in the induction of unique aspects of B-cell function. The biochemical events that might mediate B-cell growth, differentiation to Ig secretion, or switch recombination are unknown. Moreover, the interplay of IL-2 with other cytokines in regulating B-cell function is complicated and the specific biochemical and molecular events involved have not been delineated. Finally, the questions of whether IL-2 is required for specific events in B-cell biology or whether it provides a non-specific positive influence on B-cell function whose impact is regulated by costimulating cellular interactions and cytokines, remain to be resolved. Although many questions remain to be answered, the available data clearly indicate that IL-2 is a powerful inducer of activation, growth, and differentiation of IL-2 receptor-expressing B cells.

## REFERENCES


1. Morgan DA, Ruscetti FW, Gallo R. Selective in vivo growth of T lymphocytes from normal bone marrows. Science 1976; 193:1007–1008.
2. Smith KA. Interleukin 2. Annu Rev Immunol 1984; 2:319–333.
3. Taniguchi T, Matsui H, Fujita T *et al.* Structure and expression of a cloned cDNA for human interleukin-2. Nature 1983; 302:305–310.
4. Bazan J. A novel family of growth factor receptors: a common binding domain in the growth hormone, prolactin, erythropoetin, and IL-6 receptors, and in the p75 IL-2 receptor β chain. Biochem Biophys Res Commun 1989; 164:788–796.
5. Kishimoto T, Taga T, Akira S. Cytokine signal transduction. Cell 1994; 76:253–262.
6. McKay DB. Unraveling the structure of IL-2. Science 1992; 257:412–413.
7. Paul WE, Seder RA. Lymphocyte responses and cytokines. Cell 1994; 76; 241–251.
8. Boulay J-L, Paul WE. The interleukin-4 family of lymphokines. Curr Opin Immunol 1992; 4:294–298.
9. Boulay J-L, Paul WE. The interleukin-4-related lymphokines and their binding to hematopoietin receptors. J Biol Chem 1992; 267:20525–20528.
10. Boulay J-L, Paul WE. Hematopoietin sub-families: classification based on size, gene organization, and secondary structures. Curr Biol 1993; 3:573–581.
11. Cherwinski H, Schumacher J, Brown KD, Mosmann T. Two types of mouse helper T cell clone. III. Further differences in lymphokine synthesis between Th1 and Th2 clones revealed by RNA hybridization, functionally monospecific bioassays and monoclonal antibodies. J Exp Med 1987; 166:1229–1244.
12. Fiorentino DF, Bond MW, Mosmann TR. Two types of mouse T helper cell. IV. Th2 clones secrete a factor that inhibits cytokine production by Th1 clones. J Exp Med 1989; 170:2081–2095.
13. Mosmann TR, Cherwinski H, Bond MW *et al.* Two types of mouse helper T cell clone. II Definition according to profiles of lymphokine activities and secreted proteins. J Immunol 1986; 136:2348–2357.
14. Mosmann TR, Coffman RL. Two types of mouse helper T-cell clone: implications for immune regulation. Immunol Today 1987; 8:223–226.
15. Maeda-Yoshimoto K, Hirano T, Miyajima H *et al.* Suppression of IgE production in unseparated spleen cell cultures. Cell Immunol 1994; 153:277–286.
16. Reynolds DS, Boom WH, Abbas AK. Inhibition of B lymphocyte activation by interferon-gamma. J Immunol 1987; 139:767–773.
17. Justement LB, Krieger J, Cambier JC. Production of multiple lymphokines by the A20.1 B cell lymphoma after cross-linking of membrane Ig by immobilized anti-Ig. J Immunol 1989; 143:881–889.
18. Minami Y, Kono T, Miyazaki T, Taniguchi T. The IL-2 receptor complex: its structure, function, and target genes. Annu Rev Immunol 1993; 11:245–267.
19. Taniguchi T, Minami Y. The IL-2/IL-2 receptor system: a current overview. Cell 1993; 73:5–8.

20. Cosman D, Ceretti DP, Larsen A *et al.* Cloning, sequencing and expression of human interleukin-2 receptor. Nature 1984; 312:768–771.
21. Leonard WJ, Depper JM, Crabtree GR *et al.* Molecular cloning and expression of cDNAs for the human interleukin-2 receptor. Nature 1984; 311:626–631.
22. Nikaido T, Shimizu A, Ishida N *et al.* Molecular cloning of the cDNA encoding human interleukin-2 receptor. Nature 1984; 311:631–635.
23. Hatakeyama M, Tsudo M, Minamoto S *et al.* Interleukin-2 receptor β chain gene: generation of three receptor forms by cloned α and β chain cDNAs. Science 1989; 244:551–556.
24. Takeshita T, Asao H, Ohtani K *et al.* Cloning of the γ chain of the human IL-2 receptor. Science 1992; 257:379–382.
25. Nakamura Y, Russell SM, Mess SA *et al.* Heterodimerization of the IL-2 receptor β and γ chain cytoplasmic domains is required for signaling. Nature 1994; 369:330–333.
26. Hatakeyama M, Mori D, Doi T, Taniguchi T. A restricted cytoplasmic region of IL-2 receptor β chain is essential for growth signal transduction but not for ligand binding and internalization. Cell 1989; 59:837–845.
27. Russell SM, Johnston JA, Noguchi M *et al.* Interaction of IL-2R β and γc chains with Jak1 and Jak3: implications for X-SCID and XCID. Science 1994; 266:1042–1045.
28. Boussiotis VA, Barber D, Nakarai T *et al.* Prevention of T cell anergy by signaling through the γc chain of the IL-2 receptor. Science 1994; 266: 1039–1042.
29. Miyazaki T, Kawahara A, Fujii H *et al.* Functional activation of Jak1 and Jak3 by selective association with IL-2 receptor subunits. Science 1994; 266:1045–1047.
30. Giri JG, Ahdieh M, Eisenman J *et al.* Utilization of the β and γ chains of the IL-2 receptor by the novel cytokine. IL-15. EMBO J 1994; 13:2822–2830.
31. Grabstein KH, Eisenman J, Shanebeck K *et al.* Cloning of a T cell growth factor that interacts with β chain of the interleukin-2 receptor. Science 1994; 264:965–968.
32. Asao H, Takeshita T, Ishii N *et al.* Reconstitution of functional interleukin 2 receptor complexes on fibroblastoid cells: involvement of the cytoplasmic domain of the γ chain in two distinct signaling pathways. Proc Natl Acad Sci USA 1993; 90:4127–4131.
33. Russell SM, Keegan AD, Hrada N *et al.* Interleukin-2 receptor γ chain: a functional component of the interleukin-4 receptor. Science 1993; 262:1880–1883.
34. Noguchi M, Nakamura Y, Russell SM *et al.* Interleukin-2 receptor γ chain: a functional component of the interleukin-7 receptor. Science 1993; 262:1877–1880.
35. Zurawski SM, Vega F, Huyghe B, Zurawski G. Receptors for interleukin 13 and interleukin 4 are complex and share a novel component that functions in signal transduction. EMBO J 1993; 12:2663.
36. Noguchi M, Yi H, Rosenblatt HM *et al.* Interleukin-2 receptor gamma chain mutation results in X-linked severe combined immunodeficiency in humans. Cell 1993; 73:147–157.
37. DiSanto JP, Dautry-Varsat A, Certain S *et al.* Interleukin-2 (IL-2) receptor γ chain mutations in X-linked severe combined immunodeficiency disease result in the loss of high-affinity IL-2 receptor binding. Eur J Immunol 1994; 24:475–479.
38. Matthews DJ, Clark PA, Herbert J *et al.* Function of the interleukin-2 receptor gamma chain on biologic responses of X-linked severe combined immunodeficient B cells to IL-2, IL-4, IL-13, and IL-15. Blood 1995; 85:38–42.

39. DiSanto JP, Muller W, Guy-Grande D *et al.* Lymphoid development in mice with a targeted deletion of the interleukin 2 receptor $\gamma$ chain. Proc Natl Acad Sci USA 1995; 92:377–381.
40. DiSanto JP, Keever CA, Small TN *et al.* Absence of interleukin 2 production in a severe combined immunodeficiency disease syndrome with T cells. J Exp Med 1990; 171:1697–1704.
41. Di Santo JP, Le Deist F, Caniglia M *et al.* Variant forms of X-linked severe combined immunodeficiency disease: one or many genes? Immunodeficiency 1993; 4:253–258.
42. Kuhn R, Rajewsky K, Muller W. Generation and analysis of interleukin-4-deficient mice. Science 1991; 254:707–710.
43. Kundig TM, Schorle H, Bachmann MF *et al.* Immune responses in interleukin-2 deficient mice. Science 1993; 262:1059–1061.
44. Sadlack B, Kuhn R, Schorle H *et al.* Development of lymphocytes in mice deficient for both interleukins-2 and -4. Eur J Immunol 1994; 24:281–284.
45. Schorle H, Holtschke T, Hunig T *et al.* Development and function of T cells in mice rendered interleukin-2 deficient by gene targeting. Nature 1991; 352:621–624.
46. Beadling C, Smith KA. Tactics for the isolation of interleukin-2 induced immediate-early genes. Semin Immunol 1993; 5:365–373.
47. Goldstein H, Kim A. Immunoglobulin secretion and phosphorylation of common proteins are induced by IL-2, IL-4, and IL-6 in the factor responsive human B cell line SKW6.4. J Immunol 1993; 151:6701–6711.
48. Asao H, Takeshita T, Nakamura M *et al.* Interleukin 2 (IL-2)-induced tyrosine phosphorylation of the IL-2 receptor p75. J Exp Med 1990; 171:637–644.
49. Hatakeyama M, Kono T, Kobayashi N *et al.* Interaction of the IL-2 receptor with the src-family kinase $p56^{lck}$: identification of novel intermolecular association. Science 1991; 252:1523–1528.
50. Horak ID, Gress RE, Lucas PJ *et al.* T-lymphocyte interleukin 2-dependent tyrosine protein kinase signal transduction involves the activation of $p56^{lck}$. Proc Natl Acad Sci USA 1991; 88:1996–2000.
51. Minami Y, Nakagawa Y, Kawahara A *et al.* Protein tyrosine kinase Syk is associated with and activated by the IL-2 receptor: possible link with the *c-myc* induction pathway. Immunity 1995; 2:89–100.
52. Torigoe T, Saragovi HU, Reed JC. Interleukin 2 regulates the activity of the lyn protein-tyrosine kinase in a B-cell line. Proc Natl Acad Sci USA 1992; 89:2674–2678.
53. Augustine J, Sutor S, Abraham R. Interleukin 2- and polyomavirus middle T antigen-induced modification of phosphatidylinositol 3-kinase activity in activated T lymphocytes. Mol Cell Biol 1991; 11:4431–4440.
54. Merida I, Diez E, Gaulton G. IL-2 binding activates a tyrosine-phosphorylated phosphatidylinositol-3-kinase. J Immunol 1991; 147:2202–2207.
55. Remillard B, Petrilla R, Maslinski W *et al.* Interleukin-2 receptor regulates activation of phosphatidylinositol 3-kinase. J Biol Chem 1991; 266:14167–14970.
56. Mills GB, Zhang N, Schmandt R *et al.* Transmembrane signaling by interleukin 2. Biochem Soc Trans 1991; 19:277–287.
57. Turner B, Rapp U, App H *et al.* Interleukin 2 induces tyrosine phosphorylation and activation of p72–74 Raf-1 kinase in a T cell line. Proc Natl Acad Sci USA 1991; 88:1227–1231.
58. Zmuidzinas A, Mamon HJ, Robert TM, Smith K. Interleukin-2-triggered Raf-1 expression, phosphorylation, and associated kinase activity increase through G1 and S in CD3-stimulated primary T cells. Mol Cell Biol 1991; 11:2794–2803.

59. Minami Y, Kono T, Yamada K *et al.* Association of p56[lck] with IL-2 receptor β chain is critical for the IL-2-induced activation of p56[lck]. EMBO J 1993; 12:759–768.
60. Satoh T, Nakafuku M, Miyajima A, Kaziro Y. Involvement of ras in signal transduction pathways from interleukin-2, interleukin-3, and granulocyte-macrophage colony stimulating factor, but not from interleukin-4. Proc Natl Acad Sci USA 1991; 88:3314–3318.
61. Satoh T, Kaziro Y. Ras in signal transduction. In: Lowy DR (ed.) Seminars in Cancer Biology. London: Academic.
62. Shibuya H, Yoneyama M, Ninomiya-Tsuji J *et al.* IL-2 and EGF receptors stimulate the hematopoetic cell cycle via different signaling pathways: demonstration of a novel role for c-myc. Cell 1992; 70:57–67.
63. Miyazaki T, Liu ZJ, Kawahara A *et al.* Three distinct IL-2 signaling pathways mediated by *bcl-2, c-myc*, and lck cooperate in hematopoietic cell proliferation. Cell 1995; 81:223–231.
64. Caligiuri M, Zmuidzinas A, Manley TJ *et al.* Functional consequences of interleukin 2 receptor expression on resting human lymphocytes. Identification of a novel natural killer cell subset with high affinity receptors. J Exp Med 1990; 171:1509–1526.
65. Mills GB, Stewart DJ, Mellors A, Gelfand EW. Interleukin 2 does not induce phosphatidylinositol hydrolysis in activated T cells. J Immunol 1986 136:3019–3025.
66. Mills GB, Cheung RK, Grinstein S, Gelfand EW. Interleukin 2-induced lymphocyte proliferation is independent of increases in cytosolic free calcium concentrations. J Immunol 1985; 134:2431–2435.
67. Mills GB, Girard P, Grinstein S, Gelfand EW. Interleukin-2 induces proliferation of T lymphocyte mutants lacking protein kinase C. Cell 1988; 55:91–100.
68. Valge VE, Wong JGP, Datlof BM *et al.* Protein kinase C is required for responses to T cell receptor ligands but not to interleukin-2 in T cells. Cell 1988; 56:101–112.
69. Kolb JP, Abadie A, Paul-Eugene N, Dugas B. Intracellular signaling events associated with the induction of DNA synthesis in human B lymphocytes. II. Different pathways triggered by IL-2 and IL-4. Cell Immunol 1993; 146:131–146.
70. Johnson KW, Davis BH, Smith KA. cAMP antagonizes interleukin-2-promoted T cell cycle progression at a discrete point in early G1. Proc Natl Acad Sci USA 1988; 85:6072–6076.
71. Vazquez A, Auffredou MT, Galanaud P, Leca G. Modulation of IL-2 and IL-4 dependent human B cell proliferation by cyclic AMP. J Immunol 1991; 146:4222–4227.
72. Finney M, Guy GR, Michell RH *et al.* Interleukin 4 activates human B lymphocytes via transient inositol lipid hydrolysis and delayed cyclic adenosine monophosphate generation. Eur J Immunol 1990; 20:151–155.
73. Croft M, Swain SL. B cell response to fresh and effector T helper cells. Role of cognate T–B interaction and the cytokines IL-3, IL-4, and IL-6. J Immunol 1991; 146:4055–4064.
74. DeKruyff RH, Mosmann RR, Umetsu DT. Induction of antibody synthesis by $CD4^+$ T cells: IL-5 is essential for induction of antigen-specific antibody responses by TH2 but not TH1 clones. Eur J Immunol 1990; 20:2219–2227.
75. Leanderson T, Julius MH. Mouse B cells do not proliferate in human interleukin 2. Eur J Immunol 1986; 16:182–187.
76. Julius MH, Paige CJ, Leanderson T, Cambier JC. Neither interleukin 2 nor

gamma interferon directly promote growth or differentiation of mouse B cells. Scand J Immunol 1987; 25:195–202.

77. Kehrl JH, Muraguchi A, Fauci AS. The effects of interleukin-1, interleukin-2, $\alpha$ interferon, and $\gamma$ interferon on human B lymphocytes. Trans Assoc Am Physicians 1984; 97:182–189.
78. Muraguchi A, Kehrl JH, Longo DL *et al.* Interleukin 2 receptors on human B cells. Implications for the role of interleukin 2 in human B cell function. J Exp Med 1985; 161:181–197.
79. Pure E, Isakson PC, Paetkau V *et al.* Interleukin-2 does not induce murine B cells to secrete Ig. J Immunol 1982; 129:2420–2425.
80. Chan MA, Dosch HM. Human IgE response: virus-activated IgE secretors are interleukin-2-dependent cells. Int Arch Allergy Appl Immunol 1989; 89:90–97.
81. Gallagher G, Willdridge J. Evidence that interleukin 2 actively promotes both cell division and immunoglobulin secretion in human B cells. Int Arch Allergy Appl Immunol 1988; 86:337–342.
82. Liegson HJ, Marrack P, Kappler JW. B cell helper factors. I. Requirement for both interleukin 2 and another 40,000 molecular wt factor. J Exp Med 1981; 154:1681–1693.
83. Liebson HJ, Marrack P, Kappler JW. B cell helper factors. II. Synergy among three helper factors in the response of T cell- and macrophage-depleted B cells. J Immunol 1982; 129:1398–1402.
84. Jaworski MA, Shiozawa C, Diener E. Triggering of affinity-enriched B cells. Analysis of B cell stimulation by antigen-specific helper factor or lipopolysaccharide. J Exp Med 1982; 155:248–263.
85. Delovitch TL, Kaufman K, Gorczynski RD, Sinclair GD. In vitro analysis of allogeneic lymphocyte interaction. VIII. Characterization of helper components of allogeneic effect factor (AEF) that activate $Lyb5^+$ and $Lyb5^-$ B cells to respond to thymus-dependent and thymus-independent antigens. J Immunol 1983; 131:2246–2253.
86. Parker DC. Separable helper factors support B cell proliferation and maturation to Ig secretion. J Immunol 1982; 129:469–474.
87. Yoshizaki K, Nakagawa T, Kaieda T *et al.* Induction of proliferation and Ig production in human B leukemic cells by anti-immunoglobulins and T cell factors. J Immunol 1982; 128:1296–1301.
88. Zubler RH, Lowenthal JW, Erard F *et al.* Activated B cells express receptors for, and proliferate in response to, pure interleukin 2. J Exp Med 1984; 160:1170–1183.
89. Ortega G, Robb RJ, Shevach EM, Malek TR. The murine IL-2 receptor. I Monoclonal antibodies that define distinct functional epitopes on activated T cells and react with activated B cells. J Immunol 1984; 133:1970–1975.
90. Uchiyama T, Broder S, Waldmann TA. A monoclonal antibody (anti-Tac) reactive with activated functionally mature human T cells. J Immunol 1981; 126:1393–1397.
91. Fotedar R, Diener E. The role of recombinant IL-2 and IL-1 in murine B cell differentiation. Lymphokine Res 1988; 7:393–402.
92. Brooks KH, Vitetta ES. Recombinant IL-2 but not recombinant interferon-gamma stimulates both proliferation and IgM secretion in a $Ly\text{-}1^+$ clone of neoplastic murine B cells (BCL1). J Immunol 1986; 137:3205–3210.
93. Kishi H, Inui S, Muraguchi A *et al.* Induction of IgG secretion in a human B cell clone with recombinant IL-2. J Immunol 1985; 134:3104–3107.
94. Arima N, Daitoku Y, Hidaka S *et al.* Interleukin 2 acts directly on a Tac-positive cloned B cell line established from a patient with adult T cell leukemia. J Immunol 1985; 135:2474–2477.

95. Armitage RJ, Cawler JC. Normal and certain leukaemic B cells express IL-2 receptors without in vitro activation. Clin Exp Immunol 1986; 63:298–302.
96. Faure GC, Bene MC, Bolle-Chanel MH. Expression of CD25 (Tac antigen) in lymphoid leukemias and non-Hodgkin lymphomas. Eur J Haematol 1987; 38:26–30.
97. Foa R, Giovarelli M, Jemma C *et al.* Interleukin 2 (IL-2) and interferon-gamma production by T lymphocytes from patients with B-chronic lymphocytic leukemia: evidence that normally released IL-2 is absorbed by the neoplastic B cell population. Blood 1985; 66:614–619.
98. Murphy JJ, Malkovska V, Hudson L, Millard RE. Expression of functional interleukin 2 receptors on chronic lymphocytic leukemia B lymphocytes is modulated by recombinant interleukin 2. Clin Exp Immunol 1987; 70:182–191.
99. Panayotides P, Lenkei R, Porwit A, Reizenstein P. Malignant B cells have receptors for and respond to interleukin-2. Med Oncol Tumor Pharmocother 1986; 3:255–263.
100. Perri RT, Kay NE. Malignant chronic lymphocytic leukemia B cells express interleukin 2 receptors but fail to respond to interleukin 2's proliferative signal. Leukemia 1987; 1:127–130.
101. Wormann B, Anderson JM, Ling ZD, LeBien TW. Structure/function analyses of IL-2 binding proteins on human B cell precursor acute lymphoblastic leukemias. Leukemia 1987; 1:660–666.
102. Panayotides P, Porwit A, Lenkei R, Reizenstein P. Interleukin-2 can induce proliferation of leukemic B cells in prolymphocytic leukemia. Eur J Haematol 1987; 38: 274–278.
103. Sugamura K, Fujii M, Kobayshi N *et al.* Retrovirus-induced expression of interleukin 2 receptors on cells of human B cell lineage. Proc Natl Acad Sci USA 1984; 81:7441–7445.
104. Tomita S, Ambrus JL Jr, Volkman DJ *et al.* Human T cell leukemia/lymphoma virus I infection and subsequent cloning of normal human B cells. Direct responsiveness of cloned cells to recombinant interleukin 2 by differentiation in the absence of enhanced proliferation. J Exp Med 1985; 162:393–398.
105. Ford RJ, Yoshimura L, Morgan J *et al.* Growth factor-mediated tumor cell proliferation in hairy cell leukemia. J Exp Med 1985; 162:1093–1098.
106. Engel P, Ingles J, de la Calle O, Gallart T. Cellular activation without proliferation to B cell growth factor and interleukin 2 in chronic lymphocytic leukaemia B cells stimulated with phorbol ester plus calcium ionophore. Clin Exp Immunol 1989; 76:61–67.
107. Fluckinger AC, Rossi JF, Bussel A *et al.* Responsiveness of chronic lymphocytic leukemia B cells activated via surface Igs or CD40 to B-cell tropic factors. Blood 1992; 80:3173–3181.
108. Giovarelli M, Foa R, Benetton G *et al.* Release of interleukin-2-like material by B-chronic lymphocytic leukemia cells. An autocrine or paracrine model of production and utilization? Leukocyte Res 1988; 12:201–209.
109. Kabelitz D, Pfeffer K, von Steldern D *et al.* In vitro maturation of B cells in chronic lymphocytic leukemia. I. Synergistic action of phorbol ester and interleukin 2 in the induction of Tac antigen expression and interleukin 2 responsiveness in leukemic B cells. J Immunol 1985; 135:2876–2881.
110. Karray S, DeFrance T, Merle-Beral H *et al.* Interleukin 4 counteracts the interleukin 2-induced proliferation of monoclonal B cells. J Exp Med 1988; 168:85–94.
111. Lantz O, Grillot-Courvalin C, Schmitt C *et al.* Interleukin 2-induced proliferation of leukemic human B cells. J Exp Med 1985; 161:1225–1230.

112. Touw I, Lowenberg B. Interleukin 2 stimulates chronic lymphocytic leukemia colony formation in vitro. Blood 1985; 66:237–240.
113. Touw I, Delwel R, Bolhuis R *et al.* Common and pre-B acute lymphoblastic leukemia cells express interleukin 2 receptors, and interleukin 2 stimulates in vitro colony formation. Blood 1985; 66:556–561.
114. Matsuoka M, Hattori T, Kawano F *et al.* Expression of Tac antigen on human immature B-cell lineage leukemic cells. Leukocyte Res 1986; 10:597–603.
115. Bentaboulet M, Allouche M, Tsapis A *et al.* Characterization of interleukin-2 receptors expressed on acute leukemic B cells. Blood 1987; 70:954–959.
116. Karray S, Merle-Beral H, Vazquez A *et al.* Functional heterogeneity of B-CLL lymphocytes: dissociated responsiveness to growth factors and distinct requirements for a first activation signal. Blood 1987; 70:1105–1110.
117. Jelinek DF, Lipsky PE. Comparative activation requirements of human peripheral blood, spleen and lymph node B cells. J Immunol 1987; 139:1005–1013.
118. Jelinek DF, Lipsky PE. The roles of interleukin 2 and interferon-γ in human B cell activation, growth, and differentiation. Eur J Immunol 1986; 16:925–932.
119. Jelinek DF, Splawski JB, Lipsky PE. Human peripheral blood B lymphocyte subpopulations: functional and phenotypic analysis of surface IgD positive and negative subsets. J Immunol 1986; 136:83–92.
120. Miyawaki T, Suzuki T, Butler JL, Cooper MD. Interleukin-2 effects on human B cells activated in vivo. J Clin Immunol 1987; 7:277–287.
121. Bich-Thuy Lt, Queen C, Fauci AS. Interferon-gamma induces light chain synthesis in interleukin 2 stimulated human B cells. Eur J Immunol 1986; 16:547–550.
122. Bich-Thuy Lt, Fauci AS. Direct effect of interleukin 2 on the differentiation of human B cells which have not been preactivated in vitro. Eur J Immunol 1985; 15:1075–1079.
123. Gearing A, Thorpe R, Bird C, Spitz M. Human B cell proliferation is stimulated by interleukin 2. Immunol Lett 1985; 9:105–108.
124. Ralph P, Jeong G, Welte K *et al.* Stimulation of immunoglobulin secretion in human B lymphocytes as a direct effect of high concentrations of IL-2. J Immunol 1984; 133:2442–2445.
125. Romagnani S, Del Prete G, Guidizi MG *et al.* Direct induction of human B-cell differentiation by recombinant interleukin-2. Immunology 1986; 58:31–35.
126. Kehrl JH, Muraguchi A, Goldsmith PK, Fauci AS. The direct effects of interleukin 1, interleukin 2, interferon-α, interferon-γ, B-cell growth factor, and a B-cell differentiation factor on resting and activated human B cells. Cell Immunol 1985; 96:38–48.
127. Mond JJ, Thompson C, Finkelman FD *et al.* Affinity purified interleukin 2 induces proliferation of large but not small B cells. Proc Natl Acad Sci USA 1985; 82:1518–1521.
128. Grillot-Courvalin C, Labaume S, Brouet JC. Differentiation by interleukin of a subpopulation of human B cells. Scand J Immunol 1986; 23:679–684.
129. Begley CG, Burton JD, Tsudo M *et al.* Human B lymphocytes express the p75 component of the interleukin 2 receptor. Leukemia Res 1990; 14:263–271.
130. Franz A, Bryant A, Farrant J. Staphylococcal enterotoxin B upregulates interleukin-2 receptor β chain expression on tonsillar B cells. Eur J Immunol 1993; 23:2696–2699.
131. Jung LK, Hara T, Fu SM. Detection and functional studies of p60–65 (Tac antigen) on activated human B cells. J Exp Med 1984; 160:1597–1602.
132. Tanaka T, Saiki O, Doi S *et al.* Expression of novel interleukin 2 binding molecules and their functional roles in human B cell differentiation. J Clin Invest 1988; 82:316–321.

133. Tanaka T, Saiki O, Doi S *et al.* Novel receptor-mediated internalization of interleukin 2 in B cells. J Immunol 1988; 140:866–870.
134. Saiki O, Tanaka T, Doi S, Kishimoto S. Expression and the functional role of p70/75 interleukin 2-binding molecule in human B cells. J Immunol 1988; 140:853–858.
135. Hashimoto N, Nabholz M, MacDonald HR, Zubler RH. Dissociation of interleukin 2-dependent and -independent B cell proliferation with monoclonal anti-interleukin 2 receptor antibody. Eur J Immunol 1986; 16:317–320.
136. Moll H, Emmrich F, Simon MM. Recombinant human interleukin 2 directly provides signals for the proliferation and functional maturation of murine B lymphocytes. Immunobiology 1985; 169:447–454.
137. Pike BL, Raubitschek A, Nossal GJ. Human interleukin 2 can promote the growth and differentiation of single hapten-specific B cells in the presence of specific antigen. Proc Natl Acad Sci USA 1984; 81:7917–7921.
138. Birkeland ML, Simpson L, Isakson PC, Pure E. T-independent and T-dependent steps in the murine B cell response to antiimmunoglobulin. J Exp Med 1987; 166:506–519.
139. Purkerson JM, Newberg M, Wise G *et al.* Interleukin 5 and interleukin 2 cooperate with interleukin 4 to induce IgG1 secretion from anti-Ig-treated B cells. J Exp Med 1988; 168:1175–1180.
140. Pecanha LM, Snapper CM, Finkelman FD, Mond JJ. Dextran-conjugated anti-Ig antibodies as a model for T cell-independent type 2 antigen-mediated stimulation of Ig secretion in vitro. I. Lymphokine dependence. J Immunol 1991; 146:833–839.
141. Forman MS, Pure E. T-independent and T-dependent B lymphoblasts: helper T cells prime for interleukin 2-induced growth and secretion of immunoglobulins that utilize downstream heavy chains. J Exp Med 1991; 173:687–697.
142. DeKruyff RH, Rizzo LV, Umetsu DT. Induction of immunoglobulin synthesis by CD4+ T cell clones. Semin Immunol 1993; 5:421–430.
143. Grabstein KH, Maliszewski CR, Shanebeck K *et al.* The regulation of T cell-dependent antibody formation in vitro by CD40 ligand and IL-2. J Immunol 1993; 150:3141–3147.
144. Poudrier J, Owens T. CD54/intracellular adhesion molecule 1 and major histocompatibility complex II signaling induces B cells to express interleukin 2 receptors and complements help provided through CD40 ligation. J Exp Med 1994; 179:1417–1427.
145. Snapper CM *et al.* Interferon gamma induction of Ig secretion. J Immunol 1995; submitted.
146. Takatsu K, Tominaga A, Harada N *et al.* T cell-replacing factor/interleukin 5: molecular and functional properties. Immunol Rev 1988; 102:107–135.
147. Nakanishi K *et al.* Both B151-T cell replacing factor 1 and IL-5 regulate Ig secretion and IL-2 receptor expression on a cloned B lymphoma line. J Immunol 1988; 140:1168–1174.
148. Loughnan MS, Takatsu K, Harada N, Nossal GJV. T-cell-replacing factor (interleukin 5) induces expression of interleukin 2 receptors on murine splenic B cells. Proc Natl Acad Sci USA 1987; 84:5399–5403.
149. Poudrier J, Owens T. The acquisition of cytokine responsiveness by murine B cells: a role for antigen and IL-5 in the induction of IL-2 receptors. Immunology 1994; 81:373–380.
150. Purkerson JM, Isakson PC. Isotype switching in anti-immunoglobulin-activated B lymphoblasts: differential requirements for interleukin 4 and other lymphokines to elicit membrane vs. secreted IgG1. Eur J Immunol 1991; 21:707–714.

151. McFadden HJ, Koshland ME. Interleukin 2- and interleukin 5-induced changes in the binding of regulatory factors to the J-chain gene promoter. Proc Natl Acad Sci USA 1991; 88:11027–11031.
152. Karasuyama H, Rolink A, Melchers F. Recombinant interleukin 2 or 5, but not 4 or 3, induces maturation of resting mouse B lymphocytes and propagates proliferation of activated B cell blasts. J Exp Med 1988; 167:1377–1390.
153. Takatsuki F, Okano A, Suzuki C *et al.* Human recombinant IL-6/B cell stimulatory factor 2 augments murine antigen-specific antibody responses in vitro and in vivo. J Immunol 1988; 141:3072–3077.
154. Coffman RL, Lebman DA, Shrader B. Transforming growth factor beta specifically enhances IgA production by lipopolysaccharide-stimulated murine B lymphocytes. J Exp Med 1989; 170:1039–1044.
155. Kim PH, Kagnoff MF. Transforming growth factor-beta 1 is a costimulator for IgA production. J Immunol 1990; 144:3411–3416.
156. Casey LS, Lichtman AH, Boothby M. IL-4 induces IL-2 receptor p75 beta-chain gene expression and IL-2-dependent proliferation in mouse T lymphocytes. J Immunol 1992; 148:3418–3426.
157. Nakanishi K *et al.* IL-2 inhibits IL-4-dependent IgE and IgG1 production in vitro and in vivo. Int Immunol 1995; 7:259–268.
158. Brunswick M, Finkelman FD, Highet PF *et al.* Picogram quantities of anti-Ig antibodies coupled to dextran induce B cell proliferation. J Immunol 1988; 140:3364–3372.
159. Snapper CM, Mooman MA, Rosas FR *et al.* IL-3 and GM-CSF strongly induce Ig secretion by sort-purified murine B cells activated through the membrane Ig, but not CD40, signaling pathway. J Immunol 1995; 154:5842–5850.
160. Sadlack B, Merz, Schorle H *et al.* Ulcerative colitis-like disease in mice with a disrupted interleukin-2 gene. Cell 1993; 75:253–261.
161. Burton JD, Bamford RN, Peters C *et al.* A lymphokine, provisionally designated interleukin T and produced by a human adult T-cell line, stimulates T-cell proliferation and the induction of lymphokine-activated Killer cells. Proc Natl Acad Sci USA 1994; 91:4935–4939.
162. Drexler HG, Brenner MK, Coustan-Smith E *et al.* Analysis of signal transduction in B chronic lymphocytic leukemia cells. Blood 1988; 71:1461–1469.
163. Hivroz C, Grillot-Courvalin C, Brouet JC, Seligmann M. Heterogeneity of responsiveness of chronic lymphocytic leukemic B cells to B cell growth factor or interleukin 2. Eur J Immunol 1986; 16:1001–1004.
164. Moberts R, Hoogerbrugge H, van Agthoven T *et al.* Proliferative response of highly purified B chronic lymphocytic leukemia cells in serum free culture to interleukin-2 and tumor necrosis factors alpha and beta. Leukocyte Res 1989; 13:973–980.
165. Emilie D, Karray S, Merle-Beral H *et al.* Induction of differentiation in human leukemic B cells by interleukin 2 alone: different effect on the expression of mu and J chain genes. Eur J Immunol 1988; 18:1479–1483.
166. Malkovska V, Murphy J, Hudson L, Bevan D. Direct effect of interleukin 2 on chronic lymphocytic leukaemia B cell functions and morphology. Clin Exp Immunol 1987; 68:677–684.
167. Nakagawa T, Nakagawa N, Volkman DJ, Fauci AS. Sequential synergistic effect of interleukin 2 and interferon-gamma on the differentiation of a Tac-antigen-positive B cell line. J Immunol 1986; 136:164–168.
168. Jelinek DF, Lipsky PE. Inhibitory influence of IL-4 on human B cell responsiveness. J Immunol 1988; 141:164–173.
169. Mingari MC, Gerosa F, Carra G *et al.* Human interleukin-2 promotes

proliferation of activated B cells via surface receptors similar to those of activated T cells. Nature 1984; 312:641–643.

170. Mittler R, Rao P, Olini G *et al.* Activated human B cells display a functional IL-2 receptor. J Immunol 1985; 134:2393–2399.

171. Nakagawa T, Nakagawa N, Ambrus JL Jr, Fauci AS. Differential effects of interleukin 2 vs B cell growth factor on human B cells. J Immunol 1988; 140:465–469.

172. Tsudo M, Uchiyama T, Uchino H. Expression of Tac antigen on activated normal human B cells. J Exp Med 1984; 160:612–617.

173. Callaghan M, Whelan A, Feighery C, Bresnihan B. IL-2 enhances polyclonal IgM but not IgM-rheumatoid factor synthesis by activated human peripheral blood B cells. Clin Exp Immunol 1993; 93:212–217.

174. Devos R, Jayaram B, Vandenabeele P, Fiers W. Recombinant interleukin 2 induces immunoglobulin secretion in Staphylococcus aureus Cowan strain I activated human B cells. Immunol Lett 1985; 11:101–105.

175. Jelinek DF, Lipsky PE. Enhancement of human B cell proliferation and differentiation by tumor necrosis factor-alpha and interleukin 1. J Immunol 1987; 139:2970–2976.

176. Punnonen J, Eskola J. Recombinant interleukin 2 induces proliferation and differentiation of human B lymphocytes. Acta Pathol Microbiol Immunol Scand, Section C, Immunology 1987; 95:167–172.

177. Teranishi T, Hirano T, Lin BH. Demonstration of the involvement of interleukin 2 in the differentiation of Staphylococcus aureus Cowan 1-stimulated B cells. J Immunol 1984; 133:3062–3067.

178. Xia X, Lee HK, Clark SC, Choi YS. Recombinant interleukin (IL) 2-induced human B cell differentiation is mediated by autocrine IL-6. Eur J Immunol 1989; 19:2275–2281.

179. Almerigogna F, Bagiotti R, Giudizi GM *et al.* Different reactivity of activated human B cell to B-cell growth factor and interleukin 2 in the costimulation assay with anti-IgM antibody and in the preactivation assay with Staphylococcus bacteria. Cell Immunol 1985; 95:358–367.

180. Defrance T, Vanbervliet B, Aubry JP, Banchereau J. Interleukin 4 inhibits the proliferation but not the differentiation of activated human B cells in response to interleukin 2. J Exp Med 1988; 168:1321–1337.

181. Maher DW, Pike BL, Boyd AW. The response of human B cells to interleukin 4 is determined by their stage of activation and differentiation. Scand J Immunol 1991; 33:631–640.

182. Mingari MC, Gerosa F, Moretta A *et al.* B cell growth factor activity of immunoaffinity-purified and recombinant human interleukin 2. Eur J Immunol 1985; 15:193–196.

183. Morikawa K, Oseko F, Morikawa S *et al.* Recombinant human IL-5 augments immunoglobulin generation by human B lymphocytes in the presence of IL-2. Cell Immunol 1993; 149:390–401.

184. Nakagawa T, Hirano T, Nakagawa N *et al.* Effect of recombinant IL-2 and γ-IFN on proliferation and differentiation of human B cells. J Immunol 1985; 134:959–966.

185. Schwarting R, Welte K, Chiorazzi N *et al.* Biochemical characterization and purification of human B cell stimulatory factor (BSF). Eur J Immunol 1985; 15:632–637.

186. Ueda Y, Sakane T, Tsunematsu T. Hyperreactivity of activated B cells to B cell growth factor in patients with systemic lupus erythematosus. J Immunol 1989; 143:3988–3993.

187. Nakagawa T, Nakagawa N, Goldstein H *et al.* Demonstration that human B cells respond differently to interleukin 2 and B cell differentiation factor based on their stages of maturation. J Immunol 1986; 137:3175–3182.
188. Armitage RJ, Macduff BM, Spriggs MK, Fanslow WC. Human B cell proliferation and Ig secretion induced by recombinant CD40 ligand are modulated by soluble cytokines. J Immunol 1993; 150:3671–3680.
189. Freedman AS, Boyd AW, Berrebi A *et al.* Expression of B cell activation antigens on normal and malignant B cells. Leukemia 1987; 1:9–15.
190. Kehrl JH, Muraguchi A, Falkoff RJ *et al.* Activation and immunoregulation of human B lymphocytes. Uremia Invest 1984; 8:157–166.
191. Almerigogna F, Giudizi MG, Biagiotti R *et al.* Analysis of the B-cell growth-promoting activity of human IL-4, the co-stimulatory assay with anti-immunoglobulin antibodies. Comparison with the B-cell growth-promoting activity of other lymphokines. Immunology 1989; 67:244–250.
192. Romagnani S, Giudizi GM, Almerigogna F *et al.* Analysis of the role of interferon-gamma, interleukin 2 and a third factor distinct from interferon-gamma and interleukin 2 in human B cell proliferation. Evidence that they act at different times after B cell activation. Eur J Immunol 1986; 16:623–629.
193. Romagnani S, Giudizi GM, Maggi E *et al.* Synergy of B cell growth factor and interleukin 2 in the proliferation of activated human B cells. Eur J Immunol 1985; 15:1158–1164.
194. Splawski JB, Jelinek DF, Lipsky PE. Immunomodulatory role of interleukin 4 on the secretion of immunoglobulin by human B cells. J Immunol 1989; 142:1569–1575.
195. Stuber F, Ernst M, Flad HD, Gross WL. Interleukin 2 as an inducer of proliferation in Klebsiella-stimulated human B cells. Clin Immunol Immunopathol 1989; 52:386–391.
196. Suzuki T, Cooper MD. Comparison of the expression of IL-2 receptors by human T and B cells: induction by the polyclonal mitogens, phorbol myristate acetate, and anti-(mu) antibody. J Immunol 1985; 134:3111–3119.
197. Waldmann TA *et al.* Expression of interleukin 2 receptors on activated human B cells. J Exp Med 1984; 160:1450–1466.
198. Peckham DW, Mower DA, Ashman RF. Analysis of high and low responses to Staphylococcus aureus and interleukin 2 in human B lymphocytes. J Clin Immunol 1993; 13:424–438.
199. Zupo S, Dono M, Azzoni L *et al.* Evidence for differential responsiveness of human $CD5^+$ and $CD5^-$ cell subsets to T cell-independent mitogens. Eur J Immunol 1991; 21:351–359.
200. Callard RE, Smith SH. Interleukin 2 and low molecular weight B cell growth factor are T cell-replacing factors for different subpopulations of human B cells. Eur J Immunol 1988; 18:1635–1638.
201. Defrance T, Vanbervliet B, Durand L *et al.* Proliferation and differentiation of human $CD5^+$ and $CD5^-$ B cell subsets activated through their antigen receptors or CD40 antigens. Eur J Immunol 1992; 22:2831–2839.
202. Nonoyama S, Farrington ML, Ochs HD. Effects of IL-2 on immunoglobulin production by anti-CD40-activated human B cells: synergistic effect with IL-10 and antagonistic effect with IL-4. Clin Immunol Immunopathol 1994; 72:373–379.
203. Armerding D, Hren A. Phorbol ester, prostaglandin E2, forskolin and okadaic acid differentially modulate interleukin-4-versus interleukin-2-dependent immunoglobulin induction in human cellular models, in contrast to other selected modifiers of cellular activation. Int Arch Allergy Immunol 1993; 101:143–152.

204. Armitage RJ, Macduff BM, Eisenman J *et al.* IL-15 has stimulatory activity for the induction of B cell proliferation and differentiation. J Immunol 1995; 154:483–490.
205. Rousset F, Garcia E, Banchereau J. Cytokine-induced proliferation and immunoglobulin production of human B lymphocytes triggered through their CD40 antigen. J Exp Med 1991; 173:705–710.
206. Fluckiger AC, Garrone P, Durand I *et al.* Interleukin 10 upregulates functional high affinity IL-2 receptors on normal and leukemic B lymphocytes. J Exp Med 1993; 178:1473–1481.
207. Splawski JB, Fu SM, Lipsky PE. Immunomodulatory role of CD40 in human B cell differentiation. J Immunol 1993; 150:1276–1285.
208. Delfraissy JF, Wallon C, Galanaud P. Interferon-alpha can synergize with interleukin 2 for human in vitro antibody response. Eur J Immunol 1988; 18:1379–1384.
209. Llorente L, Mitjavila F, Crevon MC, Galanaud P. Dual effects of interleukin 4 on antigen-activated human B cells induction of proliferation and inhibition of interleukin 2-dependent differentiation. Eur J Immunol 1990; 20: 1887–1892.
210. Llorente L, Crevon MC, Karray S *et al.* Interleukin (IL) 4 counteracts the helper effect of IL-2 on antigen-activated human B cells. Eur J Immunol 1989; 19:765–769.
211. Flores-Romo L, Millsum MJ, Gillis S *et al.* Immunoglobulin isotype production by cycling human B lymphocytes in response to recombinant cytokines and anti-IgM. Immunology 1990; 69:342–347.
212. Jumper MD, Splawski JB, Lipsky PE. Ligation of CD40 induces sterile transcripts of multiple H chain isotypes in human B cells. J Immunol 1994; 152:438–445.
213. McKenzie AN *et al.* Interleukin-13, a T-cell-derived cytokine that regulates human monocyte and B-cell function. Proc Natl Acad Sci USA 1993; 90:3735–3739.
214. Minty A *et al.* Interleukin-13 is a new human lymphokine regulating inflammatory and immune responses. Nature 1993; 362:248–250.
215. Zurawski G, de Vries JE. Interleukin 13, an interleukin 4-like cytokine that acts on monocytes and B cells, but not T cells. Immunol Today 1994; 15:19–26.
216. Bertolini JN, Benson EM. The role of human interleukin-6 in B-cell isotype regulation and differentiation. Cell Immunol 1990; 125:197–209.
217. Nawata Y, Stall AM, Herzenberg LA *et al.* Surface immunoglobulin ligands and cytokines differentially affect proliferation and antibody production by human $CD5^+$ and $CD5^-$ B lymphocytes. Int Immunol 1990; 2:603–614.
218. Tadmori W, Feingersh D, Clark SC, Choi YS. Human recombinant IL-3 stimulates B cell differentiation. J Immunol 1989; 142:1950–1955.
219. Hornung N, Degiannis D. Up-regulation by cyclosporine (CsA) of the in vitro release of soluble CD23 (sCD23) and of the in vitro production of IL-6 and IgM. Scand J Immunol 1993; 38:287–292.
220. Splawski JB, McAnally LM, Lipsky PE. IL-2 dependence of the promotion of human B cell differentiation by IL-6 (BSF-2). J Immunol 1990; 144: 562–569.
221. Jochems GJ, Bende RJ, Klein MR *et al.* Expression of the IL-6 gene induces differentiation of a human monoclonal EBV-transformed B cell line. Hum Ab Hyb 1993; 4:124–133.
222. Pene J. Regulatory role of cytokines and CD23 in the human IgE antibody synthesis. Int Arch Allergy Appl Immunol 1989; 90:32–40.

223. Armitage RJ, Goff LK. Functional interactions between B cell populations defined by CD23 expression. Eur J Immunol 1988; 18:1753–1760.
224. Jelinek DF, Braaten JK. The role of interleukin 12 in human B lymphocyte proliferation and differentiation. J Immunol 1995; 154:1606–1613.
225. Bertolini JN, Sanderson CJ, Benson EM. Human interleukin-5 induces staphylococcal A Cowan 1 strain-activated human B cells to secrete IgM. Eur J Immunol 1993; 23:398–402.
226. van Vlasselaer P, Gascan H, de Waal Malefyt R, de Vries JE. IL-2 and a contact-mediated signal provided by TCR alpha beta + or TCR gamma delta + CD4+ T cells induce polyclonal Ig production by committed human B cells. Enhancement by IL-5, specific inhibition of IgA synthesis by IL-4. J Immunol 1992; 148:1674–1684.
227. Shirakawa F, Tanaka Y, Eto S *et al.* Requirement of macrophages (monocytes) for the induction of interleukin 2 receptors on B lymphocytes. J Immunol 1986; 136:3288–3291.
228. Itoh K, Inoue T, Ito K, Hirohata S. The interplay of interleukin 10 and interleukin 2 in humoral immune responses: IL-10 synergizes with IL-2 to enhance responses of human B lymphocytes in a mechanism which is different from upregulation of CD25 expression. Cell Immunol 1994; 157:478–488.
229. Zola H, Flego L, Weedon H. Expression of membrane receptor for tumour necrosis factor on human blood lymphocytes. Immunol Cell Biol 1993; 71:281–288.
230. Rieckmann P, D'Alessandro F, Nordan RP *et al.* IL-6 and tumor necrosis factor-alpha. Autocrine and paracrine cytokines involved in B cell function. J Immunol 1991; 146:3462–3468.
231. Spiegelberg HL, Falkoff RJ, O'Connor RD, Beck L. Interleukin-2 inhibits the interleukin-4-induced human IgE and IgG4 secretion in vivo. Clin Exp Immunol 1991; 84:400–405.
232. Carlsson M, Sundstom C, Bengtsson M *et al.* Interleukin 4 strongly augments or inhibits DNA synthesis and differentiation of B-type chronic lymphocytic leukemia cells depending on the co-stimulatory activation and progression signals. Eur J Immunol 1989; 19:913–921.
233. Brams P, Royston I, Boerner P. In vitro priming of human lymphocytes. I. IL-2 and IL-4 requirements. Hum Ab Hyb 1993; 4:47–56.
234. Callard RE, Smith SH, Scott KE. The role of interleukin 4 in specific antibody response by human B cells. Int Immunol 1991; 3:157–163.
235. Fernandez-Botran R, Sanders Vm, Vitetta ES. Interactions between receptors for interleukin 2 and interleukin 4 on lines of helper T cells (HT-2) and B lymphoma cells (BCL1). J Exp Med 1989; 169:379–391.
236. Watanabe S, Kondo M, Takatsu K *et al.* Involvement of the interleukin-2 receptor gamma subunit in interleukin-4-dependent activation of mouse hematopoietic cells and splenic B cells. Eur J Immunol 1995; 25:126–131.
237. Splawski JB, Jelinek DF, Lipsky PE. Delineation of the functional capacity of human neonatal lymphocytes. J Clin Invest 1991; 78:545–553.
238. Coffman RL, Ohara J, Bond MW *et al.* B cell stimulatory factor 1 enhances the IgE response of lipopolysaccharide-activated B cells. J Immunol 1986; 136:4538–4541.
239. Kim PH, Kagnoff MF. Transforming growth factor-β-1 increases IgA isotype switching at the clonal level. J Immunol 1990; 145:3773–3778.
240. Lebman DA, Coffman RL. Interleukin 4 causes isotype switching to IgE in T cell-stimulated clonal B cell cultures. J Exp Med 1988; 168:853–862.
241. Vitetta ES, Ohara J, Meyers CD *et al.* Serological, biochemical, and functional

identity of B cell-stimulatory factor 1 and B cell differentiation factor for IgG1. J Exp Med 1985; 162:1726–1731.
242. Renz H, Mazer BD, Gelfand E. Differential inhibition of T and B cell function in IL-4-dependent IgE production by cyclosporine A and methylprednisolone. J Immunol 1990; 145:3641–3646.
243. Henry CS, Kuribayashi K, Kern DE, Gillis S. Interleukin-2 augments natural killer cell activity. Nature 1981; 291:335–338.
244. Snapper CM, Yamaguchi H, Moorman MA *et al.* Natural killer cells induce activated murine B cells to secrete Ig. J Immunol 1993; 151:5251–5260.
245. Amigorena S, Bonnerot C, Fridman WH, Tiellaud J-L. Recombinant interleukin 2-activated natural killer cells regulate IgG2a production. Eur J Immunol 1990; 20:1781–1787.
246. Calvert JE, Johnstone R, Duggan-Keen MF, Bird P. Immunoglobulin G subclasses secreted by human B cells in vitro in response to interleukin-2 and polyclonal activators. Immunology 1990; 70:162–167.
247. Amoroso K, Lipsky PE. Frequency of human B cells that differentiate in response to anti-CD3 activated T cells. J Immunol 1990; 145:3155–3161.
248. Hirohata S, Jelinek DF, Lipsky PE. T cell-dependent activation of B cell proliferation and differentiation by immobilized monoclonal antibodies to CD3. J Immunol 1988; 140:3726–3744.
249. Amerding D, van Reijsen FC, Hren A, Mudde GC. Induction of IgE and IgG1 in human B cell cultures with staphylococcal superantigens: role of helper T cell interaction, resistance to interferon-gamma. Immunobiology 1993; 188: 259–273.
250. Splawski JB, Lipsky PE. Cytokine regulation of immunoglobulin secretion by neonatal lymphocytes. J Clin Invest 1991; 88:967–977.
251. McIlraith MJ, Splawski JB, Lipsky PE. Cytokine regulation of human B cell differentiation. FASEB J 1991; 5:A603.
252. McIlraith MJ, Dewey M, Splawski JB, Lipsky PE. Examination of the effect of cytokines on Ig heavy chain class switching in human B cells. FASEB J 1992; 6:A1126.
253. Chang CC, Aversa G, Punnonen J *et al.* Brequinar sodium, mycophenolic acid, and cyclosporine A inhibit different stages of IL-4 or IL-13 induced human IgG4 and IgE production in vitro. Ann N Y Acad Sci 1993; 696:108–122.
254. Gauchat JF, Lebman DA, Coffman RI *et al.* Structure and expression of germline ϵ transcripts in human B cells induced by interleukin 4 to switch to IgE production. J Exp Med 1990; 172:463–473.
255. Jabara HH, Schneider LC, Shapira SK *et al.* Induction of germ-line and mature Cϵ transcripts in human cells stimulated with rIL-4 and EBV. J Immunol 145:3468–3473.
256. Stavnezer-Nordgren J, Sirlin S. Specificity of immunoglobulin heavy chain switch correlates with activity of germline heavy chain genes prior to switching. EMBO J 1986; 5:95–102.
257. Yancopoulos GD, DelPhino RA, Zimmerman KA *et al.* Secondary genomic rearrangement events in pre-B cells: Vh DJh replacement by a LINE-1 sequence and directed class switching. EMBO J 1986; 12:3259–3266.
258. Wakatsui Y, Strober W. Effect of downregulation of germline transcripts on immunoglobulin A isotype differentiation. J Exp Med 1993; 178:129–138.
259. Jung S, Rajewski K, Radbruch A. Shutdown of class switch recombination by deletion of a switch region control element. Science 1993; 259:984–987.
260. Kitani A, Stober W. Regulation of Cγ subclass germ-line transcripts in human peripheral blood B cells. J Immunol 1993; 151:3478–3488.

261. Cunningham-Rundles C, Kazbay K, Hassett J *et al.* Enhanced humoral immunity in common variable immunodeficiency after long-term treatment with polyethylene glycol-conjugated interleukin-2. N Eng J Med 1994; 331:918–921.

# 8 Interleukin-4 and Interleukin-13

**JAN E. DE VRIES and JUHA PUNNONEN**
*DNAX Research Institute of Molecular and Cellular Biology, Palo Alto, California, USA*

## INTRODUCTION

Early studies have shown that supernatants of activated T cells provide help for B-cell differentiation and antibody production[1]. More recently, it has become clear that cytokines produced by activated T-helper cells are required for B-cell expansion and differentiation, immunoglobulin (Ig) isotype switching and antibody production[2]. Both mouse and human $CD4^+$ T-helper cells can be divided into at least three major subsets according to their cytokine production profiles[3]. T-helper type 1 (Th1) cells produce, among other cytokines, relatively high levels of interleukin-2 (IL-2), interferon gamma (IFN-$\gamma$) and no IL-4 or IL-5, whereas T-helper type 2 (Th2) cells generally secrete high levels of IL-4, IL-5 and IL-13 and no, or low levels of, IL-2 and IFN-$\gamma$ following antigen-specific stimulation. The third T-helper cell subset, Th0, produces both Th1 and Th2 cytokines. The differences in cytokine production profiles between the Th1 and Th2 subsets are also reflected in the functions of these cells. Th1 cells are predominantly involved in delayed hypersensitivity reactions and, through the production of IFN-$\gamma$, in the activation of macrophages to eliminate intracellular pathogens, whereas Th2 cells are more efficient in giving help to B cells for antibody production. In addition to cytokines, contact-mediated signals are necessary for productive T–B-cell interactions, resulting in Ig isotype switching and antibody production[4].

In this chapter we restrict ourselves to reviewing the roles of IL-4 and IL-13 in human Ig synthesis and Ig isotype switching, but on some occasions references relevant to mouse data are made. It has, however, to be noted that both cytokines, like all other cytokines, are pleiotropic and can modulate the functions of many other cell types than B cells, including T cells, natural killer (NK) cells, monocytes/macrophages, granulocytes, mast cells, and epithelial and endothelial cells.

*Cytokine Regulation of Humoral Immunity: Basic and Clinical Aspects.* Edited by Clifford M. Snapper.

## MOLECULAR CHARACTERISTICS OF IL-4 AND IL-13

IL-4 was originally identified as a cytokine capable of inducing proliferation and antibody production by preactivated mouse B cells[5,6]. A mouse IL-4 cDNA was isolated from a mouse T-cell library as a cDNA encoding a unique mouse interleukin which expressed B-cell, T-cell and mast cell stimulating activities[7,8]. Subsequently, a cDNA encoding human IL-4 was isolated by cross-hybridization from an activated human T-cell clone cDNA library[9]. The mature human IL-4 (hIL-4) protein consists of 129 amino acids, and has a molecular mass of 15–19 kDa, depending on its degree of glycosylation. Human IL-4 has 2 potential *N*-linked glycosylation sites and three disulfide bonds.

The mouse IL-13 cDNA (originally designated P600) was first isolated in 1989 by Brown *et al.*[10]. Isolation of the human IL-13 cDNA revealed that it encoded a 132 amino acid protein with four potential *N*-linked glycosylation sites and five cysteine residues, of which four are available to form disulfide pairs[11,12]. Human IL-13 protein is predominantly secreted as an unglycosylated species of ~10 kDa. Both human IL-4 and IL-13 are mapped to the long arm of chromosome 5 q31-1, which is the same area in which the genes for IL-3, IL-5, IL-9 and granulocyte/macrophage colony-stimulating factor (GM-CSF) are located[13,14]. The close proximity and similarities in structure of these cytokine genes suggests that they evolved by gene duplication events. Despite the low homology between the primary structures of IL-4, IL-5, IL-13 and GM-CSF, their tertiary structures are comparable. All have a four-helix anti-parallel α-helical core similar to IL-2, M-CSF and growth hormone[15]. For example, human IL-4 and IL-13 share only ~30 per cent homology at the protein level, but all 25 residues which contribute to the hIL-4 hydrophobic structural core are conserved, or have conservative reconstitutions in hIL-13[16]. In addition, mouse IL-13 was also shown to be a highly α-helical protein, similar to human IL-4[16,17].

## THE IL-4 AND IL-13 RECEPTOR

IL-4 receptors are widely distributed. Every hematopoietic and non-hematopoietic cell type tested thus far has been found to express low numbers (<3000 sites per cell) of high-affinity receptors with a $K_d$ varying from 40 to 130 pM[18,19]. A cDNA encoding a 130-kDa human IL-4-binding protein (IL-4 receptor α chain) consisting of 800 amino acids in its mature form has been isolated[20,21]. The extracellular domain of the IL-4R α chain consists of 207 amino acids and contains six cysteine residues and six potential *N*-linked glycosylation sites. The human IL-4R has the typical conserved WSXWS motif and a region which is homologous to type III fibronectin, which are both characteristic for the cytokine receptor family, to which the β chain of the IL-2R, and the receptors for IL-3, IL-5, IL-6, IL-7, GM-CSF and EPO, belong. These receptors are glycoproteins with a single membrane-spanning domain, and with N-termini oriented out of the cells[22].

Recently, it has been shown that the IL-2 receptor γ chain is part of the IL-4 receptor complex[23,24]. This γ chain, which is also a common component of the IL-7, IL-9 and IL-15 receptors[25] (and therefore is called the common γ chain ($\gamma_c$)) enhances the affinity of the 130-kDa IL-4R α chain for IL-4. The IL-4R α chain gene is mapped to chromosome 16 p12.1–11.2, whereas the $\gamma_c$ chain is located on the X-chromosome[26].

An IL-13-binding protein has not been characterized yet. However, competitive binding studies have indicated that IL-4 and IL-13 bind to different, complex receptors, but that these receptors have a common component, which is required for signal transduction[16,27]. Whether the IL-2$\gamma_c$ is part of the IL-13R complex remains to be determined. Interestingly, recent studies have shown that anti-human IL-4Rα monoclonal antibodies (mAbs), which block the binding of IL-4 and biological effects of IL-4 on certain cell types, including B cells, also blocked the binding and biological effects of IL-13, indicating that the IL-4R α chain is a functional component of the IL-13R complex[28,29].

In contrast to IL-4R, IL-13R seems to have a more restricted distribution. For example, human T cells and T-cell clones, which are responsive to IL-4, do not bind radiolabelled IL-13 and do not respond to IL-13, indicating that these cells do not have functional IL-13R[16,30,31]. Therefore, in contrast to IL-4, IL-13 does not act as an autocrine growth factor for T cells. In addition, mouse B cells may also lack functional IL-13R, since these cells failed to respond to IL-13 in test situations where IL-4 was effective in inducing IgE production (R. Coffman *et al.*, unpublished).

## PRODUCTION OF IL-4 AND IL-13

IL-4 and IL-13 are produced by $CD4^+$ T cells and at lower levels by $CD8^+$ T cells. IL-4 and IL-13 are also secreted by activated mast cells and basophils[5,32–34]. Both human IL-4 and IL-13 are produced at high levels by activated Th2 clones, but, in contrast to IL-4, human IL-13 is also produced, albeit at lower levels, by activated $CD4^+$ Th1-like clones. In addition, a proportion of human $CD8^+$ T-cell clones produce IL-4 and IL-13 following activation[31]. Optimal levels of IL-13 mRNA are already induced after 2 h of activation. At this time point, IL-13 protein production can also be detected. Steady-state levels of hIL-13 mRNA expression, reflecting ongoing IL-13 protein production, can still be observed 72 h after activation of human T-cell clones. These kinetics of IL-13 mRNA expression and IL-13 protein production are different from those of IL-4 mRNA and protein synthesis, which are transiently induced. Generally, no detectable levels of IL-4 mRNA can be observed 24 h after activation of human T-cell clones. In addition, only minimal accumulation of IL-4 protein production was measured beyond this time point[31]. Based on these data, it seems that IL-13 is produced early, and, in contrast to IL-4, over prolonged periods of time by various human T-helper cell subsets following activation.

## IL-4 IS REQUIRED FOR Th2 CELL DEVELOPMENT

The mechanisms controlling Th1 or Th2 cell development are beginning to be elucidated both *in vitro* and *in vivo*. IL-4, present during initial antigen presentation, gives rise to IL-4-producing T-cell populations following restimulation, whereas it inhibits the development of IFN-γ-producing Th1 cells (reviewed in reference 35). Although IL-4 sets the stage for Th2 cell development, it is presently not clear whether Th1 and Th2 cells arise from a common precursor cell. In addition, the cellular source of IL-4, which needs to be present during priming of naive $CD4^+$ T-helper cells by antigen, still needs to be identified. Mast cells and basophils activated via their IgE or IgG receptor have been proposed as initial sources of IL-4 for Th2 cell development. However, this does not seem to be the case, because IL-4-deficient mice reconstituted with only $CD4^+$ T cells from congenic wild-type animals were able to produce antigen-specific IgE[36]. Another IL-4 source may be a rare population of splenic $CD4^+$, $NK1.1^+$ T cells, which produce IL-4 rapidly after injecting mice with anti-CD3 mAbs or staphylococcal enterotoxin B[37]. Whether IL-13, which does not directly act on T cells, can direct Th2 cell development remains to be established. Based on the observation that IL-13, like IL-4, downregulates IL-12 and IFN-α production by human monocytes[30], it may be possible that IL-13 also directs Th2 development, since both IL-12 and IFN-α have been shown to direct Th1 cell development[38–40]. The observation that IL-4 favors Th2 development has direct consequences for B-cell functions, since Th2 cells are major producers of IL-4 and IL-13, both of which are important regulators of B-cell activities.

## EFFECTS OF IL-4 AND IL-13 ON HUMAN B-CELL PHENOTYPE AND FUNCTION

### IL-4 AND IL-13 MODULATE B-CELL PHENOTYPE

CD23 is the low-affinity receptor for IgE (FcεRII). It exists in two different forms, FcεRIIa and FcεRIIb, which are generated through the use of different transcription sites and alternative RNA splicing, and which have identical extracellular domains[41]. Normal B cells express low levels of FcεRIIa, which are enhanced by IL-4 or IL-13. IL-4 and IL-13 also induce the expression of

FcεRIIb[42]. CD23 can be released in a soluble form (sCD23), which can enhance IL-4-induced IgE synthesis *in vitro*, but only when suboptimal concentrations of IL-4 are used[43,44]. However, recombinant sCD23 has no B-cell growth-promoting activity *in vitro*[45]. Anti-CD23 mAbs strongly block IL-4-induced human IgE synthesis *in vitro*[46], and antigen-induced IgE synthesis in mice *in vivo*[47], suggesting a role for CD23 in the regulation of IgE synthesis. However, the latter *in vivo* data are difficult to reconcile with the observation that mice with disrupted CD23 genes have normal IgE responses[48].

In contrast to FcεRII, IL-4 has been demonstrated to downregulate expression of FcγRII on lipopolysaccharide (LPS)-activated murine B cells[49]. Interestingly, IFN-γ, which antagonizes several effects of IL-4, did not reverse IL-4-induced inhibition of FcγRII expression. Consistent with these results, IL-4 was shown to inhibit binding of antigen IgE complexes to murine B cells[50]. Therefore, IL-4 may also eznhance humoral immune responses by suppressing immune complex-mediated inhibitory effects on B-cell activation. Moreover, IL-4 has also been shown to induce Thy-1 expression on murine B cells, which was associated with enhanced IgE production *in vivo*[51,52].

IL-4 and IL-13 also upregulate the expression of class II MHC antigens, CD71 (transferrin receptor) and CD72 on B cells. Furthermore, IL-4 upregulates the expression of CD40, which acts as a costimulatory molecule for B-cell proliferation and differentiation[53,54], surface IgM[55] and B7-1 (CD80)[56], which is the ligand for the T-cell costimulatory molecules CD28 and CTLA4[57,58]. These effects of IL-4 and IL-13 on expression of B-cell surface molecules suggest that they may facilitate T–B-cell interactions and antigen presentation by B cells to T cells.

## IL-4 AND IL-13 INDUCE B-CELL PROLIFERATION

Both IL-4 and IL-13 induce proliferation of human B cells activated by anti-IgM, anti-CD40 mAbs, or transfectants expressing CD40L[11,12,27,59–61]. IL-4 and IL-13 are equally effective in inducing proliferation of B cells activated through their CD40 molecules by anti-CD40 mAbs, or CD40L-expressing transfectants. However, IL-13-induced proliferation of human B cells activated by anti-IgM mAbs was considerably lower than that induced by IL-4[11]. IL-4 also induces proliferation of antigen-activated human B cells[62]. Paradoxically, IL-4 also has inhibitory effects on B-cell proliferation. It inhibits IL-2-induced B-cell proliferation *in vitro*[63,64] and it induces apoptosis in normal and leukemic human B-cell precursors[65–67].

## IL-4 AND IL-13 INDUCE IgG4 AND IgE PRODUCTION

Early studies have shown that IL-4 induces IgG1 and IgE production by mouse B cells *in vitro*[68,69]. IL-4 is also important for murine IgE synthesis *in vivo*, since administration of anti-IL-4 mAbs strongly blocked IgE synthesis in response to parasite infections[70,71]. In addition, mice with disrupted IL-4 genes have normal T- and B-cell development, but, in contrast to their wild-type counterparts, they failed to produce detectable levels of IgE following nematode infections, indicating that IL-4 seems to be the only cytokine capable of inducing IgE synthesis in mice[72]. However, IgG1 can be detected in IL-4-deficient mice, but the levels are strongly reduced, indicating that IgG1 switching occurs independently of IL-4, but that IL-4 has enhancing effects on IgG1 switching, or on IgG1-producing B cells. IL-4 is not required for the production of other Ig isotypes, because IL-4-deficient mice have normal levels of IgM, IgG2a, IgG3 and IgA.

hIL-4 induces IgG4 and IgE production by human B cells derived from blood, tonsils, spleens and cord blood[45,73–77]. The finding that cord blood B cells can be induced to switch to IgE production by exogenous IL-4 indicates that these cells, in contrast to what has been proposed previously[78], are mature in their capacity to switch to IgE in response to the appropriate signals. In contrast to adult peripheral blood mononuclear cells (PBMNCs), cord blood MNCs failed to produce IL-4 following activation *in vitro*. This lack or suppression of IL-4 production by cord blood T cells may account for the absence of IgE in cord blood and in newborns. IL-4 also induces IgE production by Epstein–Barr virus (EBV)-transformed B cells and Burkitt's lymphoma cells in the presence of activated $CD4^+$ T-cell clones[79]. The fact that IL-4, in the presence of activated $CD4^+$ T-helper cells, also induces IgG4 and IgE production by naive $sIgD^+$ B cells indicates that IL-4 indeed induces Ig isotype switching and that the production of these Ig isotypes does not reflect the preferential outgrowth of IgG4/IgE-committed B cells[76,80]. Recently, we demonstrated that IL-13 has similar effects. Like IL-4, it induces IgG4 and IgE synthesis in cultures of unfractionated PBMNCs, as well as by highly purified $sIgD^+$ B cells cultured in the presence of activated $CD4^+$ T-cell clones, or their membranes[27,81]. Neutralizing anti-IL-4 mAbs failed to inhibit IL-13-induced IgE synthesis, indicating that IgE synthesis was not mediated through induction of IL-4 production by T cells and that IL-13 acts independently from IL-4. However, IL-13 generally is 2–5-fold less effective than IL-4 in inducing IgE synthesis *in vitro*. No additive or synergistic effects were observed when both IL-4 and IL-13 were used at optimal concentrations[81]. These data suggest that IL-13, in addition to IL-4, may play an important role in induction and maintenance of IgE synthesis by B cells in atopic patients. However, the relative contribution of IL-4 and IL-13 to IgE production in atopic disease remains to be determined.

Interestingly, in contrast to IL-4, IL-13 does not seem to act on mouse B cells. As mentioned above, mouse IL-13 was ineffective in assays in which IL-4 induced IgG1 and IgE production (R. Coffman, unpublished). These data are compatible with the observation that IL-4-deficient mice are not capable of producing IgE following parasite infections[72] and exclude the possibility that the lack of IgE production in these mice could be due to strongly impaired Th2 cell development and IL-13 production[82].

Whether IL-4 and IL-13 indeed are responsible for enhanced IgE synthesis in atopic patients still needs to be formally proven. However, strong indirect evidence suggests that IL-4 is associated with enhanced IgE synthesis in atopic disease. PBMNCs of atopic patients with high serum IgE levels produce more IL-4 and less IFN-γ following activation *ex vivo* than PBMNCs of healthy controls[83]. Furthermore, PBMNCs of some patients spontaneously produced IL-4 *in vitro*, a phenomenon never observed with PBMNCs of normal donors[83]. Both IL-4 and IL-5 are detected in bronchoalveolar T lymphocytes after local allergen challenge in atopic asthma patients, but not in BAL cells of healthy donors[84]. Similarly, IL-4 and IL-5 are also detected in allergen-induced late-phase cutaneous reactions in atopic individuals[85]. Taken together, these data suggest that IL-4 production in atopic patients is enhanced. This notion is further supported by data which showed that allergen-specific $CD4^+$ T-cell clones from atopic individuals, but not from healthy donors, generally belong to the Th2 subset producing high levels of IL-4, IL-5 and IL-13 and low, or no detectable, levels of IFN-γ after activation[86–89]. Co-cultivation of these Th2 clones with B cells results in IgE synthesis, which is strongly, but not completely, blocked by anti-IL-4 mAbs[73,75,90], indicating that endogenous IL-4 production by these Th2 clones predominantly accounts for their IgE-inducing effects, whereas the remaining activity is probably mediated by IL-13. These high levels of IL-4 and IL-13 production by allergen-specific Th2 cells, together with the low levels of IFN-γ production, most likely contribute to enhanced IgE synthesis observed in atopic patients.

## THE ROLE OF CD40L–CD40 INTERACTION IN Ig ISOTYPE SWITCHING

In addition to cytokines, contact-mediated costimulatory signals provided by activated $CD4^+$ T-helper cells are required for productive T–B-cell interactions, resulting in Ig switching and Ig production. The interaction between the CD40L induced on the T-helper cells after activation and CD40 constitutively expressed on B cells appears to be necessary for Ig isotype switching to occur. The ligands for both murine and human CD40 have been cloned from cDNA libraries constructed from activated T cells[61,91–93]. These cDNAs encode a 33-kDa type II glycoprotein with significant homology to tumor necrosis factor alpha (TNF-α) and TNF-β. Transfectants expressing CD40L induce naive $sIgD^+$ human B cells to proliferate and differentiate into IgG4- and IgE-producing cells in the presence of IL-4 or IL-13, indicating that the signals provided by the CD40L and IL-4 or IL-13 are sufficient for induction of IgG4 and IgE switching[61,91–93]. CD40L–CD40 interactions are also required for Ig isotype switching *in vivo*. Patients suffering from the X-linked hyper-IgM syndrome (HIS) have normal or enhanced levels of IgM, but they fail to produce significant levels of the other Ig isotypes. This defect in Ig isotype switching *in vivo* was due to mutations in the patients' CD40L genes, which result in defective CD40L expression on activated T cells. However, the B cells of these patients are normal, as they could be induced to switch to IgG4 and IgE synthesis in the presence of anti-CD40 mAbs, or CD40L transfectants and IL-4 or IL-13[94–97].

In addition to CD40L, other membrane-bound molecules expressed on activated T cells can provide costimulatory signals for induction of IL-4-dependent IgE synthesis. mAbs specific for the 26-kDa membrane form of TNF-α (mTNF-α) expressed on $CD4^+$ T cells early after activation, and anti-TNF receptor (p55) mAbs, inhibit IL-4-induced T-cell-dependent IgG4 and IgE synthesis, indicating that mTNF-α, in addition to CD40L, is another T-cell activation molecule associated with productive T–B-cell interactions, resulting in Ig isotype switching[98]. However, the signals delivered through mTNF-α–p55 interactions are quantitatively different from those provided by anti-CD40 mAbs, since anti-p55 mAbs, in contrast to anti-CD40 mAbs, fail to induce B-cell proliferation. It has been shown that a proportion of HIV-infected $CD4^+$ T cells express high levels of mTNF-α constitutively[99]. In the presence of IL-4, these $HIV^+$ T cells induce polyclonal B-cell activation *in vitro*, which is inhibited by anti-TNF-α or anti-TNF-R mAbs. This TNF-α-mediated T-helper activity was shown to be independent of CD40L, suggesting that additional ligands for CD40, or alternative pathways for polyclonal human B-cell activation, exist. Based on these *in vitro* findings, it has been proposed that mTNF-α–TNF-R interactions may play a role in polyclonal B-cell activation observed in HIV-infected patients[99].

Recently, it has been demonstrated that some T-cell clones established from HIS patients, who have well-defined mutations in their CD40L genes, and who fail to express functional CD40L, can induce IgE synthesis in the presence of IL-4 *in vitro*[100]. This IgE switching occurred independently of both CD40L and TNF-α, indicating that other, yet to be defined, accessory molecules, different from CD40L, can provide a costimulatory signal for IL-4-dependent IgE synthesis. Whether this molecule represents a second ligand for CD40 was, however, not assessed in this study. These data, indicating that human Ig isotype switching can take place without CD40L involvement, are consistent with studies in CD40L-deficient mice, which demonstrated that these mice underwent Ig isotype switching following immunization with thymus-independent antigens[101].

## INDUCTION OF HUMAN IgE SYNTHESIS IN SCID-hu MICE

Severe combined immunodeficiency (SCID) mice have a genetic defect in their recombinase system, and as a consequence they have no detectable mature T and B cells. Because of this immunodeficiency, SCID mice easily accept xenografts, and therefore provide an excellent model for human cell and organ transfer experiments. SCID mice transplanted subcutaneously with small pieces of human fetal bone (as a source of fetal bone marrow) and fetal thymus develop a functional human thymus growing on top of the bone containing normal human bone marrow. These thymus–bone structures contain >90 per cent human cells, with 50–75 per cent thymocytes, 10–15 per cent mature CD8+ and 15–20 per cent mature CD4+ T cells, 6–10 per cent B cells and 3–7 per cent CD14+ macrophages[102]. Administration of hIL-4 resulted in human B-cell maturation as judged by enhancement of CD23, CD40, class II MHC and sIgM expression in all SCID-hu mice tested. More importantly, in approximately 50 per cent of the SCID-hu mice considerable levels of human IgE production could be induced by IL-4, whereas control mice treated with saline remained human IgE negative[102]. These data indicate that productive interactions between human T and B cells resulting in IgE isotype switching and IgE synthesis are induced by IL-4 administration, proving the point that IL-4 induces human IgE synthesis *in vivo*.

## MODULATION OF IL-4 INDUCED IgE SYNTHESIS BY CYTOKINES

Several cytokines can modulate IL-4-induced IgE synthesis. IFN-α[46], IFN-γ[46], transforming growth factor beta (TGF-β)[103], IL-8[104] and IL-12[105] all inhibit human IgE synthesis *in vitro*, by mechanisms which are still ill-defined. However, with the exception of TGF-β, the inhibitory effects of these cytokines seem to be indirectly mediated through suppression of the CD4+ T-helper cell function[103,106]. TGF-β also inhibits T-cell-independent IgE synthesis induced by IL-4 in the presence of anti-CD40 mAbs[103]. More recent studies indicated that IFN-γ and IFN-α also have direct, but transient, inhibitory effects on IL-4-induced germline ϵ transcription (which is required for subsequent IgE switching; see below) in purified B cells, or B-cell lines (Cocks *et al.*, submitted). These results suggest that these interferons may inhibit IgE synthesis by both direct and indirect mechanisms. IL-10 inhibits IL-4-induced IgE synthesis by human PBMNCs, but it does not have any suppressive effects when highly purified B cells are co-cultured with activated CD4+ T cells or anti-CD40 mAbs[107]. IL-4-induced IgE synthesis by freshly isolated PBMNCs is monocyte dependent, but monocytes that had been preincubated with IL-10 were ineffective in providing help for T-cell-dependent IgE synthesis, indicating that the inhibitory effects of IL-10 were indirectly mediated by suppressing a yet to be defined accessory cell function of monocytes. IFN-γ and IFN-α also inhibit IgE production *in vivo* both in mice[2,40] and in humans[108,109]. Other cytokines can enhance IL-4-induced IgE synthesis. IL-5[44], IL-6[110] and TNF-α[103] all enhance IL-4-induced human IgE production. The increased IgE synthesis observed in the presence of TNF-α was associated with enhanced expression of IL-4-induced germline ϵ mRNA, which together with its growth-promoting effects on B cells may account for the enhanced IgE synthesis observed *in vitro*[102]. The enhancing effects of IL-5 were only observed when suboptimal concentrations of IL-4 were used[44], whereas IL-6 also enhances IgE synthesis induced by optimal IL-4 concentrations. The IgE-enhancing effects of IL-6 are probably due to the B-cell differentiation and growth-promoting activities of this cytokine[111].

## IL-4 AND IL-13 INDUCE GERMLINE ε mRNA EXPRESSION

Murine germline Ig heavy chain transcripts initiate upstream of their corresponding switch regions and it has been proposed that synthesis of germline transcripts opens up the chromatin structure of the specific switch regions, making them accessible to a putative common recombinase system (reviewed in reference 112; see also Chapter 5).

Analysis of human B-cell cultures indicated that induction of IgE switching is always preceded by transcription of germline ε mRNA[79,80]. We never observed IgE production in the absence of germline ε RNA expression. Human germline ε RNA comprises, in addition to the Cε exon, an I (initiate) ε (Iε) exon, located 3.5 kb upstream from the ε heavy chain constant region (Cε) and 5′ from the ε switch (Sε) region[80]. IL-4 induces germline ε transcripts in normal human B cells, EBV-transformed B-cells and Burkitt's lymphoma cells[79,80,103,113–115]. Germline ε mRNA expression in purified human B cells is already detectable within 2 h after incubation with IL-4. However, IL-4 alone fails to induce productive ε mRNA transcripts, which requires costimulatory signals provided by T-helper cells, anti-CD40 mAbs or CD40L transfectants[61,79–81,113–115]. IL-4-induced productive ε mRNA in PBMNCs is first detected 6–7 days after onset of the cultures, just before IgE protein synthesis is detectable, whereas maximal expression occurs around day 14[80]. The levels of germline ε mRNA expression correlate with the levels of subsequent IgE synthesis. In addition, modulation of germline ε transcription by cytokines, such as TGF-β, which has inhibitory effects, or TNF-α, which has enhancing effects, showed a similar modulation of IL-4-induced IgE synthesis *in vitro*[103], demonstrating a strong functional relationship between germline ε mRNA expression and subsequent IgE production.

The absolute requirement of germline transcripts for isotype switching in mice *in vivo* was demonstrated by disruption of the Iγ1 or Iγ2b encoding regions by gene targeting, which completely prevented class switching to γ1 and γ2b, respectively[116,117]. Like IL-4, IL-13 is able to induce germline ε transcription in human B cells, which is consistent with its capacity to induce IgE synthesis[81]. The levels of IL-13-induced germline ε transcription were always lower than those induced by IL-4, but they were strongly upregulated by anti-CD40 mAbs, or by CD40L-expressing transfectants (Cocks *et al.*, submitted). The presence of these costimulatory signals also resulted in the induction of productive ε mRNA expression. No additive or synergistic effects on germline ε transcription were observed when IL-4 and IL-13 were added together at optimal concentrations. In contrast to IL-4, IL-13 failed to induce germline ε transcripts in EBV-transformed B cells or Burkitt's lymphoma cells, which is due to the absence of functional IL-13 receptors on these cells (Cocks *et al.*, submitted). The mechanisms regulating germline ε transcription by IL-4 or IL-13 in normal B cells appear to be similar, because anti-CD40 mAbs, IFN-γ, TNF-α and TGF-β modulated both IL-4- and IL-13-induced germline ε transcription in a comparable fashion (Punnonen *et al.*, J Immunol, in press).

## EFFECTS OF IL-4 AND IL-13 ON IMMATURE HUMAN B CELLS

Early B-cell precursors express IL-4 receptors[118], but studies on the effects of IL-4 on these cells have given contradictory results. IL-4 has been shown to induce growth and differentiation of human pre-B cells[119], whereas other studies demonstrated that IL-4 has either no[120] or an inhibitory [121,122] effect on pre-B-cell proliferation. These different results may be due to the fact that IL-4 may have different effects on different subpopulations of B-cell precursors, and it has been suggested that the effects of IL-4 on pre-B cells depend on the combinations of different stimuli acting on a given cell[121].

Human surface (s)$\mu^-$, $CD10^+$, $CD19^+$ pre-B cells isolated from fetal bone marrow (BM) spontaneously differentiate into immature s$\mu^+$ B cells *in vitro*[120]. In addition, immature B cells derived from human fetal spleen, liver, BM[121,123] or thymus[124] undergo Ig isotype switching and differentiation into Ig-secreting cells in the presence of IL-4 and anti-CD40 mAbs or activated $CD4^+$ T cells. More recently, it was demonstrated that s$\mu^-$, $CD10^+$, $CD19^+$ pre-B cells derived from human fetal BM differentiate with high frequencies into Ig-secreting cells when co-cultured with activated, cloned $CD4^+$ T cells and IL-4[125]. These data indicate that ε switching machinery is operational in early B cells, suggesting that commitment to IgE synthesis may occur at a very early stage of B-cell ontogeny.

IL-13 also induces IgE switching by human immature B cells derived from fetal BM[126]. IL-4 and IL-13 also induce germline ε mRNA synthesis in immature human B cells freshly isolated from fetal BM (J. Punnonen *et al.*, J Immunol, in press). Similar mechanisms appear to regulate IL-4- and IL-13-induced IgE synthesis in immature B cells, because, as shown for mature B cells, IL-6 had enhancing, whereas IFN-α, IFN-γ, TGF-β and IL-12 had inhibitory, effects on both IL-4- and IL-13-induced IgE synthesis in the presence of cloned $CD4^+$ T-helper cells[126]. The levels of Ig produced in response to IL-13 were consistently 5–15-fold lower than those induced by IL-4, irrespective of whether anti-CD40 mAbs or $CD4^+$ T cells were used to costimulate the immature B cells. However, IL-13-induced proliferation of immature B cells was only slightly lower than that induced by IL-4[126]. The reason for the lower capacity of IL-13 to induce Ig synthesis remains to be determined. Answers to these questions await characterization of the IL-13R and information about its expression on B cells in different maturation stages.

Although IL-4R is expressed on pre-B cells and IL-4 affects the function of these cells, IL-13 appears to directly activate B cells only after they have passed the pre-B-cell stage in B-cell ontogeny, because IL-13 failed to induce phenotypic changes in human pre-B cells *in vitro*[126], whereas IL-4, in contrast, induced high levels of CD23 expression on a proportion of cultured s$\mu^-$ pre-B cells, and it consistently enhanced the expression of CD40 and HLA-DR on these cells.

## INHIBITION OF HUMAN IgE SYNTHESIS BY AN IL-4 MUTANT PROTEIN

### INHIBITION OF IL-4- AND IL-13-INDUCED IgE SYNTHESIS *IN VITRO*

Recently, a human IL-4 mutant protein was generated in which the tyrosine residue at position 124 of human IL-4 was replaced by aspartic acid. This mutant protein (IL-4.Y124D) binds with high affinity to IL-4R without receptor activation, suggesting that it could be used as a potential IL-4R antagonist[16,127]. Indeed, IL-4.Y124D inhibited, in a dose-dependent fashion, IL-4- and IL-13-induced proliferation of the TF-1 cell line[16] and IL-4- or IL-13-induced human B-cell proliferation[27]. In addition, IL-4- and IL-13-induced IgG4 and IgE synthesis by human PBMNCs, or highly purified sIgD$^+$ B cells cultured in the presence of anti-CD40 mAbs, was blocked efficiently. In general, more than 95 per cent inhibition of IgE production was observed at a 20–50-fold excess of the IL-4R antagonist[27]. Interestingly, the IL-4 mutant protein was even more effective in inhibiting IL-13 synthesis, which generally required only a 5–20-fold excess of the antagonist to obtain >95 per cent inhibition. The IL-4 mutant protein had only minimal agonistic activity at very high concentrations[27]. Thus, this IL-4 mutant protein is a potent inhibitor of both IL-4- and IL-13-induced IgE production by PBMNCs *in vitro*, which is consistent with the notion that the IL-4R and IL-13R are complex receptors which share a common subunit which is involved in signal transduction[16].

### INHIBITION OF *IN VIVO* HUMAN IgE SYNTHESIS

In order to determine whether the IL-4 mutant protein could also inhibit IgE synthesis *in vivo*, we tested its capacity to block ongoing human IgE synthesis in SCID-hu mice transplanted with fetal human thymus and bone marrow. These SCID-hu mice can spontaneously produce considerable levels of human IgM, IgG and IgA, probably in response to environmental antigens. In addition, approximately one-third of these mice have significant levels of human IgE. SCID-hu mice with comparable serum levels of human IgE were selected for treatment. The IL-4 mutant protein was continuously delivered by subcutaneously implanted micro-osmotic pumps for a period of 3 weeks. At termination of the treatment the levels of human IgE in the circulation were reduced by >90 per cent, whereas the circulating levels of human IgG were not significantly affected by IL-4.Y124D administration. In addition, the human IgG and IgE levels in control SCID-hu mice treated with saline remained unaltered. More importantly, despite the fact that IL-4.Y124D at high concentrations has low agonistic activity *in vitro*, no detectable agonistic activity, as judged by induction of CD23 expression on B cells, was observed *in vivo*[102]. The results indicate that the IL-4 mutant protein is also effective in reducing ongoing human IgE responses *in vivo*. These results suggest that this IL-4R and IL-13R antagonist may have potential therapeutic utility in reducing serum IgE levels in atopic patients.

## CONCLUDING REMARKS

IL-4 and IL-13 are structurally related cytokines, which are predominantly, but not exclusively, produced by Th2 cells. The overlapping biological activities of IL-4 and IL-13 reflect the commonly observed redundancy of cytokines in the immune system and may function as a fail-safe mechanism. Cytokines are uniformly pleiotropic and they can have shared biological activities, because of the usage of common receptor components required for signaling, as described here for IL-4 and IL-13. However, despite their many similarities and utilization of a shared receptor component, there are differences in IL-4 and IL-13 activities, which indicate that each of these cytokines in fact may play a unique role in the immune response.

IL-4 and IL-13 both have comparable effects on human B cells and monocytes. They both inhibit the production of proinflammatory cytokines, chemokines, IL-10, IL-12 and IFN-$\alpha$ by monocytes, whereas they enhance IL-1 receptor antagonist production[30,128]. IL-4 and IL-13 both have growth-promoting effects on activated human B cells and are, thus far, the only cytokines inducing IgG4 and IgE switching and synthesis *in vitro*. IL-4 and IL-13 activate immature B cells, and IL-4 also has direct stimulatory effects on $s\mu^-$ pre-B cells. The major differences between IL-4 and IL-13 are determined by the fact that IL-13, in contrast to IL-4, lacks T-cell regulatory effects, and that mouse IL-13 fails to induce IgE synthesis by mouse B cells in culture systems in which IL-4 is effective. IL-4 directs the development of Th2 cells both *in vitro* and *in vivo*, and downregulates the generation of IFN-$\gamma$-producing T cells[35]. IL-13 does not act on T cells and therefore cannot have direct effects on $CD4^+$ T-cell development. However, since IL-13, like IL-4, downregulates the production of IL-12 and IFN-α by monocytes/macrophages, cytokines which induce Th1 responses, IL-13 may also favor Th2 cell development. The present data indicate that IL-4 and IL-13 play a fundamental role in immune and inflammatory responses, and in the regulation of B-cell maturation and differentiation, particularly in directing IgG4 and IgE isotype switching. Th2 cell development and overproduction of IL-4 and IL-13 are probably responsible for the enhanced IgE synthesis in atopic individuals. Based on these observations, it is clear that counteracting these activities may provide an efficient way to intervene in atopic diseases.

## ACKNOWLEDGMENTS

We would like to thank Drs Gregorio Aversa, José Carballido, Benjamin Cocks, Hughes Gascan and Jean François Gauchat for their contributions, Bruce Bennett and Jean Chang for their assistance and Jo Ann Katheiser for expert secretarial help.

The DNAX Research Institute of Molecular and Cellular Biology is supported by Schering-Plough.

## REFERENCES

1. Schimpl A, Wecker E. Replacement of T-cell function by a T-cell product. Nature 1972; 237:15–17.
2. Coffman RL, Seymour BWP, Lebman DA *et al.* The role of helper T cell products in mouse B cell differentiation and isotype regulation. Immunol Rev 1988; 102:5–28.
3. Mosmann TR, Coffman RT. Th1 and Th2 cells: different patterns of lymphokine secretion lead to different functional properties. Annu Rev Immunol 1989; 7:145–173.
4. Clark EA, Ledbetter JA. How B and T cells talk to each other. Nature 1994; 367:425–428.
5. Howard M, Farrar J, Hilfiker M *et al.* Identification of a T cell-derived β cell growth factor distinct from interleukin 2. J Exp Med 1982; 155:914–923.
6. Isakson PC, Pure E, Vitetta ES, Krammer PH. Pure T cell-derived B cell differentiation factor(s). Effect on the isotype switch of murine B cells. J Exp Med 1982; 155:734–748.
7. Lee F, Yokota T, Meyerson P *et al.* Isolation and characterization of a mouse interleukin cDNA clone that expresses B-cell stimulatory factor 1 activities and T-cell and mast-cell-stimulating activities. Proc Natl Acad Sci USA 1986; 83:2061–2065.
8. Noma Y, Sideras P, Naito T *et al.* Cloning of cDNA encoding the murine IgG1 induction factor by a novel strategy using SP6 promoter. Nature 1986; 319:640–646.
9. Yokota T, Otsuka T, Mosmann T *et al.* Isolation and characterization of a human interleukin cDNA clone, homologous to B-cell stimulatory factor 1, that

expresses B-cell and T-cell stimulating activities. Proc Natl Acad Sci USA 1986; 83:5894–5899.

10. Brown KD, Zurawski S, Mosmann TR, Zurawski G. A family of small inducible proteins secreted by leukocytes are members of a new superfamily that include leukocytes and fibroblast-derived inflammatory agents, growth factors and indicators of various activation processes. J Immunol 1989; 142:679–687.
11. McKenzie ANJ, Culpepper JA, de Waal Malefyt R *et al.* Interleukin-13, a novel T cell-derived cytokine that regulates monocyte and B cell function. Proc Natl Acad Sci USA 1993; 90:3735–3739.
12. Minty A, Chalon P, Derocq JM *et al.* Interleukin-13 is a new human lymphokine regulating inflammatory and immune responses. Nature 1993; 362:248–250.
13. McKenzie ANJ, Li X, Largaespada DA *et al.* Structural comparison and chromosomal localization of the human and mouse IL-13 genes. J Immunol 1993; 150:5436–5444.
14. Morgan JG, Dolganov GM, Robbins SE *et al.* The selective isolation of novel cDNAs encoded by the regions surrounding the human interleukin 4 and 5 genes. Nucleic Acids Res 1992; 20:5173–5179.
15. Pandit J, Bohm A, Jancarik J *et al.* Three-dimensional structure of dimeric human recombinant macrophage colony-stimulating factor. Science 1992; 258:1358–1362.
16. Zurawski SM, Vega Jr F, Huyghe B, Zurawski G. Receptors for interleukin-13 and interleukin-4 are complex and share a novel component that functions in signal transduction. EMBO J 1993; 12:3899–3905.
17. Powers R, Garrett DS, March CJ *et al.* Three-dimensional solution of human interleukin-4 by multidimensional heteronuclear magnetic resonance spectroscopy. Science 1992; 256:1673–1675.
18. Park LS, Friend D, Sassenfeld HM, Urdal DL. Characterization of the human B cell stimulatory factor 1 receptor. J Exp Med 1987; 166:476–488.
19. Cabrillat H, Galizzi JP, Djossou O *et al.* High affinity binding of human interleukin 4 to cell lines. Biochem Biophys Res Commun 1987; 149:995–1001.
20. Idzerda RL, March CJ, Mosley B *et al.* Human interleukin 4 receptor confers biological responsiveness and defines a novel receptor superfamily. J Exp Med 1990; 171:861–873.
21. Galizzi JP, Zuber CE, Harada N *et al.* Molecular cloning of a cDNA encoding the human interleukin 4 receptor. Int Immunol 1990; 2:669–675.
22. Miyajima A, Kitamura T, Harada N *et al.* Cytokine receptors and signal transduction. Annu Rev Immunol 1992; 10:295–331.
23. Kondo M, Takeshita T, Ishii N *et al.* Sharing of the interleukin-2 (IL-2) receptor $\gamma$ chain between receptors for IL-2 and IL-4. Science 1993; 262:1874–1877.
24. Russell SM, Keegan AD, Harada N *et al.* Interleukin-2 receptor $\gamma$ chain: a functional component of the interleukin-4 receptor. Science 1993; 262:1880–1883.
25. Noguchi M, Nakamura Y, Russell SM *et al.* Interleukin-2 receptor $\gamma$ chain: a functional component of the interleukin-7 receptor. Science 1993; 262:1877–1880.
26. Noguchi M, Yi H, Rosenblatt HM *et al.* Interleukin-2 receptor gamma chain mutation results in X-linked severe combined immunodeficiency in humans. Cell 1993; 73:147–157.
27. Aversa G, Punnonen J, Cocks BG *et al.* An IL-4 mutant protein inhibits both IL-4 or IL-13-induced human IgG4 and IgE synthesis and B cell proliferation: support for a common component shared by IL-4 and IL-13 receptors. J Exp Med 1993; 178:2213–2218.
28. Tony HP, Shen BJ, Reusch P, Sebald W. Design of human interleukin-4

antagonists inhibiting interleukin-4-dependent and interleukin-13-dependent responses in T-cells and B-cells with high-efficiency. Eur J Biochem 1994; 225:659–665.

29. Zurawski SM, Chomarat P, Djossou O *et al.* The primary binding subunit of the human interleukin-4 receptor is also a component of the interleukin-13 receptor. J Biol Chem 1995; 270:13869–13878.
30. Zurawski G, de Vries JE. Interleukin 13, an interleukin 4-like cytokine that acts on monocytes and B cells, but not on T cells. Immunol Today 1994; 15:19–26.
31. de Waal Malefyt R, Abrams JS, Zurawski SM *et al.* Differential regulation of IL-13 and IL-4 production by human $CD8^+$ and $CD4^+$ Th0, Th1 and Th2 T cell clones and EBV-transformed B cells. Int Immunol 1995; 7:1405–1416.
32. Brunner T, Heusser CH, Dahinden CA. Human peripheral blood basophils primed by interleukin 3 (IL-3) produce IL-4 in response to immunoglobulin E receptor stimulation. J Exp Med 1993; 177:605–611.
33. Bradding P, Feather IH, Howath PH *et al.* Interleukin 4 is localized to and released by human mast cells. J Exp Med 1992; 176:1381–1386.
34. Burd PR, Thompson WC, Max EE, Mills FC. Activated mast cells produce IL-13. J Exp Med 1995; 1373–1380.
35. O'Garra A, Murphy K. T-cell subsets in autoimmunity. Curr Opin Immunol 1993; 5:880–886.
36. Schmitz J, Thiel A, Kuhn R *et al.* Induction of interleukin 4 (IL-4) expression in T helper (Th) cell is not dependent on IL-4 from non-Th cells. J Exp Med 1994; 179:1349–1353.
37. Yoshimoto T, Paul WE. $CD4^+$, $NK1.1^+$ T cells promptly produce interleukin 4 in response to *in vivo* challenge with anti-CD3. J Exp Med 1994; 179:1285–1295.
38. Hsieh C-S, Macatonia SE, Tripp CS *et al.* Development of TH1 $CD4^+$ T cells through IL-12 produced by *Listeria*-induced macrophages. Science 1993; 260:547–550.
39. Manetti R, Parronchi P, Giuduzu MG *et al.* Natural killer cell stimulatory factor (interleukin 12 [IL-12]) induces T helper type 1 (Th1)-specific immune responses and inhibits the development of IL-4-producing Th cells. J Exp Med 1993; 177:1199–1204.
40. Finkelman FD, Svetic A, Gresse I *et al.* Regulation by interferon alpha of immunoglobulin isotype selection and lymphokine production in mice. J Exp Med 1991; 174:1179–1188.
41. Yokota T, Otsuka T, Mosmann T *et al.* Isolation and characterization of a human interleukin cDNA clone, homologous to mouse B-cell stimulatory factor 1, that expresses B-cell- and T-cell-stimulating activities. Proc Natl Acad Sci USA 1986; 83:5894–5898.
42. Defrance T, Aubry JP, Rousset F *et al.* Human recombinant interleukin 4 induces Fcϵ receptors (CD23) on normal human B lymphocytes. J Exp Med 1987; 165:1459–1468.
43. Bonnefoy JY, Defrance T, Peronne C *et al.* Human recombinant interleukin 4 induces normal B cells to produce soluble CD23/IgE-binding factor analogous to that spontaneously released by lymphoblastoid B cell lines. Eur J Immunol 1988; 18:117–122.
44. Pène J, Rousset F, Briere F *et al.* Interleukin 5 enhances interleukin 4-induced IgE production by normal human B cells. The role of soluble CD23 antigen. Eur J Immunol 1988; 18:929–936.
45. Uchibayashi N, Kikutani H, Barsumian EL *et al.* Recombinant soluble Fcϵ receptor II (Fcϵ RII/CD23) has IgE binding activity but no B cell growth promoting activity. J Immunol 1989; 142:3901–3908.

46. Pène J, Rousset F, Briere F *et al.* IgE production by normal human lymphocytes is induced by interleukin 4 and suppressed by interferons gamma and alpha and prostaglandin E2. Proc Natl Acad Sci USA 1988; 85:6880–6884.
47. Flores-Romo L, Shields J, Humbert Y *et al.* Inhibition of an *in vivo* antigen-specific IgE response by antibodies to CD23. Science 1993; 261:1038–1041.
48. Fujiwara H, Kikutani H, Suematsu S *et al.* The absence of IgE antibody-mediated augmentation of immune responses in CD23-deficient mice. Proc Natl Acad Sci USA 1994; 91:6835–6839.
49. Snapper CM, Hooley JJ, Atasoy U *et al.* Differential regulation of murine B cell FcγRII expression by $CD4^+$ T helper subsets. J Immunol 1989; 143:2133–2141.
50. Laszlo G, Dickler HB. IL-4 induces loss of B lymphocyte Fc gamma R II ligand binding capacity. J Immunol 1988; 141:3416–3421.
51. Snapper CM, Hornbeck PV, Atasoy U *et al.* Interleukin 4 induces membrane Thy-1 expression on normal murine B cells. Proc Natl Acad Sci USA 1988; 85:6107–6111.
52. Snapper CM, Hooley JJ, Barbieri S, Finkelman FD. Murine B cells expressing Thy-1 after *in vivo* immunization selectively secrete IgE. J Immunol 1990; 144:2940–2945.
53. Clark EA, Ledbetter JA. Activation of human B cells mediated through two distinct cell surface differentiation antigens, Bp35 and Bp50. Proc Natl Acad Sci USA 1986; 83:4494–4508.
54. Gordon J, Millsum MJ, Guy GR, Ledbetter JA. Resting B lymphocytes can be triggered directly through the CDw40 (Bp50) antigen. A comparison with IL-4-mediated signaling. J Immunol 1988; 140:1425–1430.
55. Shields JG, Armitage RJ, Jamieson BN *et al.* Increased expression of surface IgM but not IgD or IgG on human B cells in response to IL-4. Immunology 1989; 66:224–227.
56. Valle A, Aubry JP, Durand I, Banchereau J. IL-4 and IL-2 upregulate the expression of antigen B7, the B cell counter structure to T cell CD28: an amplification mechanism for T–B cell interactions. Int Immunol 1991; 3:229–235.
57. Linsey PS, Clark EA, Ledbetter JA. The T cell antigen, CD28, mediates adhesion with B cells by interacting with the activation antigen, B7/BB-1. Proc Natl Acad Sci USA 1990; 87:5031–5035.
58. Linsley PS, Brady W, Urnes M *et al.* CTLA-4 is a second receptor for the B cell activation antigen B7. J Exp Med 1991; 174:561–569.
59. DeFrance T, Vanbervliet B, Aubry J-P *et al.* B cell growth-promoting activity of recombinant human interleukin 4. J Immunol 1987; 139:1135–1141.
60. Banchereau J, de Paoli P, Vallé A *et al.* Long term human B cell lines dependent on interleukin 4 and anti-CD40. Science 1991; 251:70–72.
61. Cocks B, de Waal Malefyt R, Galizzi J-P *et al.* IL-13 induces proliferation and differentiation of human B cells activated by the CD40 ligand. Int Immunol 1993; 5:657–663.
62. Llorente L, Mitjavila F, Crevon MC, Galanaud P. Dual effects of interleukin 4 on antigen-activated human B cells: induction of proliferation and inhibition of interleukin 2-dependent differentiation. Eur J Immunol 1990; 20:1887–1892.
63. Defrance T, Vanbervliet B, Aubry JP, Banchereau J. Interleukin 4 inhibits the proliferation but not the differentiation of activated human B cells in response to interleukin 2. J Exp Med 1988; 168:1321–1337.
64. Jelinek DF, Lipsky PE. Inhibitory influence of IL-4 on human B cell responsiveness. J Immunol 1988; 141:164–173.
65. Hofman FM, Brock M, Taylor CR, Lyons B. IL-4 regulates differentiation and proliferation of human precursor B cells. J Immunol 1988; 141:1185–1190.

66. Pandrau D, Sealand S, Duvert V *et al.* Interleukin 4 inhibits *in vitro* proliferation of leukemic and normal human B cell precursors. J Clin Invest 1992; 90:1697–1706.
67. Manabe A, Coustan-Smith E, Kumagai M *et al.* Interleukin-4 induces programmed cell death (apoptosis) in cases of high-risk acute lymphoblastic leukemia. Blood 1994; 83:1731–1737.
68. Coffman RL, Ohara J, Bond MW *et al.* B cell stimulatory factor-1 enhances the IgE response of lipopolysaccharide activated B cells. J Immunol 1986;4538–4541.
69. Snapper CM, Paul WE. Interferon-gamma and B cell stimulatory factor-1 reciprocally regulate Ig isotype production. Science 1987; 236:944–947.
70. Finkelman FD, Katona IM, Urban JF *et al.* Suppression of *in vivo* polyclonal IgE responses by mononuclear antibody to the lymphokine BSF-1. Proc Natl Acad USA 1986; 83:9675–9681.
71. Finkelman FD, Holmes J, Katona IM *et al.* Lymphokine control of *in vivo* immunoglobulin isotype selection. Annu Rev Immunol 1990; 8:303–309.
72. Kühn R, Rajewski K, Müller W. Generation and analysis of interleukin-4 deficient mice. Science 1991; 254:707–710.
73. Pène J, Rousset F, Briere F *et al.* IgE production by normal human B cells induced by alloreactive T cell clones is mediated by IL-4 and suppressed by IFN-gamma. J Immunol 1988; 141:1218–1224.
74. Del Prete G, Maggi E, Parronchi P *et al.* IL-4 is an essential factor for the IgE synthesis induced *in vitro* by human T cell clones and their supernatants. J Immunol 1988; 140:4193–4198.
75. Lundgren M, Persson U, Larsson P *et al.* Interleukin-4 induces synthesis of IgE and IgG4 in human B cells. Eur J Immunol 1989; 19:1311–1315.
76. Gascan H, Gauchat JF, Roncarolo MG *et al.* Human B cell clones can be induced to proliferate and switch to IgE and IgG4 synthesis by IL-4 and a signal provided by activated $CD4^+$ T cell clones. J Exp Med 1991; 173:747–750.
77. Pastorelli G, Rousset F, Pène J *et al.* Cord blood B cells are mature in their capacity to switch to IgE-producing cells in response to interleukin-4 *in vitro*. Clin Exp Immunol 1990; 82:114–119.
78. Andersson U, Bird AG, Britton S, Palacios R. Humoral and cellular immunity in human studied at the cell level from birth to two years of age. Immunol Rev 1981; 57:5–10.
79. Gauchat JF, Gascan H, de Waal Malefyt R, de Vries JE. Regulation of germ-line epsilon transcription and induction of epsilon switching in cloned EBV-transformed and malignant human B cell lines by cytokines and $CD4^+$ T cells. J Immunol 1992; 148:2291–2299.
80. Gauchat JF, Lebman DA, Coffman RL *et al.* Structure and expression of germline epsilon transcripts in human B cells induced by interleukin 4 to switch to IgE production. J Exp Med 1990; 172:463–473.
81. Punnonen J, Aversa G, Cocks BG *et al.* Interleukin-13 induces interleukin-4-independent IgG4 and IgE synthesis and CD23 expression by human B cells. Proc Natl Acad Sci USA 1993; 90:3730–3734.
82. Kopf M, Le Gros G, Bachmann M *et al.* Disruption of the murine IL-4 gene blocks Th2 cytokine responses. Nature 1993; 362:245–248.
83. Rousset F, Robert J, Andary M *et al.* Shifts in interleukin-4 and interferon-$\gamma$ production by T cells of patients with elevated serum IgE levels and the modulatory effects of these lymphokines on spontaneous IgE synthesis. J Allergy Clin Immunol 1991; 87:58–69.
84. Robinson DS, Hamid Q, Ying S *et al.* Predominant Th2-like bronchoalveolar T lymphocyte population in atopic asthma. N Engl J Med 1992; 326: 295–304.

85. Kay AB, Ying S, Varney V *et al.* Messenger RNA expression of the cytokine gene cluster, interleukin-3 (IL-3), IL-4, IL-5 and GM-CSF, in allergen-induced late phase cutaneous reaction in atopic subjects. J Exp Med 1991; 173:777–778.
86. Wierenga EA, Snoek M, de Groot C *et al.* Evidence of compartmentalization of functional subsets of CD2+ T lymphocytes in atopic patients. J Immunol 1990; 144:4651–4656.
87. Parronchi P, Macchia D, Piccini M-P *et al.* Allergen- and bacterial antigen-specific T-cell clones established form atopic donors show a different profile of cytokine production. Proc Natl Acad Sci USA 1991; 88:4538–4542.
88. Yssel H, Johnson KE, Schneider PV *et al.* T cell activation-inducing epitopes of the house dust mite allergen *Der p* I. Proliferation and lymphokine production patterns by *Der p* I-specific CD4+ T cell clones. J Immunol 1992; 148:738–745.
89. Fasler S, Aversa G, Terr A *et al.* Peptide-induced anergy in allergen-specific human Th2 cells results in lack of cytokine production and B cell help for IgE synthesis: reversal by IL-2, not by IL-4 or IL-3. J Immunol, in press.
90. De Kruyff R, Turner T, Abrams JA *et al.* Induction of human IgE synthesis by CD4+ T cell clones. J Exp Med 1989; 170:1477–1486.
91. Armitage RJ, Fanslow WC, Stockbine L *et al.* Molecular and biological characterization of a murine ligand for CD40. Nature 1992; 357:80–82.
92. Hollenbaugh D, Grosmaire LS, Kullas CD *et al.* The human T cell antigen gp39, a member of the TNF gene family, is a ligand for the CD40 receptor: expression of a soluble form of gp39 with B cell co-stimulatory activity. EMBO J 1992; 11:4313–4321.
93. Spriggs MK, Armitage RJ, Strockbine L *et al.* Recombinant human CD40 ligand stimulates B cell proliferation and immunoglobulin E secretion. J Exp Med 1992; 176:1543–1550.
94. Aruffo A, Farrington M, Hollenbaugh D *et al.* The CD40 ligand, gp39, is defective in activated T cells from patients with X-linked hyper-IgM syndrome. Cell 1993; 72:291–300.
95. Korthauer U, Graf D, Mages HW *et al.* Defective expression of T cell CD40 ligand cause X-linked immunodeficiency with hyper-IgM. Nature 1993; 361:539–541.
96. Di Santo JP, Bonnefoy JY, Gauchat JF *et al.* CD40 ligand mutations in X-linked immunodeficiency with hyper-IgM. Nature 1993; 361:541–543.
97. Allen CR, Armitage RJ, Conley ME *et al.* CD40 ligand gene defects responsible for X-linked hyper-IgM syndrome. Science 1993; 259:990–993.
98. Aversa G, Punnonen J, de Vries JE. The 26-kD transmembrane form of tumor necrosis factor alpha on activated CD4+ T cell clones provides a costimulatory signal for human B cell activation. J Exp Med 1993; 177:1575–1585.
99. Macchia D, Almerigogna F, Parronchi P *et al.* Membrane tumour necrosis factor-alpha is involved in the polyclonal B-cell activation induced by HIV-infected human T cells. Nature 1993; 363:464–466.
100. Life P, Gauchat JF, Schnuringer V *et al.* T cell clones form an X-linked hyper IgM patient induce IgE synthesis *in vitro* despite expression of non-functional CD40 ligand. J Exp Med 1994; 180:1775–1784.
101. Xu J, Foy TM, Laman JD *et al.* Mice deficient for the CD40 ligand. Immunity 1994; 1:423–431.
102. Carballido JM, Schols D, Namikawa R *et al.* *In vivo* treatment with IL-4 inducing B cell maturation and IgE synthesis in SCID-hu mice. Suppression of ongoing IgE synthesis by an IL-4 receptor antagonist protein. Submitted.
103. Gauchat J-F, Aversa GG, Gascan H, de Vries JE. Modulation of IL-4 induced germline $\epsilon$ RNA synthesis in human B cells by tumor necrosis factor-$\alpha$, anti-

CD40 monoclonal antibodies or transforming growth factor-β correlates with levels of IgE production. Int Immunol 1992; 4:397–406.

104. Kimata H, Yoshida A, Ishioka C *et al.* Interleukin 8 (IL-8) selectively inhibits immunoglobulin E production induced by IL-4 in human B cells. J Exp Med 1992; 176:1227–1231.

105. Kiniwa M, Gately M, Gubler U *et al.* Recombinant interleukin-12 suppresses the synthesis of immunoglobulin E by interleukin-4 stimulated human lymphocytes. J Clin Invest 1992; 90:262–266.

106. Zhang K, Clark EA, Saxon A. CD40 stimulation provides an IFN-γ independent and IL-4 dependent differentiation signal directly to human B cells for IgE production. J Immunol 1991; 146:1836–1842.

107. Punnonen J, de Waal Malefyt R, Van Vlasselaer P *et al.* IL-10 and viral IL-10 prevent IL-4-induced IgE synthesis by inhibiting the accessory cell function of monocytes. J Immunol 1993; 151:1280–1289.

108. Souillet G, Rousset F, de Vries JE. Alpha-interferon treatment of patients with hyper IgE syndrome. Lancet 1989; 1:1384–1389.

109. King CL, Gallin JI, Malech HL *et al.* Regulation of immunoglobulin production in hyperimmunoglobulin E recurrent-infection syndrome by interferon-γ. Proc Natl Acad Sci USA 1989; 86:10085–10089.

110. Vercelli D, Jabara HH, Arai K-I *et al.* Endogenous interleukin 6 plays an obligatory role in interleukin 4-dependent human IgE synthesis. Eur J Immunol 1989; 19:1419–1424.

111. Muraguchi A, Hirano T, Tang B *et al.* The essential role of B cell stimulatory factor 2 (BSF-2/IL-6) for the terminal differentiation of B cells. J Exp Med 1988; 167:332–344.

112. Coffman RL, Lebman DA, Rothman P. Mechanism and regulation of immunoglobulin isotype switching. Adv Immunol 1993; 54:29–270.

113. Jabara HH, Schneider LC, Shapira SK *et al.* Induction of germ-line and mature C epsilon transcripts in human B cells stimulated with rIL-4 and EBV. J Immunol 1990; 145:3468–3473.

114. Ichiki T, Takahashi W, Watanabe T. The effect of cytokines and mitogens on the induction of C epsilon germline transcripts in a human Burkitt lymphoma B cell line. Int Immunol 1992; 4:747–754.

115. Zhang K, Mills FC, Saxon A. Switch circles form IL-4-directed epsilon class switching from human B lymphocytes. Evidence for direct, sequential and multiple step sequential switch from mu to epsilon Ig heavy chain gene. J Immunol 1994; 152:3427–3435.

116. Jung S, Rajewsky K, Radbruch A. Shutdown of class switch recombination by deletion of a switch region control element. Science 1993; 259:984–987.

117. Zhang J, Bottaro A, Li S *et al.* A selective defect in IgG2b switching as a result of targeted mutation of the I gamma 2b promoter and exon. EMBO J 1993; 12:3529–3537.

118. Law CL, Armitage RJ, Villablanca JG, LeBien TW. Expression of interleukin-4 receptors on early human B-lineage cells. Blood 1991; 79:703–710.

119. Hofman FM, Brock M, Taylor CR, Lyons B. IL-4 regulates differentiation and proliferation of human precursor B cells. J Immunol 1988; 141:1185–1190.

120. Villablanca JG, Anderson JA, Mosely M *et al.* Differentiation of normal human pre-B cells *in vitro*. J Exp Med 1990; 172:325–334.

121. Rennick D, Yang G, Müller-Sieberg C *et al.* Interleukin 4 (B cell stimulatory factor 1) can enhance or antagonize the factor-dependent growth of hemopoietic progenitor cells. Proc Natl Acad Sci USA 1987; 84:6889–6895.

122. Pandrau D, Sealand S, Duvert V *et al.* Interleukin 4 inhibits *in vitro* proliferation

of leukemic and normal human B cell precursors. J Clin Invest 1992; 90:1697–1706.

123. Punnonen J, Aversa GG, Vandekerckhove B *et al.* Induction of isotype switching and Ig production by $CD5^+$ and $CD10^+$ human fetal B cells. J Immunol 1992; 148:3398–3404.
124. Punnonen J, de Vries JE. Characterization of a novel $CD2^+$ human thymic B cell subset. J Immunol 1993; 151:100–110.
125. Punnonen J, Aversa G, de Vries JE. Human pre-B cells differentiate into immunoglobulin-secreting plasma cells in the presence of interleukin-4 and activated $CD4^+$ T cells or their membranes. Blood 1993; 82:2781–2789.
126. Punnonen J, de Vries JE. IL-13 induces proliferation, Ig isotype switching, and Ig synthesis by immature fetal B cells. J Immunol 1994; 152:1094–1102.
127. Kruse N, Tony HP, Sebald W. Conversion of human interleukin-4 into high affinity antagonist by a single amino acid replacement. EMBO J 1991; 11:3237–3244.
128. de Waal Malefyt R, Figdor C, Huijbens R *et al.* Effects of IL-13 on phenotype, cytokine production, and cytotoxic function of human monocytes: comparison to IL-4 and modulation by IFN-γ or IL-10[1]. J Immunol 1993; 151:6370–6381.

# 9 Interleukin-5

**KIYOSHI TAKATSU**
*University of Tokyo, Tokyo, Japan*

## INTRODUCTION

Interleukin 5 (IL-5) is a dimeric cytokine produced by T cells, mast cells and eosinophils. Murine (m) IL-5 was originally described as an activity that induced antigen-primed B cells to differentiate into antigen-specific IgG antibody-producing cells[1–3] (T-cell-replacing factor, TRF) and stimulated IgM secretion by BCL1 B-cell tumor cells (B-cell differentiation factor-μ, BCDFμ)[4,5]. IL-5 was also recognized as an activity that stimulated proliferation of activated B cells (B-cell growth factor II, BCGFII)[6]. In addition, IL-5 has been found to enhance IgA synthesis by B cells that have switched to IgA (IgA-enhancing factor, IgA-EF)[7–10] and support the proliferation and differentiation of eosinophils (eosinophil-differentiation factor, EDF)[11]. Thus, the various designations of mIL-5 as TRF, BCDFμ, BCGFII, IgA-EF and EDF reflect its functional multiplicity. Human (h) IL-5, like mIL-5, is also a stimulator of eosinophil function in that it induces the production of eosinophils from bone marrow progenitors, enhances survival of, and primes, eosinophils *in vitro*[11] and stimulates the release of chemical mediators from eosinophils and basophils. As will be discussed below, IL-5, IL-3 and granulocyte-macrophage colony-stimulating factor (GM-CSF) display a variety of overlapping actions in the production and activation of eosinophils on the basis of their utilizing a common β chain in their respective receptors[12].

The IL-5 receptor (IL-5R) consists of two distinct membrane proteins, α and β. IL-5Rα alone specifically binds IL-5, but with low affinity[13,14]. While the β chain does not by itself bind IL-5, it associates with IL-5Rα to form a high-affinity IL-5R[15–18]. The β chain is the common β chain (βc) for the IL-5, IL-3 and GM-CSF receptors[19]. Thus, the βc also associates with IL-3Rα and GM-CSFRα, which specifically bind IL-3 and GM-CSF, respectively, to form high-affinity receptors for IL-3 and GM-CSF[20–24]. The βc is not only required for high-affinity binding, but is also essential for signal transduction. As mentioned, this provides a molecular basis for the overlapping effects of IL-5, IL-3 and GM-CSF, especially on eosinophil function[2,11,19]. As discussed in

*Cytokine Regulation of Humoral Immunity: Basic and Clinical Aspects.* Edited by Clifford M. Snapper.

Chapter 13, IL-5, IL-3 and GM-CSF also share the ability to stimulate Ig secretion by murine B cells activated through their antigen receptor.

A key question regarding the action of IL-5 in responsive cells has been the molecular mechanism of the signal transduction cascade after its high-affinity binding to the functional IL-5R. Here I will review the normal structure and function of IL-5 and its receptor system in B-cell development, proliferation and differentiation, and discuss the nature and consequences of defects in its operation.

## STRUCTURE OF IL-5

Both mIL-5 and hIL-5 have been characterized by cloning, sequencing and expression[25–27]. Mouse IL-5 mRNA is expressed in $CD4^+$ type 2 helper T cells (Th2) and mast cells[28–30]. Human IL-5 mRNA is also expressed in T cells[31], as well as in non-T cells such as Epstein–Barr virus (EBV)-transformed B cells[32], Reed–Sternberg cells in Hodgkin's disease[33], and activated eosinophils found at sites of inflamed tissue[34]. Both mIL-5 and hIL-5 have a molecular mass of 45–60 kDa when expressed in mammalian cells, but this changes to 22–30 kDa after treatment with a reducing agent[35,36]. This indicates that IL-5 is a disulfide-linked dimer; it has been shown that two conserved cysteine residues crosslink the dimer in an anti-parallel arrangement[37]. Dimerization is essential for conferring biological activity to IL-5, since monomeric IL-5, produced by reduction and alkylation of IL-5[38] or by mutating the cysteine residue to threonine[39], fails to exert biological activity. The crystal structure of hIL-5 reveals an intimate dimer configuration in which each domain contains secondary structural elements from both chains[40]. The core of IL-5 is composed of two left-handed bundles of four α-helices, laid end to end, and two short anti-parallel β-strands packed on opposite sides of the dimer. The formation of four α-helix bundles and two β-sheets appears to be required for IL-5 to be active, as for other cytokines. Receptor binding sites for IL-5 are located at the C-terminus of each monomer[41].

## FUNCTIONAL PROPERTIES OF IL-5 ON B CELLS

### REGULATION OF B-CELL PROLIFERATION

It has been shown that IL-5 induces DNA synthesis of murine chronic leukemic B cells (BCL1) and dextran sulfate-stimulated splenic B cells[6,42]. It has been suggested that IL-5 plays a role in the development of a subpopulation of B cells termed Ly-1 B cells (also known as $CD5^+$ or B1 cells, see Chapter 3) but this issue has not been resolved[43,44]. B cells develop from pluripotent hematopoietic stem cells resident in the bone marrow. These pluripotent cells also generate myeloid and erythroid elements[45]. B-cell development in the bone marrow comprises various stages whereby progenitor cells initially do not express Ig molecules on their surface. Decisive commitment to the B-cell lineage occurs with V–D–J recombination that brings variable (V), diversity (D) and joining (J) segments of Ig heavy chain (IgH) genes together to create a complete V gene[46]. IgH genes are formed by rearranging $V_H$, $D_H$, and $J_H$ elements to create first $D_HJ_H$ and then $V_HD_HJ_H$ DNA segments[46]. Pro-B cells contain the germline, unrearranged pattern of Ig heavy chain (IgH) genes and express a characteristic B-cell lineage surface phenotype that allows for IgH gene rearrangement with the expression of cytoplasmic $\mu$ chains (pre-B cells). The coexpression of surrogate light chains with rearranged IgH chains on the cell surface of pre-B cells[47] allows for their proliferation, rearrangement of their light (L) chain genes[48] and subsequent expression of surface IgM (sIgM) giving rise to mature B cells.

IL-5 can support the development of early B cells. Specifically, addition of IL-5 to culture allowed for the development of $CD5^+$ precursor B cells from long-term bone marrow cultures grown in the presence of stromal cells[49]. Most of these IL-5- and stromal-cell-dependent Ly-$1^+$ precursor B-cell lines showed a germline configuration of the IgH genes, and expressed CD45R, Lyb-2, BP-1 and IL-2R$\alpha$, but did not express cytoplasmic (c)IgM, Mac-1 and Thy-1[49–52]. They also expressed high-affinity IL-5R and could differentiate to pre-B cells, with rearranged IgH genes, that express C$\mu$, $\lambda$5 and c-*fms* mRNA. Culture of these pre-B cell lines on ST2 stromal cells and GM-CSF, however, resulted in their development of Ly-$1^+$ and Mac-$1^+$ macrophages which lost expression of surface $\mu$ chain[52]. These converted myeloid lines had the same $J_H$ rearrangement pattern as their pre-B lymphoid parents. As reported, several pre-B-cell lines have been shown to differentiate either to Ly-$1^+$ B cells or to macrophage/monocytes[53]. These observations support evidence for a close relationship between the myeloid and Ly-$1^+$ B-cell pathways of differentiation, and indicate that IL-5-dependent clones are Ly-$1^+$ multipotential intermediates in the differentiation process from pro-B to B cells, or to macrophages. We have also established an IL-5-dependent and stromal-cell-independent pre-B cell line, T88-M[49], whose growth is sensitive to IFN-$\gamma$ and transforming growth factor beta (TGF-$\beta$), but not to cyclosporin A[54,55]. All IL-5-dependent early B cell lines can also grow in the presence of IL-3.

## REGULATION OF B-CELL DIFFERENTIATION

The effect of IL-5 on Ig production has been investigated in detail in the mouse. Mouse IL-5 stimulates polyclonal IgM, IgG1 and/or IgA production, depending upon the presence of additional stimuli[56]. IL-5 stimulates polyclonal IgM production in BCL1 and in *in vivo* activated B-cell blasts, by inducing an increase in the level of mRNA for the secreted forms of the μ, γ1 and α chains[56,57]. Relatively low concentrations (30 ng/ml) of cyclosporin A can significantly inhibit IL-5-induced IgM production by BCL1 cells without affecting IL-5-induced proliferation[55], suggesting that a calcineurin-dependent pathway is involved in IL-5 signaling. Mouse IL-5 markedly increases the frequencies of both proliferating and antibody-secreting clones[58,59]. Using the BCg3R-1d transfected cell line, which produces antibody specific for phosphocholine and expressing the T15 idiotype, a region of between −250 and −125 base pairs, lying 5′ of the Ig transcription start site, has been identified that is necessary for the induction of increased μ mRNA levels by phosphocholine-coupled antigen plus IL-5[60].

It has been reported that hIL-5 enhances IgA or IgM synthesis of human peripheral blood B cells stimulated with *Staphylococcus aureus* Cowan I (SAC)[27,61]. Human IL-5 augments Ig production by SAC- or pokeweed mitogen-stimulated human B blasts in the presence of IL-2 and also increases the secretory form of μ chain mRNA expression[62]. Although IL-5 has been reported to barely induce IgM and IgG production in B cells from human peripheral blood[63], human peripheral blood B cells, stimulated with *Moraxella catarrhalis* (Mcat), although not SAC, synthesized IgM in response to hIL-5 in the absence of IL-2[64]. These data may provide evidence for a direct role of IL-5 in human B-cell terminal differentiation. The nature of the activation signal may be critical in determining human B-cell responsiveness to hIL-5.

## REGULATION OF Ig ISOTYPE SELECTION

It is well established that T-cell-derived cytokines can selectively regulate Ig isotype production. Early studies revealed that mIL-5 could stimulate antigen-specific and polyclonal IgA production by antigen-primed B cells and lipopolysaccharide (LPS)-stimulated B cells, respectively[9,10,65–70]. This raised the question of whether IL-5 was able to induce class switching from μ to α chain expression. IL-5 was shown to act on surface IgA-positive ($sIgA^+$) B cells, but not on $sIgA^-$ B cells, to induce IgA production, indicating that its IgA-inducing effect was not at the level of an IgM to IgA class switch[9,69]. Mouse IL-5 was shown to augment IgA secretion by $sIgA^+$ B cells without significantly increasing cellular outgrowth[9,10,69]. We demonstrated that IL-5 slightly enhanced [$^3$H]thymidine incorporation by sorted $sIgA^+$ B cells compared to control cultures. Further, cell recoveries in IL-5-containing cultures were greater than in control cultures irrespective of the presence of LPS[10], suggesting that IL-5 may enhance IgA secretion at least in part through mediating prolonged survival of $sIgA^+$ B cells.

TGF-β1 has been shown to enhance IgA production of LPS-stimulated mouse B cells[9,10,71–73], although it inhibits the production of other Ig isotypes (see Chapter 12). TGF-β1 can synergize with IL-5 for enhanced IgA production. TGF-β acts on LPS-stimulated sIgA⁻ cells to induce class switching from μ to α chains. This is associated with a TGF-β-mediated increase in the expression of sterile α chain transcripts[74,75] (see Chapter 5). TGF-β can also synergize with IL-5 for IgA expression by enhancing IL-5R expression[10], thus increasing the ability of IL-5 to stimulate IgA secretion by B cells that have already switched to α chain expression[9,10]. That TGF-β in fact induces switching from μ to α chains is strongly supported by its ability to stimulate the appearance of germline Cα transcripts, induce IgA-specific switch circular DNA[76,77], and increase the frequency of IgA-secreting cells at the clonal level[72,78]. TGF-β has been shown to increase the frequency of switch recombination through successive recombination from Sμ to Sγ to Sα[79]. IL-2 also synergizes with TGF-β to augment IgA production by LPS-activated B cells without affecting the total number of $sIgA^+$ cells[74,75], in contrast to IL-5, which causes a significant increase in the number of $sIgA^+$ B cells (up to 17 per cent) in LPS+ TGF-β-stimulated B-cell cultures. IL-5 fails to induce either germline Cα transcripts or the formation of IgA-specific switch circular DNA (Sonoda *et al.*, in preparation). TGF-β enhances not only IgA but can also stimulate IgG2b, and to a lesser extent IgG3 production, by LPS-stimulated B cells[10,80]. In contrast to IgA, IL-5 does not synergize with TGF-β for IgG2b or IgG3 synthesis. The addition of anti-TGF-β antibody to LPS-stimulated cultures decreases the production of IgG2b and IgG3[10,80], which are the major isotypes induced by LPS stimulation. The ability of TGF-β to act directly on $mIgM^+mIgG2b^-$ B cells to stimulate IgG2b production, stimulate an increase in IgG2b-secreting cells, and selectively increase the steady-state levels of germline γ2b RNA[80], strongly suggests that TGF-β is a switch factor for IgG2b, as well as IgA (see also Chapter 12).

IL-5 also promotes IgG1 and IgE secretion by activated B cells stimulated with IL-4[67]. Although the role of IL-4 was to stimulate μ to γ1 chain or μ to ϵ chain switching (see Chapter 8), IL-5 induced a marked accumulation of productive, but not germline, γ1 and ϵ chain transcripts in LPS + IL-4-stimulated B cells[81], indicating that it acted to enhance B-cell maturation of post-switched cells. IL-5 was also shown to enhance steady-state levels of productive γ1 RNA in B cells stimulated with dextran-conjugated anti-IgD antibodies (αδ-dex) and IL-4[82]. In this system, IL-5 was shown to be necessary for induction of Sμ–Sγ1 DNA rearrangement in αδ-dex + IL-4-activated cells but it has little effect on rearrangement in the absence of IL-4, which was necessary for induction of germline γ1 RNA[82]. These observations suggested that IL-5 may enhance IgG1 and/or IgE production through stimulatory effects on switch recombination, transcription of rearranged γ1 and ϵ chain loci, and/or stability of the VDJ-Cγ1 and VDJ-Cϵ mRNA.

## GENES AND STRUCTURE OF THE IL-5 RECEPTOR

### MOLECULAR CONSTITUTION OF IL-5 RECEPTOR

IL-5 binds to a specific cell surface receptor (IL-5R) that consists of two distinct membrane proteins, α and β[83]. The α chain (IL-5Rα) is specific to IL-5, whereas the β chain is also common (βc) to IL-3 and GM-CSF. Anti-mIL-5R monoclonal antibodies (mAbs) H7 and R52.120 (R52) that recognize the IL-5Rα and βc, respectively, have been prepared[84,85]. H7 mAb specifically inhibits IL-5-induced proliferation, while R52 mAb partially inhibits both IL-5- and IL-3-induced proliferation of a pre-B-cell line. Murine IL-5Rα is constitutively expressed on more than 70 per cent of peritoneal B cells, most of which are Ly-1 (CD5)$^+$, and on 4–8 per cent of splenic B cells, most of which are Ly-1$^-$[86]. In contrast to IL-5Rα, the βc, recognized by R52 mAb, is expressed not only on IL-5-dependent cell lines, but also on IL-3-dependent cell lines[87].

cDNAs encoding membrane-bound forms for both mIL-5Rα and hIL-5Rα have been isolated[13–15,18]. cDNAs coding for soluble forms of both mIL-5Rα and hIL-5Rα chains have also been isolated. The IL-5Rα is a type I membrane protein with an extracellular domain, a glycosylated extracellular domain, a single transmembrane segment, and a cytoplasmic tail. The entire nucleotide sequences of mouse and human IL-5Rα cDNA show considerable similarity and the amino acid sequences demonstrate ~70 per cent homology (Figure 9.1). Both the membrane-bound and the soluble forms of the mIL-5Rα transcripts are expressed in spleen cells, peritoneal exudate cells and IL-5-dependent cell lines (Figure 9.2)[51,88]. The external domain of IL-5Rα contains two motifs that are characteristics of a set of receptors for cytokines, growth hormone and prolactin. These motifs show a particular spacing of four cysteine residues in the N-terminal half of the receptor and a tryptophan–serine–(X)–tryptophan–serine (where X is any amino acid) motif located close to the transmembrane domain[89]. In addition, the external region comprises three tandemly repeated sets of a fibronectin type III domain. The cytoplasmic domain of IL-5Rα shows no homology with signaling molecules such as kinases, phosphatases, nucleotide-binding proteins and *src* homology domains. IL-5Rα contains a proline-rich region (Pro–Pro–X–Pro)v[13] on the cytoplasmic side, near the transmembrane domain, that is well conserved between IL-5Rα and the receptors for IL-3, GM-CSF, prolactin and growth hormone. This region shows homology with a part of the actin-binding domain of β-spectrin[90]. The proline-rich region contains a Pro–X–Pro sequence that exists in the membrane-proximal, box 1, region of other members of the cytokine receptor family[91]. In addition to the Pro–X–Pro motif, the critical proline-rich sequence of IL-5Rα also contains a Pro–X–X–Pro motif that is conserved among various SH3-binding proteins[92].

The mIL-5Rα genomic gene was isolated and its entire nucleotide

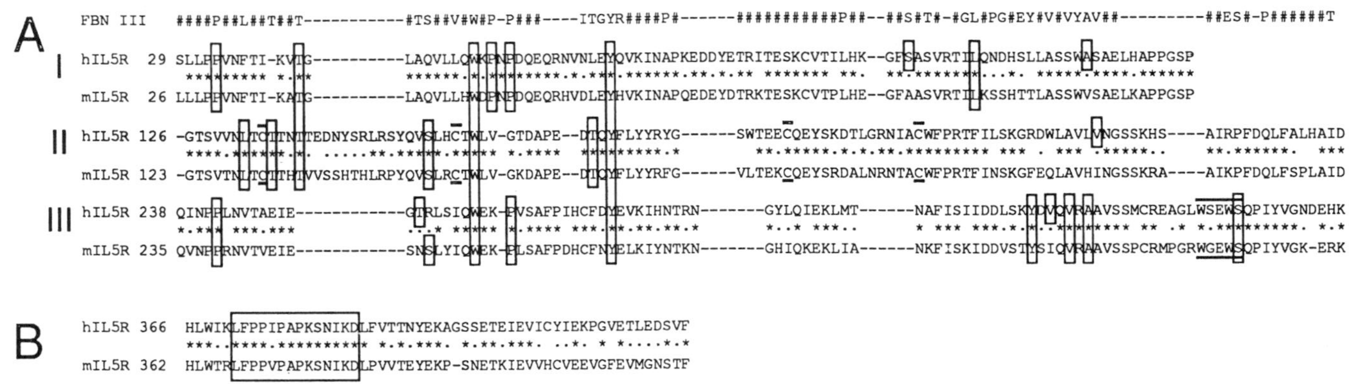


**Figure 9.1** Alignment of human and murine IL-5Rα amino acid sequence. (A) Alignment of human and murine IL-5Rα extracellular region with a consensus sequence of a FBN III module. Nonconserved amino acid residues and gaps are indicated by # and −, respectively. (B) Comparison of the amino acid sequences from the cytoplasmic domain of IL-5Rα between human and mouse. Identical and related amino acids between the hIL-5Rα and mIL-5Rα are shown by asterisks and dots, respectively

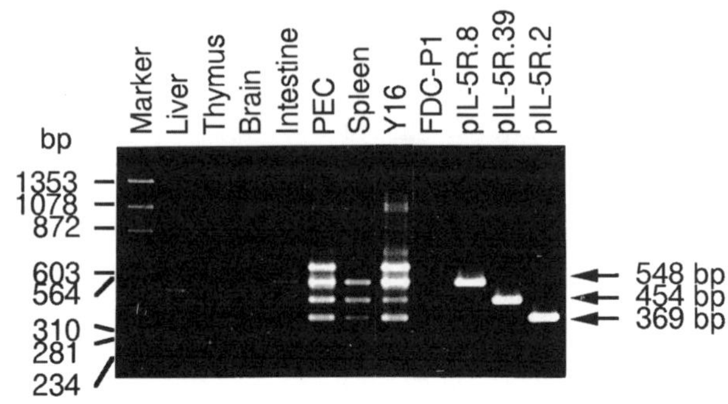


**Figure 9.2** Expression of sIL-5Rα transcripts in various tissues. Poly(A)$^+$ RNA from the tissues and cell lines or plasmid DNA was subjected to PCR amplification. Y16, IL-5-dependent line; FDC-P1, IL-3-dependent line; pIL-5R.8, plasmid DNA containing cDNA encoding the membrane-bound form of mIL-5Rα cDNA; pIL-5R.39 and pIL-5R.2, plasmid DNA containing cDNA encoding the soluble form of mIL-5Rα cDNA

sequence has been determined[93]. The mIL-5Rα genomic gene is divided into 11 exons and 10 introns and spans more than 35 kb (Figure 9.3)[93]. The consensus sequences for splicing junctions, 5′-GT and 3′-AG, are found at the boundaries of all 10 introns. The nucleotide sequences of all exons are in agreement with that of the mIL-5Rα cDNA. Comparison of the exon–intron

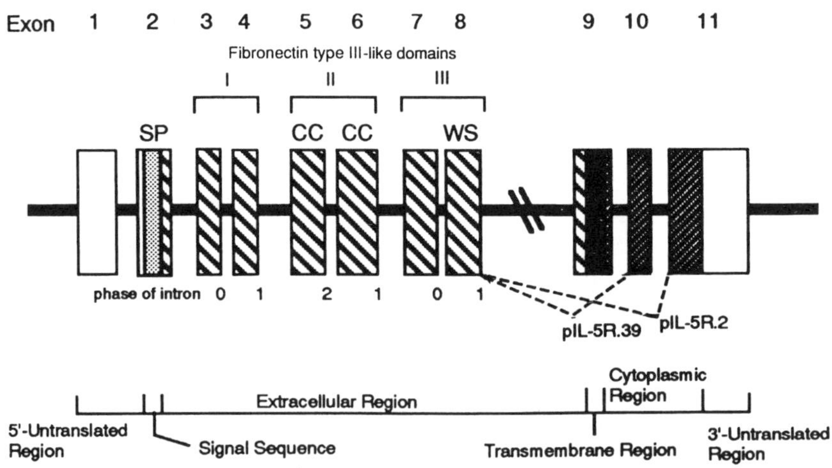


**Figure 9.3** Organization of the genomic mIL-5Rα chain. Each box indicates an exon. Dotted, horizontal, closed, and hatched regions in exons indicate a signal peptide, an extracellular region, a transmembrane region, and a cytoplasmic region, respectively. The cysteine residues are indicated by CC and WSXWS motif is shown as WS. Dashed lines indicate alternative splicing to generate the soluble forms of mIL-5Rα

boundaries of the murine IL-5Rα gene with those of other members of the cytokine receptor family reveals a conserved evolutionary structure. The gene organization reveals a pattern of considerable structural homology with genomic genes for IL-2Rβ, AIC2A and AIC2B, IL-4R, IL-7R, and EpoR. The soluble forms of mIL-5Rα (s-mIL-5Rα) appear to be produced through alternative splicing: (1) exon 8 spliced to exon 11 with deletion of exons 9 and 10; or (2) exon 8 spliced to exon 10 with deletion of exon 9. The mIL-5Rα and hIL-5Rα genes map to the distal half of chromosome 6[93,94] and to chromosome 3 (3p24–3p26), respectively[95].

Recombinant IL-5Rα has a molecular mass of 60 kDa and binds IL-5 with low affinity. The IL-5-nonbinding but IL-3-dependent cell line FDC-P1, when transfected with IL-5Rα cDNA, binds IL-5 with both high and low affinity and proliferates in response to IL-5[13]; this indicates that IL-5Rα-negative FDC-P1 cells constitutively express βc that confers high-affinity binding when expressed with mIL-5Rα. Purified recombinant s-mIL-5Rα retains the ability to bind IL-5 with low affinity, possibly comparable to that of membrane-bound mIL-5Rα[83,85]. However, it fails to inhibit the proliferation of IL-5-responsive cells. Stimulation of cells which constitutively express βc alone with IL-5 plus s-mIL-5Rα fails to induce cell proliferation, suggesting that s-mIL-5Rα–mIL-5 complexes can neither interact with βc nor trigger biological responses. These results are in sharp contrast to those obtained with an IL-6–IL-6Rα (p80) system, in which the IL-6–sIL-6Rα complex can trigger biological responses[96]. s-mIL-5Rα is not detected in normal mouse sera, but is detected in the sera of aged NZB and NZW mice (Table 9.1) (see Chapter 17).

In the human, two forms of s-hIL-5Rα (s1hIL-5Rα and s2hIL-5Rα) are generated by a mechanism that is different from that seen in the mouse[97]. Both recombinant s-hIL-5Rα and a fusion protein consisting of hIL-5Rα linked to an Fc domain of Ig (hIL-5Rα-Fc) bind hIL-5 with high affinity and inhibit the biological activities of hIL-5[92]. s-hIL-5Rα appears to bind dimerized hIL-5 in a 1 : 1 ratio. These observations support the possibility

**Table 9.1** Levels of sIL-5Rα in mouse biological fluids

| Sample | *n* | Amount of sIL-5Rα (ng/ml) |
|---|---|---|
| Normal Balb/c serum | 4 | <0.5 |
| Normal C3H/He serum | 4 | <0.5 |
| BCL1 serum | 6 | 27.8 ± 1.9 |
| MOPC104E ascites | 3 | 25.0 ± 6.2 |
| X5563 ascites | 3 | <0.5 |
| NZB serum (10–12 months) | 3 | 2.8 ± 1.6 |
| NZW serum (10–12 months) | 3 | 2.1 ± 1.1 |

Results represent the means ± SD.

that s-hIL-5Rα may act as a potent regulator for hIL-5. s-hIL-5Rα has not been detected in human biological fluids. The differences between s-mIL-5Rα and s-hIL-5Rα, both in their mechanism of production and ligand-binding affinity, suggests different functional roles for s-hIL-5Rα and s-mIL-5Rα.

Anti-mIL-5R mAb/R52 downregulates the number and $K_d$ of the high-affinity mIL-5R and inhibits the growth of IL-5- and IL-3-dependent cell lines and FDC-P1[85,87]. Anti-mIL-3R mAb also inhibits the growth of IL-5-responsive cell lines. Both R52 and anti-mIL-3R mAbs immunoprecipitate an identical polypeptide with approximate molecular mass of 130 kDa, whereas they do not react with mIL-5Rα. Functional IL-5R can be reconstituted in CTLL by transfection of cDNAs for IL-5Rα and AIC2B protein[13,16,17], which is a component of IL-3Rβ[20,21]. Thus, IL-5Rβ has been shown to be AIC2B. The β chain of IL-5R, AIC2B, is the common β chain (βc) of receptors for IL-3 and GM-CSF (Figure 9.4)[21,24]. The βc also associates with IL-3Rα and GM-CSFRα to form high-affinity receptors for IL-3 and GM-CSF, respectively. The βc is required not only for high-affinity

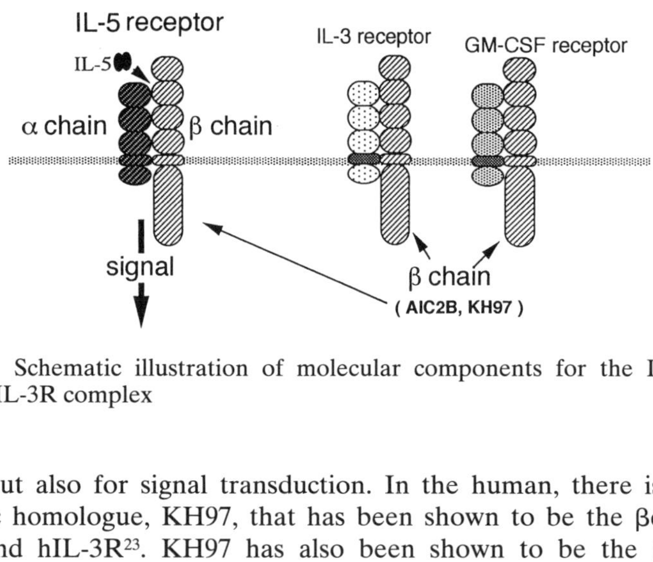


**Figure 9.4** Schematic illustration of molecular components for the IL-5R, GM-CSFR and IL-3R complex

binding, but also for signal transduction. In the human, there is only one murine βc homologue, KH97, that has been shown to be the βc of hGM-CSFR[22] and hIL-3R[23]. KH97 has also been shown to be the βc for the human IL-5R through co-transfection studies with hIL-5Rα in FDC-P1 or CTLL[17,18]. The βc has a relatively large cytoplasmic domain (~440 amino acid residues) which shows no homology with signaling molecules such as kinases, phosphatases, nucleotide-binding proteins and *src* homology domains. Studies using a series of cytoplasmic deletion mutants of the human βc have revealed that there are at least two distinct regions in the cytoplasmic domain of βc that are required for mediating growth-enhancing signal transduction[98,99].

## CRITICAL CYTOPLASMIC REGIONS OF IL-5Rα AND βc FOR IL-5-MEDIATED SIGNALING

Although the cytoplasmic domains of the α chains and of the βc have no homology with signaling molecules such as kinases, phosphatases, nucleotide-binding proteins and *src*-homology domains, it has been well established that IL-5, IL-3 and GM-CSF induce rapid tyrosine phosphorylation of cellular proteins[100–102] as well as transcription of nuclear protooncogenes[103]. Transfectants expressing βc and a mutant IL-5Rα which lacks the entire cytoplasmic domain are unable to transduce the IL-5 signal for proliferation, indicating that the cytoplasmic region of IL-5Rα also has an important role in transmitting a growth signal through the IL-5R[17]. To identify region(s) critical for the IL-5-mediated signal transduction, four different mutant cDNAs of IL-5Rα have been created, each of which has a deletion of six amino acid residues in its cytoplasmic domain[104]. Regardless of the cytoplasmic deletions, all four different transfectants express similar levels of high-affinity IL-5R on their cell surface, with $K_d$ values equivalent to that using wild-type IL-5Rα. Further, these mutated IL-5Rα proteins are processed properly with the correct size, indicating that mutations induced in the cytoplasmic domain of IL-5Rα do not affect the interactions of IL-5Rα with IL-5 or the βc, thus allowing reconstitution of the high-affinity IL-5R. Transfectants expressing mutant IL-5Rα that have deletions in the C-terminal region that is unique to IL-5Rα can proliferate well upon stimulation with IL-5[104]. By contrast, transfectants expressing the mutant IL-5Rα having a deletion in the region rich in proline residues (Pro–Pro–X–Pro) do not respond to IL-5, indicating that the region rich in proline residues is essential for IL-5-mediated growth signal transduction. The proximal region, downstream from the proline-rich area, has been shown to be important, though not essential.

A single amino acid substitution in the proline-rich region of IL-5Rα does not significantly affect IL-5 responsiveness. Substitution of Pro$^{352}$ and Pro$^{353}$ for Ala, or Pro$^{353}$ and Pro$^{355}$ for Ala, result in transfectants showing a proliferative response to IL-5. Substitution of Pro$^{352}$ and Pro$^{355}$ for Ala leads only to a slightly impaired proliferative response to IL-5. Substitution of all three proline residues for Ala results in complete loss of IL-5-induced proliferation[104]. These results indicate that the existence, in IL-5Rα, of one of these three proline residues is adequate for IL-5 signal transduction. In addition, Pro$^{352}$ and Pro$^{355}$, in the proline-rich region, appear to have more critical function in the cytoplasmic domain of IL-5Rα than does Pro$^{353}$.

The interaction between proline-rich sequences of various proteins and the SH3 domains of adapter proteins has attracted considerable attention as a possible mechanism for signal transduction through growth factor receptors[92,105,106]. The proline-rich region of IL-5Rα contains a Pro–X–Pro sequence that exists in the membrane-proximal, box 1, region of other members of the cytokine receptor family[107]. The βc also contains a box 1 region. A truncated mutant of the βc that lacks the box 1 region does not transduce GM-CSF-induced growth signals in BaF3 cells[99], suggesting that the box 1 region of the βc is also important in IL-5-mediated signal transduction (Figure 9.5). In the case of the IL-6R gp130 subunit, mutation of two proline residues in the Pro–X–Pro sequence results in a complete loss of receptor activity[102]. In addition to the Pro–X–Pro motif, the critical proline-rich sequence of IL-5Rα also contains a Pro–X–X–Pro motif that is

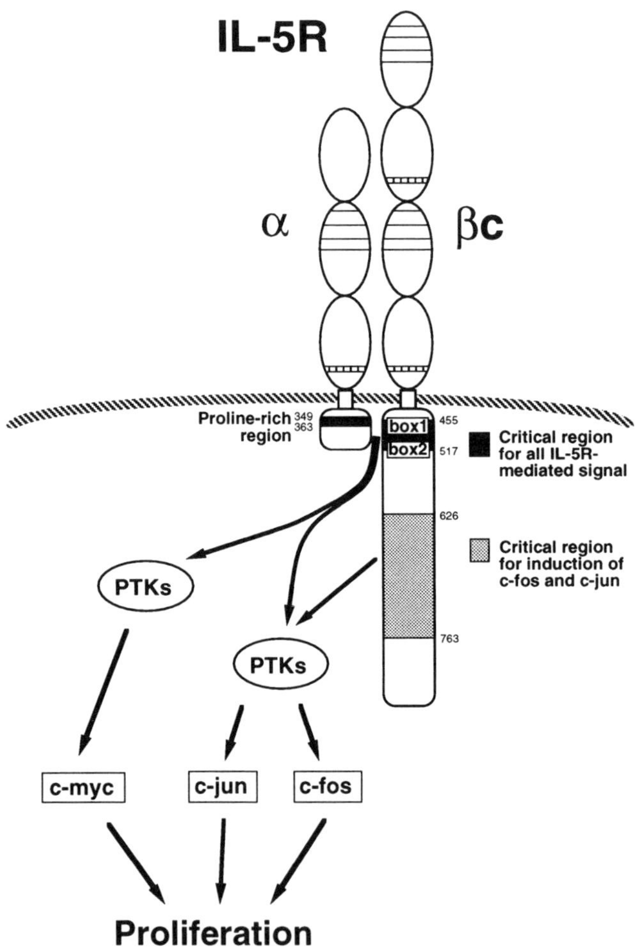


**Figure 9.5** Functional unit of IL-5Rα and the βc. Functional IL-5R consists of IL-5Rα and βc. Critical regions in IL-5Rα (proline-rich residues) and the βc (box 1 and box 2) for IL-5 signaling are shown by the closed square. PTK, protein tyrosine kinase

conserved among various SH3-binding proteins[92]. In contrast, based on our analysis of substitution mutations of IL-5Rα[104], neither of the proline residues of the Pro–X–Pro sequence is required for growth signal transduction. However, one of the proline residues in the well-conserved cytoplasmic region common to IL-5R, IL-3R and GM-CSFR (from $Leu^{350}$ to $Pro^{355}$ in mIL-5Rα) does appear to be required for interaction with the βc for growth signal transduction. This is demonstrated by the pAvA mutation, which does not greatly affect receptor-mediated growth signal transduction.

The interaction of the proline-rich sequence of IL-5Rα and SH3 domains may not be critical for transduction of IL-5-mediated signals, for the following two reasons. First, the proline-rich sequence of IL-5Rα lacks the additional proline residue usually found one or two residues N-terminally of the Pro–X–X–Pro motif[105]. Second, substitutions of either of the two proline residues of the Pro–X–X–Pro motif with alanine, which is expected to greatly reduce the binding affinity to a target SH3 domain[92,106], does not impair IL-5-mediated signal transduction. Instead, the proline residues in the critical region of IL-5Rα may contribute to the flexibility of its cytoplasmic domain, which is important for signal transduction, or may be important for the interaction with certain intracellular signalling protein(s) which do not have an SH3 domain, such as members of the Jak tyrosine kinase family. Further studies will be required to explore the functional differences of the proline-rich residues among IL-5Rα, IL-3Rα and GM-CSFRα.

## ROLE OF THE CYTOPLASMIC DOMAIN OF IL-5Rα IN DIMERIZATIONS OF THE βc

In addition to growth factor receptors having intrinsic tyrosine kinase activity, cytokine receptors such as growth hormone receptor[108], gp130 of IL-6R[107], G-CSFR[109], erythropoietin receptor[110] and IL-2R[111,112] are activated by homodimerizations or heterodimerizations of receptor complexes. As described above, all functions of the cytoplasmic domain of IL-5Rα in signal transduction depend on the short-stretch proline-rich region. It is, therefore, reasonable to speculate that IL-5Rα contributes to signal transduction solely by promoting, through its cytoplasmic proline-rich regions, the dimerization of the βc. To evaluate this hypothesis, two chimeric receptors with transmembrane portions from IL-5Rα (ααβ mutant) or the βc (αββ mutant) consisting of the extracellular domain of IL-5Rα with the cytoplasmic domain of the βc have been generated[104]. FDC-P1 transfectants of these two chimeric receptors exhibit high-affinity IL-5-binding sites and are capable of proliferating in response to IL-5 (Figure 9.6). CTLL transfectants only stably expressing both αββ mutant and βc show IL-5-dependent growth, indicating that αββ alone is not functional. As it is considered that IL-5 binding induces heterodimerization (heteromultimerization) of extracellular domains of IL-5Rα and βc,

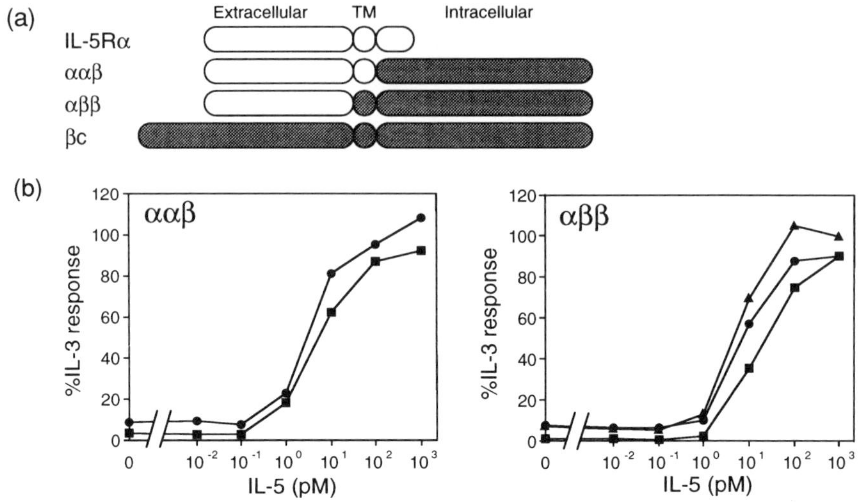


**Figure 9.6** (a) Schematic representation of the chimeric receptors between IL-5Rα and the βc. Open and shaded boxes originate from IL-5Rα and the βc, respectively. (b) Proliferation of FDC-P1 transfectants expressing the chimeric receptors. Transfectants were incubated for 48 h in the presence of various concentrations of IL-5 and incorporated [$^3$H]thymidine was measured. The results are expressed as the percentage of [$^3$H]thymidine incorporation in the same cells incubated with 100 units/ml of IL-3

resulting in homodimerization of the cytoplasmic domain of βc, the IL-5-dependent growth signals appear to be transduced by dimerization (multimerization) of the cytoplasmic domain of the βc without that of IL-5Rα.

## IL-5-RECEPTOR-MEDIATED SIGNALING

### TYROSINE PHOSPHORYLATION AND PROTOONCOGENE EXPRESSION MEDIATED THROUGH THE IL-5 RECEPTOR

Ample evidence has been provided that tyrosine phosphorylation of membrane receptors and cellular proteins is important for the regulation of receptor-mediated signal transduction. Tyrosine phosphorylation of cellular proteins has been reported in IL-5-, IL-3- and GM-CSF-stimulated cells[113–118]. The patterns of protein tyrosine phosphorylation in response to these cytokines appear to display no differences, most likely reflecting the fact that the βc which is indispensable for their signal transduction is shared among the receptors for IL-3, IL-5 and GM-CSF. The importance of tyrosine phosphorylation in IL-5 signal transduction is underscored by experiments using the tyrosine kinase inhibitor herbimycin A. Treatment of IL-5-dependent cell lines with herbimycin A causes the inhibition of not only protein tyrosine phosphorylation, but also cell growth induced by IL-5. In the wild-type IL-5Rα transfectants, several tyrosine-phosphorylated cellular proteins (130–140, 120, 95, 70, 55, 50, 42 kDa) are observed within 10 min of stimulation with IL-5[97,103]. A tyrosine-phosphorylated protein with a molecular mass of 130–140 kDa that appears 20 min following stimulation with IL-5 has been shown to be the βc[113]. IL-5 fails to induce phosphorylated cellular proteins in transfectants having a deletion in the region rich in proline residues[104,113].

Induction of nuclear protooncogene expression has also been well established to be critical for cytokine signal transduction[103]. In the wild-type IL-5Rα transfectants, expressions of c-*fos*, c-*jun* and c-*myc* protooncogene mRNA are rapidly induced upon stimulation with IL-5[104]. In contrast, the protooncogene expressions are not induced in transfectants having a deletion in the region rich in proline residues, in response to stimulation with IL-5.

## THE IL-5-INDUCED TYROSINE PHOSPHORYLATION OF SH2/SH3 DOMAIN-CONTAINING PROTEINS

Several tyrosine-phosphorylated effector molecules controlling growth have been identified in association with growth factor receptors carrying intrinsic protein tyrosine kinase activity. These effector molecules are phospholipase C-γ (PLC-γ), phosphatidylinositol-3 (PI-3) kinase, and Ras-associated GPTase-activating protein (GAP)[119]. They contain *src*-homology 2 (SH2) and/or *src*-homology 3 (SH3) domains, the former of which binds to phosphorylated tyrosine on protein[120], while the latter has been suggested to be responsible for the targeting of signaling molecules to specific subcellular locations[121]. Immunoprecipitation followed by immunoblot analysis revealed that IL-5 induces marked tyrosine phosphorylations of a p85 subunit of PI-3 kinase, Vav, HS1 and Shc within 5 min (Figure 9.7)[113]. In contrast, IL-5 does not induce tyrosine phosphorylation of PLC-γ or GAP. No tyrosine phosphorylations of any of these SH2/SH3-containing proteins are observed in transfectants having a deletion in the region rich in proline residues.

It has been clarified[122] that the tyrosine-phosphorylated Shc protein functions as an adapter because of its association with Grb2, another adapter protein[123]. Grb2 binds to both Shc and mSos through its SH2 and SH3 domains, respectively. mSos is a Ras nucleotide-exchange protein and activates Ras[124]. Ras has been shown to work downstream of tyrosine kinases in the growth signaling pathway[124–126]. It has been demonstrated that herbimycin A decreases both the increase of Ras–GTP and cell proliferation in response to IL-3 and GM-CSF[99], suggesting that tyrosine kinase(s) is

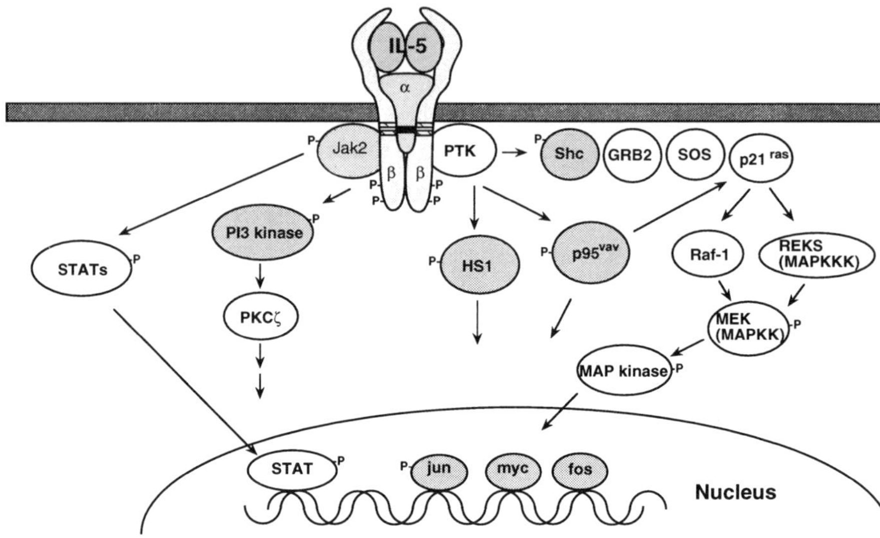


**Figure 9.7** Schematic representation of IL-5-induced tyrosine phosphorylation. Cellular proteins tyrosine phosphorylated in response to IL-5 are shown by shading

involved in the pathway for activation of Ras by these cytokines. IL-5 may facilitate this pathway for signaling.

The $p95^{Vav}$(Vav), a protooncogene product specifically expressed in hematopoietic cells, contains a single SH2 and two SH3 domains as well as sequence motifs commonly found in transcription factors, such as the helix–loop–helix, leucine zipper and zinc-finger motifs, and nuclear localization signals, in addition to being homologous with guanine nucleotide releasing factors (GRFs)[127,128]. We observed that Vav was rapidly tyrosine phosphorylated upon stimulation with IL-5[113]. Vav has also shown to be tyrosine phosphorylated upon crosslinkage of the antigen receptors on T and B cells[128,129]. Recently, Gulbins *et al.*[128] demonstrated that both the tyrosine phosphorylation of Vav and the Vav-associated GRF activity of Ras are enhanced after T-cell receptor (TCR) crosslinking. They proposed the concept that Vav is a tyrosine kinase-regulated GRF which is important in TCR-initiated signal transduction through activation of Ras. The tyrosine phosphorylation of Vav in response to IL-5 may be associated with the increase in the active form of Ras. It is also possible that, as expected from its structural homology, Vav plays other crucial roles as a transcription factor in the IL-5-induced gene expression associated with cell growth.

The *HS1* gene is expressed specifically in cells of hematopoietic lineage[130]. The N-terminal moiety of the HS1 protein has three copies of a 37 amino acid repeating motif, each of which contains a helix–turn–helix motif. The C-terminal one has a potential α-helix containing an amphipathic region. In addition, an SH3 motif is present near the C-terminus. The HS1 is a major substrate of protein tyrosine kinase(s) (PTK) activated by ligation of B-cell antigen receptor, IgM and IgD[131]. Both Vav and HS1 might be involved in the formation of such a DNA-binding complex.

PI-3 kinase consists of an 85-kDa regulatory subunit and a 110-kDa catalytic subunit. The p85 regulatory subunit harbors two tyrosine phosphate binding domains and SH2 domains. Further, the majority of the tyrosine residues in PI-3 kinase serve as the substrates for various PTKs both *in vivo* and *in vitro*[132]. Although it is unclear what role tyrosine phosphorylation of the p85 regulatory subunit plays in PI-3 kinase activation, this phosphorylation may indicate the interaction of PI-3 kinase with a tyrosine-phosphorylated PTK such as Lyn through its SH2 domain.

## THE ACTIVATION OF Jak2 AND BRUTON'S TYROSINE KINASES BY IL-5 STIMULATION

The fact that tyrosine phosphorylation of cellular proteins, including βc, can be rapidly induced after IL-5 stimulation indicates the association of PTK with IL-5R. However, no tyrosine kinase activity was detected in the immunoprecipitates using anti-βc or anti-IL-5Rα mAb of the lysates from IL-5-stimulated Y16 cells.

A new family of cytoplasmic PTKs called Janus kinases (alternatively referred to as 'just another kinase' family) consisting of Jak1, Jak2, Jak3 and Tyk2, has been described and cloned[133–138]. In addition to a kinase domain, these proteins are characterized by the presence of a second kinase-like domain and the absence of SH2, SH3 and membrane-spanning domains. Jak kinases associate with the box 1 regions of the members of the cytokine receptor family. It has been reported that the Jak family kinases induce tyrosine phosphorylation and translocation of signal transducers and activators of transcription (STATs), as well as their translocation into the nucleus, upon stimulation with interferons or IL-6[139–142]. The Tyk2 has been implicated in IFN-α receptor signal transduction[134], and a variety of different cytokines, including erythropoietin, growth hormone, IL-3, IL-6, GM-CSF, G-CSF and IFN-γ, has been found to induce tyrosine phosphorylation and kinase activation of Jak2[134,135,142–144]. More recently, IL-2 and IL-4 were shown to induce tyrosine phosphorylation and kinase activation of Jak3[137,138].

IL-5 stimulation rapidly (within 10 s) induces tyrosine phosphorylation and kinase activation of Jak2[104,113]. In transfectants expressing the mutant IL-5Rα, having a deletion in the region rich in proline residues, tyrosine phosphorylation of Jak2 is barely detectable in response to IL-5. We propose two models for the mechanism of activation of the IL-5R complex. In one model, IL-5 induces multimerization of IL-5Rα and dimerization of the cytoplasmic domain of the βc. The proline-rich regions of the cytoplasmic domain of IL-5Rα interact directly or indirectly with the βc, and this interaction is essential for either dimerization or conformational change of the cytoplasmic domain of the βc. This dimerization of the βc brings the two Jak2 kinases, which are associated with the box 1 region of the βc, in sufficiently close proximity to allow for their cross-phosphorylation with resultant activation of these two Jak2 kinases. In the second model, the proline-rich region of IL-5Rα interacts with an intracellular protein kinase, such as Jak2 or other members of the Jak family. The IL-5Rα-associated kinase and the βc-associated Jak2 kinase cross-phosphorylate and activate each other. At present, we have no definite evidence for supporting either of these two models.

Recently, Larner *et al.*[145] demonstrated that treatment of human peripheral blood monocytes or basophils with IL-3, IL-5, IL-10 or GM-CSF activated DNA-binding proteins whose tyrosine residues are phosphorylated. They suggested that these cytokines as well as IFN-α and IFN-γ can modulate gene expression through activation of putative transcription factors by tyrosine phosphorylation. The Jak2 tyrosine kinase at least may play an important role in the activation of transcription factors involved in IL-5-mediated signal transduction.

The Bruton's tyrosine kinase, Btk, has been cloned as a B-cell-specific cytosolic tyrosine kinase and identified as the molecule involved in X-linked human agammaglobulinemia (XLA)[146,147]. A single conserved residue within the N-terminal unique region of Btk has been shown to be mutated in XID mice[148,149]. Since we observed that B cells derived from XID mice show defective responses to IL-5, we examined the effects of IL-5 on Btk activity using an immune complex kinase assay. Stimulation of Y16 cells for 5–20 min with IL-5 led to a significant enhancement in Btk kinase activity (two to three times higher than that of unstimulated controls) as detected in anti-Btk immunoprecipitates[113]. No enhancement of Btk activity was detected in IL-5-stimulated transfectants expressing mutants of IL-5Rα which lack the entire region of the cytoplasmic domain. The Btk protein, which belongs to a newly identified family of non-receptor tyrosine kinases, may have the potential to interact in a novel way with protein(s) involved in the IL-5R-mediated signaling pathway. The discovery of cellular molecule(s) that can interact with Btk, through its N-terminal unique region, should shed light on the complex signaling requirements of B-cell differentiation in response to cytokines, including IL-5.

## B-CELL-SPECIFIC DEFECT IN IL-5 RESPONSIVENESS IN XID MICE

Murine X-linked immunodeficiency (XID) results in a failure of B cells to become phenotypically and functionally diverse[150]. B cells from XID mice show a decrease in the overall number of B cells, low levels of circulating IgM and IgG3, and a high surface IgM to IgD ratio[150], do not respond to thymus-independent type 2 (TI-2) antigens[150], and have abnormal responses to a variety of activation signals through Ig receptors[151], CD40[152] and cytokine receptors[153,154]. XID mice have fewer IL-5R$^+$ B cells than normal mice[153]. In particular, there is a remarkable decrease in the number of peritoneal IL-5R$^+$ B cells among the Ly-1 B-cell population. Furthermore, the frequency of precursors of IL-5-responsive B cells in XID mice is approximately 100-fold lower than that of normal mice. Interestingly, sorted IL-5R$^+$ B cells from XID mice display a low response to IL-5. However, eosinophils obtained from IL-5-injected XID mice express both α and βc of IL-5R and respond to IL-5 with prolonged *in vitro* survival to an extent similar to that observed for eosinophils from wild-type mice[153]. These results indicate that low responsiveness to IL-5 in XID mice is restricted to B-lineage cells and that IL-5-mediated signaling cascades in eosinophils are somehow different from those in B cells. These results raise two possibilities which may account for the B-cell-specific abnormality of IL-5 responsiveness in XID mice. One possibility is that IL-5Rα expressed on XID B cells is non-functional. Alternatively, IL-5Rα$^+$ XID B cells may have a defect in the IL-5R-mediated signaling pathway.

To evaluate both of the above possibilities, we generated IL-5Rα transgenic (5Rα-Tg) mice carrying the mIL-5Rα gene ligated to the human IgH enhancer and mouse $V_H$ promoter[155]. In these transgenic mice, the majority of B cells expressed IL-5Rα and showed enhanced responsiveness to IL-5 for Ig production and proliferation. 5Rα-Tg mice carrying the *xid* gene (XRD-5Rα-Tg mice) were generated by crossing C57BL/6.*xid* female mice with 5Rα-Tg male mice. FACS (fluorescence activated cell sorting) analysis revealed that IL-5Rα was expressed on the majority of spleen B cells and B220-positive bone marrow cells from XID-5Rα-Tg mice, indicating that expression of the *xid* gene had no effect on the induced expression of IL-5Rα. Numbers of Ly-1$^{dull+}$ and B220$^{dull+}$ B cells in both the XID-5Rα-Tg and XID mice were strikingly reduced (Figure 9.8). As the Ly-1$^{dull+}$ and B220$^{dull+}$ B cells that coexpress mIL-5Rα are considered to be Ly-1 B cells in the wild-type mice, our results indicate that the absence of Ly-1 B cell population in XID mice is not due to decreased expression of IL-5Rα.

Determination of the levels of each Ig isotype in sera by ELISA revealed that the concentrations of serum IgM in both XID-5Rα-Tg and XID mice were lower than in female non-XID mice, while serum IgG1 levels were comparable to those of the female littermates[155]. The serum levels of circulating IgG2a, IgG2b and IgA of XID-5Rα-Tg, as well as those of XID, mice were within normal range, but the IgG3 levels of these animals were lower than those of female littermates. XID-5Rα-Tg mice immunized with TNP-Ficoll produce no significant anti-TNP IgM antibodies, as in the case of XID mice. These results indicate that the induced expression of IL-5Rα in XID mice has no effect on

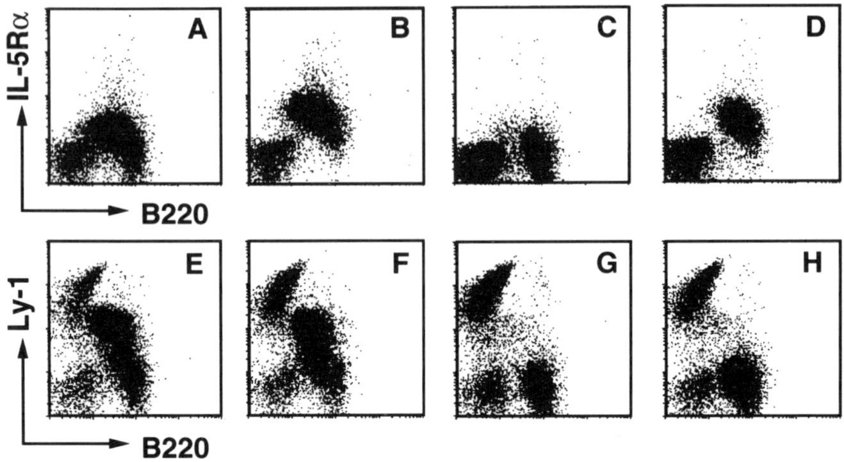


**Figure 9.8** XID-5Rα-Tg mice lack Ly-1-positive B cells in peritoneal cavity. Peritoneal exudate cells from phenotypically normal female mice (A, E), 5Rα-Tg female mice (B, F), XID male mice (C, G), and XID-5Rα-Tg male mice (D, H) were stained with biotinylated H7 (anti-mIL-5Rα mAb) and FITC-labeled RA3-6B2 (anti-B220 mAb) (A, B, C, D) or biotinylated anti-Ly-1 mAb and FITC-labeled RA3-6B2 (anti-B220 mAb) (E, F, G, H). The cells in the lymphoid gate were analyzed by flow cytometry

the abnormal B-cell development caused by the *xid* mutation. B cells from XID-5Rα-Tg mice, like B cells from XID mice, do not respond to IL-5, although most B cells from XID-5Rα-Tg mice expressed IL-5Rα.

Proliferative responses of B cells from XID, XID-5Rα-Tg and normal mice to 10 μg/ml of LPS were indistinguishable, while XID B cells show lower responsiveness to LPS than normal B cells at lower concentrations (less than 1.0 μg/ml) of LPS, as reported[147,148]. These cells failed to respond to 0.1 μg/ml of LPS, a concentration at which normal B cells respond moderately. Interestingly, proliferative responses were induced when B cells from XID-5Rα-Tg mice, but not from XID mice, were cultured with mIL-5 and a low dose of LPS. This proliferative response was specific to IL-5, because B cells from XID-5Rα-Tg mice did not respond to IL-2, IL-4, IL-6, IFN-γ or TGF-β, with or without 0.1 μg/ml of LPS. B cells from XID-5Rα-Tg, but not from XID, mice also respond to mIL-5 in the presence of PMA. Intriguingly, B cells from XID-5Rα-Tg mice can produce significant amounts of IgM, IgG1 and IgG3 when co-cultured with mIL-5 plus LPS (Figure 9.9). These results indicate that the B-cell-specific defect of XID B cells in terms of IL-5 responsiveness is due to an abnormality in IL-5 signaling and that this may be overcome in part by costimulation and suboptimum doses of LPS or phorbol ester (PMA) (Figure 9.10).

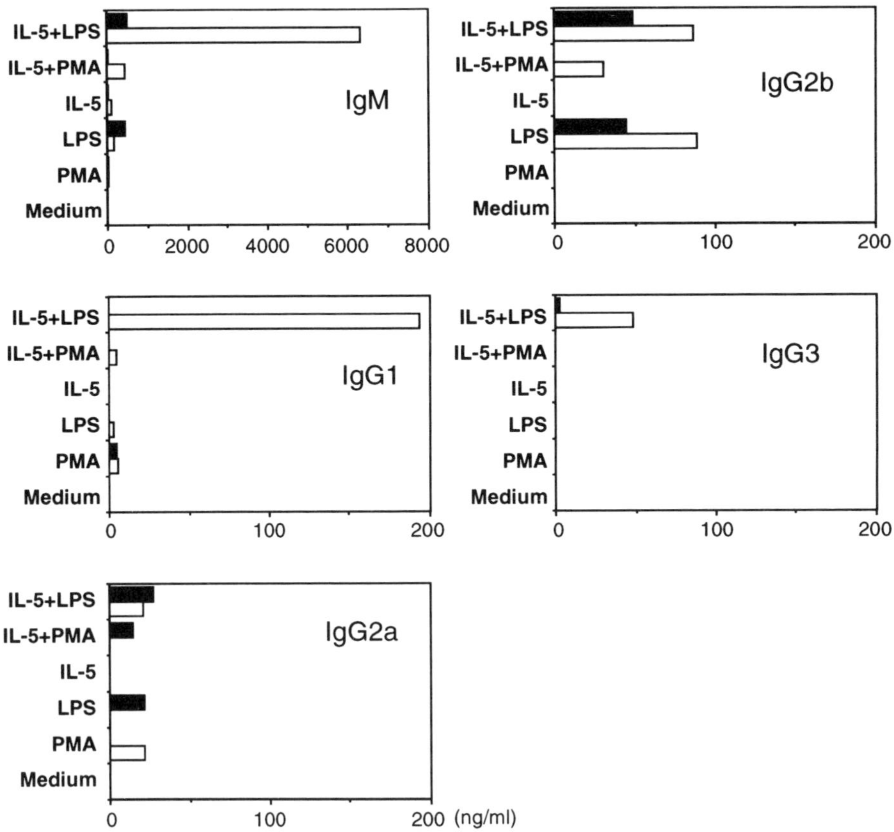


**Figure 9.9** Ig secretion from B cells in response to IL-5 and costimuli. B cells from XID mice (closed column) and XID-5Rα-Tg mice (open column) were cultured under the indicated conditions for 7 days. After the culture, the amount of each Ig isotype in the culture supernatant was determined by ELISA. The concentrations of added stimuli were as follows: IL-5 at 1000 U/ml, LPS and PMA at 0.1 μg/ml

As we discussed above, XID mice show an amino acid substitution of Btk which may partially inhibit Btk function[148,149,156]. The substitution of Arg at position 28 for Cys of Btk in XID mice may adversely affect recognition of an as yet unidentified Btk-associated protein, resulting in the alteration of IL-5R-mediated signaling in B cells from both XID and XID-5Rα-Tg. Other IL-5 signaling pathways have also been proposed in light of the normal responsiveness of eosinophils from XID mice to IL-5[143]. In humans, it has been reported that *btk* mRNA is expressed in B cells and myeloid cells, but not in T cells[146,147], while *btk*-related tyrosine kinase genes, *itk* and *tek(II)*, have been shown to be expressed in myeloid cells, but not in B cells[157,158]. The

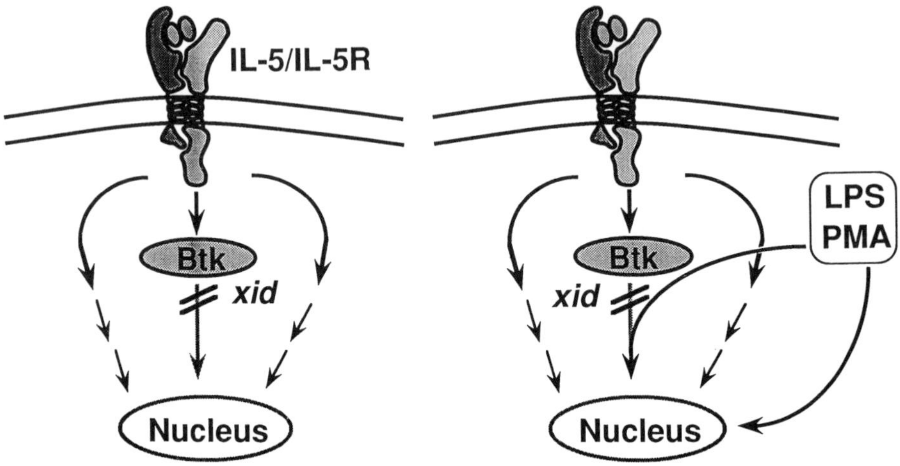


**Figure 9.10** Models for two IL-5 signaling pathways in conjunction with Btk activation. In B cells, Btk activation may play a role in transducing IL-5 signals to other signaling molecules. B cells from XID mice may not transduce IL-5 signals properly. In XID-5Rα-Tg B cells, IL-5 signaling may be bypassed by Btk-related pathway in the presence of LPS or PMA. This latter IL-5 signaling pathway may operate in eosinophils

expression of the *btk*-related tyrosine kinase genes in myeloid cells could explain the responsiveness of XID eosinophils to IL-5. The discovery of cellular molecule(s) that can interact with Btk, through its N-terminal unique region, should shed light on analysis of the B-cell-specific defect in XID mice.

## INTERPRETATIONS

### FUNCTIONAL PROPERTIES OF IL-5

Two issues of current interest to our laboratory is the role of IL-5 in preventing apoptosis of B cells, and its role in stimulating Ig isotype switching. As discussed above, IL-5 appears to sustain survival of TGF-β/LPS-stimulated B cells in *in vitro* culture. Further, we and others have evidence that IL-5 partially prevents the anti-IgM-induced apoptosis of WEHI-231 cells and *in vitro* apoptosis of eosinophils. Determining the role of IL-5 in Ig isotype switching will require additional model systems for evaluating the molecular mechanisms involved in this process.

In this chapter, I have not focused on the role of IL-5 in eosinophilopoiesis and activation of eosinophils. However, there is considerable evidence supporting the idea that IL-5 has a critical role in the pathogenesis of asthmatic diseases. The development of animal models for asthma is required in order to evaluate the role of IL-5 in asthmatic disease. Mice made genetically deficient in expression of the IL-5 or IL-5Rα gene may provide us with useful tools for clarifying the exact role of IL-5 in B-cell and eosinophil development and triggering.

## IL-5R-MEDIATED SIGNALING PATHWAYS

IL-3, IL-5 and GM-CSF make up a subfamily of cytokines displaying a variety of overlapping actions during hematopoiesis. These three hematopoietic factors bind to distinct specificity-determining α receptor components, but share βc as a common signal transducer; the unique distributions of the individual α subunits will determine which hematopoietic cells are capable of responding to each of these factors. Given that IL-5, IL-3 and GM-CSF also have certain unique functional effects, it remains to be determined how the IL-5 signal is transduced differently from that of GM-CSF or IL-3. The signals generated by these cytokines may be equivalent, and the different functions of these cytokines are due to the stage of development of the cells expressing the receptors. Alternatively, different signal-transducing molecules, which generate a specific signal for each cytokine, may be associated with the respective ligand-binding α subunit of each receptor. These possibilities are not mutually exclusive.

The α subunits of the IL-5R, IL-3R and GM-CSFR have a conserved region on the cytoplasmic side of the transmembrane domain. This region appears to be important for interaction of IL-5Rα with the cytoplasmic domain of the βc. The membrane-proximal proline-rich sequences and the adjacent downstream proline-rich region of the cytoplasmic domain of the IL-5Rα are essential and important, respectively, for IL-5-mediated signal transduction involved in mediating the growth-promoting effect[17,104]. These two regions are well conserved among IL-5Rα, IL-3Rα and GM-CSFRα, prolactin and growth hormone receptors and are speculated to play a critical role in transducing common growth signals. The C-terminal regions of the α chains of IL-5R, IL-3R and GM-CSFR are different from each other. These regions may contribute to the transduction of ligand-specific signals. Deletions in the C-terminal region of the cytoplasmic domain of IL-5Rα do not, however, affect growth signal transduction ability. In our preliminary data, IL-5 but not GM-CSF can induce Ig production by transfectants expressing both IL-5Rα and GM-CSFRα together with βc, although both IL-5 and GM-CSF can induce proliferation of transfectants (Shiiba *et al.*, unpublished data). To evaluate the role of the C-terminal region in the unique aspects of IL-5R-mediated signaling, experiments using transfectants expressing chimeric receptors composed of the extracellular domain, transmembrane domain and cytoplasmic regions of the IL-5Rα, up to the adjacent regions of the proline-rich regions, and the C-terminal region of the GM-CSFRα, will be required.

We have been particularly interested in the tyrosine phosphorylation of Shc and HS1 proteins and in the activation of Jak2 and Btk kinases. As tyrosine phosphorylation of Ras–GAP is not induced by IL-5 stimulation, enhanced activity of Ras may not be caused by tyrosine phosphorylation of GAP in response to IL-5 stimulation. Therefore, activation of Ras upon IL-5 stimulation is, at least in part, due to the modulation of Shc by the tyrosine kinase(s) activated by IL-5 ligation. Our finding on the tyrosine phosphorylation of HS1 upon IL-5 stimulation indicates that HS1 may transduce a signal generated by IL-5 ligation directly into the genetic loci involved in IL-5-induced cell growth. The kinase activities of Btk can be significantly enhanced in IL-5-responsive cell lines in response to IL-5. This suggests that the involvement of Btk in IL-5R-mediated signaling and the abnormal expression of Btk in XID B cells may be coupled with an impaired IL-5 responsiveness. The Btk protein could have the potential to interact in a novel way with protein(s) involved in the IL-5R-mediated signaling pathway. Search for cellular molecule(s) that can interact with Btk through its N-terminal unique region should shed light on the complex signaling requirements of B-cell differentiation in response to cytokines, including IL-5.

It is also important to clarify the differences in signal transduction pathways between B cells and eosinophils in response to IL-5. Eosinophils from XID mice respond to IL-5 with prolonged survival, while B cells from XID mice do not respond to IL-5. These results strongly suggest that there are at least two different signaling pathways for IL-5; one operating in B cells and the other in eosinophils. If we can find specific inhibitors for IL-5R-mediated signaling in eosinophils, they would represent good candidates for anti-asthmatic drugs.

## ACKNOWLEDGMENTS

I am grateful to my collaborators for their tremendous contribution during the course of these studies, including the sharing of data. This work was supported in part by a Grant-in-Aid for Scientific Research for Special Project Research, Cancer Bioscience from the Ministry of Education, Science, and Culture; by Special Coordination Funds for promoting Science and Technology from the Japanese Ministry of Science and Technology; and by a grant from Mochida Memorial Foundation of Medical and Pharmaceutical Science.

## REFERENCES

1. Takatsu K. Interleukin-5 receptor. Curr Opin Immunol 1992; 3:299–304.
2. Takatsu K, Takai S, Hitoshi Y. Interleukin 5 and its receptor system: implications in the immune response and inflammation. Adv Immunol 1994; 57:145–190.

3. Takatsu K, Tanaka K, Tominaga A *et al.* Antigen-induced T cell-replacing factor (TRF) III. Establishment of T cell hybridoma producing TRF and analysis of released TRF. J Immunol 1980; 125:2646–2653.
4. Isakson P, Pure E, Vitetta ES, Krammer PH. T cell-derived B cell differentiation factors: effect of the isotype switch of murine B cells. J Exp Med 1981; 155:734–748.
5. Pure E, Isakson PC, Takatsu K *et al.* Induction of B cell differentiation by T cell factor I. Stimulation of IgM secretion by products of a T cell hybridoma and a T cell line. J Immunol 1981; 127:1953–1958.
6. Swain SL, Howard M, Kappler J *et al.* Evidence for two distinct classes of murine B cell growth factors with activities in different functional assays. J Exp Med 1982; 158:822–835.
7. Coffman RL, Shrader B, Carty J *et al.* A mouse T cell product that preferentially enhances IgA production. I. Biologic characterization. J Immunol 1987; 139:3685–3690.
8. Harriman GR, Kunimoto DY, Elliott JF *et al.* The role of IL-5 in IgA B cell differentiation. J Immunol 140:3033–3039.
9. Sonoda E, Matsumoto R, Hitoshi Y *et al.* Transforming growth factor β and interleukin 5 acts additively for IgA production. J Exp Med 1989; 170:1415–1420.
10. Sonoda E, Hitoshi Y, Yamaguchi N *et al.* Differential regulation of IgA production by TGF-β and IL-5: TGF-β induces surface IgA-positive cells bearing IL-5 receptor, whereas IL-5 promotes their survival and maturation into IgA-secreting cells. Cell Immunol 1992; 140:158–172.
11. Sanderson CJ. Interleukin-5, eosinophils, and disease. Blood 1992; 79:3101–3109.
12. Lopez AF, Elliott MJ, Woodcock J, Vadas MA. GM-CSF, IL-3 and IL-5: cross-competition on human haemopoietic cells. Immunol Today 1992; 13:495.
13. Takaki S, Tominaga A, Hitoshi Y *et al.* Molecular cloning and expression of the murine interleukin-5 receptor. EMBO J 1990; 9:4367–4374.
14. Murata Y, Takaki S, Migita M *et al.* Molecular cloning and expression of the human interleukin-5 receptor. J Exp Med 1992; 175:341–351.
15. Devos P, Plaetinck G, der Heyden JV *et al.* Molecular basis of a high affinity murine interleukin-5 receptor. EMBO J 1991; 10:2133–2137.
16. Takaki S, Mita S, Murata Y *et al.* Identification of the second subunit of the murine interleukin 5 receptor: interleukin-3 receptor-like protein, AIC2B is a component of the high affinity interleukin-5 receptor. EMBO J 1991; 10:2833–2838.
17. Takaki S, Murata Y, Kitamura T *et al.* Reconstitution of the functional receptors for murine and human interleukin 5. J Exp Med 1993; 177:1523–1529.
18. Tavernier J, Devos R, Cornelis S *et al.* A human high affinity interleukin-5 receptor (IL5R) is composed of an IL5-specific α chain and a β chain shared with the receptor for GM-CSF. Cell 1991; 66:1175–1184.
19. Miyajima A, Kitamura T, Harada N *et al.* Cytokine receptors and signal transduction. Annu Rev Immunol 10:295–331.
20. Gorman DM, Itoh N, Kitamura T *et al.* Cloning and expression of a gene encoding an interleukin 3 receptor-like protein: identification of another member of the cytokine receptor gene family. Proc Natl Acad Sci USA 1990; 87:5459–5463.
21. Hara T, Miyajima A. Two distinct functional high affinity receptors for mouse interleukin-3 (IL-3). EMBO J 1992; 11:1875–1884.
22. Hayashida K, Kitamura T, Gorman DM *et al.* Molecular cloning of a second subunit of the receptor for human granulocyte-macrophage colony-stimulating

factor (GM-CSF): reconstitution of a high-affinity GM-CSF receptor. Proc Natl Acad Sci USA 1990; 87:9655–9659.
23. Kitamura T, Sato N, Arai K, Miyajima A. Expression cloning of the human IL-3 receptor cDNA reveals a shared β subunit for human IL-3 and GM-CSF receptors. Cell 1991; 66:1165–1174.
24. Park LS, Martin U, Sorensen R *et al.* Cloning of the low-affinity murine granulocyte-macrophage colony-stimulating factor receptor and reconstitution of a high-affinity receptor complex. Proc Natl Acad Sci USA 1992; 89:4295–4299.
25. Kinashi T, Harada N, Severinson E *et al.* Cloning of complementary DNA for T-cell replacing factor and identity with B-cell growth factor II. Nature 1986; 324:70–73.
26. Azuma C, Tanabe T, Konishi M *et al.* Cloning of cDNA encoding human T-cell replacing factor (Interleukin-5) and comparison with the murine homologue. Nucleic Acids Res 1986; 14:9149–9158.
27. Yokota T, Coffman RL, Hagiwara H *et al.* Isolation and characterization of lymphokine cDNA clones encoding mouse and human IgA-enhancing factor and eosinophil colony-stimulating factor activities: relationship to interleukin 5. Proc Natl Acad Sci USA 1987; 84:7388–7392.
28. Tominaga A, Matsumoto M, Harada N *et al.* Molecular properties and regulation of mRNA expression for murine T cell-replacing factor, (TRF)/interleukin 5 (IL-5). J Immunol 1988; 140:1175–1181.
29. Mosmann TR, Coffman RL. TH1 and TH2 cells: different patterns of lymphokine secretion lead to different functional properties. Annu Rev Immunol 1989; 7:145–173.
30. Plaut M, Pierce JH, Watson CJ *et al.* Mast cell lines produce lymphokines in response to cross-linkage of FceRI or calcium ionophores. Nature 1989; 339:64–67.
31. Honjo T, Takatsu K. Interleukin 5. In: Sporn MA, Roberts AB (eds) (Handbook of Experimental Pharmacology, Vol. 95/I, Peptide Growth Factors and Their Receptors I). Peptide Growth Factors and Their Receptors Heidelberg: Springer-Verlag, 1990, pp. 609–632.
32. Bauman AA, Paul CC. Interleukin-5 is an autocrine growth factor for Epstein–Barr virus-transformed B lymphocytes. Blood 1992; 79:1763–1767.
33. Samoszuk M, Nansen L. Detection of interleukin-5 messenger RNA in Reed–Sernberg cells of Hodgkin's disease with eosinophilia. Blood 1990; 75:13–16.
34. Desreumaux P, Janin A, Colombel JE *et al.* Interleukin 5 messenger RNA expression by eosinophils in the intestinal mucosa of patients with Coeliac disease. J Exp Med 1992; 175:293–296.
35. Tominaga A, Takahashi T, Kikuchi Y *et al.* Role of carbohydrate moiety of IL-5. Effect of tunicamycin on the glycosylation of IL-5 and the biologic activity of deglycosylated IL-5. J Immunol 1990; 144:1345–1352.
36. Tsujimoto M, Adachi H, Kodama S *et al.* Purification and characterization of recombinant human interleukin 5 expressed in Chinese hamster ovary cells. J Biochem (Tokyo) 1989; 106:23–28.
37. Minamitake Y, Kodama S, Katayama T *et al.* Structure of recombinant human interleukin 5 produced by Chinese hamster ovary cells. J Biochem (Tokyo) 1990; 107:292–297.
38. Takahashi T, Yamaguchi N, Mita S *et al.* Structural comparison of murine T-cell (B151K12)-derived T-cell-replacing factor (IL-5) with rIL-5: dimer formation is essential for the expression of biological activity. Mol Immunol 1990; 9:911–920.
39. McKenzie ANJ, Ely B and Sanderson CJ. Mutated interleukin-5 monomers are biologically-inactive. Mol Immunol 1991; 28:155–158.

40. Milburn MV, Hassell AM, Lambert MH *et al.* A novel dimer configuration revealed by the crystal structure at 2.4 Å resolution of human interleukin-5. Nature 1993; 363:172–176.
41. McKenzie ANJ, Barry SC, Strath M, Sanderson CJ. Structure–function analysis of interleukin-5 utilizing mouse/human chimeric molecules. EMBO J 1991; 10:1193–1199.
42. Harada N, Kikuchi Y, Tominaga A *et al.* BCGFII activity on activated B cells of a purified murine T cell-replacing factor (TRF) from a T cell hybridoma (B151K12). J Immunol 1985; 134:3944–3951.
43. Herzenberg LA, Stall AM, Lalor PA *et al.* The LY-1 B cell lineage. Immunol Rev 1986; 93:81–102.
44. Kantor AB. The development and repertoire of B-1 cells (CD5 B cells). Immunol Today 1991; 12:389–391.
45. Kincade PW. Formation of B lymphocytes in fetal and adult life. Adv Immunol 1981; 31:177–245.
46. Alt FW, Blackwell TK, Yancopoulos GD. Development of the primary antibody repertoire. Science 1987; 238:1079–1087.
47. Rolink A, Melchers F. Molecular and cellular origin of B lymphocyte diversity. Cell 1991; 66:1081–1094.
48. Tonegawa S. Somatic generation of antibody diversity. Nature 1983; 302:575–581.
49. Tominaga A, Mita S, Kikuchi Y *et al.* Establishment of IL-5 dependent early B cell lines by long-term bone marrow cultures. Growth Factors 1989; 1:135–146.
50. Takatsu K, Tominaga A. Interleukin-5 and its receptor. Growth Factor Res 1991; 3:87–102.
51. Takatsu K, Takaki S, Hitoshi Y *et al.* Cytokine receptors on CD5 B cells: IL-5 and its receptor. Ann N Y Acad Sci 1992; 651:229–241.
52. Katoh S, Tominaga A, Migita M *et al.* Conversion of normal Ly-1-positive B lineage cells into Ly-1-positive macrophages in long-term bone marrow cultures. Dev Immunol 1990; 1:113–125.
53. Klinken SP, Alexander WS, Adams JM. Hemopoietic lineage switch: v-raf oncogene converts Eμ-myc transgenic B cells into macrophages. Cell 1988; 53:857–867.
54. Hitoshi Y, Mita S, Tominaga A *et al.* Interferon-gamma inhibits the proliferation but not the differentiation of murine B cells in response to IL-5. Int Immunol 1989; 1:185–190.
55. Mita S, Kikuchi Y, Hitoshi Y *et al.* Cyclosporin A preferentially inhibits the differentiation of murine B cells in response to IL-5 and its restoration by IL-6. Kumamoto Med J 1993; 42:63–72.
56. Takatsu K, Tominaga A, Harada N *et al.* T cell-replacing factor (TRF)/interleukin 5 (IL-5): molecular and functional properties. Immunol Rev 1988; 102:107–135.
57. Matsumoto M, Tominaga A, Harada N, Takatsu K. Role of T cell-replacing factor (TRF) in the murine B cell differentiation: induction of increased levels of secreted type IgM mRNA. J Immunol 1987; 138:1826–1833.
58. Alderson MR, Pike BL, Harada N *et al.* Recombinant T cell-replacing factor (interleukin 5) acts with antigen to promote the growth and differentiation of single hapten-specific B lymphocytes. J Immunol 1987; 139:2656–2660.
59. Karasuyama H, Rolink A, Melchers F. Recombinant interleukin 2 or 5, but not 3 or 4, induces maturation of resting mouse B lymphocytes and propagate proliferation of activated B cell blasts. J Exp Med 1988; 167:1377–1390.
60. Webb SF, Das C, Eaton S *et al.* Novel protein–DNA interactions associated with increased immunoglobulin transcription in response to antigen plus interleukin-5. Mol Cell Biol 1991; 115:5197–5205.

61. Bertolini JN, Sanderson CJ, Benson EM. Human interleukin-5 induces staphylococcal A Cowan I strain-activated human B cells to secrete IgM. Eur J Immunol 1993; 23:398–402.
62. Morikawa K, Oseki F, Morikawa S *et al.* Recombinant human IL-5 augments immunoglobulin generation by human B lymphocytes in the presence of IL-2. Cell Immunol 1993; 149:390–401.
63. Clutterbuck E, Shields JG, Gordon J *et al.* Recombinant human interleukin 5 is an eosinophil differentiation factor but has no activity in standard human B cell growth factor assays. Eur J Immunol 1987; 17:1743–1750.
64. Huston DP, Moore JP, Huston MM. Human B cells express IL-5 receptor mRNA and respond to IL-5 with enhanced IgM production under selective mitogenic stimulation. J Immunol 1993; 150:182A.
65. Beagley KW, Eldridge JH, Kiyono H *et al.* Recombinant murine IL-5 induces high rate IgA synthesis in cycling IgA-positive Peyer's patch B cells. J Immunol 1988; 141:2035–2042.
66. Coffman RL, Shrader B, Carty J *et al.* A mouse T cell product that preferentially enhances IgA production. I. Biologic characterization. J Immunol 1987; 139:3685–3690.
67. McKenzie DT, Filutowitz H, Swain SL, Dutton RW. Purification and partial sequence analysis of murine B cell growth factor II (interleukin 5). J Immunol 1987; 139:2661–2668.
68. Harriman GR, Kunimoto DY, Elliott JF *et al.* The role of IL-5 in IgA B cell differentiation. J Immunol 1988; 140:3033–3039.
69. Matsumoto R, Matsumoto M, Mita S *et al.* Interleukin 5 induces maturation but not class switching of surface IgA-positive B cells into IgA-secreting cells. Immunology 1989; 66:32–38.
70. Schoenberck S, McKenzie DT, Kagnoff MF. Interleukin 5 is a differentiation factor for IgA B cells. Eur J Immunol 1992; 19:965–969.
71. Coffman RL, Lebman DA, Shrader B. Transforming growth factor β specifically enhances IgA production by lipopolysaccharide-stimulated B lymphocytes. J Exp Med 1989; 170:1039–1043.
72. Kim P-H, Kagnoff MF. Transforming growth factor-β1 is a costimulator for IgA production. J Immunol 1990; 145:3774–3778.
73. Snapper CM, Yamada H, Smoot D *et al.* Comparative *in vitro* analysis of proliferation, Ig secretion, and Ig switching by murine marginal zone and follicular B cells. J Immunol 1993; 150:2737–2745.
74. Lebman DA, Nomura DY, Coffman RL, Lee FD. Molecular characterization of germline immunoglobulin A transcripts produced during transforming growth factor type β-induced isotype switching. Proc Natl Acad Sci USA 1990; 87:3962–3966.
75. Lebman DA, Coffman RL. The effects of IL-4 and IL-5 on the IgA response by murine Peyer's patch B cell subpopulations. J Immunol 1990; 141:2050–2056.
76. Matsuoka M, Yoshida K, Maeda T *et al.* Switch circular DNA formed in cytokine-treated mouse splenocytes: evidence for intermolecular DNA deletion in immunoglobulin class. Cell 1990; 62:135–142.
77. Iwasato T, Shimizu A, Honjo T, Yamagishi H. Circular DNA is excised by immunoglobulin class switch recombination. Cell 1990; 62:143–149.
78. Whitmore AC, Prowse DM, Haughton G, Arnold LW. Ig isotype switching in B lymphocytes. The effect of T cell-derived interleukins, cytokines, cholera toxin, and antigen on isotype switch frequency of a cloned B cell lymphoma. Int Immunol 1991; 3:95–103.
79. Iwasato T, Arakawa H, Shimizu A *et al.* Biased distribution of recombination sites within S regions upon immunoglobulin class switch recombination induced

by transforming growth factor β and lipopolysaccharide. J Exp Med 1992; 175:1539–1546.
80. McIntyre TM, Klinman DR, Rothman P *et al.* Transforming growth factor β1 selectively stimulates immunglobulin G2b secretion by lipopolysaccharide-activated murine B cells. J Exp Med 1993; 177:1031–1037.
81. Purkerson JM, Isakson PC. Interleukin 5 (IL-5) provides a signal that is required in addition to IL-4 for isotype switching to immunoglobulin (Ig) G1 and IgE. J Exp Med 1992; 175:973–982.
82. Mandler R, Chu CC, Paul WE *et al.* Interleukin 5 induces Sμ-Sγ1 DNA rearrangement in B cells activated with dextran-anti-IgD antibodies and interleukin 4: a three component model for Ig class switching. J Exp Med 1993; 178:1577–1586.
83. Mita S, Tominaga A, Hitoshi Y *et al.* Characterization of high-affinity receptors for interleukin 5 on interleukin 5-dependent cell lines. Proc Natl Acad Sci USA 1989; 86:2311–2315.
84. Yamaguchi N, Hitoshi Y, Mita S *et al.* Characterization of the murine IL-5 receptors by using monoclonal anti-receptor antibody. Int Immunol 1990; 2:181–187.
85. Rolink AG, Melchers F, Palacios R. Monoclonal antibodies reactive with the mouse interleukin 5 receptor. J Exp Med 1989; 169:1693–1701.
86. Hitoshi Y, Yamaguchi N, Mita S *et al.* Distribution of interleukin-5 receptor-positive B cells: expression of IL-5-receptor on Ly-1 (CD5)-positive B cells. J Immunol 1990; 144:4218–4225.
87. Mita S, Takaki S, Hitoshi Y *et al.* Molecular characterization of the β chain of the murine interleukin 5 receptor. Int Immunol 1991; 3:665–672.
88. Kikuchi Y, Migita M, Takaki S *et al.* Biochemical and functional characterization of soluble form of IL-5 receptor α (sIL-5Rα): development of ELISA system for detection of sIL-5Rα. J Immunol Methods 1994; 167:289–298.
89. Bazan JF. Structural design and molecular evolution of a cytokine receptor superfamily. Proc Natl Acad Sci USA 1990; 87:6934–6938.
90. Yamaguchi N, Hitoshi Y, Mita S *et al.* Characterization of the murine interleukin 5 receptor by using a monoclonal antibody. Int Immunol 1990; 2:181–187.
91. Murakami M, Narazaki M, Hibi M *et al.* Critical cytoplasmic region of the interleukin 6 signal transducer gp130 is conserved in the cytokine receptor family. Proc Natl Acad Sci USA 1991; 88:11349–11353.
92. Ren R, Mayer BJ, Cicchetti P, Baltimore D. Identification of a ten-amino acid proline-rich SH3 binding site. Science 1993; 259:1157–1161.
93. Imamura F, Takaki S, Akagi K *et al.* Structure of genomic DNA for detection of sIL-5Rα DNA Cell Biol 1994; 13:283–292.
94. Gough NM, Raker S. Localization of the IL-5 receptor gene to the distal half of murine chromosome 6 using recombinant inbred strains of mice. Genomics 1992; 12:855–856.
95. Isobe M, Kumura Y, Murata Y *et al.* Localization of the gene encoding human interleukin-5 receptor (IL-5R) chromosome region, 3p24–3p26. Genomics 1992; 14:755–758.
96. Kishimoto T, Akira S, Taga T. Cytokine signal transduction. Cell 1994; 76:253–262.
97. Devos R, Guisez Y, Cornelis S *et al.* Recombinant soluble human interleukin-5 (hIL-5) receptor molecules: cross-linking and stoichiometry of binding to IL-5. J Biol Chem 1993; 268:6581–6587.
98. Sato N, Sakamaki S, Terada N *et al.* Signal transduction by the high-affinity GM-CSF receptor: two distinct cytoplasmic regions of the common β subunit

responsible for different signaling. EMBO J 1993; 12:4181–4189.
99. Sakamaki K, Miyajima I, Kitamura T, Miyajima A. Critical cytoplasmic domains of the common β subunit of the human GM-CSF, IL-3 and IL-5 receptor for growth signal transduction and tyrosine phosphorylation. EMBO J 1992; 11:3541–3549.
100. Isfort RJ, Ihle JN. Multiple hematopoietic growth factors signal through tyrosine phosphorylation. Growth Factors 1990; 2:213–220.
101. Morla AO, Schreurs J, Miyajima A, Wang JYJ. Hematopoietic growth factors activate the tyrosine phosphorylation of distinct sets of proteins in interleukin-3-dependent murine cell lines. Mol Cell Biol 1988; 8:2214–2218.
102. Murata Y, Yamaguchi N, Hitoshi Y *et al.* Interleukin 5 and interleukin 3 induce serine and tyrosine phosphorylations of several cellular proteins in an interleukin 5-dependent cell line. Biochem Biophys Res Commun 1990; 173:1102–1108.
103. Conscience JF, Verrier B, Martin G. Interleukin-3-dependent expression of the c-*myc* and c-*fos* proto-oncogenes in hematopoietic cell lines. EMBO J 1986; 5:317–323.
104. Takaki S, Kanazawa H, Shiiba M, Takatsu K. Critical cytoplasmic domain of the IL-5R α chain and its function in IL-5-mediated growth signal transduction. Mol Cell Biol 1994; 12:7404–7413.
105. Yu H, Chan JK, Feng S *et al.* Structural basis for the binding of proline-rich peptides to SH3 domains. Cell 1994; 76:933–945.
106. Gout I, Dhand R, Hiles ID *et al.* The GTPase dynamin binds to and is activated by a subset of SH3 domains. Cell 1993; 75:25–36.
107. Murakami M, Hibi M, Nakagawa N *et al.* IL-6-induced homodimerization of gp 130 and associated activation of a tyrosine kinase. Science 1993; 260:1808–1810.
108. de Vos AM, Ultsch M, Kossiakoff AA. Human growth hormone and extracellular domain of its receptor: crystal structure of the complex. Science 1992; 255:306–312.
109. Ishizaka-Ikeda E, Fukunaga R, Wood WI *et al.* Signal transduction mediated by growth hormone receptor and its chimeric molecules with the granulocyte colony-stimulating factor receptor. Proc Natl Acad Sci USA 1993; 90:123–127.
110. Watowich SS, Yoshimura A, Longmore GD *et al.* Homodimerization and constitutive activation of the erythropoietin receptor. Proc Natl Acad Sci USA 1992; 89:2140–2144.
111. Nakamura Y, Russell SM, Mess SA *et al.* Heterodimerization of the interleukin-2 receptor β and γ cytoplasmic domains is required for signalling. Nature 1994; 369:330–333.
112. Nelson BH, Lord JD, Greenburg PD. Cytoplasmic domains of the interleukin-2 receptor β and γ chains mediate the signal for T-cell proliferation. Nature 1994; 369:333–336.
113. Satoh S, Katagiri T, Takaki S *et al.* IL-5 receptor-mediated tyrosine phosphorylation of SH2/SH3-containing protein and regulations of Btk and JAK2 kinases. J Exp Med 1994; 180:2101–2111.
114. Torigoe T, O-Connor R, Fagard R *et al.* Interleukin-3 regulates the activity of the LYN protein-tyrosine kinase in myeloid-committed leukemic cell lines. Blood 1992; 80:617–624.
115. Corey S, Eguinoa A, Theall KP *et al.* Granulocyte macrophage-colony stimulating factor stimulates both association and activation of phosphoinositide 3OH-kinase and src-related tyrosine kinase(s) in human myeloid derived cells. EMBO J 1993; 12:2681–2690.
116. Mui ALF, Kay RJ, Humphries RK, Krystal K. Ligand-induced phosphorylation of the murine interleukin 3 receptor signals its cleavage. Proc Natl Acad Sci

USA 1992; 89:10812–10816.
117. Duronio V, Lewis IC, Federsppiel B *et al.* Tyrosine phosphorylation of receptor β subunits and common substrates in response to interleukin-3 and granulocyte-macrophage colony-stimulating factor. J Biol Chem 1992; 267:21856–21863.
118. Hanazono Y, Chiba S, Sasaki K *et al.* c-fps/fes protein-tyrosine kinase is implicated in a signaling pathway triggered by granulocyte-macrophage colony-stimulating factor and interleukin-3. EMBO J 1993; 12:1641–1646.
119. Koch CA, Anderson D, Moran MF *et al.* SH2 and SH3 domains: elements that control interactions of cytoplasmic signaling proteins. Science 1991; 252:668–674.
120. Matsuda MB, Mayer BG, Hanafusa H. Identification of domains of the v-*crk* oncogene product sufficient for association with phosphotyrosine-containing proteins. Mol Cell Biol 1991; 11:1607–1613.
121. Bar-Sagi D, Rotin D, Batzer A *et al.* SH3 domains direct cellular localization of signaling molecules. Cell 1993; 74:83–91.
122. Pelicci G, Lanfrancone L, Grignani F *et al.* A novel transforming protein (SHC) with an SH2 domain is implicated in mitogenic signal transduction. Cell 1992; 70:93–104.
123. Egan SE, Giddings BW, Brooks MW *et al.* Association of Sos Ras exchange protein with Grb2 is implicated in tyrosine kinase signal transduction and transformation. Nature 1993; 363:45–51.
124. Duronio V, Welham MJ, Abraham S *et al.* p21ras activation via hemopoietic receptors and c-*kit* requires tyrosine kinase activity but not tyrosine phosphorylation of $p21^{ras}$ GTPase-activating protein. Proc Natl Acad Sci USA 1992; 89:1587–1591.
125. Smith MR, DeGudicubus SJ, Stacey DW. Requirement for c-*ras* proteins during viral oncogene transformation. Nature 1986; 320:540–543.
126. Satoh T, Nakafuku M, Miyajima A, Kaziro Y. Involvement of $p21^{ras}$ protein in signal-transduction pathways from interleukin 2, interleukin 3 and granulocyte/macrophage colony-stimulating factor, but not from interleukin 4. Proc Natl Acad Sci USA 1991; 88:3314–3318.
127. Katzav S, Cleveland JL, Heslop HE, Pulido D. Loss of the amino-terminal helix-loop-helix domain of the vav proto-oncogene activates its transforming potential. Mol Cell Biol 1991; 11:1912–1920.
128. Gulbins E, Coggeshall KM, Baier G *et al.* Tyrosine kinase-stimulated guanine nucleotide exchange activity of Vav in T cell activation. Science 1993; 260:822–825.
129. Gold M, Law DA, DeFranco AL. Stimulation of protein tyrosine phosphorylation by the B-lymphocyte antigen receptor. Nature 1990; 345:810–813.
130. Kitamura D, Kaneko H, Miyagoe Y *et al.* Isolation and characterization of a novel human gene expressed specifically in the cells of hematopoietic lineage. Nucleic Acids Res 1989; 17:9367–9379.
131. Yamanashi Y, Fukui Y, Wongsasant B *et al.* Activation of Src-like protein-tyrosine kinase Lyn and its association with phosphatidyl-inositol 3-kinase upon B-cell antigen receptor-mediated signaling. Proc Natl Acad Sci USA 1992; 89:1118–1122.
132. Gout I, Dhand R, Panayotou G *et al.* Expression and characterization of the p85 subunit of the phosphatidylinositol 3-kinase complex and a related p85b protein by using the baculovirus expression system. Biochem J 1992; 288:395–402.
133. Ihle JN, Witthuhn BA, Quelle FW *et al.* Signaling by the cytokine receptor superfamily: JAKs and STATs. TIBS 1994; 19:222–227.
134. Velazquez L, Fellous M, Stark GR, Pellegrini S. A protein tyrosine kinase in the interferon α/β signaling pathway. Cell 1992; 70:313–322.

135. Argetsinger LS, Campbell GS, Yang X *et al.* Identification of JAK2 as a growth hormone receptor-associated tyrosine kinase. Cell 1993; 74:237–244.
136. Stahl N, Yancopoulos GD. The alphas, betas and kinases of cytokine receptor complexes. Cell 1993; 74:587–590.
137. Johnston JA, Kawamura M, Kirken RA *et al.* Phosphorylation and activation of the Jak-3 Janus kinase in response to interleukin-2. Nature 1994; 370:151–153.
138. Witthuhn BA, Silvennoinen O, Miura O *et al.* Involvement of the Jak-3 Janus kinase in signalling by interleukin 2 and 4 in lymphoid and myeloid cells. Nature 1994; 370:153–157.
139. Lütticken C, Wegenka UM, Yuan J *et al.* Association of transcription factor APRF and protein kinase Jak1 with the interleukin-6 signal transducer gp130. Science 1994; 263:89–92.
140. Shuai K, Stark GR, Prezioso VR, Darnell JE Jr. A single phosphotyrosine residue of Stat91 required for gene activation by interferon-γ. Science 1993; 261:1736–1739.
141. Akira S, Nishio Y, Inoue M *et al.* Molecular cloning of APRF, a novel IFN-stimulated gene factor 3 p91-related transcription factor involved in the gp130-mediated signaling pathway. Cell 1994; 77:63–71.
142. Stahl N, Boulton TG, Farruggella T *et al.* Association and activation of Jak-Tyk kinases by CNTF-LIF-OSM-IL-6 β receptor components. Science 1994; 263:92–95.
143. Witthuhn BA, Quelle FW, Silvennoinen O *et al.* JAK2 associates with the erythropoietin receptor and is erythropoietin. Cell 1993; 74:227–236.
144. Silvennoinen O, Witthuhn BA, Quelle FW *et al.* Structure of the murine Jak2 protein-tyrosine kinase and its role in interleukin 3 signal transduction. Proc Natl Acad Sci USA 1993; 90:8429–8433.
145. Larner AC, David M, Feldman GM *et al.* Tyrosine phosphorylation of DNA binding proteins by multiple cytokines. Science 1993; 261:1730–1733.
146. Tsukada S, Saffran DC, Rawlings DJ *et al.* Deficient expression of a B cell cytoplasmic tyrosine kinase in human X-linked agammaglobulinemia. Cell 1993; 72:279–290.
147. Vetrie D, Vorechovsky I, Sideras P *et al.* The gene involved in X-linked agamma-globulinaemia is a member of the src family of protein-tyrosine kinases. Nature 1993;361:226–233.
148. Rawlings D, Saffran DC, Tsukada S *et al.* Mutation of unique region of Bruton's tyrosine kinase in immunodeficient Xid mice. Science 1993; 261:358–360.
149. Thomas JD, Sideras P, Smith CIE *et al.* Colocalization of X-linked agamma-globulinemia and X-linked immuno-deficiency genes. Science 1993; 261:355–358.
150. Scher I. CBA/N immune defective mice: evidence for the failure of a B cell subpopulation to be expressed. Immunol Rev 1982; 64:117–136.
151. Hayakawa K, Hardy RR, Herzenberg LA. Peritoneal Ly-1 B cells: genetic control, autoantibody production, increased lambda light chain expression. Eur J Immunol 1986; 16: 450–456.
152. Hasbold J, Klaus GGB. B cells from CBA/N mice do not proliferate following ligation of CD40. Eur J Immunol 1994; 24:152–157.
153. Hitoshi Y, Sonoda E, Kikuchi Y *et al.* Interleukin-5 receptor positive B cells, but not eosinophils are functionally and numerically influenced in the mice carried with X-linked immunodeficiency. Int Immunol 1993; 5:1183–1190.
154. Go NF, Castle BE, Barrett R *et al.* Interleukin 10, novel B cell stimulatory factor: unresponsiveness of X chromosome-linked immunodeficiency B cells. J Exp Med 1990; 172:1625–1631.
155. Koike M, Kikuchi Y, Tominaga A *et al.* Defect of IL-5-receptor-mediated signaling in B cells of X-linked immunodeficient (XID) mice. Int Immunol 1995; 7:21–30.

156. Tsukada S, Rawlings DJ, Witte ON. Role of Bruton's tyrosine kinase in human and murine B cell immunodeficiency. Curr Opin Immunol 1994; 6:623–630.
157. Siliciano JD, Morrow TA, Desiderio SV. *Itk*, a T-cell-specific tyrosine kinase gene inducible by interleukin 2. Proc Natl Acad Sci USA 1992; 90:669–673.
158. Mano H, Mano K, Tang B *et al.* Expression of a novel form of *Tec* kinase in hematopoietic cells and mapping of the gene to chromosome 5 near *Kit*. Oncogene 1993; 8:417–424.

# 10 Interleukin-6

**TOSHIO TANAKA, YOSHINORI KATADA, MASAKI SUEMURA and TADAMITSU KISHIMOTO**
*Osaka University Medical School, Osaka, Japan*

## INTRODUCTION

Interleukin-6 (IL-6) was originally defined as a B-cell differentiation factor which enhanced immunoglobulin (Ig) synthesis by cloned B-cell lines[1–3]. Since the cloning of the IL-6 gene[4], striking progress has been made over the last 10 years in our understanding of IL-6 biology. Like many other cytokines, IL-6 demonstrates both functional redundancy and pleiotropy, and plays a distinct role in the inflammatory process by acting on multilineage cells[5]. Abnormal synthesis of IL-6 appears to contribute to the pathogenesis of several kinds of diseases, including multiple myeloma, atrial myxoma, rheumatoid arthritis and other diseases[6,7]. Thus, neutralization of IL-6 activity in such diseases could be of clinical value. In this chapter we will give a general overview of the structure and function of IL-6 and its receptor, with a particular focus on its biological actions on B cells.

## GENERAL CONCEPTS

### IDENTIFICATION OF IL-6

B cells in response to antigen challenge differentiate into antibody-secreting cells in the presence of T cells and macrophages. In the early 1970s soluble factors from T cells and macrophages were shown to partially replace the function of these cells[8–10]. At least two factors, B-cell growth factor (BCGF) and B-cell differentiation factor (BCDF), were shown to be involved in this process; the former induced B-cell growth or enhanced anti-IgM-induced B-cell growth and the latter stimulated Ig secretion by activated B cells[3]. B-cell-stimulating factor 2 (BSF2; formerly BCDF) was identified as a factor in the culture supernatants of phytohemagglutinin (PHA) or antigen-stimulated peripheral mononuclear cells which enhanced Ig production by Epstein–Barr virus (EBV)-transformed B-cell lines[1,2]. Subsequently, BSF2 was shown to augment Ig secretion by cloned B-cell lines, at least in part by augmenting the secretory form of Ig-specific mRNA in these cells[11]. BSF2 was then purified to

*Cytokine Regulation of Humoral Immunity: Basic and Clinical Aspects.* Edited by Clifford M. Snapper.

homogeneity from the supernatant of a human T-cell leukemia virus type 1-transformed T-cell line, and its partial amino acid sequence was determined[12]. In 1986 the nucleotide sequence of the cDNA for BSF2 was determined[4].

## IL-6 PROTEIN

IL-6 is a glycoprotein with a molecular mass of 20–30 kDa. Human IL-6 consists of 211 amino acids (AA), including a 28 AA signal peptide. There is a homology of 42 per cent at the AA level between human IL-6 and mouse IL-6, but the central portion spanning residues 42–102 is more conserved, where the four cysteine residues of the protein are perfectly aligned[13]. The same motif of cysteines is also found in human and mouse granulocyte colony-stimulating factor (G-CSF)[14].

## SYNTHESIS OF IL-6

IL-6 is synthesized by many cells in response to appropriate stimuli[6,7,15]. These cells include monocytes/macrophages, T and B cells, fibroblasts, keratinocytes, endothelial cells, stroma cells, mesangial cells, glial cells, chondrocytes, osteoblasts, smooth muscle cells, granulocytes and mast cells. In some tumors or tumor-derived cell lines, autocrine IL-6 is found to play a key role in cell growth. IL-6 production is regulated positively or negatively in response to various stimuli. Thus: (1) lipopolysaccharide (LPS) enhances IL-6 synthesis by monocytes and fibroblasts[16]; (2) IL-1, tumor necrosis factor (TNF), interferon beta (IFN-β) and platelet-derived growth factor (PDGF) enhance IL-6 production in fibroblasts[17–19]; (3) IFN-γ induces IL-6 production by macrophages and endothelial cells[20,21]; (4) IL-4 stimulates IL-6 synthesis in keratinocytes, and endothelial cells[22,23], whereas it inhibits IL-6 production in monocytes, fibroblasts and synoviocytes[24–27]; (5) IL-10 and IL-13 are potent inhibitors of IL-6 production by macrophages and monocytes[28–31]; and (6) transforming growth factor beta (TGF-β) suppresses IL-6 production by human monocytes[32] but it enhances its production by intestinal epithelial cells[33]. Thus, a variety of cytokines regulate IL-6 production. It is also clear that second-messenger agonists such as diacylglycerol, phorbol ester, forskolin, isobutylmethyl/xanthine and calcium ionophore can stimulate IL-6 gene expression[34,35]. In B cells, cross-linking to CD40 (described in detail later)[36,37], and *Staphylococcus* Cowan I are reported to induce IL-6 production[38]. IL-4 alone or in the presence of anti-CD40 antibody (Ab) is also capable of stimulating IL-6 synthesis[36,39]. Moreover, it has been shown that incubation of B-lymphoid cells with phorbol ester results in synthesis of IL-6[40].

## REGULATION OF IL-6 GENE EXPRESSION

The chromosomal genes for human and mouse IL-6 have been isolated[41,42]. Both human and mouse IL-6 genes consist of five exons and four introns. The genes for human and mouse IL-6 are located on chromosomes 7 and 5, respectively. Besides the sequence similarity in the coding region, the 3′ untranslated and the 5′ flanking regions are highly conserved between the human and mouse genes. The 3′ untranslated region contains ATTTA sequences which are commonly found in the 3′ untranslated regions of mRNAs for cytokines and protooncogenes, and are believed to be associated with mRNA stability[43]. The 350 bp upstream of the transcription start site are highly conserved between human and mouse IL-6 genes and transcriptional regulatory elements have been identified in this region. Three regulatory regions have been shown to be involved in stimulating IL-6 gene expression[44]. These are a 14 bp NF-IL-6 binding site, a 23 bp IL-6 multiresponsive element (MRE) and a 12 bp NFκB binding site. NF-IL-6 was originally identified as a nuclear factor binding to a 14-bp sequence (ACATTGCACAATCT) within an IL-1-responsive element in the IL-6 gene[45]. The cloned NF-IL-6 contains a region homologous to the C-terminal portion of C/EBP, the first nuclear factor proposed to contain a leucine zipper structure[46]. NF-IL-6 recognizes the same nucleotide sequences as C/EBP with different affinities and the consensus sequence is T(T/G)NNGNNAA(T/G). These consensus sequences are found to exist in the 5′ flanking regions of cytokine genes such as IL-1, IL-6, IL-8 and G-CSF, in liver-specific genes and in the regulatory regions for Ig, indicating that NF-IL-6 is a pleiotropic mediator of many inducible genes in acute-phase, immune and inflammatory responses[6,7,15,45]. Recently, mice with a disrupted NF-IL-6 gene were created by the homologous recombination technique[47]. These mice were highly susceptible to infection by *Listeria monocytogenes*, relative to their wild-type counterparts, although synthesis of cytokines involved in macrophage activation, such as TNF and IFN-γ, and nitric oxide formation were not impaired. Moreover, macrophages from NF-IL-6-targeted mice were severely defective in anti-tumor cytotoxicity, indicating that NF-IL-6 plays a crucial role in macrophage bactericidal and tumoricidal activities.

## BIOLOGICAL ACTIVITIES OF IL-6

The cloning of the IL-6 gene and the consequent availability of large amounts of recombinant IL-6 has led to the discovery of multiple functions for IL-6 on responding cell populations[5,6,15]. IL-6 was originally identified as a T-cell-derived lymphokine(s) that induced final maturation of B cells into antibody-producing cells[1,2]. However, a series of subsequent studies have revealed that this cytokine functions not only in the immune system but also in the hematopoietic, endocrine, hepatic and even neural systems. IL-6 promotes proliferation of many cells, including myeloma/hybridoma/plasmacytomas, T cells, EBV-transformed B cells, mesangial cells, keratinocytes and hematopoietic cell[48–54]. It inhibits growth of myeloid leukemic cell lines and breast carcinoma cell lines[55,56]. IL-6 induces neural differentiation of PC12 cells[57], cytotoxic T-cell differentiation[58,59], megakaryocyte maturation[60,61], and production of acute-phase proteins in hepatocytes[62,63]. It is also associated with osteoporosis through its ability to activate osteoclasts[64].

## IL-6 TRANSGENIC MICE

To determine the functions of IL-6 *in vivo*, transgenic mice carrying the human IL-6 genomic genes were generated[65]. A massive plasmacytosis in thymus, lymph nodes and spleen and an infiltration of plasma cells into lung, liver and kidney were found. There was a striking increase of serum IgG1, 120–400-fold, whereas the other classes of Igs (IgM, IgG2a, IgG2b, IgG3 and IgA) remained within three times of Ig concentrations in normal mice. Moreover, development of mesangioproliferative glomerulonephritis and an increase in megakaryocytes in bone marrow were found.

## IL-6-DEFICIENT MICE

To better understand the unique function of IL-6 *in vivo*, IL-6-deficient (IL-$6^{-/-}$) mice were created in which the IL-6 gene was disrupted by homologous recombination[66,67]. IL-$6^{-/-}$ mice developed normally. Thymocytes and peripheral T cells revealed normal expression patterns of T-cell receptor $\alpha$, $\beta$, $\gamma$ and $\delta$ chain, CD4, CD8, Pgp1 and heat-stable antigen (HSA), although absolute numbers of thymocytes and peripheral T cells were consistently reduced by 20–40 per cent. B cells in the bone marrow and spleen of IL-$6^{-/-}$ mice expressed B220, IgM, IgD and CD23 within normal ranges, and total serum Ig concentrations in IL-$6^{-/-}$ mutants were similar to those observed in their normal littermates. Moreover, no differences were observed between IL-$6^{-/-}$ and IL-$6^{+/+}$ mice in plasma cell number and serum concentrations of natural Ab in 8–12-week-old mice. However, numbers of IgA-producing cells were reduced at mucosae, and grossly deficient local Ab responses were observed after mucosal challenge with vaccinia virus or ovalbumin. IL-$6^{-/-}$ mice failed to control vaccinia virus infection and infection with *Listeria monocytogenes*, a facultative intracellular bacterium. The T-cell-dependent Ab response against vesicular stomatitis virus was also impaired. The inflammatory acute-phase response after tissue damage or infection is also severely compromised in IL-$6^{-/-}$ mice. These data indicate that IL-6 synthesis stimulated by injury or infection is important for inducing activation of liver cells, macrophages and lymphocytes, but is not essential for the maintenance of basal levels of Ig and generation of plasma cells.

## IL-6 RECEPTOR AND ITS SIGNALING PATHWAY

The molecular basis for the pleiotropy and redundancy of various cytokines has begun to emerge with recent progress in the cloning of cytokine receptors, their associated molecules and their signal transducers, and analyses of their signaling pathways[68].

At the present time, several cytokine receptor families can be identified on the basis of homologies in their structure[69,70]. Most of the cytokine receptors, including IL-2Rβ, IL-2Rγ(γc), IL-3R, IL-4R, IL-5R, IL-6R, IL-7R, IL-9R, G-CSFR, GM-CSFR and IL-6 signal transducer (gp 130), fall into the *type 1 cytokine receptor family*. The type 1 cytokine receptor family exhibits an extracellular domain which consists of two fibronectin type 3 domains with a set of four spaced cysteines and WSXWS motifs in the membrane-distal and membrane-proximal domain. The *type 2 cytokine receptor family* includes IL-10 and interferon receptors and has one or two similar domains in the extracellular portion, with a set of spaced cysteines but without the WSXWS motif.

The IL-6R is an 80 kDa molecule and exists in two forms on responding cells; high affinity ($K_d$ = 10 pM) and low affinity (700 pM)[71]. IL-6 can exert its function by binding either to membrane IL-6R or to the soluble form of IL-6R, leading to the homodimerization of gp 130[72].

As discussed in a number of chapters in this book, the redundancy observed in the action of various cytokines can be explained, in part, by the shared association of a number of signal-transducing structures with various groups of cytokine receptors. These common signal transducers include gp 130, βc and γc[70,73]. The gp 130 molecule was initially shown to be a signal transducer which is commonly used for IL-6R, oncostatin-MR, leukemia inhibitory factor (LIF)R, ciliary neurotrophic factor (CNTF)R and perhaps IL-11R. Similarly, βc is shared with IL-3R, IL-5R and GM-CSFR, and γc is utilized for signaling with IL-2, IL-4, IL-7 and perhaps IL-9 and IL-13 in association with their unique receptors. Recently, mutations or deletions of γc genes were shown to underly the pathogenesis of the X-linked severe combined immunodeficiency, in which the patient's maturation of T cells is defective[74]. Complexes of IL-6 and CNTF with the soluble form of their respective receptors are capable of inducing cell signaling. By contrast, soluble forms of receptors for other cytokines inhibit cytokine signal transduction, by inhibiting ligand binding to its specific membrane receptor. These data indicate that the transmembrane and intracytoplasmic domains of both IL-6R and CNTFR are not required for transmitting their signals and that these complexes, even in the soluble form, are believed to trigger the formation of homo-dimers or heterodimers of gp 130[75]. By contrast, the cytoplasmic portions of other cytokine receptors appear to be essential for signal transduction, along with their respective common signal transducers such as βc or γc.

The characteristic pleiotropy of cytokines may also be explained by the recent discovery of (at least) two signaling pathways of cytokine receptors[76]. The first involves the activation of the Janus kinase (Jak) family of cytoplasmic tyrosine kinases upon receptor oligomerization after binding of cytokine. Activated Jaks phosphorylate the receptor as well as cytoplasmic proteins belonging to a family of transcription factors called the signal transducer and activators of transcription (STATs) (in the case of the IL-6 system, acute-phase response factor (APRF) or STAT3)[77], leading to the activation of the target gene(s). The second pathway is mediated through stimulation of the Ras-dependent mitogen-activated protein (MAP) kinase cascade initiated by the interaction of phosphorylated Shc with Grb2. Grb2 then binds tightly to Sos through an SH3 domain, and in so doing activates Ras. Activated Ras induces the activation of a serine–threonine–tyrosine phosphorylation cascade in which Raf, MAPK/ERK and MAP kinases are sequentially phosphorylated. This second pathway finally leads to the stimulation of the transcription factor(s) (such as NF-IL-6 in the case of the IL-6 signaling pathway)[45]. These activated transcriptional factors then stimulate and/or inhibit targeted gene activation.

## IL-6 AND B CELLS

### B-CELL DIFFERENTIATION

IL-6 acts late in the B-cell differentiation pathway, consistent with the finding that IL-6R is expressed on activated B cells but not resting B cells[78]. IL-6 induces IgM, IgG and IgA production without affecting B-cell growth[79,80]. The role of IL-6 has also been demonstrated in polysaccharide-specific Ig production[81], tetanus toxoid-specific Ig production[82], and the primary Ab response to influenza A[83]. *In vivo* antigen-stimulated lymphoblastoid B cells differentiate into Ab-producing cells *in vitro* in response to IL-6[84]. IL-6 enhanced the *in vivo* secondary anti-sheep red blood cell (SRBC) Ab production in mice[85]. These results clearly demonstrate that IL-6 functions as a B-cell differentiation factor *in vitro* as well as *in vivo*.

### STIMULATION OF IgE SYNTHESIS

IL-6 has been shown to play a key role in IgE synthesis. Induction of IgE class switching by purified B cells requires two stimulants; the class switching factor IL-4 (or IL-13) (see Chapter 8), and an activator of the switching machinery to effect DNA switch recombination of the IL-4 (or IL-13) targeted $C_H\epsilon$ gene[86] (Figure 10.1a) (see Chapter 5). IL-4 induces expression of the $C_H\epsilon$ germline transcript, made up of the spliced product of the intervening exon (I$\epsilon$) and C$\epsilon$[87]. This germline transcript is not translated into protein, and thus is also called a sterile transcript (see Chapter 5). Although the exact role of this transcript in the switching process remains to be determined, it is believed that its appearance is essential for the targeted S–S recombination, since the disruption of I exon (I$\gamma$1) causes failure of class

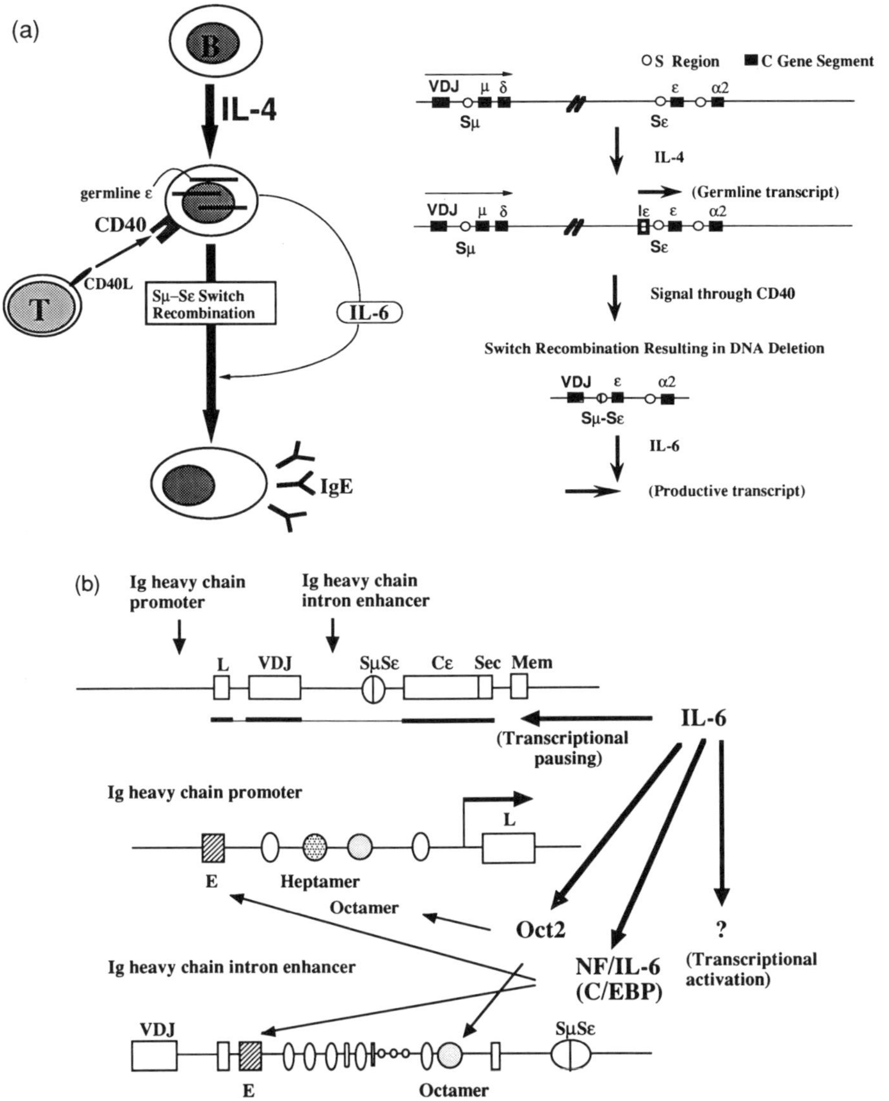


**Figure 10.1** Role of IL-6 in IgE synthesis. (a) B cells, when stimulated with CD40L and IL-4, are activated to produce IL-6. IL-4 induces expression of the germline transcript of the Cε gene and signaling through the CD40 molecule leads to Sμ–Sε recombination. Then endogenously produced IL-6 acts on switched B cells, resulting in the expression of the secretory form of the productive transcript of the Cε gene. (b) IL-6 induces expression of the secretory form of the productive transcript of the Cε gene through activation of Ig gene transcription by stimulating Oct2 and/or C/EBP related molecule(s) which bind to octamer, heptamer or the E box located at the Ig promoter and the intron enhancer sequences, respectively. Moreover, IL-6 has been demonstrated to cause transcription pausing/termination, leading to a selective expression of the secretory form of Ig

switching to γ1[88]. The second signal has been shown to be generated by LPS[89], EBV infection[90] or activated T cells[91]. Recently, it has been shown that a key *physiological* second signal is generated through CD40[92], which is expressed on B cells, and which belongs to the TNF/NGFR (nerve growth factor receptor) family[93]. Signaling through CD40, in concert with IL-4, leads to switch (S)μ–Sε recombination with the consequent expression of productive RNA transcripts consisting of VDJ and Cε. The molecule which physiologically interacts with and activates through CD40 is the recently cloned CD40 ligand (CD40L), or gp 39[94,95] (see Chapters 2 and 4). Recently, it has been shown that mutations or deletions of CD40L genes result in X-linked hyper-IgM immunodeficiency, in which patients' serum levels of IgG, IgA and IgE are decreased or absent[96–100].

To reveal the molecular mechanisms through which IL-6 enhances Ig synthesis, the CD40-dependent IgE-inducing system was employed[92,101,102]. Purified resting B cells were stimulated with anti-CD40 Ab plus IL-4 in the absence or presence of IL-6 or neutralizing anti-IL-6 Ab, and IgE synthesis was measured. IL-6 augmented and anti-IL-6 Ab strongly suppressed IgE synthesis. Indeed, IL-6 synthesis itself was induced by the incubation of B cells with anti-CD40 or IL-4 alone, with greater synthesis being observed with the two stimulants. It has been suggested that the CD40-mediated induction of IL-6 synthesis is secondary to the activation of NFκB, resulting in IL-6 gene activation[103], but how IL-4 stimulates IL-6 gene expression remains to be determined. The expression of $C_H\epsilon$ germline transcripts was not modulated by IL-6 or anti-IL-6 Ab, but that of productive transcripts of the $C_H\epsilon$ gene was enhanced by IL-6 and inhibited by anti-IL-6 Ab in anti-CD40 + IL-4-stimulated B cells. Moreover, utilizing the recently described and novel technique of digestive-circularization polymerase chain reaction DC-PCR[104] to measure Sμ–Sε DNA rearrangement events, it was found that IL-6 did not affect Sμ–Sε DNA recombination, indicating that IL-6 acts on switched B cells and stimulates an increase in productive transcripts[102]. Moreover, by using a human B-cell line in which IL-6 enhances IgG1 synthesis, it has been shown that IL-6 not only stimulates the transcriptional activation of the Ig genes but also contributes to the selection of γ1s and γ1m polyadenylation sites by transcription pausing/termination[105]. Recently, the transcriptional activation of Ig genes by IL-6 was shown to be associated with induction of the B-cell-enriched transcription factor Oct-2[106], which recognizes an octamer motif, ATGCAAAT, the most conserved sequence in the Ig promoters and enhancers[107–109]. In addition, NF-IL-6, which binds to the E boxes, the conserved sequence present in the Ig promoters and enhancers, has also been suggested to play a role in activating the Ig gene[110] (Figure 10.1b). These results thus indicate that IL-6 primarily acts as a B-cell differentiation factor, and enhances Ig synthesis by switched B cells, without affecting the process of switching itself.

Recently, however, an IL-4 responsive region has been described in the Ig heavy chain germline $\epsilon$ promoter containing Stat-4 (or NF-IL-4), C/EBP family and NFκB binding sites[111]. The mouse $\gamma 1$ germline promoter also contains Stat-4 and C/EBP family binding sites[112]. As mentioned earlier, *in vivo* overexpression of IL-6 leads to a selective increase in serum IgG1 concentrations. The ability of IL-6 to stimulate NF-IL-6, which shows homology to C/EBP, could account for this selective IgG1 expression on the basis of IL-6 induction of germline $C_H\gamma 1$ transcripts *in vivo*.

### GROWTH OF B-CELL TUMORS

IL-6 is a potent growth factor for hybridoma/plasmacytoma/myeloma cells; as little as 2 pg/ml of IL-6 can induce 50 per cent maximal proliferation in myeloma cell lines[19,113]. This concentration of IL-6 is 100-fold less than that required for Ig induction in B cells. IL-6 also promotes the proliferation of EBV-infected human B cells and permits their growth at low cell densities[114].

## IL-6 AND DISEASE

### MULTIPLE MYELOMA/PLASMACYTOMAS

Since IL-6 is a potent growth factor for myeloma/plasmacytoma cells, it is possible that IL-6 is involved in the *generation* of myeloma/plasmacytoma. A close association between the occurrence of plasma cell neoplasias and chronic inflammation has been observed. The study of freshly prepared myeloma cells from bone marrow demonstrated that IL-6 is an autocrine growth factor for human myelomas. This was based on the following evidence: (1) IL-6 augments *in vitro* growth of myeloma cells; (2) myeloma cells produce IL-6; and (3) anti-IL-6 Ab inhibits the spontaneous growth of myeloma cells[49]. Although others have demonstrated IL-6 mRNA expression in the bone marrow stromal cells from most of the myeloma patients, but not in purified myeloma cells[115], it is clear that dysregulation of IL-6 synthesis is involved in the generation of myeloma cells. Viral insertion of IL-6 and IL-6R genes into murine cells has been reported to induce plasmacytoma or myelomas[116,117]. A murine plasmacytoma cell line, MPC11, constitutively produces IL-6 due to the insertion of an intracisternal A particle (IAP) retrotransposon 18 bp 5′ of the transcriptional start site of the IL-6 gene. Similarly, enhanced expression of IL-6R was found in a murine plasmacytoma cell line, P3U1, in which the intracytoplasmic region of the IL-6R was replaced with part of the long terminal repeat (LTR) of the IAP gene. An autocrine growth mechanism is also suggested in EBV-transformed B cells[50,51,118]. EBV infection appears to play a pathogenic role in the development of Burkitt lymphoma. The continuous proliferation of EBV-infected B cells seems to depend on autocrine secretion of cytokines, including IL-1 and IL-6[119]. Although the mechanism through which EBV infection induces IL-6 gene activation remains to be determined, LMP-1, an EBV product associated with transformation of B cells, utilizes the same molecules (LAP-1) as the CD40-mediated signal transducer (CD40 bp)[120,121] and it has been demonstrated that the stimulation of CD40 leads to IL-6 production[36]. A possible autocrine role of IL-6 has also been reported in non-Hodgkin's lymphomas, chronic lymphocytic leukemias, and acute myeloid leukemias[122–124].

## INFLAMMATORY AND AUTOIMMUNE DISEASES

The first example of a disease associated with IL-6 overproduction was *cardiac myxoma*, a benign intra-atrial heart tumor[125]. Patients with cardiac myxomas frequently display hypergammaglobulinemia and various autoantibodies, and an increase in serum levels of acute-phase proteins. Since these symptoms disappear after resection of the tumor, it was considered that the myxoma cells or their products were responsible for the development of these changes. Indeed, it has been shown that cultured myxoma cells constitutively produce a large amount of IL-6[126].

Similarly, abnormal IL-6 synthesis was observed in patients with *Castleman's disease*[127], a benign hyperplastic lymphadenopathy characterized by large lymphoid follicles with intervening sheets of plasma cells. B blastoid cells in the germinal centers of such hyperplastic lymph nodes were found to synthesize IL-6. Again, clinical improvement and a decrease in the serum level of IL-6 was observed after resection of the involved lymph node.

*Rheumatoid arthritis* (RA) is a chronic disease of continuous growth of synovial cells leading to inflammation of the joints with polyclonal plasmacytosis, presence of autoantibodies, and increases in acute-phase proteins and platelets. These symptoms may also be explained by overproduction of IL-6[128]. In fact, elevated levels of IL-6 were detected in the synovial fluid from affected joints and sera of patients with active RA[129,130]. Several other cytokines, including IL-1 and TNF-α, which are potent IL-6 inducers, are also overproduced in the synovia of RA patients[131]. Thus, proinflammatory cytokines appear to be involved in the pathogenesis of RA.

*Mesangial proliferative glomerulonephritis* (MPG) is characterized by proliferation of mesangial cells. IL-6 is reported to be a mesangial cell growth factor and to be produced by renal mesangial cells in patients with MPG[53,132]. There is a correlation between the level of urine IL-6 and the progressive stage of MPG.

Constitutive production or overproduction of IL-6 has also been demonstrated in renal cell carcinoma, ovarian carcinoma, pleural mesothelioma, parotid gland adenoma, pheochromocytoma, and glioblastoma[133–138]. Patients with these malignancies often exhibit paraneoplastic symptoms, including thrombocytosis, hypercalcemia and elevated acute-phase reactants, indicating that IL-6 may play a role in the autocrine growth of tumors as well as in the generation of paraneoplastic symptoms. High-level expression of local or systemic IL-6 mRNA or protein has been reported in many other diseases.

## CLINICAL APPLICATION OF IL-6

The ability of IL-6 to affect a wide array of biological functions *in vitro* as well as *in vivo*, and the implication that dysregulation of IL-6 synthesis locally or systemically is associated with the pathogenesis of many diseases, have generated considerable interest in either the clinical application of IL-6 or strategies to neutralize IL-6 activity for the treatment of various diseases.

### TREATMENT USING IL-6

Based on the ability of IL-6 to stimulate multilineage hematopoiesis and maturation of megakaryocytes, this cytokine may be useful in the treatment of idiopathic or chemical- or radiation-induced *myelosuppression* and *thrombocytopenia*[139,140]. It has recently been shown that treatment of human hematopoietic progenitor cells with IL-6 and stem cell factor (SCF) in the presence of soluble IL-6R can maintain and expand such progenitor cells to a striking degree, suggesting the possible application of this treatment to *ex vivo* expansion of $CD34^+$ cells for bone marrow transplantation[141].

Several kinds of cytokines are now undergoing clinical trials in *cancer treatment*[142]. Since IL-6 has been shown to induce cytotoxic T cells, through the activation of helper cells, *in vitro* as well as *in vivo*, and enhances antibody-dependent cellular cytotoxity (ADCC) by human peripheral blood mononuclear cells, IL-6 is expected to exert an anti-tumor effect in human malignancies. Phase 1 trials are now in progress[142].

Injection of IL-6 subcutaneously at a dose of 1–25 μg/kg induces a significant increase (200 per cent) in platelet counts. Bone marrow biopsies reveal no significant effect of IL-6 on the numbers of megakaryocytes, indicating that IL-6 induces megakaryocyte maturation. Leukocyte counts and their differentials are not affected by IL-6 treatment, whereas a dose-dependent decrease (20 per cent) in numbers of erythrocytes and hemoglobin is observed. After chemotherapy IL-6 can reduce the severity of thrombocytopenia. Acute-phase proteins such as CRP (C-reactive protein), fibrinogen and haptoglobulin are induced within 24 h after IL-6 administration. However, no increase of bone marrow plasma cells or peripheral B cells is found, and there is no significant qualitative or quantitative change in Ig patterns. Immunologic tests reveal that expression of intercellular adhesion molecule-1 (ICAM-1) and CD25 is augmented on peripheral mononuclear cells. So far no objective anti-tumor response has been found in a phase I monotherapy trial.

## STRATEGIES TO NEUTRALIZE IL-6 ACTIVITY

Klein and colleagues reported that injection of mouse anti-IL-6 Abs into terminal-stage, *multiple myeloma* patients with extramedullary myeloma cell proliferation could inhibit myeloma cell growth, and decrease serum IL-6 activity and CRP levels[143]. The clinical improvement was maintained throughout treatment and no major side-effects were found. Repeatable injection of mouse Abs appeared to decrease the inhibitory activity for myeloma cells due to neutralization of the mouse Ab by the patient's immune system or escape of the IL-6 dependency of the myeloma cells. Clinical trials using humanized anti-IL-6R Abs for myelomas and plasmacytomas are now in progress.

In *Castleman's disease*, affected lymph nodes produce IL-6 and this overproduction of IL-6 induces systemic symptoms. Indeed, resection of all affected lymph nodes completely abolishes these symptoms; however, in many cases it is difficult to remove all of them. It has been reported that anti-IL-6 Abs could control disease activity in patients with Castleman's disease[144]. Anti-TNF-α Abs have been shown to be effective in the treatment of RA[145,146]. Similarly, anti-IL-6 or anti-IL-6R may have potential benefit for the treatment of RA.

## CYTOKINES AND CHEMICALS MODULATING IL-6 SYNTHESIS

$CD4^+$ T-helper cells can be classified into two types: Th1 cells and Th2 cells[147,148] (see Chapter 6). Th1 cells produce IL-2 and IFN-γ as their signature cytokines, and Th2 cells synthesize IL-4, IL-5, IL-6, IL-9, IL-10 and IL-13. Since IFN-γ is a mediator for activation of macrophages and monocytes, generation of Th1 cells is associated with cellular immunity and inflammation. In contrast, Th2 cells are efficient mediators of Ig production (humoral immunity). As described earlier, IL-6 is synthesized by many cell types, and different mechanisms regulating IL-6 expression are found. For example, IL-4 is a strong inducer of IL-6 production by B cells[36,39], whereas IL-4 inhibits IL-6 production (and IL-1 and TNF-α production) by monocytes[23,26]. IL-10 and IL-13 also inhibit the production of these proinflammatory cytokines (IL-1, IL-6 and TNF-α) by monocytes[28–31], but IFN-γ induces their expression[20]. Since IL-6 plays an important role in both types of immunity, such a precise regulation is perhaps required. Although how IL-4 regulates IL-6 expression (by activating or suppressing transcriptional factors) remained to be determined, Th2 cells in association with B cells can stimulate Ig synthesis by inducing IL-6 production by B cells and, Th1 cells in association with monocytes/macrophages, stimulate an inflammatory response (Figure 10.2). Thus strategies to control IL-6 production in particular cells by cytokines may have therapeutic potential. Generation of Th2 cells or inhibition of proinflammatory cytokine production by IL-4, IL-10 or IL-13 might provide the rationale for the clinical use either systemically or locally at the site of inflammation in chronic inflammatory diseases such as RA without inhibiting Ig synthesis.

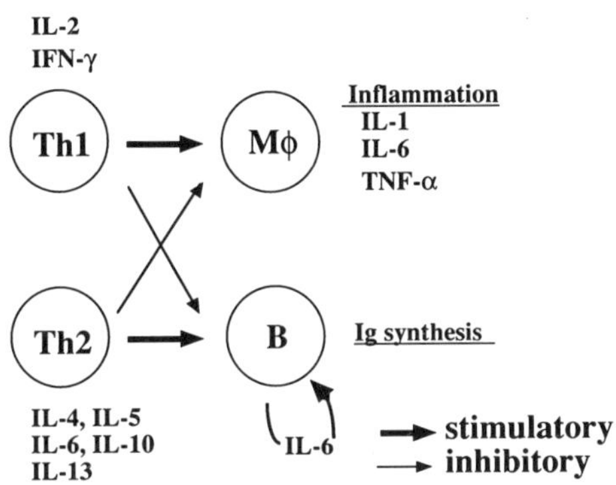


**Figure 10.2** Essential role of IL-6 in both inflammatory response and Ig production. Interaction of B cells with Th2 cells induces Ig production via B-cell stimulatory cytokines and membranous attachment, including CD40–CD40L. IL-4 and signaling through CD40 causes IL-6 production by B cells, which enhances Ig synthesis. In contrast, interaction of macrophages or monocytes with Th1 cells induces proinflammatory cytokine synthesis such as IL-1, IL-6 and TNF-α. Since IL-6 plays an important role in both responses, there is a fine mechanism which stimulates IL-6 production

Corticosteroids and estrogens are potent suppressants of IL-6 production[149]. The inhibitory effects of corticosteroids on myeloma growth seem to be mediated by a decrease of IL-6 expression. Retinoic acid, IFN-α and IL-4 have been shown to suppress myeloma cell or plasmacytoma cell growth by blocking the IL-6–IL-6R autocrine loop[150–152].

## CONCLUSION AND FUTURE DIRECTIONS

IL-6, originally found to be a B-cell differentiation factor, is a typical cytokine with multiple biological activities in hematopoiesis, immune reactions and acute-phase reactions. Functional redundancy of IL-6 with other cytokines is based on the existence of a common signal transducer, gp 130, and multiple functions are mediated through several kinds of signal pathways. In the mouse, IL-6 deficiency (knockout mouse by disrupted IL-6 gene) or abnormal expression of IL-6 (transgenic mouse) are shown to cause several symptoms and signs and induce 'disease states'. Indeed, in the human abnormal expression and dysregulation of IL-6 are involved in the pathogenesis of certain diseases. Although in most diseases apparently more than one cytokine is involved and the clinical manifestations result from the dysregulated cytokine network, modulation of IL-6 *in vivo* might be useful for the therapy of certain diseases. If the cause(s) of dysregulation of IL-6 expression could be discovered, more specific immunotherapy controlling IL-6 production would be anticipated.

In B cells IL-6 is shown to act primarily as a late-acting B-cell differentiation factor which induces the secretory form of Ig, in either an autocrine or paracrine fashion, through transcriptional activation of Ig genes and transcriptional pausing by switched B cells. Under certain conditions it also promotes B-cell growth. IL-6 is a myeloma and plasmacytoma growth factor, and overproduction of IL-6 causes hyperimmunoglobulinemia. However, several issues concerning IL-6 action remain to be resolved, as follows:

1. Molecular mechanisms regulating IL-6-mediated Ig gene activation and transcriptional pausing.
2. Whether or not IL-6 may also act as a class switching factor by modulating expression of germline transcripts.
3. Molecular mechanisms regulating IL-6 synthesis by B cells and malignant B-cell neoplasias.
4. IL-6 signaling in B cells; particularly the mechanism through which IL-6 induces myeloma or plasmacytoma cell growth.

In the near future these issues should be resolved, and the development of more effective therapies in certain B-cell diseases associated with IL-6 is expected.

## REFERENCES


1. Muraguchi A, Kishimoto T, Miki Y *et al.* T cell-relapsing factor (TRF)-induced IgG secretion in human B blastoid cell line and demonstration of acceptors for TRF. J Immunol 1981; 127:412–416.
2. Teranishi T, Hirano T, Naomichi A, Onoue K. Human helper T cell factor(s) (ThF). II. Induction of IgG production in B lymphoblastoid cell lines and identification of T cell-relapsing factor-(TRF) like factors. J Immunol 1982; 128: 193–198.
3. Kishimoto T. Factors affecting B cell growth and differentiation. Annu Rev Immunol 1985; 3:133–157.
4. Hirano T, Yasukawa K, Harada H *et al.* Complementary DNA for a novel human interleukin (BSF-2) that induces B lymphocytes to produce immunoglobulin. Nature 1986; 324:73–76.
5. Kishimoto T. The biology of interleukin-6. Blood 1989; 74: 1–10.

6. Akira S, Taga T, Kishimoto T. Interleukin-6 in biology and medicine. Adv Immunol 1993; 54:1–78.
7. Akira S, Hirano T, Taga T, Kishimoto T. Biology of multifunctional cytokines: IL-6 and related molecules (IL-1 and TNF). FASEB J 1990; 4:2860–2867.
8. Dutton RW, Falkoff R, Hirst JA *et al.* Is there evidence for a nonantigen specific diffusable chemical mediator from the thymus cell in the initiation of the immune response? Prog Immunol 1971; 1:355–368.
9. Schimple A, Wecker E. Replacement of T cell function by a T cell product. Nature 1972; 237:15–17.
10. Kishimoto T, Ishizaka K. Regulation of antibody response *in vitro*. VII. Enhancing soluble factors for IgG and IgE antibody response. J Immunol 1973; 111:1194–1205.
11. Kikutani H, Taga T, Akira S *et al.* Effect of B cell differentiation factor (BCDF) on biosynthesis and secretion of immunoglobulin molecules in human B cell lines. J Immunol 1985; 134:990–995.
12. Hirano T, Taga T, Nakano N *et al.* Purification to homogenity and characterization of human B-cell differentiation factor (BCDF or BSFp-2). Proc Natl Acad Sci USA 1985; 85:5490–5494.
13. Van Snick J, Cayphas S, Szikora JP *et al.* cDNA cloning of murine interleukin-HP1: homology with human interleukin-6. Eur J Immunol 1988; 18:193–198.
14. Leutz A, Damm K, Sterneck E *et al.* Molecular cloning of the chicken myelomonocytic growth factor (cMGF) reveals relationship to interleukin-6 and granulocyte colony stimulating factor. EMBO J 1989; 8:175–181.
15. Akira S, Kishimoto T. IL-6 and NF-IL6 in acute phase response and viral infection. Immunol Rev 1992; 127:25–50.
16. Helfgott DC, May LT, Sthoeger Z *et al.* Bacterial lipopolysaccharide (endotoxin) enhances expression and secretion of β2 interferon by human fibroblasts. J Exp Med 1987; 166:1300–1309.
17. Kohase M, Henriksen-DeStefano D, May LT *et al.* Induction of β2-interferon by tumor necrosis factor: a homeostatic mechanism in the control of cell proliferation. Cell 1986; 45:659–666.
18. Walther Z, May LT, Sehgal PB. Transcriptional regulation of the interferon-β2/B cell differentiation factor BSF-2/hepatocyte-stimulating factor gene in human fibroblasts by other cytokines. J Immunol 1988; 140:974–977.
19. Van Damme J, Opdenakker G, Simpson RJ *et al.* Identification of the human 26-kD protein, interferon β2, as a cell hybridoma/plasmacytoma growth factor induced by interleukin-1 and tumor necrosis factor. J Exp Med 1987; 165:914–919.
20. Sanceau J, Beranger F, Gaudelet C, Wieetzerbin J. IFN-γ is an essential cosignal for triggering IFN-β2/BSF-2 gene expression in human monocytic cell lines. Ann NY Acad Sci 1989; 557:130–143.
21. Leeuwenberg JFM, Von Asmuth EJC, Jeuhomme TMA, Buurman WA. IFN-γ regulates the expression of the adhesion molecule ELAM-1 and IL-6 production by human endothelial cells *in vitro*. J Immunol 1990; 145:2110–2114.
22. Howell G, Pham P, Taylor D *et al.* Interleukin 4 induces interleukin 6 production by endothelial cells: synergy with interferon-γ. Eur J Immunol 1991; 21:97–101.
23. Colottia F, Sironi M, Borre A *et al.* Interleukin 4 amplifies monocyte chemotactic protein and interleukin 6 production by endothelial cells. Cytokine 1992; 4:24–28.
24. Te Velde AA, Huijibens RJF, Hieje K *et al.* Interleukin-4 (IL-4) inhibits secretion of IL-1β, tumor necrosis factor-α and IL-6 by human monocytes. Blood 1990; 76:1392–1397.

25. Gibbons R, Martinez O, Matli M *et al.* Recombinant IL-4 inhibits IL-6 synthesis by adherent peripheral blood cells *in vitro*. Lymphokine Res 1990; 9:283–293.
26. Cheung DL, Hart PH, Vitti GF *et al.* Contrasting effects of interferon-γ and interleukin-4 on the interleukin-6 activity of stimulated human monocytes. Immunology 1990; 71:70–75.
27. Lee J, Swischer SG, Minehart EH *et al.* Interleukin-4 downregulates interleukin-6 production in human peripheral blood mononuclear cells. J Leukocyte Biol 1990; 47:475–479.
28. Fiorentino DF, Zlotnik A, Mosmann TR *et al.* IL-10 inhibits cytokine production by activated macrophages. J Immunol 1990; 147:3815–3822.
29. De Waal Malefyt R, Abrams J, Bennett B *et al.* Interleukin 10 (IL-10) inhibits cytokine synthesis by human monocytes: an autoregulatory role of IL-10 produced by monocytes. J Exp Med 1991; 174:1209–1220.
30. Doherty TM, Kastelein R, Menon S *et al.* Modulation of murine macrophage function by IL-13. J Immunol 1993; 151:7151–7160.
31. de Waal Malefyt R, Fidgor CG, Hujibens R *et al.* Effects of IL-13 on phenotype, cytokine production, and cytotoxic function of human monocytes: comparison with IL-4 and modulation by IFN-gamma or IL-10. J Immunol 1993; 151:6370–6381.
32. Musso T, Espinoza-Delgado J, Pulkki K *et al.* Transforming growth factor beta downregulates interleukin-1-induced IL-6 production by human monocytes. Blood 1990; 76:445–453.
33. McGee DW, Beagley KW, Aicher WK, McGee JR. Transforming growth factor-β enhances interleukin-6 secretion by intestinal epithelial cells. Immunology 1992; 77:7–12.
34. Sehgal PB, Walther Z, Tamm I. Rapid enhancement of β2-IFN/BSF-2 gene expression in human fibroblasts by diacylglycerols and the calcium ionophore A23187. Proc Natl Acad Sci USA 1987; 84:3633–3667.
35. Zhang Y, Lin JX, Vilcek J. Synthesis of interleukin 6 (interferon-b2/B cell stimulatory factor 2) in human fibroblasts is triggered by an increase in intracellular cyclic AMP. J Biol Chem 1988; 263:6177–6182.
36. Clark EA, Shu GL. Association between IL-6 and CD40 signaling: IL-6 induces phosphorylation of CD40 molecule. J Immunol 1990; 145:1400–1406.
37. Westendorf JJ, Ahmann GJ, Armitage RJ *et al.* CD40 expression in malignant plasma cells: role in stimulation of autocrine IL-6 secretion by a human myeloma cell line. J Immunol 1994; 152:117–128.
38. Horii Y, Muraguchi A, Suematsu S *et al.* Regulation of BSF-2/IL-6 production by human mononuclear cells. J Immunol 1988; 141:1529–1535.
39. Smeland EB, Blomhoff HK, Funderud S *et al.* Interleukin 4 induces selective production of interleukin 6 from normal human B lymphocytes. J Exp Med 1989; 170:1463–1468.
40. Hutchins D, Chen B, Steel M. Production and regulation of interleukin-6 in human B lymphoid cells. Eur J Immunol 1990; 20:961–968.
41. Yasukawa K, Hirano T, Watanabe Y *et al.* Structure and expression of human B cell stimulatory factor-2 (BSF-2/IL-6) gene. EMBO J 1987; 6:2939–2945.
42. Tanabe O, Akira S, Kamiya T *et al.* Genomic structure of the murine IL-6 gene. High degree of conservation of potential regulatory sequences between mouse and human. J Immunol 1988; 141:3875–3881.
43. Shaw G, Kamen R. A conserved AU sequence from the 3′ untranslated region of GM-CSF mRNA mediates selective mRNA degradation. Cell 1986; 46:659–667.
44. Isshiki H, Akira S, Tanabe O *et al.* Constitutive and IL-1 inducible factors interact with the IL-1 responsive element in the IL-6 gene. Mol Cell Biol 1990; 10:2757–2764.

45. Akira S, Isshiki H, Sugita T *et al.* A nuclear factor for IL-6 expression (NF-IL6) is a member of a C/EBP family. EMBO J 1990; 9:1897–1906.
46. Landschuz WH, Johnson PF, McKnight SL. The leucine zipper: a hypothetical structure common to a new class of DNA binding proteins. Science 1988; 240:1759–1764.
47. Tanaka T, Akira S, Yoshida K *et al.* Targeted disruption of the NF-IL6 gene discloses its essential role in bacteria killing and tumor cytotoxicity by macrophages. Cell 1995; 80:353–361.
48. Vink A, Coulie PG, Warnier G *et al.* Mouse plasmacytoma growth *in vivo*. Enhancement by interleukin-6 and inhibition by antibodies directed against IL-6 or its receptor. J Exp Med 1990; 172:997–1000.
49. Kawano M, Hirano T, Matsuda T *et al.* Autocrine generation and requirement of BSF-2/IL-6 for human multiple myelomas. Nature 1988; 332:83–85.
50. Tosato G, Tanner J, Jones KD *et al.* Identification of interleukin-6 as an autocrine growth factor for Epstein–Barr virus-immortalized B cells. J Virol 1990; 64:3033–3041.
51. Yokoi T, Miyawaki T, Yachie A *et al.* Epstein–Barr virus-immortalized B cells produce IL-6 as an autocrine growth factor. Immunology 1990; 70:100–105.
52. Shimizu S, Hirano T, Yoshioka R *et al.* Interleukin-6 (B-cell stimulatory factor-2)-dependent growth of a Lennert's lymphoma-derived T-cell line (KT-3). Blood 1988; 72:1826–1828.
53. Horii Y, Muraguchi A, Iwano M *et al.* Involvement of interleukin-6 in mesangial proliferative glomerulonephritis. J Immunol 1989; 143:3949–3955.
54. Grossman RM, Krueger J, Yourish D *et al.* Interleukin 6 is expressed in high levels in psoriasis skin and stimulates proliferation of cultured human keratinocytes. Proc Natl Acad Sci USA 1989; 86:6367–6371.
55. Shabo Y, Lotem J, Rubinstein M *et al.* The myeloid blood cell differentiation-inducing protein MGI-2A is interleukin 6. Blood 1988; 72:2070–2073.
56. Chen L, Mory Y, Zilberstein A, Revel M. Growth inhibition of human breast carcinoma and leukemia/lymphoma cell lines by recombinant interferon β2. Proc Natl Acad Sci USA 1988; 85:8037–8041.
57. Satoh T, Nakamura S, Taga T *et al.* Induction of neural differentiation in PC12 cells by B cell stimulatory factor 2/interleukin 6. Mol Cell Biol 1988; 8:3546–3549.
58. Okada M, Kitahara M, Kishimoto S *et al.* IL-6/BSF-2 functions as a killer helper factor in the *in vitro* induction of cytotoxic T cells. J Immunol 1988; 141:1543–1549.
59. Takai Y, Wong GG, Clark SC *et al.* B cell stimulatory factor-2 is involved in the differentiation of cytotoxic T lymphocytes. J Immunol 1988; 140:508–512.
60. Ishibashi T, Kimura H, Shikawa Y *et al.* Interleukin 6 is a potent thrombopoietic factor *in vivo* in mice. Blood 1989; 74:1241–1244.
61. Asano S, Okano A, Ozawa K *et al.* *In vivo* effects of recombinant human interleukin-6 in primates: stimulated production of platelets. Blood 1990; 75:1602–1605.
62. Gauldie J, Richards C, Haarnish D *et al.* Interferon β2/B cell stimulating factor type 2 shares identity with monocyte-derived hepatocyte stimulating factor and regulates the major acute phase protein response in liver cells. Proc Natl Acad Sci USA 1987; 84:7251–7255.
63. Andus T, Geiger T, Hirano T *et al.* Recombinant human B cell stimulatory factor 2 (BSF-2/IFN-β) regulates fibronogen and albumin mRNA levels in Fao-9 cells. FEBS Lett 1987; 221:18–22.
64. Kurihara N, Bertolini D, Suda T *et al.* IL-6 stimulates osteoclast-like multinucleated cell formation in long term human marrow cultures by inducing IL-1 release. J Immunol 1990; 144:4226–4230.

65. Suematsu S, Matsuda T, Aozasa K *et al.* IgG1 plasmacytosis in interleukin-6 transgenic mice. Proc Natl Acad Sci USA 1989; 86:7547–7551.
66. Kopf M, Baumann H, Freer G *et al.* Impaired immune and acute-phase responses in interleukin-6-deficient mice. Nature 1994; 368:339–342.
67. Ramsay AJ, Husband AJ, Ramshaw IA *et al.* The role of interleukin-6 in mucosal IgA antibody responses *in vivo*. Science 1994; 264:561–563.
68. Paul WE. Pleiotropy and redundancy; T cell-derived lymphokines in the immune response. Cell 1989; 57:521–526.
69. Taga T, Kishimoto T. Cytokine receptors and signal transduction. FASEB J 1993; 7:3387–3396.
70. Kishimoto T, Taga T, Akira S. Cytokine signal transduction. Cell 1994; 76:253–262.
71. Yamasaki K, Taga T, Hirata Y *et al.* Cloning and expression of the human interleukin-6 (BSF-2/IFNβ) receptor. Science 1988; 241:825–828.
72. Hibi M, Murakami M, Saito M *et al.* Molecular cloning and expression of an IL-6 signal transducer, gp130. Cell 1990; 63:1149–1157.
73. Miyajima A, Kitamura T, Harada N *et al.* Cytokine receptors and signal transduction. Annu Rev Immunol 1992; 10:295–331.
74. Noguchi M, Yi H, Rosenblatt HM *et al.* Interleukin-2 receptor γ chain mutation results in X-linked severe combined immunodeficiency in humans. Cell 1993; 73:147–157.
75. Murakami M, Hibi M, Nakagawa N *et al.* IL-6-induced homodimerization of gp 130 and associated activation of a tyrosine kinase. Science 1993; 260:1808–1810.
76. Ihle JN, Witthuhn BA, Quelle FW *et al.* Signaling by the cytokine receptor superfamily:Jaks and STATs. Trends Biochem Sci 1994; 19:222–227.
77. Akira S, Nishio Y, Inoue M *et al.* Molecular cloning of APRF, a novel IFN-stimulated gene factor 3 p91-related transcription factor involved in the gp 130-mediated signaling pathway. Cell 1994; 77:63–71.
78. Taga T, Kawanishi T, Hardy RR *et al.* Receptors for B cell stimulatory factor 2 (BSF-2): quantitation, specificity, distribution, and regulation of their expression. J Exp Med 1987; 166:967–981.
79. Muraguchi A, Hirano T, Tang B *et al.* The essential role of B cell stimulatory factor 2 (BSF-2/IL-6) for the terminal differentiation of B cells. J Exp Med 1988; 167:332–344.
80. Beagley KW, Eldridge JH, Lee F *et al.* Interleukins and IgA synthesis: human and murine interleukin 6 induce high rate IgA secretion in IgA-committed B cells. J Exp Med 1989; 169:2133–2148.
81. Ambrosino DM, Delaney NR, Shamberger RC. Human polysaccharide-specific B cells are responsive to pokeweed mitogen and IL-6. J Immunol 1990; 144:1221–1226.
82. Brieva JA, Martin RA, Martinez-Maza O *et al.* Interleukin-6 is essential for antibody secretion by human *in vivo* antigen-induced lymphoblastoid B cells. Cell Immunol 1990; 130:303–310.
83. Hilbert DM, Cancro MP, Scherle PA *et al.* T cell derived IL-6 is differently required for antigen-specific antibody secretion by primary and secondary B cells. J Immunol 1989; 143:4019–4024.
84. Lue C, Kiyono H, McGhee JR *et al.* Recombinant human interleukin-6 (rhIL-6) promotes the terminal differentiation of *in vivo*-activated human B cells into antibody-secreting cells. Cell Immunol 1991; 132:423–432.
85. Takatstuki F, Okano A, Suzuki C *et al.* Interleukin 6 perfusion stimulates reconstitution of the immune and hematopoietic systems after 5-fluorouracil treatment. Cancer Res 1990; 50:2885–2890.
86. Purkerson J, Isakson P. A two signal model for regulation of immunoglobulin isotype switching. FASEB J 1992; 6:3245–3250.

87. Gauchat JF, Lebman DA, Coffman RL *et al.* Structure and expression of germline ϵ transcripts in human B cells induced by interleukin 4 to switch to IgE production. J Exp Med 1990; 172:463–474.
88. Jung S, Rajewsky K, Radbruch A. Shutdown of class switch recombination by deletion of a switch region control element. Science 1993; 259:984–987.
89. Coffman RL, Ohara J, Bond MH *et al.* B cell stimulatory factor-1 enhances IgE response of lipopolysaccharide-activated B cells. J Immunol 1986; 136:4538–4544.
90. Thyphronitis G, Tsokos GC, June CH *et al.* IgE secretion by Epstein–Bar virus-infected purified human B lymphocytes is stimulated by interleukin-4 and suppressed by interferon-γ. Proc Natl Acad Sci USA 1989; 86:5580–5584.
91. Lebman DA, Coffman RL. Interleukin-4 causes isotype switching to IgE in T cell-stimulated clonal B cell cultures. J Exp Med 1988; 168:853–862.
92. Jabara HH, Fu SM, Geha RS, Vercelli D. CD40 and IgE: synergism between anti-CD40 MAb and IL-4 in the induction of IgE synthesis by highly purified B cells. J Exp Med 1990; 172:1861–1864.
93. Stamenkovic I, Clark EA, Seed B. A B-lymphocyte activation molecule related to the nerve growth factor receptor and induced by cytokines in carcinomas. EMBO J 1989; 8:1403–1410.
94. Armitage RJ, Fanslow WC, Strockbine L *et al.* Molecular cloning and biological characterization of a murine ligand for CD40. Nature 1992; 357:80–82.
95. Gauchat JF, Aubry JP, Mazzei G *et al.* Human CD40-ligand: molecular cloning, cellular distribution and regulation of expression by factors controlling IgE production. FEBS Lett 1993; 315:259–266.
96. Korthauer U, Graf D, Mages HW *et al.* Defective expression of T-cell CD40 ligand causes X-linked immunodeficiency with hyper-IgM. Nature 1993; 361:539–541.
97. DiSanto JP, Bonnefoy JY, Gauchat JF *et al.* CD40 ligand mutations in X-linked immunodeficiency with hyper-IgM. Nature 1993; 361:541–543.
98. Allen RC, Armitage RJ, Conley ME *et al.* CD40 ligand gene defects responsible for X-linked hyper-IgM syndrome. Science 1993; 259:990–993.
99. Aruffo A, Farrington M, Hollenbaugh D *et al.* The CD40 ligand, gp 39, is defective in activated T cells from patients with X-linked hyper-IgM syndrome. Cell 1993; 72:291–300.
100. Fuleihan R, Ramesh N, Loh R *et al.* Defective expression of the CD40 ligand in X chromosome-linked immunoglobulin deficiency with normal or elevated IgM. Proc Natl Acad Sci USA 1993; 90:2170–2173.
101. Vercelli D, Jabara HH, Arai K *et al.* Endogenous interleukin-6 plays an obligatory role in interleukin-4 dependent human IgE synthesis. Eur J Immunol 1989; 19:1419–1424.
102. Katada Y *et al.* Interleukin-6 augments IgE synthesis by acting on switched B cells. In preparation.
103. Berberich I, Shu GL, Clark EA. Cross-linking CD40 on B cells rapidly activates nuclear factor-kB. J Immunol 1994; 153:4357–4366.
104. Chu CC, Paul WE, Max EE. Quantitation of immunoglobulin mu-gamma 1 heavy chain switch region recombination by a digested-circularization polymerase chain reaction method. Proc Natl Acad Sci USA 1992; 89:6978–6982.
105. Raynal MC, Liu Z, Hirano T *et al.* Interleukin 6 induces secretion of IgG1 by coordinated transcriptional activation and differential mRNA accumulation. Proc Natl Acad Sci USA 1989; 86:8024–8028.
106. Natkunam Y, Zhang X, Liu Z, Chen-Kiang S. Simultaneous activation of Ig and Oct-2 synthesis and reduction of surface MHC class II expression by IL-6. J Immunol 1994; 153:3476–3484.

107. Staudt LM, Singh H, Sen R *et al.* A lymphoid-specific protein binding to the octamer motif of immunoglobulin genes. Nature 1986; 323:640–643.
108. Staudt LM, Clerc RG, Singh H *et al.* Cloning of lymphoid-specific cDNA encoding a protein binding the regulatory octamer DNA motif. Science 1988; 241:577–580.
109. Landolfi NF, Capra JD, Tucker PW. Interaction of cell-type specific nuclear proteins with immunoglobulin VH promoter region sequences. Nature 1986; 323:548–551.
110. Staudt LM, Lenardo MJ. Immunoglobulin gene transcription. Annu Rev Immunol 1991; 9:373–398.
111. Delphin S, Stavnezer J. Characterization of an interleukin 4 (IL-4) responsive region in the immunoglobulin heavy chain germline e promoter: regulation by NF-IL-4, a C/EBP family member and NF-kB/p50. J Exp Med 1995; 181:181–192.
112. Xu M, Stavnezer J. Regulation of transcription of immunoglobulin germ-line $\gamma$1 RNA: analysis of the promoter/enhancer. EMBO J 1992; 11:145–155.
113. Nordan R, Potter M. A macrophage-derived factor required by plasmacytomas for survival and proliferation *in vitro*. Science 1986; 233:566–569.
114. Tosato G, Seaman KB, Goldman ND *et al.* Monocyte-derived human B-cell growth factor identified as interferon-$\beta$2 (BSF2/IL-6). Science 1988; 239:502–504.
115. Klein B, Zhang XG, Jourdan M *et al.* Paracrine rather than autocrine regulation of myeloma-cell growth and differentiation by interleukin-6. Blood 1989; 73:518–526.
116. Blankenstein T, Qin Z, Li W, Diamanstein T. DNA rearrangement and constitutive expression of the interleukin 6 gene in a mouse plasmacytoma. J Exp Med 1990; 171:965–970.
117. Sugita T, Totsuka M, Saito M *et al.* Functional murine interleukin 6 receptor with intracisternal A particle gene product at its cytoplasmic domain: its possible role in plasmacytomagenesis. J Exp Med 1990; 171:2001–2009.
118. Scala G, Quinto T, Ruocco MR *et al.* Expression of an exogenous interleukin-6 gene in human Epstein–Barr virus B cell growth advantage and tumorgenicity. J Exp Med 1990; 172:61–68.
119. Scala G, Kuang YD, Hall RE *et al.* Accessory cell function of human B cells. I. Production of both interleukin-1 like activity and an interleukin-1 inhibitory factor by an EBV-transformed B cell line. J Exp Med 1985; 159:1637–1652.
120. Hu HM, O'Rourke K, Boguski MS, Dixit VM. A novel RING finger protein interacts with the cytoplasmic domain of CD40. J Biol Chem 1994; 269:30069–30072.
121. Mosialos G, Birkenbach M, Yalamanchili R *et al.* The Epstein–Barr virus transforming protein LMP1 engages signaling proteins for the tumor necrosis factor receptor family Cell 1995; 80:389–399.
122. Bioddi A, Rossi V, Bassan R *et al.* Constitutive expression of the interleukin-6 gene in chronic lymphocytic leukemia. Blood 1989; 73:1279–1284.
123. Freeman GJ, Fredman AS, Rabinowe SN *et al.* Interleukin 6 gene expression in normal and neoplastic B cells. J Clin Invest 1989; 83:1512–1518.
124. Oster W, Cicco NA, Klein H *et al.* Participation of the cytokines interleukin-6, tumor necrosis factor-alpha, and interferon-beta secreted by acute myelogenous leukemia blasts in autocrine and paracrine leukemia growth control. J Clin Invest 1989; 84:451–457.
125. Hirano T, Taga T, Yasukawa K *et al.* Human B cell differentiation factor defined by an anti-peptide antibody and its possible role in autoantibody production. Proc Natl Acad Sci USA 1987; 84:228–231.

126. Jourdan M, Battaille R, Seguin J *et al.* Constitutive production of interleukin-6 and immunoloic features in cardiac myxomas. Arthritis Rheum 1990; 33:398–402.
127. Yoshizaki K, Matsuda T, Nishimoto N *et al.* Pathological significance of interleukin 6 (IL-6/BSF-2) in Castleman's disease. Blood 1989; 74:1360–1367.
128. Hirano T, Matsuda T, Turner M *et al.* Excessive production of interleukin 6/B cell stimulatory factor-2 in rheumatoid arthritis. Eur. J Immunol 1988; 18:1797–1801.
129. Houssiau FA, Devogelaer JP, Van Damme J *et al.* Interleukin-6 in synovial fluid and serum of patients with rheumatoid arthritis and other inflammatory arthritides. Arthritis Rheum 1988; 31:784–788.
130. Guerne PA, Zuraw BL, Vaughan JH *et al.* Synovium as a source of interleukin 6 *in vitro*. Contribution to local and systemic manifestations of arthritis. J Clin Invest 1989; 83:585–592.
131. Firestein GS, Alvaro Gracia JM, Maki R, Alvaro Gracia JM. Quantitative analysis of cytokine gene expression in rheumatoid arthritis. J Immunol 1990; 144:3347–3353.
132. Ruef C, Budde K, Lacy J *et al.* Interleukin 6 is an autocrine growth factor for mesangial cell. Kidney Int 1990; 38:249–257.
133. Miki S, Iwato M, Miki Y *et al.* Interleukin-6 (IL-6) functions as an *in vitro* autocrine growth factor in renal cell carcinomas. FEBS Lett 1989; 250:607–610.
134. Watson JM, Sensintaffar JL, Berek JS, Martinez-Maza O. Constitutive production of interleukin 6 by ovarian cancer cell lines and by primary ovarian tumor cultures. Cancer Res 1990; 50:6959–6965.
135. Schmitter D, Lauber B, Fagg B, Stahel RA. Hematopoietic growth factors secreted by seven human pleural mesothelioma cell lines: interleukin-6 production as a common feature. Int J Cancer 1992; 51:196–201.
136. Gallo O, Bani D, Toccafondi G *et al.* Characterization of a novel cell line from pleomorphic adenoma of the parotid gland with myoepithelial phenotype and producing interleukin-6 and an autocrine growth factor. Cancer 1992; 70:559–568.
137. Fukumoto S, Matsumoto T, Harada S *et al.* Pheochromocytoma with pyrexia and marked inflammatory signs: a paraneoplastic syndrome with possible relation to interleukin-6 production. J Clin Endocrinol Metab 1991; 73:877–881.
138. Van Meir E, Sawamura Y, Diserens AC *et al.* Human glioblastoma cells release interleukin 6 *in vivo* and *in vitro*. Cancer Res 1990; 50:6683–6688.
139. Burstein SA, Downs T, Friese P *et al.* Thrombocytosis in normal and sublethally irradiated dogs: response to human interleukin 6. Blood 1992; 80:420–428.
140. Herodin F, Mestries JC, Janodet D *et al.* Recombinant glycosylated human interleukin-6 accelerates peripheral blood platelet count recovery in radiation-induced bone marrow depression in baboons. Blood 1992; 80:688–695.
141. Sui X, Tsuji K, Tanaka R *et al.* gp 130 and c-Kit signalings synergize for ex vivo expansion of human primitive hemopoietic progenitor cells. Proc Natl Acad Sci USA 1995; 92:2859–2863.
142. Aulitzky WE, Schuler M, Peschel C, Huber C. Interleukins: clinical pharmacology and therapeutic use. Drugs 1994; 48:667–677.
143. Klein B, Wijdenes J, Zhang XG *et al.* Murine anti-interleukin-6 monoclonal antibody therapy for a patient with plasma cell leukemia. Blood 1991; 78:1198–1204.
144. Beck JT, Hsu SM, Wijdenes J *et al.* Alleviation of systemic manifestations of Castleman's disease by monoclonal anti-interleukin-6 antibody. New Engl J Med 1994; 330:602–604.
145. Elliott MJ, Maini RN, Feldmann M *et al.* Treatment of rheumatoid arthritis with

chimeric monoclonal antibodies to tumor necrosis factor alpha. Arthritis Rheum 1993; 36:1681–1690.

146. Elliott MJ, Maini RN, Feldmann M *et al.* Randomised double-blind comparison of chimeric monoclonal antibody to tumor necrosis factor α (cA2) versus placebo in rheumatoid arthritis. Lancet 1994; 344:1105–1110.
147. Mosmann TR, Cherwinski H, Bond MW *et al.* Two types of murine helper T cell clone. I. Definition according to profiles of lymphokine activities and secreted proteins. J Immunol 1986; 136:2348–2357.
148. Paul WE, Seder RA. Lymphocyte responses and cytokines. Cell 1994; 76:241–251.
149. Ray A, LaForge KS, Sehgal PB. On the mechanism for efficient repression of the interleukin-6 promoter by glucocorticoids: enhancer, TATA box, and RNA start site (Inr motif) occlusion. Mol Cell Biol 1989; 9:5537–5547.
150. Sidell N, Taga T, Hirano T *et al.* Retinoic acid-induced growth inhibition of a human myeloma cell line via down-regulation of IL-6 receptors. J Immunol 1991; 146:3809–3814.
151. Heslep HE, Bianchi AC, Cordingley FT *et al.* Effects of interferon alpha on autocrine growth factor loops in B lymphoproliferative disorders. J Exp Med 1990; 172:1729–1734.
152. Ogata A, Nishimoto N, Shima Y *et al.* Inhibitory effect of all-trans retinoic acid on growth of freshly isolated myeloma cells via interference with interleukin-6 signal transduction. Blood 1994; 84:3040–3046.

# 11 Interleukin-10

**FRANCINE BRIERE, FLORENCE MALISAN, CHRISTINE SERVET-DELPRAT and JACQUES BANCHEREAU**
*Schering-Plough, Laboratory for Immunological Research, Dardilly, France*

## INTRODUCTION

Interleukin-10 (IL-10) was identified in 1989 as a factor produced by the T-helper cell subset (Th2) which inhibits cytokine synthesis by Th1 cells[1]. IL-10 has also been characterized independently as a product of murine CD5+ B-cell lymphomas able to support the survival of mast cell clones[2] and to enhance the proliferation of thymocytes[3]. As Th2 cells more specifically control humoral responses[4], effects of IL-10 on B lymphocytes have been readily tested and demonstrated[5,6]. Effects of IL-10 on B-cell growth and differentiation were particularly expected, inasmuch as the Epstein–Barr virus (EBV), which transforms B lymphocytes, carries a gene, BCRF1, whose product is 84 per cent homologous to human IL-10; hence its name viral IL-10 (vIL-10). This chapter analyzes the function of IL-10 in B-cell pathophysiology.

## PRODUCTION OF IL-10

### B CELLS AS A SOURCE OF IL-10

In the mouse, IL-10 is secreted by activated Th2 clones, mast cell lines, macrophages, keratinocytes[7], B lymphomas[3] and activated peritoneal B cells[2]. In the human, IL-10 is produced by T cells, monocytes, carcinoma and melanoma cell lines[7] and CD40-activated $CD5^+$ and $CD5^-$ human B lymphocytes[8]. Significantly, addition of IL-4 to activated B-cell cultures results in decreased IL-10 secretion but increased IL-6 production[8]. Peripheral blood B lymphocytes and monocytes, but not T cells, from patients with systemic lupus erythematosus (SLE), rheumatoid arthritis (RA) and Sjögren's syndrome spontaneously secrete IL-10[9].

EBV-transformed B-cell lines produce large amounts of hIL-10[10–12], whereas viral IL-10 is detected in only a minority of EBV-transformed B-cell lines. B cells are induced to produce significant amounts of hIL-10 after EBV

*Cytokine Regulation of Humoral Immunity: Basic and Clinical Aspects.* Edited by Clifford M. Snapper.

transformation, but hIL-10 neutralizing antibodies do not prevent the establishment of EBV-transformed cell lines[10], though they slow their growth considerably. While B lymphocytes infected with EBV display rare vIL-10 transcripts a few hours after infection[12], vIL-10 is mostly expressed as a 'late' viral gene during the lytic phase of virus replication[13]. Yet vIL-10 may play a role early during the transformation process by EBV, as anti-sense oligonucleotides for vIL-10 mRNA added at the time of viral infection have been shown to prevent subsequent B-cell transformation[12]. However, this observation is challenged by the powerful transforming capacity of EBV mutants whose BCRF1 gene has been deleted[14].

### IL-10 IN BIOLOGICAL FLUIDS AND NATURAL ANTI-IL-10 ANTIBODIES

Human IL-10 is not present in the serum of healthy individuals but it may be detected in biological fluids under various pathological circumstances. In particular, hIL-10 was found in the serum of 47/101 patients with active non-Hodgkin's lymphomas, while it was detected in only 3/52 patients with partial or complete response[15]. IL-10 occurrence in the serum of patients with intermediate- or high-grade lymphomas is associated with a poor survival. Recent studies have indicated that IL-10 is produced by the lymphoma cells themselves (Blay, personal communication), as also observed with AIDS lymphomas[16]. The ability of B lymphocytes to produce and respond to IL-10 suggests that this cytokine may act directly as an autocrine growth factor for certain human B-lymphoid malignancies. Interestingly, SCID mice that develop EBV lymphoproliferative disease after injection of human blood lymphocytes have high levels of serum human IL-10 originating from the $EBV^+$ tumor cells[17]. IL-10 has also been detected in the serum of patients suffering from early-stage multiple myelomas, particularly those with solitary myelomas[18]. However, IL-10 is not detectable in the serum of patients with advanced myelomatous disease. In contrast to IL-6, the presence of IL-10 is associated with a good prognosis. The ascites of patients with ovarian and other intra-abdominal cancers also contain IL-10[19].

Autoantibodies specific for various cytokines have been detected in certain human serum samples[20]. In recent studies, anti-IL-10 autoantibodies have been detected at a low frequency, as only 6 out of 2000 tested sera scored positive. Interestingly, the IgG anti-IL-10 autoantibodies inhibited IL-10-induced proliferation of a mouse pro-B-cell line (Ba/F3) transfected with the human IL-10 receptor[21].

## B-CELL SURVIVAL

Murine IL-10, like mIL-4, augments expression of MHC class II antigens on small resting mouse splenic B cells and is a viability maintenance factor for these cells in culture[5]. Murine and viral IL-10 do not enhance MHC class II expression on B cells from X-linked immune deficient (XID) mice, though both IL-10s sustain the viability of those cells[5], which suggests a certain complexity in the IL-10 receptors and/or in the signaling pathway. Human IL-10 was also found to enhance the survival of splenic B lymphocytes during a 15-day culture period, an effect associated with enhanced expression of bcl-2 protein[22]. However, in our studies, hIL-10 does not modify expression of HLA class II antigens on human resting tonsillar B cells, possibly because of their already high level of constitutive HLA class II expression, and nor does it permit their increased short-term survival.

In contrast, addition of IL-10 to cultures of some samples of chronic lymphocytic leukemia (CLL) was found to decrease viable cell recovery. Flow cytomeric analysis, DNA gel electrophoresis and Giemsa staining revealed that IL-10 induces BCLL cells to die from apoptosis. Addition of IL-2, IL-4, interferon gamma (IFN-$\gamma$) and anti-CD40 monoclonal antibody (mAb) prevents the IL-10-mediated apoptosis of BCLL cells. The proapoptotic effect of IL-10 is limited to some BCLL samples; cells from non-Hodgkin's lymphomas and hairy cell leukemias were not found to undergo apoptosis after IL-10 treatment[23]. Normal human B lymphocytes activated with *Staphylococcus aureus* Cowan (SAC) particles were found to undergo apoptosis in response to IL-10[24].

## B-CELL GROWTH

Human IL-10 can enhance the proliferation of human B cells at all their different maturation stages. Fetal bone marrow B-cell precursors ($CD10^+sIg^-$), freshly isolated or precultured on stromal cells, proliferate when activated through their CD40 antigen in the presence of IL-3, and further addition of IL-10 and IL-7 potentiates this effect[25].

hIL-10 also enhances the DNA replication of mature B lymphocytes stimulated through their antigen receptors (surface Ig) either with insolubilized anti-IgM antibody or with SAC particles[6]. The costimulation is of lower magnitude than that observed with either IL-2 or IL-4. In contrast, when B cells are stimulated by crosslinking of their CD40 antigen (with either anti-CD40 antibody and mouse L cells transfected with Fc$\gamma$RII/CD32 or mouse L cells transfected with CD40 ligand), hIL-10 markedly enhances B-cell growth and is as effective as IL-4 over a 10-day period. hIL-10 induces a 10–25-fold multiplication of B cells within 2 weeks. IL-4 and IL-10 are additive in those systems, their combination resulting in a 60–100-fold expansion of the number of viable B cells. This signal is the most efficient tested so far, and during these two weeks even surpasses the proliferation induced by EBV infection[6]. IL-10 also costimulates with IL-2 for the proliferation of B cells activated through CD40, an effect which is particularly striking, as CD40-activated B cells respond poorly to IL-2. This correlates with an increased Tac/CD25 expression and high-affinity IL-2 receptors on CD40-activated normal B lymphocytes or BCLL cells[23]. hIL-10 enhances EBV-induced B-cell proliferation, whereas IL-2 and IL-4 have no effect[10]. Interestingly, hIL-10 produced endogeneously upon EBV transformation plays a role in the growth of these B cells, as demonstrated by the addition of hIL-10 neutralizing antibodies, which reduces considerably the EBV-induced B-cell proliferation[10].

Among mature B cells, subsets can be identified which differentially express specific surface molecules and which correspond to discrete stages of antigen-dependent B-cell immunopoiesis[26]. In particular, naive B cells express sIgD, while sIgD$^-$ B cells are composed of two major subsets which include germinal center B cells and memory B cells[27–29]. IL-10 enhances equally well the DNA synthesis of the three different B-cell subsets, be they stimulated through their antigen receptor or their CD40 antigen[29] (Liu and Brière, unpublished observations).

LPS or anti-δ-dextran-activated mouse splenic B cells do not enhance their proliferation in response to IL-10[5,30], yet prolonged administration of neutralizing anti-IL-10 antibodies to mice results in depletion of CD5$^+$ B cells. However, this effect may be indirect, acting through increased IFN-γ levels which inhibit CD5$^+$ B-cell growth[31].

## B-CELL DIFFERENTIATION

### HUMAN B LYMPHOCYTES

*In vitro*, hIL-10 induces SAC-preactivated human tonsillar B lymphocytes to produce high levels of IgM, IgG and IgA. Whereas IL-2 scores as the most potent cytokine for enhancing SAC-induced DNA synthesis, IL-10 appears to be the most efficient for induction of Ig synthesis by such cells[6]. The differentiation effect of IL-10 is particularly striking when B cells have been stimulated through their CD40 antigen. With IL-10, unseparated CD40-activated B cells produce large amounts of IgM, IgA, IgG1, IgG2 and IgG3, but usually neither IgG4 nor IgE[6,32]. The IL-10-induced B-cell differentiation does not require intense crosslinking of the CD40 antigen, as soluble anti-CD40 mAbs and IL-10 are sufficient to induce Ig secretion[33,34]. Morphological studies have shown that cells differentiate into plasmablasts with an extended endoplasmic reticulum network, including cisternae full of Igs[35,36]. Eventually, CD40-activated B cells stop proliferating after several days of culture in the presence of IL-10, probably as a consequence of a terminal differentiation. Combination of IL-10 with IL-2 or IL-3 induces, respectively, SAC-preactivated B cells or T-cell-preactivated B cells to terminally differentiate into plasma cells when secondarily cultured onto peculiar microenvironments such as RA synoviocytes[37] or bone marrow stroma[38]. Significantly, IL-10 induces, in some cases, CD40-activated BCLL cells to differentiate into plasma cells producing IgG, IgA and IgM[39].

Interestingly, IL-10 is capable of enhancing Ig synthesis by isotype-committed B cells. In particular, in response to IL-10, CD40-activated memory B cells produce considerable amounts of IgG and IgA, whereas germinal center B cells secrete lower levels of Igs (Liu and Brière, unpublished observations). Finally, CD40 triggering and IL-10 play an important role in antigen specific antibody production by antigen-primed memory B cells[34]. In this context, the spontaneous *in vitro* secretion of Igs by SLE mononuclear cells is inhibited by anti-IL-10. This effect was further observed *in vivo* in SCID mice which were injected with mononuclear cells from SLE patients, since anti-IL-10 mAb strongly inhibited the production of autoantibodies and that of total IgG[40].

## MOUSE B LYMPHOCYTES

*In vitro*, IL-10 inhibits proliferation and IL-5-dependent Ig production by high-density mouse splenic B cells stimulated by thymo-independent antigens but does not inhibit T cell-induced Ig production[30,41]. IL-10 appears to be a switch factor for activated murine B cells that would act by a mechanism that differs from those turned on by IL-4, IFN-$\gamma$ and transforming growth factor beta (TGF-$\beta$) (Snapper, personal communication). *In vivo* data suggest that IL-10 could also have a potentiating effect in mouse B-cell differentiation. Continuous administration of neutralizing anti-IL-10 antibodies to mice results in reduced serum IgM and IgA but increased serum IgG2a and IgG2b, depletion of peritoneal B cells, and a defective response to bacterial antigens such as phosphorylcholine and $\alpha$1,3-dextran[31]. Furthermore, IL-10 mRNA is upregulated 100-fold in spleen cells during the primary immune response of mice to goat anti-mouse IgD antibody, which strongly activates humoral immunity[42]. However, IL-10-deficient mice do not display alteration in T- and B-lymphocyte development and have normal levels of the various serum isotypes[43]. Furthermore, when these animals develop chronic enterocolitis, they display increased serum IgA levels as a consequence of numerous plasma cells infiltrating into the inflamed mucosa. The explanations for these discrepancies are not clear and may involve the well-recognized redundancy that exists within the cytokine system[44]. It is possible that a developing mouse embryo will compensate for the loss of a critical cytokine gene by amplifying expression of a gene that codes for a protein of comparable function.

Neutralizing IL-10 may be beneficial in B-cell-mediated autoimmune disease such as SLE. NZB/W F1 mice, which spontaneously develop an SLE-like syndrome with lethal immune complex-dependent glomerulonephritis, display a delayed onset of autoimmunity when treated with anti-IL-10, and conversely injection of IL-10 accelerates the disease process[45].

## ISOTYPE SWITCHING

### POLYCLONAL ACTIVATION OF B LYMPHOCYTES

In the murine system, different signals, such as antigen receptor engagement with dextran-conjugated anti-IgD antibodies as well as lipopolysaccharide (LPS), efficiently induce naive B cells to secrete secondary isotypes in response to cytokines. In contrast, in humans, only triggering of CD40 has been extensively studied for its role in isotype switch. CD40 triggering alone is not sufficient to induce human B lymphocytes to secrete Ig in significant amounts. However, one can stimulate differentiation of human B cells by triggering CD40 in the presence of SAC particles, without exogenous factors. Indeed, the Ig response by naive $sIgD^+$ B cells activated through CD40 together with SAC particles is exclusively restricted to the IgM isotype, while isotype-committed $sIgD^-$ B cells produce high amounts of IgG and IgA under these culture conditions[46]. SAC particles have been shown to activate B cells through protein A-induced triggering of B-cell receptor[47]. However, this is unlikely to explain the CD40/SAC-induced differentiation, because cotriggering of B cells through CD40 and their B-cell receptor (with anti-$\kappa^+$ anti-λ or anti-CD79β/Igβ) does not result in Ig secretion (our unpublished observations). Additional studies are therefore required to determine the B-cell surface molecule(s) that SAC particles activate.

The physiological relevance of the interaction between CD40 on B lymphocytes and CD40 ligand expressed on activated T cells in isotype switch has been clearly demonstrated *in vivo*, in humans. Indeed, patients suffering from the hyper-IgM syndrome are incapable of mounting an efficient secondary immune response because of mutations in the gene encoding for CD40 ligand. At the present time, there is no evidence that human B lymphocytes may be induced to switch isotype using either LPS or antigen receptor triggering. Yet minor CD40-independent pathways of isotype switch may exist, as patients with hyper-IgM syndrome present minor amounts of IgG and IgE, and T-cell clones from such patients can induce peripheral blood B cells to produce IgG, IgA[48] and IgE[49].

### IL-10 AND SWITCH TO IgG

The studies suggesting that IL-10 acts as a switch factor have essentially been performed by our group and are based on the analysis of IgG and IgA secretion by human naive $sIgD^+$ B cells stimulated through their CD40 antigen. Our initial studies demonstrated that highly purified $sIgD^+$ tonsillar B lymphocytes cultured in a CD40 system (composed of an anti-CD40 mAb presented by a CD32-transfected fibroblastic cell line) secreted large amounts of IgM as well as significant amounts of IgG when IL-10 was added to the cultures[46].

An isotype switch towards IgG in response to IL-10 was further suggested by the detailed analysis of IgG subclasses by different B-cell subsets. Supernatants of *memory* B cells stimulated through their CD40 antigen, and in the presence of SAC particles, contained IgG1 (65 per cent of total IgG), IgG2 (25 per cent) and IgG3 (10 per cent) (IgG4 was rarely measurable). Addition of IL-10 to CD40-activated *naive* $sIgD^+$ B cells induced specifically the secretion of IgG1 and IgG3 in roughly equivalent quantities, which could be further increased by addition of SAC. Addition of IL-10 to CD40-activated memory B cells increased IgG1 (2-fold), IgG2 (2-fold) and more particularly IgG3 (9–10-fold), thus suggesting a different action of IL-10 on these two subsets of B lymphocytes (Table 11.1). A significant contribution of contaminating memory B cells within the naive B-cell population is unlikely, inasmuch as functional IgG transcripts are difficult to identify using polymerase chain reaction (PCR) analysis[27]. Furthermore, if this were the case, IL-10 should induce the population of naive B cells to secrete IgG2. Finally, naive B cells of various origins could be induced to secrete IgG1 and IgG3 when stimulated through their CD40 antigen together with IL-10: cord blood B cells, adult blood B cells, adult spleen B cells and B lymphocytes of patients suffering from hyper-IgM syndrome (Figure 11.1)[32]. Note that extensive CD40 crosslinking is required for the induction of isotype switch towards IgG, as soluble CD40 antibody could induce human peripheral blood $sIgD^-$ memory B cells, but not $sIgD^+$ B cells, to secrete IgG in response to IL-10[34,50]. Ligation of CD40 on unseparated B cells isolated from peripheral blood induced $\gamma1$, $\gamma3$ and $\gamma2$ germline transcripts after 7 days of culture in the absence of exogenous cytokines[51]. It is not yet known whether IL-10 alone induces specifically $\gamma1$ and $\gamma3$ germline transcripts and/or increases those induced by CD40 ligation. As CD40 ligation also turns on IL-10 gene transcription[52] and IL-10 secretion by B cells[8], the respective roles of CD40 and IL-10 in the induction of Ig germline transcripts remain to be elucidated.

**Table 11.1** Immunoglobulin synthesis by CD40-activated human B-cell subsets in response to IL-10

| | | (μg/ml) | | | | | |
|---|---|---|---|---|---|---|---|
| B-cell subsets | IL-10 | IgG1 | IgG2 | IgG3 | IgG4 | IgA | IgM |
| Follicular mantle B cells | – | < | < | < | < | < | 0.2 |
| | + | 1.2 | < | 1.45 | < | 1.3 | 20 |
| Germinal center B cells | – | < | < | < | < | < | 0.3 |
| | + | 3 | 1 | 0.3 | < | 1.5 | 2.3 |
| Memory B cells | – | 0.7 | 0.2 | 0.1 | < | < | 0.6 |
| | + | 6.2 | 2.1 | 0.9 | 0.4 | 4.5 | 17 |

$2 \times 10^4$ B cells were co-cultured for 14 days with $5 \times 10^3$ irradiated CD40 ligand transfected L cells with or without 100 ng/ml of IL-10. Ig levels represent the mean values of triplicate experiments. Limits of sensitivities of each ELISA are 50 ng/ml, 90 ng/ml, 65 ng/ml, 30 ng/ml, 10 ng/ml and 20ng/ml for IgG1, IgG2, IgG3, IgG4, IgA and IgM respectively (< meaning below the background levels).

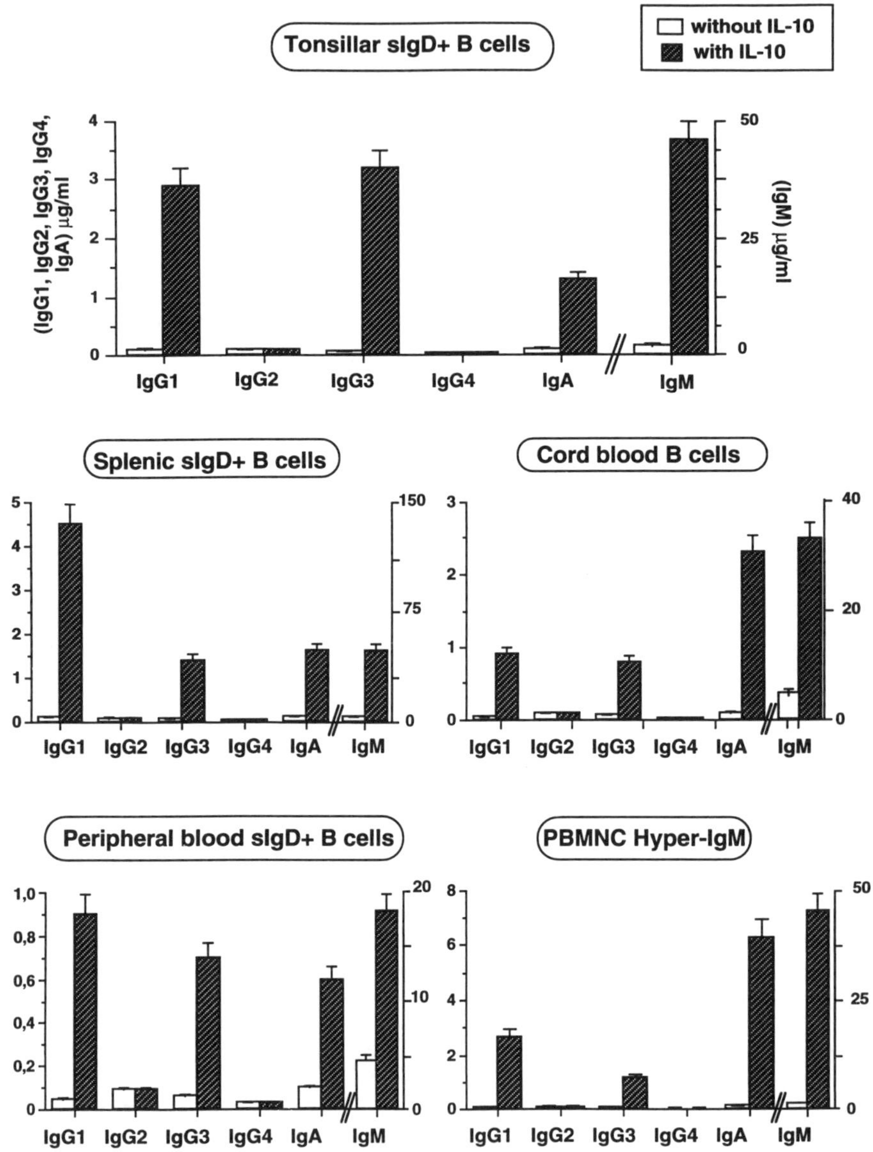


**Figure 11.1** IL-10 induces IgG1, IgG3 and IgA synthesis by CD40-activated naive B cells from various origins. sIgD+ B cells were purified by magnetic activated cell sorting when isolated from tonsils, spleen or peripheral blood, CD19+ B cells were sorted with FACSstar when isolated from cord blood, and peripheral blood mononuclear cells (PBMNC) from hyper-IgM were cultured at $5 \times 10^4$ cells/well and cultured with $5 \times 10^3$ irradiated CD40 ligand-transfected L cells with or without 100 ng/ml of human IL-10. Supernatants were harvested and IgG subclasses, IgA and IgM levels were determined by ELISA. Results are means ± SD of quadruplicate cultures

## IL-10 AND SWITCH TO IgA

In our initial studies, we observed that highly purified CD40-activated $sIgD^+$ tonsillar B lymphocytes, cultured with IL-10, secreted essentially IgM, significant amounts of IgG and low but reproducible levels of IgA[46]. Unlike IL-10, TGF-β alone did not induce Ig synthesis by normal CD40-activated naive $sIgD^+$ B cells. Addition of TGF-β strongly enhanced IL-10-induced IgA production but inhibited secretion of IgG and IgM[46]. In contrast TGF-β dramatically decreased IgA and IgG synthesis by CD40-activated $sIgD^-$ B cells (essentially memory B cells) driven by IL-10. Thus, while TGF-β acts specifically on (1) the naive B-cell subset, and (2) the IgA isotype, the presence of IL-10 is necessary for IgA to be secreted.

Analysis of α1 and α2 germline transcripts demonstrated that TGF-β alone was able to induce their expression in *Branhamella catarrhalis*-activated human B lymphocytes[53] as well as in non-activated high-density $sIgM^+sIgA^-$ human B cells[52]. With regard to induction of mature transcripts, TGF-β alone does not induce either Cα1 or Cα2 but does induce mature Cα1 transcripts in concert with IL-10[52]. Furthermore, CD40 triggering induces both germline and mature Cα1 transcripts but only germline Cα2 transcripts. The production of mature Cα2 transcripts could only be obtained by the combination of CD40 ligation, TGF-β and IL-10[52]. In conclusion, induction of Cα1 and Cα2 germline and mature transcripts is differentially regulated.

## IL-10 INDUCES DNA RECOMBINATION

To formally prove that B cells were indeed undergoing isotype switch in response to IL-10, we recently turned our attention to the detection of DNA deletion pieces. As described in detail in Chapter 5, the switch from the expression of Cμ and Cδ to the expression of downstream isotypes normally involves a recombination which deletes the intervening $C_H$ genes from the chromosome and positions the new $C_H$ gene directly 3′ of the assembled $V_H$ gene. The sites of these recombinations are in regions of tandem repeats, termed switch (S) regions, which are present 5′ of each $C_H$ gene, except Cδ. This recombination may occur in several ways but the primary mechanism for switching involves intrachromosomal recombination with looping out and deletion of the $C_H$ genes between the sites of recombination as extrachromosomal circular DNA, also referred as switch circles. DNA analysis has been performed by PCR using primers designed so that only circular DNA fragments could be amplified, followed by hybridization with an internal probe. Switch circles representing the product of a μ to γ switch were observed in DNA which was extracted from CD40-activated human $sIgD^+$ B cells cultured during 5 days in the presence of IL-10[54,55]. This demonstrates that IL-10 acts as a switch factor towards IgG through deletional rearrangement. Experiments are being done in our laboratory, in order to determine whether IL-10 may also induce a switch towards IgA through the same mechanism.

### IL-10 IS NOT A SWITCH FACTOR FOR IgE

IL-10 was found to enhance the production of IgE induced by IL-4[33] or IL-13 (personal observation) of CD40-activated naive $sIgD^+$ B cells. The inhibition by IL-10 of IL4-induced IgE production by unseparated blood mononuclear cells[56] is best explained by the strong inhibitory effect of IL-10 on monocyte-dependent T-cell activation[57]. Thus, IL-10 is capable of inducing IgG1, IgG3 and IgA secretion by CD40-activated naive B cells and also, as a potent differentiation factor, of enhancing IgE synthesis induced by IL-4/13.

## IMMUNODEFICIENCIES

### IgA DEFICIENCIES

IgA deficiency is the most common form of primary immunodeficiency in humans, with a frequency of 1 : 300 in the Caucasian population, a third of whom are susceptible to infections. The molecular basis of this disorder is mostly unknown[58] and little information is available concerning the cytokines possibly involved in this disease. Peripheral blood lymphocytes from such IgA-deficient patients cultured in the CD40 system in the presence of SAC produce IgM and IgG but no IgA[59]. Addition of IL-10 to cultures enhances the production of IgM and IgG and, most strikingly, induces the production of high amounts of IgA. The IgA-inducing effect of IL-10 is direct, as highly purified blood B cells from these patients can be induced to secrete IgA in response to CD40 engagement and IL-10. Of note is the fact that TGF-β alone was unable to induce these activated B cells to secrete IgA. Yet it is possible that IL-10 may require the presence of TGF-β for the IgA switch to occur. In keeping with this, the TGF-β mRNA levels in peripheral blood mononuclear cells from IgA-deficient patients were not different from those of healthy subjects' cells[58]. Eventually, mononuclear cells from IgA-deficient patients produced upon activation less IL-10 than those of matched controls[59]. Consistent with a profound decrease in Cα membrane transcripts, B cells from IgA-deficient patients had significantly less α germline transcripts[60] and Sμ–Sα fragments[58]. Whether, in those IgA-deficient B cells, IL-10 and/or CD40 ligation alleviate the switch defect, or allow the survival of IgA-committed B lymphocytes, remains to be addressed.

### COMMON VARIABLE IMMUNODEFICIENCIES

Common variable immunodeficiency (CVI) is an acquired disorder characterized by a failure of B cells to mature into Ig-secreting cells, resulting in reduced Ig levels in serum and recurrent bacterial infections. One study indicated that, in 6 out of 7 patients tested, IL-10 could induce B cells to secrete IgG, IgA and IgM following activation with either anti-CD40 mAb or with SAC particles[61]. However, another study indicated a wide heterogeneity in the capacity of CD40-activated CVI B cells to produce different isotypes in response to IL-10, as either IgM only, or IgM and IgG or IgM, IgG and IgA could be secreted[34]. CD40 ligand levels on activated T cells from CVI patients were found to be either normal[61] or reduced[62]. Finally, in our own studies with 13 CVI patients, CD40-activated peripheral blood mononuclear cells were induced to secrete IgG and IgA in all cases in the presence of anti-CD40 mAb and IL-10 (Brière *et al.*, unpublished). Thus, in most CVI cases, IL-10 appears to be able to overcome the inability of B cells to secrete IgG and IgA. Whether CVI is associated with defects in the IL-10 pathway remains to be determined.

## CONCLUDING REMARKS

The effects of hIL-10 on B lymphocytes have been most convincingly demonstrated on human cells whose responses (apoptosis, proliferation, differentiation or isotype switch) are dependent on their stage of maturation and/or activation. Such apparently contrasting effects of a cytokine on the different maturation stages of a given cell lineage are not specific to IL-10, inasmuch as IL-4, which promotes the growth of activated mature B cells[63], is an inhibitor of the proliferation of B-cell progenitors[64]. When considering mature B lymphocytes, IL-10 displays two major activities: induction of switch towards IgG1, IgG3 and IgA, and induction of terminal B-cell differentiation towards the plasma cell stage. This dual key function of IL-10 in B-cell immunopoiesis is found with other cytokines, as illustrated by IL-4 and IL-13, which induce B-cell growth as well as a switch towards IgG4 and IgE. In keeping with this, it is interesting to note that, in mouse, IL-4 and interferons (rather than IL-10) control IgG subclass switch. The fact that different cytokines control the IgG subclass switch in mice and humans can be related to relevant fundamental notions. There was a single IgG gene in the ancestor common to mice and humans, and it was only after evolutionary divergence that each species elaborated four IgG subclasses following two independent gene duplication events. It is therefore not surprising that different cytokines have been selected during evolution to control the regulation of molecules that have evolved independently. In this context, human and mouse IL-13 can induce human B cells to switch towards IgE, while they cannot induce mouse B cells to do so. In keeping with the differences of cytokine regulation of B-cell immunopoiesis between mice and humans, there is a major contribution of IL-10 in humans but a limited one in mice, and, similarly, a limited role of IL-5 in humans while its role in mice is well established.

The activities of IL-10 on B lymphocytes suggest several clinical applications of either IL-10 agonists or IL-10 antagonists in diseases involving B cells. Administration of IL-10 to patients suffering from IgA deficiencies and common variable immunodeficiencies may permit the alleviation of the block of B-cell differentiation, thus possibly normalizing their deficient humoral responses. In contrast, IL-10 antagonists may prove useful in the management of SLE, as well as non-Hodgkin's lymphomas. Such an antagonist may be (1) a soluble form of the receptor, (2) a neutralizing antibody specific for IL-10, (3) a chemical agent blocking the IL-10 cascade (not yet available), or (4) interferons, which have been shown to block the production of IL-10[65].

Finally, studies aimed at identifying the respective intracellular pathways transducing IL-10 proliferation and differentiation signals will hopefully enable us to better understand the mechanisms underlying these different effector functions.

## NOTE

Florence Malisan is a recipient of a grant from Foundaton Marcel Mérieux, Lyon, France and Christine Servet-Delprat is a recipient of a grant from the Ecole Normale Superieure.

## REFERENCES

1. Fiorentino DF, Bond MW, Mosmann TR. Two types of mouse T helper cell. IV. Th2 clones secrete a factor that inhibits cytokine production by Th1 clones. J Exp Med 1989; 170:2081–2095.
2. O'Garra A, Stapleton G, Dhar V *et al.* Production of cytokines by mouse B cells: B lymphomas and normal B cells produce interleukin 10. Int Immunol 1990; 2:821–832.
3. Suda T, O'Garra A, MacNeil I *et al.* Identification of a novel thymocyte growth promoting factor derived from B cell lymphomas. Cell Immunol 1990; 129:228–240.
4. Mosmann TR, Coffman RL. Heterogeneity of cytokine secretion patterns and functions of helper T cells. Adv Immunol 1989; 46:111–147.
5. Go NF, Castle B, Barrett R *et al.* Interleukin 10, a novel B cell stimulatory factor: unresponsiveness of X chromosome-linked immunodeficiency B cells. J Exp Med 1990; 172:1625–1631.
6. Rousset F, Garcia E, Defrance T *et al.* Interleukin 10 is a potent growth and differentiation factor for activated human B lymphocytes. Proc Natl Acad Sci USA 1992; 89:1890–1893.
7. Moore KW, O'Garra A, de Waal Malefyt R *et al.* Interleukin-10. Annu Rev Immunol 1993; 11:165–190.

8. Burdin N, van Kooten K, Galibert L *et al.* Endogenous IL-6 and IL-10 contribute to the differentiation of CD40-activated human B lymphocytes. J Immunol 1995; 154:2533–2544.
9. Llorente L, Richaud-Patin Y, Wijdenes J *et al.* Spontaneous production of interleukin 10 by B lymphocytes and monocytes in systemic lupus erythematosus. Eur Cytokine Network 1993; 4:421–430.
10. Burdin B, Péronne C, Banchereau J, Rousset F. Epstein–Barr virus-transformation induces B lymphocytes to produce human interleukin-10. J Exp Med 1993; 177:295–304.
11. Benjamin D, Knobloch TJ, Dayton MA. Human B-cell interleukin-10: B cell lines derived from patients with acquired immunodeficiency syndrome and Burkit's lymphoma constitutively secrete large quantities of interleukin-10. Blood 1992; 80:1289–1298.
12. Miyazaki I, Cheung RK, Dosch H-M. Viral interleukin 10 is critical for the induction of B cell growth transformation by Epstein–Barr virus. J Exp Med 1993; 178:439–447.
13. Hudson GS, Bankier AT, Satchwell SC, Barrell BG. The short unique region of the B95–8 Epstein–Barr virus genome. Virology 1985; 147:81–98.
14. Swaminathan S, Hesselton R, Sullivan J. Epstein–Barr virus recombinants with specifically mutated BCRF1 genes. J Virol 1993; 67:7406–7413.
15. Blay J-Y, Burdin N, Rousset F *et al.* Serum interleukin-10 in non-Hodgkin's lymphoma: a prognostic factor. Blood 1993; 82:2169–2174.
16. Emilie D, Touitou R, Raphael M *et al.* *In vivo* production of interleukin-10 by malignant cells in AIDS lymphomas. Eur J Immunol 1992; 22:2937–2942.
17. Baiocchi RA, Ross ME, Tan JC *et al.* Lymphomagenesis in the SCID-hu mouse involves abundant production of human interleukin-10. Blood 1995; 85:1063–1074.
18. Merville P, Rousset F, Banchereau J *et al.* Serum interleukin 10 in early stage multiple myeloma. Lancet 1992; 340:1544–1545.
19. Gotlieb WH, Abrams JS, Watson JM *et al.* Presence of interleukin 10 (IL-10) in the ascites of patients with ovarian and other intra-abdominal cancers. Cytokine 1992; 4:385–390.
20. Bendtzen K, Svenson M, Jonsson V, Hippe E. Autoantibodies to cytokines: friends or foes? Immunol Today 1990; 11:167–169.
21. Ménétrier-Caux C, Brière F, Jouvenne P *et al.* Identification of human anti-hIL10 autoantibodies in different pathologies. Submitted.
22. Levy Y, Brouet J-C. Interleukin-10 prevents spontaneous death of germinal center B cells by induction of the bcl-2 protein. J Clin Invest 1994; 93:424–428.
23. Fluckiger A-C, Garrone P, Durand I *et al.* IL-10 upregulates functional high affinity IL-2 receptors on normal and leukemic B lymphocytes. J Exp Med 1993; 178:1473–1481.
24. Itoh K, Inoue T, Ito K, Hirohata S. The interplay of interleukin-10 (IL-10) and interleukin-2 (IL-2) in humoral immune responses: IL-10 synergizes with IL-2 to enhance responses of human B lymphocytes in a mechanism which is different from upregulation of CD25 expression. Cell Immunol 1994; 157:478–488.
25. Saeland S, Duvert V, Moreau I, Banchereau J. Human B cell precursors proliferate and express CD23 after CD40 ligation. J Exp Med 1993; 178:113–120.
26. Banchereau J, Rousset F. Human B lymphocytes: phenotype, proliferation and differentiation. Adv Immunol 1992; 52:125–251.
27. Pascual V, Liu Y-J, Magalski A *et al.* Analysis of somatic mutation in five B cell subsets of human tonsil. J Exp Med 1994; 180:329–339.
28. Liu Y-J, Barthelemy C, de Bouteiller O *et al.* Memory B cells from human tonsils colonize mucosal epithelium and directly present antigen to T cells by rapid upregulation of B7.1 and B7.2. Immunity 1995; 2:239–248.

29. Lagresle C, Bella C, Defrance T. Phenotypic and functional heterogeneity of the IgD$^-$ B cell compartment: identification of two major tonsillar B cell subsets. Int Immunol 1993; 5:1259–1268.
30. Peçanha LMT, Snapper CM, Lees A *et al.* IL-10 inhibits T cell-independent but not T cell-dependent responses *in vitro*. J Immunol 1993; 150:3215–3223.
31. Ishida H, Hastings R, Kearney J, Howard M. Continuous anti-IL-10 antibody administration depletes mice of Ly-1 B cells but not conventional B cells. J Exp Med 1992; 175:1213–1220.
32. Brière F, Servet-Delprat C, Bridon J-M *et al.* Human interleukin 10 induces naive sIgD$^+$ B cells to secrete $IgG_1$ and $IgG_3$. J Exp Med 1994; 179:757–762.
33. Garrone P, Galibert L, Rousset F *et al.* Regulatory effects of prostaglandin E2 on the growth and differentiation of human B lymphocytes activated through their CD40 antigen. J Immunol 1994; 152:4282–4290.
34. Nonoyama S, Hollenbaugh D, Aruffo A *et al.* B cell activation via CD40 is required for specific antibody production by antigen-stimulated human B cells. J Exp Med 1993; 178:1097–1102.
35. Arpin C, Dechanet J, van Kooten K *et al. In vitro* generation of memory B cells and plasma cells. Science 1995; 268:720–722.
36. Rousset F, Peyrol S, Garcia E *et al.* IL10 induces the differentiation of CD40-activated B lymphocytes into plasma cells. Int Immunol 1995; 7:1243–1253.
37. Dechanet J, Rissoan MC, Banchereau J, Miossec P. Interleukin 4, but not interleukin 10, regulates the production of inflammation mediators by rheumatoid synoviocytes. Cytokine 1995; 7:176–183.
38. Merville P, Dechanet J, Grouard G *et al.* T cell-induced B cell blasts differentiate into plasma cells when cultured on bone marrow stroma with IL3 and IL10. Int Immunol 1995; 7:635–643.
39. Malisan F, Fluckiger A-C, Ho S *et al.* B-chronic lymphocytic leukemias can undergo isotype switching *in vivo* and can be induced to differentiate and switch *in vitro*. Blood 1995; in press.
40. Llorente L, Zou W, Levy Y *et al.* Role of interleukin 10 in the B lymphocyte hyperactivity and autoantibody production of human systemic lupus erythematosus. J Exp Med 1995; 181:839–844.
41. Peçanha LMT, Snapper CM, Lees A, Mond JJ. Lymphokine control of type 2 antigen response. IL-10 inhibits IL-5- but not IL-2-induced Ig secretion by T cell-independent antigens. J Immunol 1992; 148:3427–3432.
42. Svetic A, Finkelman FD, Jian YC *et al.* Cytokine gene expression after *in vivo* primary immunization with goat antibody to mouse IgD antibody. J Immunol 1991; 147:2391–2397.
43. Kühn R, Löhler J, Rennick D *et al.* Interleukin-10-deficient mice develop chronic enterocolitis. Cell 1993; 75:263–274.
44. Finkelman FD, Holmes J, Katona IM *et al.* Lymphokine control of *in vivo* immunoglobulin isotype selection. Annu Rev Immunol 1990; 8:303–333.
45. Ishida H, Muchamuel T, Sakaguchi S *et al.* Continuous administration of anti-interleukin 10 antibodies delays onset of autoimmunity in NZB/W F1 mice. J Exp Med 1994; 179:305–310.
46. Defrance T, Vanbervliet B, Brière F *et al.* Interleukin 10 and transforming growth factor β cooperate to induce anti-CD40-activated naive human B cells to secrete immunoglobulin A. J Exp Med 1992; 175:671–682.
47. Ricci M, Romagnani S, Giudizi GM *et al.* Mechanisms of human B-cell activation by *Staphylococcus Aureus*. In: Fauci AS, Ballieux RE (eds) Human B-Lymphocyte Function. New York: Raven Press 1982, pp. 17–36.
48. Nishioka Y, Lipsky PE. The role of CD40–CD40 ligand interaction in human T cell–B cell collaboration. J Immunol 1994; 153:1027–1036.

49. Life P, Gauchat J-F, Schnuriger V *et al.* T cell clones from an X-linked hyperimmunoglobulin (IgM) patient induce IgE synthesis *in vitro* despite expression of nonfunctional CD40 ligand. J Exp Med 1994; 180:1775–1784.
50. Saiki O, Tanaka T, Wada Y *et al.* Signaling through CD40 rescues IgE but not IgG or IgA secretion in X-linked immunodeficiency with hyper-IgM. J Clin Invest 1995; 95:510–514.
51. Jumper MD, Splawski JB, Lipsky PE, Meek K. Ligation of CD40 induces sterile transcripts of multiple Ig heavy chain isotypes in human B cells. J Immunol 1994; 152:438–445.
52. Kitani A, Strober W. Differential regulation of Cα1 and Cα2 germ-line and mature mRNA transcripts in human peripheral blood B cells. J Immunol 1994; 153:1466–1477.
53. Islam KB, Nilsson L, Sideras P *et al.* TGF-β1 induces germ-line transcripts of both IgA subclasses in human B lymphocytes. Int Immunol 1991; 3:1099–1106.
54. Malisan F, Brière F, Bridon J-M *et al.* IL-10 induces switch towards IgG through DNA deletional rearrangement. In: Proceedings of 9th International Congress of Immunology. San Francisco 1995; p87.
55. Malisan F, Brière F, Bridon J-M. IL-10 acts as a switch factor in human. Submitted.
56. Punnonen J, Aversa GG, Cocks BG *et al.* Interleukin-13 induces interleukin-4-independent IgG4 and IgE synthesis and CD23 expression by human B cells. Proc Natl Acad Sci USA 1993; 90:3730–3734.
57. de Waal Malefyt R, Yssel H, de Vries JE. Direct effects of IL-10 on subsets of human CD4+ T cell clones and resting T cells. J Immunol 1993; 150:4754–4765.
58. Islam KB, Baskin B, Nilsson L *et al.* Molecular analysis of IgA deficiency. Evidence for impaired switching to IgA. J Immunol 1994; 152:1442–1452.
59. Brière F, Bridon J-M, Chevet D *et al.* Interleukin 10 induces B lymphocytes from IgA deficient patients to secrete IgA. J Clin Invest 1994; 94:97–104.
60. Islam KB, Baskin B, Christensson B *et al. In vivo* expression of human immunoglobulin germ-line mRNA in normal and in immunodeficient individuals. Clin Exp Immunol 1994; 95:3–9.
61. Zielen S, Bauscher P, Hofmann D, Meuer SC. Interleukin 10 and immune restoration in common variable immunodeficiency. Lancet 1993; 342:750–751.
62. Farrington M, Grosmaire LS, Nonoyama S *et al.* CD40 ligand expression is defective in a subset of patients with common variable immunodeficiency. Proc Natl Acad Sci USA 1994; 91:1099–1103.
63. Banchereau J, de Paoli P, Vallé A *et al.* Long term human B cell lines dependent on interleukin 4 and antibody to CD40. Science 1991; 251:70–72.
64. Pandrau D, Saeland S, Duvert V *et al.* Interleukin-4 inhibits *in vitro* proliferation of leukemic and normal human B cell precursors. J Clin Invest 1992; 90:1697–1706.
65. Chomarat P, Rissoan M-C, Banchereau J, Miossec P. Interferon γ inhibits interleukin-10 production by monocytes. J Exp Med 1993; 177:523–527.

# 12 Transforming Growth Factor Beta

**JANET STAVNEZER**
*University of Massachusetts Medical School, Worcester, Massachusetts, USA*

## INTRODUCTION

This chapter will focus on the effects of transforming growth factor Beta (TGF-β) on B-cell development and differentiation, but I will also mention some effects on the T-cell lineage. The chapter begins with a very brief overview of the structure of TGF-β, its receptors and the regulation of TGF-β expression. Several recent reviews of these areas are available and will be referred to in these overview sections.

## THE TGF-β SUPERFAMILY

TGF-β is a pleiotropic cytokine having suppressive effects on growth, and both inhibitory and stimulatory effects on the differentiation of a variety of cell types. It is an important immunomodulator, having both inductive and suppressive effects on inflammation and the immune response. It is important in both the recruitment of inflammatory cells, and in inhibiting the inflammatory cell response after activation. It also plays an important role in fibrinogenesis and wound repair[1–4].

TGF-β inhibits differentiation of pre-B and B cells by inhibition of immunoglobulin (Ig) synthesis, and inhibits cytokine production by T cells[5–7]. It inhibits proliferation and cytotoxic activities of cytotoxic T lymphocytes and natural killer (NK) cells[8–10], and inhibits macrophage activity by decreasing hydrogen peroxide production and respiratory burst activity[11]. TGF-β delays the onset and reduces the severity of experimental autoimmune disease in animal models of multiple sclerosis[12] and rheumatoid arthritis (RA)[13], and is implicated in oral tolerance[14]. Mice genetically deficient in the gene for TGF-β, generated by knockout technology, die from a wasting syndrome accompanied by widespread inflammation[15–17].

By contrast, TGF-β also has stimulatory effects on differentiation of immune cells, as it increases class switching to IgA and IgG2b[18–21], and induces chemotaxis of monocytes and their secretion of IL-1, IL-6, tumor

*Cytokine Regulation of Humoral Immunity: Basic and Clinical Aspects.* Edited by Clifford M. Snapper.

necrosis factor alpha TNF-α and TGF-β, and expression of CD16 (FcγRIII)[22]. It facilitates macrophage migration into tissues by stimulating expression of integrins and matrix-degrading enzymes[23]. It is also a chemotactic factor for human $CD4^+$ and $CD8^+$ T cells[24] and human neutrophils[25]. TGF-β does not directly stimulate proliferation but indirectly can do so by, for example, stimulating the production of extracellular matrix proteins, resulting in fibrogenesis, or by stimulating production of certain cytokines, e.g. platelet-derived growth factor[2].

TGF-β belongs to a large superfamily of structurally related regulatory proteins, which include three mammalian isoforms of TGF-β, (TGF-β1, TGF-β2 and TGF-β3), activin/inhibins, and bone morphogenic proteins. The proteins of this family mediate many key events in normal growth and development of organisms as diverse as *Drosophila, Xenopus* and mammals[1,26,27]. The three mammalian isoforms of TGF-β exist as disulfide-bonded homodimers, but are also found as heterodimers in certain cell types. Each of the TGF-βs is produced as a precursor approximately 400 amino acids in length (110 kDa) with an N-terminal signal sequence, a pro-domain, and a mature C-terminal domain of 112 amino acids (25 kDa) (Figure 12.1). The TGF-β precursor protein is cleaved intracellularly but remains in a latent form with the pro-domain associated with the active signaling fragment. TGF-βs are secreted from cells in the latent form, which do not bind TGF-β receptors. The pro-domain (now called the TGF-β latency-associated peptide) remains associated with mature TGF-β until it is removed by enzymatic degradation by proteases (plasmin, cathepsin D, glycosidase), resulting in activation of TGF-β. The pro-domain can also be removed by extremes of pH or by heating[1,26–29].

The mature parts of the three TGF-β1 isoforms have 70–80 per cent sequence identity and exert similar but not identical biological activities *in vitro*, although certain cells respond selectively[30]. Furthermore, there are quantitative differences in that TGF-β1 and TGF-β3 generally elicit their effects at about a 100-fold lower concentration than does TGF-β2. The three isoforms are controlled by unique transcriptional regulatory elements and thus are likely to have different functions *in vivo*. This idea is further supported by the finding that mice in which the TGF-β1 gene is 'knocked out' die by 2 or 3 weeks of age, indicating that TGF-β2 and TGF-β3 genes cannot substitute for the TGF-β1 gene[15,16]. Each of the three isoforms is highly conserved during evolution and each has nine conserved cysteine residues. Crystallographic studies of TGF-β2 have shown that six of these cysteines are closely grouped to create a rigid structure called a cysteine knot, which holds together two pairs of anti-parallel β-sheets and three α-helices. The backbone structure of TGF-β1 is modeled to be very similar[26,27]. TGF-β1 and TGFβ2 differ in positions that have been shown to affect binding to the TGF-β receptors I and II and to the serum protein α-macroglobulin, which sequesters TGF-β[30,31].

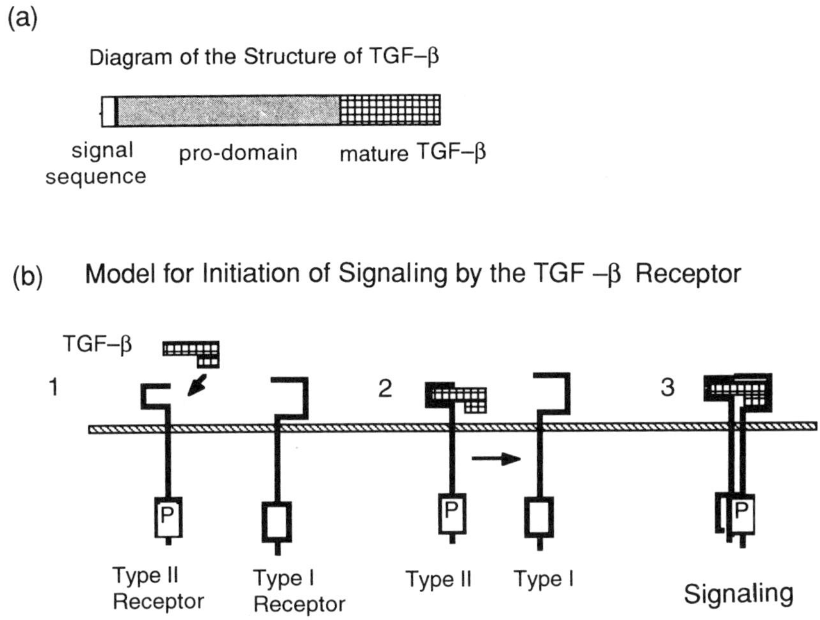


**Figure 12.1.** (a) TGF-β precursor with domains indicated. (b) Model for signalling by the TGF-β receptor as described in the text. (1) TGF-β binds to the type II receptor, which is constitutively phosphorylated. (2) The TGF-β-type II receptor complex binds to the type I receptor, which is not phosphorylated. (3) Upon formation of the trimolecular complex, the type II receptor phosphorylates the types I receptor, resulting in activation of the kinase activity of the type I receptor, and signaling. References are in the text

## TGF-β RECEPTORS AND THEIR SIGNAL TRANSDUCTION MECHANISM

The actions of TGF-β are mediated via binding to cell surface receptors. Three types of receptors exist on most cells, although often they are reduced in amounts or lacking in transformed cells. Two receptors, types I (53 kDa) and II (70 kDa), each have a small extracellular region, a single transmembrane domain and an intracytoplasmic serine/threonine kinase domain (Figure 12.1b). Type III receptors do not have signaling domains. Thus far, two glycoproteins of known structure, betaglycan and endoglin, are known to serve as type III receptors. Signaling has been shown to require the formation of a trimeric complex consisting of both the TGF-β receptors I and II and TGF-β (Figure 12.1b)[32–34]. TGF-β1 binds directly to the type II receptor, which is constitutively phosphorylated, and binding does not further increase its phosphorylation. The bound TGF-β is then recognized by the type I receptor, which appears to bind TGF-β only in association with the type II receptor. The associated type I receptor is phosphorylated by the type II receptor and is then capable of generating a signal to the cell. This signaling requires the type I receptor to have an active kinase domain[35]. Different isoforms of type I and II receptors exist, and it is postulated that the isoform of the type I receptor determines the nature of the biological response, and that the type II receptor determines ligand-bonding specificity.

The type III receptor, betaglycan, is a broadly distributed membrane proteoglycan (approximately 280 kDa) with a 100 kDa protein core to which TGF-β binds directly and with high affinity. Betaglycan serves to increase the effective affinity of the type I and II receptors for TGF-β, but does not provide a signaling function itself. Betaglycan bound to TGF-β is capable of binding to the type II receptor, which then associates with a type I receptor, resulting in the dissociation of betaglycan. Cells lacking betaglycan are quite insensitive to TGF-β2, although they remain sensitive to TGF-β1 because the affinity of the type II receptor is much greater for TGF-β1 than for TGF-β2. Betaglycan increases the affinity of the signaling receptor for TGF-β2 so that it becomes comparable to that for TGF-β1[36]. Some transformed cells may lack one or more of the receptors (reviewed in reference 27).

Activation of tonsillar B cells increases the number of high-affinity receptors expressed from approximately 200 to approximately 1200 per cell, as measured by binding of $^{125}$I-labeled TGF-β1 to cells. By the inclusion of a protein crosslinker in these assays, Kehrl *et al.*[6] demonstrated the presence of both type I and II receptors on activated tonsillar B cells.

The signaling mechanism is basically unknown, although recent evidence indicates that the type I receptor kinase domain, but not the type II receptor kinase domain, binds the immunophilin FKBP-12 and that this binding can be inhibited by FK506[37]. This binding was identified using the two-hybrid system in yeast.

## REGULATION OF SYNTHESIS AND ACTIVATION OF TGF-β

TGF-β1 has been detected by immunohistochemistry both intra- and extra-cellularly in numerous tissues throughout embyronic development and adulthood[38]. The intensity of staining varies between tissues and cells types within a given tissue. TGF-β mRNA is also synthesized in numerous cell types freshly isolated or in culture[1,39]. The immunohistologic distribution of a particular TGF-β does not always correlate with the distribution of the corresponding mRNA, a discrepancy that probably results from accumulation of the protein away from the sites of synthesis or a lack of translation of the mRNA.

The expression of active TGF-β is highly regulated, which is as expected, since so many cells can synthesize it and have receptors for it. The expression of active TGF-β has been shown to be regulated at several levels: (1) by regulation of transcription mRNA, (2) by regulation of stability of mRNA, (3) by regulation of translation of mRNA, (4) by regulation of storage of latent protein inside platelets, (5) by regulation of activation of TGF-β after secretion in the latent form, and (6) by concentration for delivery to receptors (by the type III receptor betaglycan)[40], or, alternatively, (7) by sequestration of the protein by extracellular matrix and circulating proteins, e.g. α-macroglobulin[1,27,41–43].

## TGF-β EXPRESSION IS REGULATED BY SEVERAL CYTOKINES AND CELL ACTIVATORS

TGF-β1 mRNA is induced by TGF-β1 itself at both the transcriptional and post-transcriptional levels, with the mechanisms differing among different cell types[44]. Induction of transcription by TGF-β1 involves the AP-1 (Jun/Fos) transcription factor complex in human lung adenocarcinoma cells[45]. Although AP-1 can also be induced by phorbol esters (PMAs) which activate protein kinase C (PKC), treatment of human peripheral blood T cells with phorbol ester and ionomycin only marginally increases the expression of TGF-β mRNA[46]. This suggests that the autocrine induction of TGF-β1 may involve additional factors (see below) and/or that AP-1 may not be involved in induction of transcription of TGF-β1 mRNA in all cell types. PMA treatment stabilizes TGF-β1 mRNA in a promonocyte line (U937) by about 5-fold (from a half-life of 6 h to become almost as stable as rRNA), and probably also in the erythroblast line K562, but does not appear to stabilize TGF-β1 mRNA in a fibroblast or two ephithelial cell lines[41]. Autoinduction of TGF-β2 and TGF-β3 mRNA also occurs, but with different kinetics and apparently not via induction of AP-1[47]. The three TGF-βs also regulate the expression of each other in complex patterns[44].

The cytokines IL-2 and IL-7 also regulate TGF-β mRNA production. IL-2 induces TGF-β1 mRNA expression in macrophages[48]. IL-7, a growth factor for pre-B cells, inhibits the constitutive and IL-2-induced transcription of the TGF-β gene in peritoneal macrophages and in a monocyte cell line[48]. This repression does not require protein synthesis and thus appears to be a direct effect of IL-7. IL-10 inhibits expression of active TGF-β1 when added to mouse bone marrow cultures[49].

IL-1α induces mouse splenic T cells to produce active TGF-β, but has no obvious effect on the level of TGF-β mRNA. Concanavalin (Con) A also induces production of active TGF-β in these same cultures, but the combination of IL-1α and Con A does not. The induction by IL-1α requires protein synthesis[50].

Expression of TGF-β mRNA and secretion of active TGF-β are both induced by about 10–50-fold in tonsillar T cells activated by phytohemagglutinin (PHA)[51]. TGF-β mRNA was shown to be induced maximally within 2 h, and secretion of TGF-β reaches maximal levels 3–4 days after stimulation. Both the $CD4^+$ and $CD8^+$ subsets were shown to contain TGF-β mRNA, and the T-lymphoma line Jurkat was found to constitutively secrete active TGF-β in these studies. Mouse thymic epithelial cells express TGF-β1 and 2, but not TGF-β3, on their surface, and some thymic epithelial cell lines synthesize TGF-β1 and TGF-β2, but not TGF-β3[40].

Transcription of TGF-β is also induced by the tumor suppressor protein Rb in some cell types, by interaction with at least two different transcription factors. Rb appears to interact with the transcription factor Sp1, which binds to the promoter for TGF-β1 at the multiple *retinoblastoma control elements*[52]. TGF-β2 and TGF-β3 promoters also have multiple copies of the *retinoblastoma control element*[53], although Sp1 only increases transcription driven by the TGF-β1 and TGF-β3 promoters and not the TGF-β2 promoter[54]. Rb also binds to the transcription factor ATF-2, and together these bind to the TGF-β2 promoter, and activate transcription[55]. Interestingly, TGF-β1 also regulates Rb expression (see below).

## TGF-β IS SYNTHESIZED BY B CELLS

Highly purified human peripheral blood B cells can be induced by treatment with a monoclonal antibody (mAb) to IgM to express mRNA for TGF-β, as assayed by RNA blotting. The mRNA is transiently induced, with a maximum of 2 h of treatment, and is no longer detectable by 14 h. In the absence of induction, no mRNA is detected[56]. Using the more sensitive polymerase chain reaction (PCR) assay, purified peripheral blood B cells were shown to contain mRNA for TGF-β1, and the levels were shown by a PCR assay to be up-regulated by culture with a human T-cell supernatant and an irradiated subline of the mouse EL-4 T-cell line[57]. The mRNA remained elevated for several days in the latter study, in which B cells were activated by T cells[57]. Limiting dilution analyses demonstrated that at least 85 per cent of the activated B cells expressed TGF-β mRNA[57]. The expression of TGF-β protein was not examined in either of these studies.

Activation with the polyclonal B-cell mitogen *Staphylococcus aureus* Cowan (SAC) slightly upregulates TGF-β mRNA levels in human tonsillar B cells[58], but has a much greater effect on the secretion of protein. Kehrl *et al.* demonstrated that tonsillar B cells secrete latent TGF-β, and this secretion is stimulated 7-fold by SAC[58]. If activated by acid treatment, the levels of TGF-β secreted are adequate to almost completely inhibit proliferation of these B cells, i.e. 0.5–0.8 ng/ml. However, in the absence of activation, the amount of active TGF-β in the cultures only marginally inhibits DNA synthesis, as demonstrated by the small stimulatory effect of adding antibody to TGF-β1 to the cultures[58]. Less than 10 per cent of the secreted TGF-β1 is estimated to be in the active form[6], and latent TGF-β2 is also detected in these cultures.

In the adult mouse bone marrow about 75 per cent of a population consisting of $B220^+,sIg^-$ and pre-B cells have TGF-β on their surface, as detected by immunohistochemistry[5]. Splenic mouse B cells activated with lipopolysaccharide (LPS) have been demonstrated by Snapper *et al.* (1993)[59] to secrete active TGF-β using a standard bioassay. Since the cells were cultured in bovine fetal calf serum which contains TGF-β, presumably released by platelets in the blood, it was not possible to determine the absolute amount of TGF-β. However, the authors demonstrated that LPS-activated B cells, but not untreated B cells, secrete 10 pg/ml above background levels of active TGF-β when cultured at $10^5$ cells/ml for 48 h. Whether these cells secrete an additional amount in the inactive form was not determined.

TGF-β is also secreted by human chronic lymphocytic leukemia B (BCLL) cells, some apparently in the active form, since antibody to TGF-β1 increases proliferation of these cells in culture. Treatment with anti-μ antibody induces BCLL cells to synthesize TGF-β, and the addition of PMA increases the amount secreted to 5 ng/ml[60]. This secreted TGF-β may explain the slow growth rate of BCLL, since treatment of BCLL cells with a combination of anti-μ and anti-TGF-β induces greater proliferation than treatment with anti-μ alone[60].

Mouse B-lymphoma cell lines can be stimulated by treatment with anti-IgM to secrete large amounts of active TGF-β. Specifically, Warner *et al.*[61] observed that three B-lymphoma lines, WEHI-231, CH31 and CH12, secrete 3–5 ng of active TGF-β per ml when cultured with anti-IgM (10 μg/ml) for 20 h at $2 \times 10^5$ cells/ml. This amount of TGF-β inhibits proliferation of these B lymphomas. Less than 0.6 ng/ml of active TGF-β is secreted in the absence of stimulation with anti-IgM. These investigators did not determine whether there was an additional amount of secreted TGF-β in the latent form in any of these cultures. The secreted TGF-β does not appear to cause the inhibition of proliferation induced by anti-IgM treatment of the WEHI-231 and CH31 lymphomas, because treatment with anti-TGF-β does not reverse the inhibition by anti-IgM, and because these authors obtained variants of WEHI-231 which are resistant to the antiproliferative effects of TGF-β but still sensitive to anti-Ig. The differences between the effects of anti-Ig and TGF-β on proliferation of B cells is discussed further on pp. 297–298. TGF-β has also been detected on the surface of the mouse pre-B-cell line 70Z/3, and on the surfaces of the mouse B-lymphoma lines WEHI-231 and WEHI-279[5].

Plasmacytoma-bearing mice develop a polyclonal B-cell immunodeficiency characterized by marked impairment of both antibody responses and proliferative responses to B-cell mitogens. This may be explained by the finding that the ascites of mice with plasmacytomas contain TGF-β (0.5–1 ng/ml)[62]. Cultures of total spleen cells from these mice contain about five times more TGF-β (0.1–0.2 ng/ml) than do comparable cultures from normal mice. Although the source of the TGF-β in these mice is unknown, Berg and

Lynch demonstrated that an *in vitro* plasmacytoma line secretes small amounts (0.06 ng/ml) of latent TGF-β[62].

In conclusion, it appears likely that the majority, and perhaps all, of both normal and transformed mouse and human B cells synthesize and secrete TGF-β in the latent and/or active forms. Furthermore, activation of B cells and B-cell lymphomas and leukemias increases the level of mRNA for TGF-β, expression of surface receptors for TGF-β, and production of active TGF-β. It also appears likely that most T cells can secrete TGF-β. However, almost nothing is known about the regulation of secretion of TGF-β and the production of the active versus latent forms.

## THE EFFECT OF TGF-β ON B-CELL PROLIFERATION

In several different systems, TGF-β has been found to inhibit proliferation of both normal B cells and B-cell lines without decreasing cell viability, but in other experimental systems to induce apoptosis. Both TGF-β1 and TGF-β2 inhibit the induction by SAC and IL-2 of proliferation of tonsillar B cells, as assayed by thymidine incorporation, but addition of increasing amounts of IL-2 restores the proliferation to 90 per cent of the level in the absence of TGF-β1[6,58]. TGF-β had no effect on cell viability in these experiments. TGF-β (2–10 ng/ml) inhibits by 80 per cent the proliferation of tonsillar B cells induced by antibody to CD40 + PMA[63], or by CD40L expressed on the surface of CV1/EBNA cells[64]. The addition of IL-4 partially restores the proliferation[64]. TGF-β also inhibits by greater than 95 per cent the proliferation of dense tonsillar B cells which is induced by treatments with antibody to CD20 + B-cell growth factor[63]. TGF-β inhibits proliferation of purified peripheral blood B cells induced by the EL-4 mouse T-cell line + IL-1β[65].

TGF-β (1 ng/ml; 40 pM) also completely inhibits the ability of LPS-induced mouse splenic B cells to give rise to B-cell colonies in agar[5]. TGF-β was maintained in the cultures for the entire duration of the 6-day assay, and had no effect if only present for 1 to 2 h. When TGF-β (2.5 ng/ml) is added at the initiation of cultures of dense splenic B cells induced by LPS or by anti-IgM + IL-4 + immobilized anti-class II antibody, it inhibits thymidine incorporation by 90–95 per cent at 3 days[66]. Cross and Cambier also found that TGF-β inhibits proliferation of B-cell blasts produced by prior treatment with LPS + dextran sulfate for 47 h[66]. By cell cycle analysis with acridine orange staining, they demonstrated that TGF-β causes an accumulation of splenic B cells in G1 phase, whether TGF-β is added to resting B cells or to B-cell blasts[66].

Many B-cell lines and tumors appear to be about as sensitive as normal B cells to growth inhibition by TGF-β. Treatment of the mouse B-cell lymphoma WEHI-231 with $\geq$ 1 ng/ml of TGF-β for 18–24 h inhibits thymidine incorporation by 80 per cent[61]. As described above, human BCLL cells are characterized by a slow growth rate and have been shown to synthesize TGF-β. TGF-β inhibits by 80 per cent the DNA synthesis induced by treatment with antibody to CD40[60]. As is also generally true for normal B cells, TGF-β does not completely inhibit DNA synthesis of BCLL cells, even when 10 μg of TGF-β per ml is added. Infection with Epstein–Barr virus (EBV) appears to slightly reduce the inhibitory effect of TGF-β on proliferation of human B cells[67]. In contrast, TGF-β has no effect on proliferation of the mouse pre-B leukemia line 70Z/3[5]. This is not due to a lack of response to TGF-β, because the expression of surface Igκ chains is markedly reduced by TGF-β in 70Z/3.

TGF-β must be added at the initiation of the cultures to obtain full inhibition, suggesting that it acts during the G1 phase. In experiments in which proliferation of purified peripheral blood B cells was induced with $F(ab')_2$ anti-μ + B-cell growth factor, delay of addition of TGF-β by 6 h reduced inhibition of DNA synthesis measured at 64 h from 90 per cent to 70 per cent. Delay of addition to 40 h completely eliminated the inhibition[56]. This is consistent with findings in other cell types which indicate that TGF-β arrests or delays the cell cycle in the G1 phase, but has no effect once cells have entered S phase[1,68].

Gold *et al.*[69] suggested that rather than reversibly arresting B-lymphoma cells in G1 phase, TGF-β instead delays their progression through G1, because they found that if WEHI-231 lymphoma cells are treated with TGF-β (1 ng/ml) for 76 h, and thymidine incorporation is measured at 72–76 h, DNA synthesis is only inhibited by 40 per cent[69]. They also found that if DNA synthesis was assayed in individual cells by measuring bromodeoxyuridine incorporation from 72 to 96 h after adding TGF-β, 97 per cent of the cells incorporated bromodeoxyuridine. Thus, they concluded that TGF-β does not cause cell cycle arrest, but instead delays progression through G1 phase. Furthermore, they found that inhibition of proliferation is quantitatively reversible when TGF-β is removed, even after 3 days in TGF-β. These results indicate that the mechanism of inhibition by TGF-β of proliferation differs from that of anti-Ig, whether or not TGF-β reversibly arrests or delays the cell cycle, since anti-Ig treatment of WEHI-231 cells causes an irreversible arrest in G1 phase and programmed cell death. Another difference is that LPS can prevent growth arrest caused by anti-Ig, but not that caused by treatment with TGF-β[69].

Other experiments suggest that in certain systems TGF-β can induce programmed cell death, or apoptosis. Warner *et al.*[61] found that treatment of three different B lymphomas (WEHI-231, CH12 and CH31) with TGF-β (10 ng/ml) results in arrest in G1, followed by apoptosis, which is first apparent after 24–48 h, as evidenced by appearance of a DNA ladder on agarose gels. Lomo *et al.* also found that apoptosis is stimulated in cultures of resting peripheral blood B cells treated for 48 h with TGF-β (1–10 ng/ml)[70]. These authors examined the effect of TGF-β on constitutive levels of Bcl-2, an oncoprotein that inhibits apoptosis, and found that it is not reduced by TGF-β treatment for 48 h[70]. When germinal center B cells are put into culture they undergo apoptosis. TGF-β (1 ng/ml) inhibits the rescue from apoptosis by anti-Ig treatment of mouse germinal center B cells, although it does not inhibit the rescue by antibody to CD40[71].

Several other cell types have been demonstrated to undergo apoptosis after treatment with TGF-β: cultured rabbit uterine epithelial cells[72], rat hepatocytes and rat liver *in vivo*[73], and the mouse myeloid cell line M1[74]. TGF-β induces 90 per cent of M1 cells to undergo apoptosis after 3 days of treatment. Prior to apoptosis, at days 1–2, the cells arrest in G1 phase. The induction of apoptosis in M1 cells is accompanied by a decrease in levels of *c-myc, c-myb* and *bcl-2* mRNAs and proteins, and induction of mRNA for a myeloid primary response gene (*MyD*) called *MyD118*. By stable transfection of anti-sense expression constructs for *MyD118*, Selvakumaran *et al.*[74] provided evidence suggesting that induction of this gene is necessary for induction of apoptosis in M1 cell. Overexpression of Bcl-2 prevents apoptosis induced by TGF-β in these cells, but does not prevent cell cycle arrest in G1 phase.

In conclusion, it appears that arrest of the cell cycle by TGF-β results in apoptosis in some cells, whereas in other cell types or systems the arrest is reversible. In most reports, TGF-β does not reduce the viability of pre-B cells or B cells or B-cell lines, although it appears that in a few systems apoptosis is induced after more than one day of treatment. Regulation of Bcl-2 appears to be important for determining whether cells undergo apoptosis in response to TGF-β[74].

Although TGF-β inhibits proliferation of B cells in the presence of a variety of other cytokines or B-cell activators, it appears possible that helper T cells may be able to overcome this inhibition, consistent with findings discussed above indicating that antibody to CD40 can rescue germinal center B cells from apoptosis even in the presence of TGF-β. Ehrhardt *et al.*[75] found that if splenic B cells are activated with either of two different Th2 lines and TGF-β is added on day 1, the addition of TGF-β actually increases the yield of viable B cells on day 4 by 2–3-fold, although after day 6 TGF-β treatment results in reduced cell survival. In this same report the authors found, as have others, that TGF-β added after one day of activation with LPS or anti-δ dextran reduces B-cell proliferation. IL-4 can partially rescue peripheral blood B cells from the apoptosis induced by TGF-β[70].

## MECHANISM OF INHIBITION OF PROLIFERATION BY TGF-β

TGF-β modifies the expression or activity of a number of proteins that regulate the G1 phase of the cell cycle. Treatment of CH31 mouse B-lymphoma cells with TGF-β for 20 h reduces the level of *c-myc* mRNA present in these cells[76]. TGF-β treatment for 3 h also reduces the already very low level of *c-myc* mRNA present in purified human peripheral blood B cells and slightly reduces the induction of *c-myc* mRNA by anti-Ig in these cells[56], or induced in anti-Ig-treated dense tonsillar B cells[63]. Fischer *et al.*[76] also found that treatment of CH31 cells for 5 h with TGF-β (1 ng/ml) very much reduces the amount of c-Myc protein detected.

TGF-β also appears to block the phosphorylation of Rb, an anti-oncogene that regulates cell cycle progression and is differentially phosphorylated during the cell cycle[76–78]. Hypophosphorylated Rb reversibly arrests cell cycle progression in G1, preventing entry into S phase. Fischer *et al.* demonstrated that WEHI-231 cells treated with TGF-β for 24 h mostly have the hypophosphorylated, growth-suppressive form of Rb, but if anti-sense oligonucleotide for *c-myc* (but not a non-specific oligonucleotide) is added simultaneously with TGF-β, Rb is found almost completely in the hyperphosphorylated form[76]. In these particular experiments, the anti-sense *c-myc* oligonucleotide actually increased the levels of *c-myc* mRNA and protein. The c-Myc and Rb proteins have been shown to physically associate[79].

C-Myc has also been shown to function downstream of Rb protein by co-injection experiments into osteosarcoma cells[80]. In these microinjection experiments, c-Myc was found to antagonize and to be dominant to Rb. This is consistent with the finding that downregulation of *c-myc* transcription by TGF-β is blocked by viral-transforming proteins that bind Rb (SV40 T antigen, adenovirus type 5 E1A, and human papilloma virus type 16 E7), suggesting that Rb may be an intermediary in regulation of *c-myc* by TGF-β[68,81]. Furthermore, mutations of the Rb-binding sites of E1A and SV40 T antigen abrogate the ability of these proteins to modulate the TGF-β repression of *c-myc* transcription. Transient transfection of an expression plasmid for the Rb gene can inhibit *c-myc* transcription, and the addition of TGF-β does not inhibit further[81]. The same DNA element within the *c-myc* promoter, termed TIE or TCE, is necessary for inhibition by either the transfected Rb gene or by TGF-β. Although binding of nuclear proteins to this promoter element is decreased by TGF-β treatment, it appears that the Rb protein itself does not bind to this element. TGF-β also appears able to reduce transcription of *c-myc* by a mechanism not involving Rb, since a prostrate carcinoma line with a mutant non-functional Rb gene also responds to TGF-β treatment by reduction in transcription of *c-myc* in a nuclear run-on assay[82].

TGF-β also negatively regulates cell cycle progression by its effect on another target of Rb, the transcription factor E2F, which controls transcription of several S-phase genes, including DNA polymerase α and thymidine kinase, Mv1Lu (mink lung epithelial) cells. Hypophosphorylated Rb binds and negatively regulates the activity of E2F[83]. Furthermore, treatment with TGF-β (2.5 ng/ml) for 24 h greatly reduces the levels of E2F mRNA (by at least 10-fold). Overexpression of E2F completely abrogates the 10-fold inhibition of DNA synthesis by TGF-β[84].

Recently it has been demonstrated that TGF-β inhibits activation of certain members of the family of cyclin-dependent kinases (CDKs). CDKs are a family of kinases which are activated by association with cyclins, and which catalyze transitions between phases of the cell cycle. Progression from G1 to S phase in mammalian cells involves activation of cyclin E–Cdk2, cyclin D–Cdk4, and cyclin A–Cdk2 complexes[85,86]. Cyclins D1 and E accumulate in G1, and the kinetics of cyclin A accumulation suggest a role in S phase. In mid-G1, Cdk2 associates with cyclin E, and this complex is believed to function in controlling progression through G1. The activity of Cdk2 is first evident at this time, when it may phosphorylate Rb[77]. Rb can also regulate Cdk activity[87]. TGF-β, or contact inhibition, have recently been shown to inhibit activation of cyclin E–Cdk2 in G1, resulting in the accumulation of an inactive cyclin E–Cdk2 complex and cell cycle arrest in late G1 phase[88–90]. TGF-β-treated and contact-inhibited cells contain a titratable excess of a 27- or 28-kDa protein ($p27^{Kip1}$ or $p28^{ICK}$) that binds to cyclin E–Cdk2 complexes and prevents their activation[90,91]. p27/28 appears to act stoichiometrically rather than catalytically. This inhibitory protein also binds, but less well, to the cyclin D2–Cdk4 complex. It is not understood how TGF-β regulates the levels of the 27–28-kDa inhibitor. In their discussion, Polyak *et al.*[91] point out that during cell cycle arrest, cells accumulate inactive cyclin E–Cdk2 complexes and, thus, recovery from arrest might not require synthesis of new cyclin E. This might be useful *in vivo* to allow rapid re-entry into cycle when the growth-inhibitory signals cease. Furthermore, $p27^{Kip1}$ is present in proliferating cells, where it might be involved in setting a threshold requirement for cyclin E for regulating the $G_1$ to S transition.

TGF-β also reduces synthesis of Cdk4 by reducing translation of the mRNA, resulting in a net reduction in cyclin D–Cdk4 complexes[77,92,93]. Constitutive expression of Cdk4 in Mv1Lu cells renders these cells unresponsive to TGF-β[92]. TGF-β also induces synthesis of another CDK inhibitor, $p15^{Ink4B}$, which binds to and inhibits cyclin D–Cdk4 and cyclin D–Cdk6 complexes[94]. TGF-β induces the mRNA for p15 by 30-fold in human keratinocytes. Although the above studies of the mechanism of cell cycle arrest were performed in mink lung epithelial cells, HeLa cells, and mouse or human keratinocytes, it is likely that at least some of these mechanisms also occur in B cells.

In conclusion, TGF-β appears to reversibly arrest cells in late $G_1$ phase, and also in some cases to induce apoptosis, through effects on several proteins important in cell cycle progression, interfering with activities of at least three different cyclin–Cdk complexes by at least three mechanisms. Inhibition of the cyclin–Cdk complexes appears to result in maintenance of Rb in the hypophosphorylated growth-suppressive state. The resulting hypophosphorylated Rb has inhibitory effects on transcription of several genes, including *c-myc* and perhaps E2F mRNAs, which may be necessary for transition into S phase. TGF-β can also repress *c-myc* transcription by an Rb-independent mechanism. TGF-β also represses synthesis of c-Myb and Bcl-2.

## REGULATION OF DEVELOPMENT OF B AND T CELLS

Very few data are available on whether TGF-β affects development of B cells. Rehmann and LeBien[95] reported that TGF-β reduces the frequency of appearance of surface $Ig^+$(sIg) B cells expressing Igλ chains in cultures of human fetal bone marrow pre-B cells which spontaneously differentiate in culture, but has no effect on the frequency of appearance of $sIg\kappa^+$ cells. When purified pre-B cells were cultured for 3 days, an average of 27 per cent of the cells become $s\lambda^+$, but if TGF-β (1 ng/ml) is added to the cultures, 21 per cent become $s\lambda^+$, with an average inhibition of about 30 per cent. The results were statistically significant. Rehmann and LeBien speculate that TGF-β may be involved in development of B cells *in vivo*, since the ratio of $\kappa^+$ to $\lambda^+$ cells which develop *in vivo* is greater than the ratio which develop in *in vitro* cultures in the absence of TGF-β.

Somewhat different results were obtained by Lee *et al.*[5], who found that TGF-β inhibits development of B-cell colonies by 90 per cent in 6-day cultures of mouse bone marrow B-cell precursors. The frequency of B cells expressing sIgκ in these colonies is reduced by 60 per cent relative to B cells developing in the absence of TGF-β. They did not examine λ expression. TGF-β also reduces the numbers of pre-B cells ($c\mu^+$, $\kappa^-$) recovered from the cultures. It is not known for either of these experimental models whether the effects of TGF-β are to regulate rearrangement of the light chain genes and/or to regulate RNA expression or proliferation after formation of functional light chain genes. Lee *et al.* did, however, demonstrate that either TGF-β1 or TGF-β2 can dramatically inhibit LPS- or IL-1-induced expression of sIgκ and κ mRNA in the pre-B-cell line 70Z/3. There is no effect on μ mRNA, which is not induced by LPS treatment. 70Z/3 cells have rearranged κ genes, but do not express sIg or κ mRNA unless they are induced with LPS, or a few other inducers. Thus, the effect of TGF-β on expression of sIgκ by bone marrow cells might be due to inhibition of induction of expression of κ RNA by LPS, since LPS is included in their agar cultures. It appears possible that TGF-β may be involved in the development of B cells in the bone marrow, since TGF-β is found on the surface of the majority of nucleated cells in mouse bone marrow, including B-lineage cells[5].

This hypothesis is strengthened by a recent paper which indicates that TGF-β is involved in regulation of development of T cells in the thymus. Takahama *et al.*[40] demonstrated that the differentiation of $CD4^-/CD8^{lo}$ cells into $CD4^+/CD8^+$ thymocytes requires at least one cell division in culture, and that this differentiation step is specifically retarded by addition of TGF-β1,

TGF-β2 or TGF-β3. TGF-β was shown to prevent CD4⁻/CD8^lo cells from entering S phase, and the authors speculated that this was the mechanism of inhibition of expression of CD4. Furthermore, they demonstrated that thymic epithelial cells in the subcapsular and cortical areas of the thymus (where $CD4^-/CD8^{lo}$ cells are located) express TGF-β1 and TGF-β2 on their surface. They also found that thymic epithelial lines which have TGF-β on their surface are capable of inhibiting this differentiation step *in vitro*, but those that do not express TGF-β do not inhibit. Medullary thymocyte lines do not express TGF-β on their surface. Furthermore, Takahama *et al.*[40] found that the TGF-β on the thymic epithelial lines is bound to the type III receptor, betaglycan, and that TGF-β cannot be detected in the culture supernatant of these cells. They speculate that the function of the TGF-β is to slow down development of T cells in order to allow adequate time for negative selection to prevent development of autoreactive T cells, fitting with the finding that TGF-β knockout mice suffer from an apparent autoimmune disorder with massive lymphocyte infiltration of multiple organs[15,16].

Takahama *et al.*[40] found that TGF-β alone does not affect differentiation of double-negative ($CD4^-/CD8^-$) thymocytes to $CD4^-/CD8^{lo}$ cells in single-cell suspension culture. Evidence from other groups suggests, however, that TGF-β may function at additional stages of thymocyte development, since TGF-β has been found to upregulate expression of CD8α on double-negative thymocytes cultured with IL-2 or with IL-7+TNFα[96,97].

## REGULATION OF DIFFERENTIATION OF B CELLS BY TGF-β

### EXPRESSION OF CELL SURFACE RECEPTORS

TGF-β has several effects on differentiation of mature B cells. It has been shown to inhibit expression of CD23 (FcεRII) and the transferrin receptor on mouse splenic B cells[62]. In contrast, TGF-β has been shown to increase expression of MHC class II molecules on mature B cells[62,66], and to synergize with IL-4 or interferon-γ (IFN-γ) to induce class II expression on 70Z/3 pre-B cells[5]. TGF-β alone induces a 1.5-fold increase in class II expression on resting and a 3-fold increase on LPS-activated mouse splenic B cells[66]. The induction of class II expression on resting B cells is transient with maximum expression at 18 h and return to baseline at 48 h[66].

### SYNTHESIS AND SECRETION OF Ig

TGF-β has been shown to reduce expression of Ig in many different systems. As described above, TGF-β greatly inhibits induction by LPS or IL-1 of expression of sIgκ and κ mRNA by 70Z/3 pre-B cells[5]. The induction by LPS and the inhibition by TGF-β both occur at the transcriptional level, as demonstrated by a nuclear run-on assay[98]. TGF-β does not, however, inhibit the induction by IFN-γ of κ gene transcription, or have any effect on expression of μ mRNA, which is not affected by LPS treatment of these cells.

Addition of TGF-β during activation of mouse splenic B cells with LPS for one or two days inhibits the induction of sIgκ expression, but does not reduce constitutive expression of sIgκ on splenic B cells. It has no effect on expression of surface Ig or μ or κ mRNAs in two B-cell lymphomas (WEHI-279 and WEHI-231)[5,62].

Kehrl *et al.* examined the effect of TGF-β on expression of Ig in human tonsillar B cells activated by SAC and IL-2, and found that treatment with TGF-β (2–5 ng/ml) for 4 days greatly reduces surface expression of IgM, IgD, IgA, κ and λ chains[99], and completely inhibits secretion of IgM and IgG[6,58]. Inhibition requires several days of treatment. The levels of κ mRNA are reduced within 2 days by 70 per cent and within 4 days by 85 per cent, which appears to account for the 80 per cent inhibition of κ chain biosynthesis on day 4. This inhibition occurs at the transcriptional level, as an 85 per cent reduction in the rate of transcription of κ chain RNA on day 5 after TGF-β addition is observed in nuclear run-on assays. The level of λ chain mRNA is also reduced, by 80 per cent on day 4.

Interestingly, the effect of TGF-β on μ mRNA appears to be specific for the form that encodes secreted IgM. After 4 days of treatment, the secreted form can barely be detected, whereas the overall level of μ mRNA is only reduced by 50 per cent[99]. The secreted form of mRNA detected with a Cγ1 probe is reduced by 60 per cent. Treatment with TGF-β (0.1 ng/ml) for 3 days also reduces mRNA for the secreted form of Ig α chains and secretion of IgA by about 50 per cent in the 4F2 clone of the mouse CH12.LX B lymphoma[100]. Expression of sIgA and the membrane-bound forms of α mRNA are not reduced. Simultaneous treatment of 4F2 cells with LPS (10 μg/ml) overcomes the inhibition of secretion of IgA by TGF-β. Altogether these data suggest that TGF-β inhibits production of secreted Igs of all classes, and that the inhibition of expression of surface Ig by TGF-β may be due mostly to inhibition of light chain gene transcription, rather than inhibition of synthesis of the membrane form of Ig heavy chains. The mechanism of specific inhibition of production of secreted heavy chain mRNA is unknown. Since inhibition requires several days of treatment, it appears possible that the effects are indirect.

### Mechanism of Inhibition of Ig Synthesis by TGF-β

As described above, TGF-β1 and TGF-β2 (2 ng/ml) completely inhibit production of secreted IgM and IgG by cultured tonsillar B cells stimulated with SAC and IL-2[6,58]. Kehrl *et al.*[58] demonstrated that this profound inhibition is not a secondary effect due to inhibition of cell proliferation by TGF-β, because addition of increasing amounts of IL-2 reduces the inhibition of proliferation to about 10 per cent without effect on the profound inhibition of IgM and IgG production. These results suggest that there is a divergence in the signaling pathways resulting in inhibition of cell proliferation of Ig secretion. Contrasting results were obtained by Coffman *et al.*, who examined the effect of TGF-β and IL-2 on proliferation of and secretion or Igs by LPS-activated mouse splenic B cells[18,101]. They only used IL-2 at one concentration (10 ng/ml) and found that it did not overcome the inhibition of proliferation due to TGF-β treatment, but that IL-2 partially overcame the inhibition of secretion of Igs. Nonetheless, these results are probably consistent with the conclusion that the signaling pathways induced by TGF-β which lead to inhibition of proliferation and inhibition of secretion diverge.

To investigate the mechanism of inhibition of transcription of the κ chain gene by TGF-β, Briskin *et al.*[98] asked whether binding activity of the transcription factor NKκB, which is important for induction of transcription of the Ig κ gene and is induced by LPS, is inhibited by TGF-β in an electrophoretic mobility shift assay (EMSA). They found that NFκB is induced by LPS treatment of 70Z/3 cells, but that this induction is not inhibited by TGF-β. Similarly, Kehrl *et al.*[99] found that TGF-β has no effect on the binding activity of NFκB in tonsillar B cells activated by SAC + IL-2.

Kehrl *et al.*[99] did find, however, that the binding of AP-1 to a consensus binding site is greatly reduced in activated tonsillar B cells or in unactivated BJA-B cells after treatment with TGF-β for 24 h. This is a surprising result, since it has been shown that mRNAs for a few AP-1 family members (c-Jun, JunB, and c-Fos) are induced differentially in several cell types by TGF-β, although levels of these mRNAs in B cells have not been examined[82,102,103]. Perhaps early downregulation of AP-1 binding activity is not due to regulation at the mRNA level, or different members of the Fos and Jun family are downregulated by TGF-β, as the particular AP-1 factors detected in the EMSA in the B-cell extracts were not identified. Although AP-1 has not been shown to be involved in regulation of transcription of Ig genes, AP-1 is involved in TGF-β induction of transcription of the TGF-β gene[45], and an AP-1-like sites is involved in TGF-β-mediated suppression of transcription of the transin gene[104].

The B- and T-cell-specific transcription factor Oct-2 may be a mediator of inhibition of transcription κ chain genes by TGF-β. As described above, TGF-β inhibits the induction of κ gene transcription induced by LPS in 70Z/3 cells, but not transcription of the μ gene, which is not induced by LPS. Miller *et al.*[105] showed that LPS also induces Oct-2 transcription and protein in 70Z/3 cells (but not Oct-1), and TGF-β causes a reduction in the level of Oct-2 mRNA by 19 h but does not eliminate it. They did not examine the effect of TGF-β on Oct-2 protein levels or binding to DNA, or examine the effect of TGF-β on Oct-1. Miller *et al.* suggested that Oct-2 may contribute to regulation of κ gene transcription, since TGF-β coordinately regulates both these genes, and because the induction of Oct-2 by LPS precedes the induction of κ. To explain why μ gene transcription is not inhibited by TGF-β or induced by LPS, Miller *et al.* point out that there are two adjacent Oct-binding sites in heavy chain promoters, but only one in κ chain promoters, suggesting that a higher amount of Oct-2 would be required for κ transcription, whereas the basal level might be adequate for transcription of the μ gene. These conclusions appear to disagree, however, with those of Kehrl *et al.*[99], who found that TGF-β treatment of activated tonsillar cells for one or two days does not result in inhibition of binding of Oct-1 or Oct-2 to a consensus octamer site.

A recent study on the inhibition of transcription of the IL-2 gene by TGF-β in T cells further suggests, however, that Oct proteins are involved. Brabletz *et al.*[7] demonstrated that TGF-β inhibits by 80 per cent transcription driven by the IL-2 promoter in mouse EL-4 T-lymphoma cells induced with PMA and Con A. This inhibition is due to an element in the IL-2 promoter called UPS, which contains a noncanonical octamer element that can bind Oct-1 and Oct-2 and an AP-1-like element. Binding to this latter element can be competed with by a consensus AP-1 site. They showed that mutation of either the octamer or AP-1 elements abolishes inhibition by TGF-β. Although TGF-β inhibits transcription driven by the UPS element, TGF-β does not inhibit binding of Oct-1, Oct-2, or AP-1 to the UPS element in nuclear extracts from EL-4 cells. These data suggest that TGF-β can inhibit the activity of Oct proteins by other means than reducing their binding. Transcriptional activity and binding activity are not always in perfect correspondence, since transcription factors can be activated or inactivated by modifications that do not affect their binding to DNA.

Brabletz *et al.*[7] also demonstrated that a multimerized oligonucleotide bearing an octamer element from the μ intron enhancer drives transcription that could be inhibited by TGF-β, but only by 40 per cent. Although these studies were performed in the EL-4 T-cell line, they also performed one experiment in the B-lymphoma line A20J, in which they demonstrated that the transcriptional activity of a fragment containing the μ intron enhancer could be inhibited by 75 per cent by TGF-β. They did not, however, determine which DNA sequences in the μ intron enhancer are required for this inhibition, although in an experiment whose data were not shown they found that TGF-β inhibits expression driven by a multimerized octamer element. Thus, it is tempting to speculate that an octamer element may be involved in inhibition of Ig transcription.

Although there are octamer elements in the Ig light (κ and λ) and heavy chain promoters, and in the κ and μ intron enhancers[106], they have not been identified in Ig Cλ enhancers[107,108]. However, Oct-binding sequences are quite variable, and thus not always readily recognized[109]. It is entirely possible that TGF-β also affects other factors that regulate light chain gene transcription in addition to Oct-2, since TGF-β is known to affect a surprising number of transcription factors.

One can speculate that the effects of TGF-β on inhibition of growth may also be mediated by Oct proteins, since Oct-1 is phosphorylated during the cell cycle by a $p34^{cdc2}$-related kinase, and appears to be involved in cell cycle regulation of transcription of the histone H2b gene[88,110,111]. Furthermore, it has recently been shown that Oct-2 is required for G1 progression and proliferation of B cells[112].

### Small Amounts of TGF-β Increase Secretion of Most Classes of Ig

All the above studies demonstrating that TGF-β inhibits production of secreted Ig involved adding TGF-β to the cultures at 0.1 ng/ml or more. Surprisingly, Snapper *et al.* demonstrated that low levels of TGF-β actually stimulate secretion of most antibody classes by LPS-activated purified splenic B cells[59]. This was demonstrated by the addition of anti-TGF-β antibody to cultures induced with LPS ± other cytokines required to induce isotype-specific switching, with the finding that anti-TGF-β antibody causes more than a 10-fold reduction of IgG2a, a 9-fold reduction in IgG3, and a 2–3-fold reduction in IgG1 and IgE secretion, but has no effect on IgM secretion. As described above, these authors detected picogram quantities of active TGF-β in cultures of LPS-activated B cells, but could not precisely quantitate the amount of TGF-β required for optimum synthesis of these Igs. If TGF-β is added back to cultures treated with an excess of anti-TGF-β antibody (30 μg/ml), about 0.2 ng of TGF-β per ml is adequate to restore levels of IgG3 secreted in the absence of anti-TGF-β antibody. Since TGF-β directs antibody class switching to IgA and IgG2b (see below), it could not be determined whether small amounts of TGF-β also stimulate secretion of these classes. Thus, in conclusion, although many reports have demonstrated that TGF-β, in quantities of 0.1 ng/ml or greater, inhibits production of secreted Igs of all classes, the results of Snapper *et al.*[59] indicate that very small amounts stimulate production of all classes except IgM.

## REGULATION OF ANTIBODY CLASS SWITCHING BY TGF-β

### TGF-β Induces Switching to IgA

The addition of TGF-β (with optimal amounts of 0.4–2 ng/ml) to cultures of LPS-activated splenic or Peyer's patch mouse B cells increases the frequency of detection of IgA-secreting cells and the production of IgA by 5–10-fold[18,19,113]. Prior depletion of sIgA$^+$ cells indicate that TGF-β acts on sIgA$^-$ cells. Furthermore, delay of the addition of TGF-β to 2 days after initiation of the cultures reduces the IgA produced, suggesting that TGF-β acts prior to switching[19,113]. In these first reports, the amount of IgA secreted in the TGF-β-treated cultures was quite low, less than 1 μg/ml, which is not really surprising, since TGF-β inhibits synthesis of Ig light and α heavy chain mRNAs[99,100]. However, secretion of IgA and detection of IgA-secreting cells was found to increase by 3–7-fold if IL-2 was added. To determine if the effect on switching is specific to IgA, the effect of TGF-β on secretion of IgM and IgG subclasses by LPS-activated B cells was also analyzed, and these early reports showed that TGF-β reduces secretion of IgM, IgG1 and IgG3, but has little or no effect on IgG2b or IgG2a at the doses tested. Addition of IL-2 or IL-5 does not restore secretion of IgG1, but in some, but not all, of the experiments partially restored production of IgM.

These reports did not address whether TGF-β actually increases the frequency of cells that undergo class switching to IgA, or instead increases proliferation of cells committed to switch or even cells that have already switched, but not producing enough IgA to have been removed during the preparation of sIgA$^-$ cells. To address this question, Kim and Kagnoff[114] performed limiting dilution experiments, first treating sIgA$^-$ splenic B cells with LPS and then diluting them into 160-μl cultures in the presence of TGF-β ± IL-2. TGF-β increased the frequency of clones secreting IgA by about 20-fold in the presence or absence of IL-2, without any effect on the size of the B-cell clones. These data suggest that TGF-β increases frequency of switching to IgA rather than outgrowth of cells committed to switch IgA. The total frequency of clones secreting any Ig class was reduced by 2–3-fold in cultures treated with TGF-β, in keeping with the known inhibition of cell proliferation and Ig secretion of TGF-β.

The frequency of IgA-secreting cells induced in bulk cultures with LPS + TGF-β + IL-2 or IL-5 is very low, generally less than 0.5 per cent[19,114]. Furthermore, only 1 cell in 2500 was able to be activated to become a precursor for IgA-secreting cells in the limiting dilution analyses of Kim and Kagnoff[114]. By contrast, in limiting dilution experiments in which B cells are activated with LPS + IL-4, 1 in 100 to 1 in 10 cells are precursors for IgG1-secreting cells[115,116], and, using a Th2 cell line + IL-4, it was determined that approximately 90 per cent of splenic IgM$^+$IgD$^+$ B cells can be precursors for IgG1- and for IgE-secreting cells[117]. Furthermore, in experiments in which expression of sIg is assayed, it is found that only about 2–3 per cent of splenic B cells express sIgA after stimulation with TGF-β in combination with LPS or dextran-conjugated anti-IgD (anti-δ dextran)[75,101], whereas up to 50 per cent of splenic B cells stimulated with LPS + IL-4 express sIgG1[118]. Because such a low frequency of IgA-expressing cells is induced, and because of the antiproliferation effect of TGF-β, which generally results in a significant loss of cells during these experiments, the hypothesis that TGF-β directs switching to IgA from *uncommitted* B cells has not been accepted by all investigators[119]. Investigators questioned how the large numbers of IgA-expressing cells in the Peyer's patches and mesenteric lymph nodes could be produced when TGF-β treatment appears to result in no actual increase in $IgA^+$ cells, but only an increase in their proportion. Data discussed below suggest that additional cytokines and B-cell activators may overcome the antiproliferative effects of TGF-β or may interact with TGF-β to increase switching to IgA. Furthermore, although additional cytokines and B-cell activators increase secretion of IgA in the presence of TGF-β, it is also possible that IgA secretion occurs at sites lacking active TGF-β.

To address the possibility that different methods of activating B cells may increase the yield of IgA-expressing cells, Ehrhardt *et al.*[75] tested the effect of adding TGF-β to cultures of splenic B cells induced to switch by two different Th2 cell lines. Although they found that only 2 per cent of cells express sIgA in these cultures on day 4, the antiproliferative effects of TGF-β were abrogated, so that treatment with TGF-β resulted in an increase by 13–27-fold in the final yield of $sIgA^+$ cells in the cultures. The overall cell number in these cultures increased 2–3-fold relative to the number at the initiation of the cultures. Taken together with the limiting dilution experiments, these results support the hypothesis that TGF-β directs switching to IgA rather than causing a selective survival of IgA-committed or expressing cells.

Experiments using human tonsillar B cells also support the hypothesis that TGF-β directs switching to IgA[120]. Purified $sIgD^+$ B cells in limiting dilution cultures were induced with a combination of TGF-β, SAC, antibody to CD40 presented on a line of fibroblasts bearing FcγRII, and IL-10, assaying at day 13 for wells containing IgA. It was determined that in the absence of TGF-β, 1 cell in 340 is a precursor for IgA-secreting cells, whereas if TGF-β (0.6 ng/ml) is added, 1 cell in 75 is a precursor. Thus, TGF-β increases the frequency of IgA precursors in human B cells. Anti-IgM could substitute for SAC. The much higher frequency of IgA precursors found in these experiments as compared to those using mouse splenic B cells activated with LPS + IL-2 + TGF-β[114] may be caused by the use of both CD40 antibody presented on fibroblasts and SAC. In this system, IL-10 is required for production of IgA in both limiting dilution and bulk culture experiments. No other cytokine tested, including IL-1 through IL-7, is able to substitute for IL-10. DeFrance *et al.*[120] speculate that IL-10 is required for secretion in their experimental model, since it increases production of IgM, IgG and IgA in bulk culture experiments, whereas the effect of TGF-β is to specifically increase production of IgA, and to decrease production of IgM and IgG. Thus, IL-10 appears to be acting similarly to IL-2 and IL-5 in the mouse experiments described above. Further supporting the importance of IL-10 are results reported by Kitani and Strober[121], who found that purified human B cells stimulated with TGF-β plus antibody to CD40 (presented on fibroblasts) would not switch to expression of

IgA1 or IgA2 without addition of IL-10. IL-10 is also required when SAC + TGF-β is used to induce switching to IgA1, although it does not have to be added to the cultures, since they found that SAC stimulates human B cells to synthesize IL-10. Interestingly, in these experiments Kitani and Strober found that in the presence of TGF-β and IL-10, a T-cell signal is required for induction of switching to IgA2, but that either SAC or a T-cell signal induces switching to IgA1.

Recent experiments by McIntyre *et al.*[122] demonstrate that TGF-β can induce very high frequencies of $sIgA^+$ cells (10–20 per cent) within 4 days, when purified resting splenic B cells are activated with anti-δ dextran + a CD40L–CD8α fusion protein + IL-4 + IL-5. LPS can be substituted for the CD40L chimera. Leaving out any component very much reduces the frequency of $sIgA^+$ cells. During the course of the experiment the total number of B cells increased by 12-fold, and the percentage of $sIgA^+$ cells increased by two orders of magnitude. Thus, these data further support the conclusion that TGF-β directs switching to IgA from $sIgD^+sIgM^+$ cells, and that it is likely that the negative effects of TGF-β on B-cell proliferation can be overcome by stimulation with signals that mimic antigen and the signals from Th2 cells.

TGF-β increases switching to IgA by 5–20-fold (up to 4–6 per cent of the cells by days 4–5) in two mouse B-cell lymphomas that switch preferentially to IgA even in the absence of TGF-β[123–125]. One of the cell lines, I.29μ, can be induced to switch by LPS, and the other line CH12.LX, by IL-4, but not by LPS. IL-4 appears to be acting in a non-isotype-specific manner to induce switching in CH12.LX cells. Furthermore, antibody to IL-4 inhibits switching induced by LPS in the I.29μ line. Although TGF-β increases the frequency of IgA expressing CH12.LX cells in limiting dilution experiments, it also inhibits secretion of IgA by these cells, just as it does in the 4F2 subclone of CH12.LX[100].

## Mechanism of the Induction by TGF-β of Switching to IgA

As expected from data obtained on the mechanism of switching to other antibody classes, switching to IgA was shown to be due to switch recombination, rather than to a RNA-processing mechanism, by finding of DNA circles containing excised Sμ–Sα or Sγ–Sα regions in splenic B cells treated with LPS + TGF-β[126]. Southern blots of DNA from I.29μ cells show a reduction in hybridization to the chromosomal Sμ segment in Southern blots of DNA from I.29μ cells treated with LPS + TGF-β in comparison with those treated with LPS alone[127].

## TGF-β Induces Transcription of Germline Cα RNA

Further convincing evidence for the hypothesis that TGF-β actually directs class switch recombination to IgA, rather than selecting committed cells, comes from the finding that TGF-β induces expression of RNA transcripts from unrearranged Ig Cα gene prior to switch recombination in both mouse and human B cells and B-cell lines[101,121,124,128,129]. A large body of data demonstrates that transcription of unrearranged $C_H$ genes, yielding what are called germline transcripts, is induced by cytokines which direct subsequent switching to the same $C_H$ genes[130–136]. The germline transcripts themselves do not induce class switch recombination, which is induced by unknown mechanisms by various B-cell activators (including LPS, or $T_H$ cells, or anti-δ dextran and IL-5, or SAC), but gene knockout experiments indicate that the transcripts are necessary to direct switch recombination[137–139]. IL-4 induces transcripts of unrearranged Cγ1 and Cϵ genes in mouse splenic B cells and of the Cϵ gene in human B cells. IFN-γ induces germline Cγ2a transcripts in the mouse[135,140]. In some cases this induction has been demonstrated to occur at the transcriptional level, and segments of DNA containing promoter elements for these transcripts have been characterized in reporter gene assays.

Germline $C_H$ gene transcripts all have an analogous structure, initiating 5′ to the tandem repeats of the switch region, and proceeding through the $C_H$ gene and terminating at the normal poly(A) sites for secreted or for membrane-bound heavy chain mRNAs (Figure 12.2b)[141–147]. The primary transcript is spliced to generate a mature germline RNA containing an upstream, or 5′, germline exon (I exon) spliced at the normal splice acceptor for the mature $C_H$ transcripts. After switch recombination, the segment of DNA 5′ to the switch region is deleted from the chromosome, and thus germline transcripts cannot be synthesized after class switching (Figure 12.2c). Instead, the mature α mRNAs are transcribed (Figure 12.2d).

Germline α transcripts are induced in mouse splenic B cells by treatment with TGF-β + LPS for 2 days[101]. They are undetectable in the absence of TGF-β in LPS-activated splenic B cells. Germline transcripts for both the α1 and α2 genes of human are also upregulated in activated splenic B cells within 1 day after addition of TGF-β[128,148]. Kitani and Strober[121] found that the two human α germline transcripts are differentially regulated in peripheral blood B cells treated for 2 days with TGF-β, in that SAC further upregulates the human α1 germline transcripts, but has no effect on the level of the α2 germline transcripts. However, these results are difficult to interpret, since TGF-β mRNA is induced by SAC in these B cells[121]. Germline α transcripts are constitutively present in two mouse B-cell lymphomas, I.29μ and CH12.LX, that switch preferentially to IgA when treated with LPS or IL-4, respectively[129,149]. These transcripts are upregulated 5–9-fold by TGF-β treatment of I.29μ cells, reaching a maximum at 24 h. In the presence of LPS, this induction is followed by class switching in I.29μ cells starting at day 2, with maximal switching (about 6 per cent occurring on days 3–5)[125]. The induction of germline α transcripts by TGF-β correlates

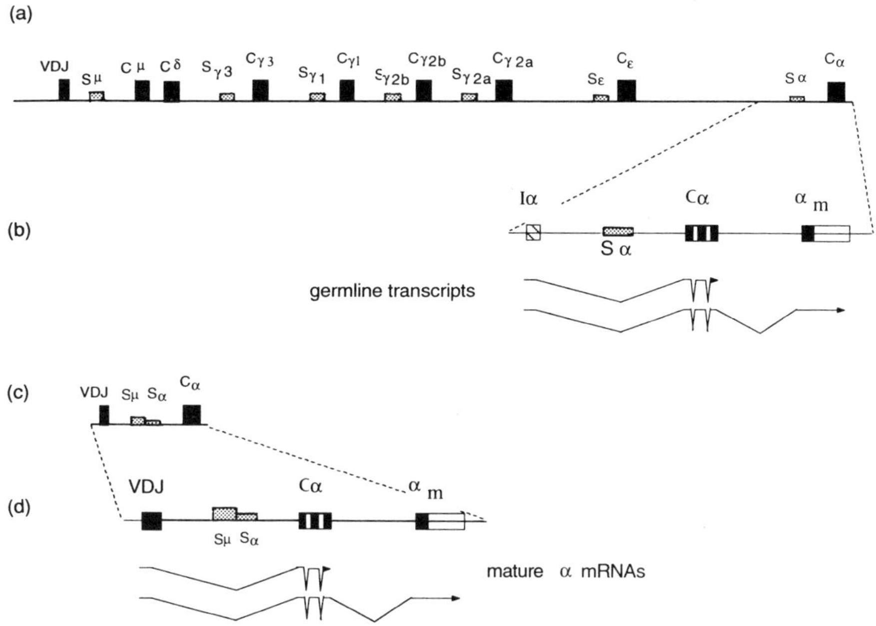


**Figure 12.2** Diagram of Ig heavy chain genes (mouse), germline α transcripts and mature α chain mRNAs. (a) Diagram of the structure of Ig heavy chain genes in cells expressing IgM/IgD. (b) Map of region transcribed in germline α transcripts, and splicing diagrams of germline α transcripts. (c) Diagram of an expressed Ig α gene produced by recombination between Sμ and Sα regions. (d) Expanded diagram of gene encoding functional Ig α chain mRNA and splicing diagrams for production of mature α chain mRNAs encoding secreted and membrane-bound α heavy chains

quantitatively with the induction of switching in the presence of LPS, since TGF-β increases switching to IgA in I.29μ cells by 5–11-fold relative to that obtained by LPS alone.

To investigate the mechanism of induction of germline α transcripts by TGF-β, nuclear run-on assays have been performed. In I.29μ cells, TGF-β increases transcription of the Iα–Sα–Cα segment by 4 h of treatment with a maximum of 5.4-fold at 12 h. Furthermore, TGF-β does not increase the stability of germline α RNA, indicating that the regulation is at the transcriptional level[124]. This finding agrees with the results for regulation of other germline transcripts. Specifically, IL-4 has been shown to induce germline ϵ RNA at the transcriptional level in the mouse pre-B-cell line, 18.81A20[150], and to induce the appearance of DNase hypersensitive sites 5′ to the start sites for germline γ1 transcripts, suggesting that IL-4 induces transcription of germline γ1 RNA in splenic B cells[151,152]. Surprisingly, experiments examining whether TGF-β induces germline αRNAs at the transcriptional level in mouse splenic B cells appeared to suggest the opposite conclusion, i.e. that TGF-β does not induce germline α transcripts at the transcriptional level, but rather increases their stability. This conclusion was based on run-on experiments in which it was found that TGF-β does not increase hybridization to a 75-bp probe for the Iα exon probe at any time from 12 to 48 h after addition[153]. The authors did not demonstrate, however, that this probe only hybridizes with germline α RNA. The signal obtained with this probe was about as intense as that obtained with an 880-bp probe for the Cα segment, suggesting that the Iα probe was hybridizing to RNA species in addition to the germline α RNA. Supporting this idea are results using a probe for the entire Iα region on a Northern blot of mouse spleen cell RNA induced by LPS + Th2 supernatant, in which it was found that the Iα probe hybridized with numerous RNA species in spleen cells, a heterogeneous smear being detected in addition to the germline α RNA[131]. Using an actinomycin D chase protocol, Lebman *et al.*[153] also examined the stability of splenic RNA hybridizing with a probe for Cα, and found that in cells treated with TGF-β + LPS, αRNA is slightly more stable than in cells treated with LPS alone (half-life of 2.8 h versus 1.7 h). This experiment, however, analyzed both germline and mature α mRNA together.

The hypothesis that TGF-β induces transcription of the germline α RNA is further supported by the demonstration that transiently transfected reporter genes driven by the 5′ flanking segment for germline α transcripts of both mouse and human can be induced by TGF-β, 3–20-fold, depending on the cell lines[154,155]. The mouse and human α1 and α2 promoters are very similar in sequence in a region extending a few hundred base pairs 5′ to the RNA initiation sites, and several putative and demonstrated transcription factor-binding sites have been identified in this promoter/enhancer segment. Binding sites for both Ets and ATF/CRE transcriptional activators are necessary for basal expression, and also contribute to TGF-β-inducible expression. A novel tandem direct repeat which is necessary for induction of transcriptional activity by TGF-β has been identified in the mouse germline α promoter, ACCACAGCCAGACCACAGGCCAGAC. Substitution mutations of this tandem repeat reduce the induction by TGF-β of the germline α promoter activity from 11.0-fold to 1.4-fold (M.J. Shi and J. Stavnezer, in preparation). This element is also present in the human α1 and α2 promoters, and results of Nilsson and Paschalis[155] suggest it is also necessary for activation by TGF-β of the human promoters. Lin and Stavnezer[154] demonstrated that two or more copies of this tandem direct repeat could transfer TGF-β inducibility to a minimal *c-fos* promoter (which does not otherwise respond to TGF-β). EMSA data indicate that nuclear proteins in I.29μ and splenic B cells bind this tandem repeat, although treatment of cells with TGF-β does not increase binding to the element[154] (M.-J. Shi and J. Stavenzer, in preparation). As pointed out above, TGF-β receptors generate a phosphorylation signal, and it is sometimes found that phosphorylation can activate the function of a transcription activator without increasing its DNA-binding activity. Although TGF-β has been shown to induce transcription of other promoters in other cell types via several different transcription factors, i.e. AP-1, ATF-2, NF-I and USF[45,55,156,157], the sequence of the responsive element in the germline α promoter differs from these, and has not been demonstrated to be involved in induction of transcription by TGF-β in other promoters. Interestingly, however, one copy of the same sequence element is present in two other promoters known to be inducible by TGF-β. It is present immediately abutting an element(s) responsive to TGF-β in the promoter for plasminogen activator protein-1[158,159], and also in the promotor for TGF-β itself[154,160], although it has not been identified in these promoters as being involved in regulation.

In conclusion, a considerable body of data supports the hypothesis that TGF-β directs antibody class switching to IgA by inducing transcription of germline α transcripts. The mechanism of this transcriptional induction is unknown, although it appears that a novel DNA element and transcriptional activator may be involved. Although TGF-β in doses required to induce switching to IgA inhibits proliferation of B cells and production of Ig by B cells under some conditions, data suggest that if an adequate combination of activators, e.g. antigen and T-cell help, is provided, the inhibitory effects are abrogated and large numbers of $IgA^+$ cells can be produced[122].

It is believed that the main sites at which switching to IgA occurs in the body are in the Peyer's patches, which are patches of lymphoid tissue in the small intestine, just below the mucosal epithelium. To investigate whether germline α transcripts are present in Peyer's patches in which switching to IgA is occurring, Weinstein and Cebra[161] orally infected germ-free mice with reovirus, since this will induce the formation of Peyer's patches and switching to IgA in these mice. Peyer's patches do not develop in germ-free mice. Weinstein and Cebra found that germline α transcripts, followed by expression of IgA, are induced by the reovirus infection. Although it is reasonable to hypothesize that this induction requires TGF-β, there are no data indicating the source of TGF-β important for induction of germline α transcripts, and TGF-β is synthesized by many cell types. Therefore, which cells produce the TGF-β involved in regulation of IgA switching and how it is regulated are topics of much current interest. Using an ELISA specific for the active form of TGF-β, Santos *et al.*[162] have recently shown that mouse Peyer's patch T cells secrete active TGF-β after stimulation with an antigen to which the mice are tolerant.

## Human IgA Deficiency

IgA deficiency is the most common form of primary immunodeficiency in humans. It has recently been shown by Islam *et al.*[163] that the peripheral blood B cells of these patients do not contain Igα mRNA and do not contain recombined Sμ–Sα DNA segments. Germline α transcripts cannot be detected in unstimulated peripheral blood cells from these patients, whereas they are detected in controls. Although peripheral blood cells in patients contain TGF-β mRNA at the same levels as in controls, when peripheral blood cells are treated in culture with TGF-β and PMA, they respond by inducing germline α transcripts to the same level as in controls[163]. Thus, the patients' cells are capable of responding if provided with active TGF-β. These data suggest that the defect in IgA deficiency might be the production of active TGF-β. Since latent TGF-β is secreted by many cell types, activation of latent TGF-β should be a very important regulatory step, and it would be interesting to determine if this process is defective in the Peyer's patches of these individuals.

### TGF-β Induces Germline γ2b Transcripts and Directs Switching to IgG2b in Mouse Splenic B Cells

In experiments examining the effect of TGF-β on switching to IgA in LPS-treated splenic B cells, Sonada *et al.* noticed that TGF-γ (0.1–1 ng/ml) also increases secretion of IgG2b and secretion of IgG3[164]. They also found an increase in the proportion of cells expressing these isotypes on their surface. McIntyre *et al.*[21] then demonstrated that TGF-β induces germline γ2b transcripts in LPS-activated splenic B cells, further supporting the conclusion that TGF-β directs switching to IgG2b. They found, however, that TGF-β decreases expression of germline γ3 transcripts, and suggested that small amounts of TGF-β may increase secretion rather than switching to IgG3 (see above, p. 306). Treatment of sorted IgG2b$^-$ cells with TGF-β (1 ng/ml) + LPS induces a 9-fold increase in IgG2b secretion relative to LPS alone at 6 days of culture. These experiments were done using C57BL/6[164] or Balb/c splenocytes[21], and it was found that LPS-activated splenic B cells from DBA/2 mice switch to IgG2b without addition of TGF-β[21]. Furthermore, addition of antibody to TGF-β decreases secretion of IgG2b by DBA/2B cells, causing McIntyre *et al.* to suggest that LPS-activated DBA/2B cells synthesize more active TGF-β than do Balb/c cells. Interestingly, TGF-β does not induce IgG2b switching in splenic B cells activated with anti-δ dextran instead of LPS. TGF-β was found to increase switching to IgG2b in CH12.LX B-lymphoma cells, which do not require LPS in order to switch[123]. A search of the promoter region for the germline γ2b transcript[141] failed to reveal sequences resembling the TGF-β response element (direct repeat element) of the germline α promoter (J. Stavnezer, unpublished).

Although the data are quite incomplete, it appears likely that TGF-β may specifically inhibit switching to IgE, because it inhibits induction of germline ϵ transcripts by IL-4 in purified human splenic B cells and in a human EBV-transformed B-cell line, and also in the mouse B lymphoma I.29μ[124,165,166]. It inhibits production of IgE by IL-4-treated peripheral blood mononuclear cells, but not the constitutive production of IgE by peripheral blood mononuclear cells from atopic individuals[165].

## CONCLUSIONS

In conclusion, TGF-β directs switch recombination to two isotypes, IgA in both mouse and human, and IgG2b in the mouse, by inducing transcription from the unrearranged Iα–Cα and Iγ2b–Cγ2b gene segments. A TGF-β-responsive element has been identified in the promoter for germline α transcripts, but the regulation of the promoter for the germline γ2b transcript by TGF-β has not been studied. A major problem in understanding how TGF-β induces switching is lack of information about the relevant sources of active TGF-β at the presumptive site of induction of germline transcripts and IgA switching, the Peyer's patches. Furthermore, since TGF-β is ubiquitous, it is highly likely that understanding the regulation of activation of TGF-β after it is synthesized will be necessary for understanding how TGF-β specifically directs switching to IgA and to IgG2b or any other of its functions.

## REFERENCES


1. Massague J. The transforming growth factor-β family. Annu Rev Cell Biol 1990; 6:587–641.
2. Moses HL, Yang EY, Pietenpol JA. TGF-β stimulation and inhibition of cell proliferation: new mechanistic insights. Cell 1990; 63:245–247.
3. McCartney-Francis NL, Wahl SM. TGF-β: a matter of life and death. J Leukocyte Biol 1994; 55:401–409.
4. Wahl SM. TGFβ: the good, the bad, and the ugly. J Exp Med 1994; 180:1587–1590.
5. Lee G, Ellingsworth LR, Gillis S *et al.* β TGFs are potential regulators of B lymphopoiesis. J Exp Med 1987; 166:1290–1299.
6. Kehrl JH, Taylor AS, Delsing GA *et al.* Further studies of the role of TGFβ in human B cell function. J Immunol 1989; 143:1868–1874.
7. Brabletz T, Pfeuffer I, Schorr E *et al.* TGFβ and cyclosporin A inhibit the inducible activity of the IL-2 gene in T cells through a noncanonical octamer-binding site. Mol Cell Biol 1993; 13:1155–1162.
8. Ranges GE, Figari IS, Espevik T, Palladino MA. Inhibition of cytotoxic T cell development by TGFβ and reversal by recombinant tumor necrosis factor α. J Exp Med 1987; 166:991–1000.
9. Lucas C, Bald LN, Fendly BM *et al.* The autocrine production of TGFβ1 during lymphocyte activation. A study with a monoclonal antibody-based ELISA. J Immunol 1990; 145:1415–1422.
10. Su HC, Leite-Morris KA, Braun L, Biron CA. A role for TGFβ1 in regulating natural killer cell and T lymphocyte proliferation responses during acute infection with lymphocytic choriomeningitis virus. J Immunol 1991; 147:2717–2727.

11. Tsunawaki S, Sporn M, Ding A, Nathan C. Deactivation of macrophages by TGFβ. Nature 1988; 334:260–262.
12. Racke MK, Dhib-Jalbut S, Cannella B *et al.* Prevention and treatment of chronic relapsing experimental allergic encephalomyelitis by TGFβ1. J Immunol 1991; 146:3012–3017.
13. Kuruvilla AP, Shah R, Hochwald GM *et al.* Protective effects of TGFβ1 on experimental autoimmune disease in mice. Proc Nat Acad Sci USA 1991; 88:2918–2921.
14. Miller A, Lider O, Roberts AB *et al.* Suppressor T cells generated by oral tolerization to myelin basic protein suppress both both in vitro and in vivo immune responses by the release of TGFβ after antigen-specific triggering. Proc Natl Acad Sci USA 1992; 89:421-425.
15. Shull MM, Ormsby I, Kier AB *et al.* Targeted disruption of the mouse TGFβ1 gene results in multifocal inflammatory disease. Nature 1992; 359:693–699.
16. Kulkarni AB, Huh C-G, Becker D *et al.* TGFβ1 null mutation in mice causes excessive inflammatory response and early death. Proc Natl Acad Sci USA 1993; 90:770–774.
17. Christ M, McCartney-Francis NL, Kulkarni AB *et al.* Immune dysregulation of TGFβ1-deficient mice. J Immunol 1994; 153:1936–1946.
18. Coffman RL, Lebman DA, Shrader B. Transforming growth factor-β specifically enhances IgA production by lipopolysaccharide-stimulated murine B lymphocytes. J Exp Med 1989; 170:1039–1044.
19. Sonoda E, Matsumoto R, Hitoshi Y *et al.* Transforming growth factor β induces IgA production and acts additively with interleukin 5 for IgA production. J Exp Med 1989; 170:1415–1420.
20. Vlasselaer Pv, Punnonen J, deVries JE. Transforming growth factor-β directs IgA switching in human B cells. J Immunol 1992; 148:2062–2067.
21. McIntyre TM, Klinman DR, Rothman P *et al.* Transforming growth factor $\beta_1$ selectively stimulates immunoglobulin G2b secretion by lipopolysaccharide-activated murine B cells. J Exp Med 1993; 177:1031–1037.
22. McCartney-Francis N, Mizel D, Wong H *et al.* TGFβ regulates production of growth factors and TGFβ by human peripheral blood monocytes. Growth Factors 1990; 4:27–35.
23. Wahl SM, Allen JB, Weeks BS *et al.* TGFβ enhances integrin expression and type IV collagenase secretion in human monocytes. Proc Natl Acad Sci USA 1993; 90:4577–4581.
24. Adams DH, Hathaway M, Shaw J *et al.* TGFβ induces human T lymphocyte migration in vitro. J Immunol 1991; 147:609–612.
25. Brandes ME, Mai UEH, Ohura K, Wahl SM. Human neutrophils express type I TGFβ receptors and chemotax to TGFβ. J Immunol 1991; 147:1600–1606.
26. Kingsley DM. The TGF-β superfamily: new members, new receptors, and new genetic tests of function in different organisms. Genes and Dev 1994; 8:133–146.
27. Miyazono K, Dijke PT, Ichijo H, Heldin C-H. Receptors for transforming growth factor-β. Adv Immunol 1994; 55:181–220.
28. Sato Y, Rifkin DB. Inhibition of endothelial cell movement by pericytes and smooth muscle cells: activation of a latent TGFβ-like molecule by plasmin during co-culture. J Cell Biol 1989; 109:309–315.
29. Flaumenhaft R, Kojima S, Abe M, Rifkin DB. Activation of latent TGFβ. Adv Pharmacol 1993; 24:51–76.
30. Burmester JK, Qian SW, Roberts AB *et al.* Characterization of distinct functional domains of transforming growth factor β. Proc Natl Acad Sci USA 1993; 90:8628–8632.

31. Cheifetz S, Hernandez H, Laiho M *et al.* Distinct transforming growth factor-β receptor subsets as determinants of cellular responsiveness of three TGF-β isoforms. J Biol Chem 1990; 265:20533–20538.
32. Wrana JL, Attisano L, Carcamo J *et al.* TGFβ signals through a heteromeric protein kinase receptor complex. Cell 1992; 71:1003–1014.
33. Franzen P, Dijke Pt, Ichijo H *et al.* Cloning of the TGFβ type I receptor that forms a heteromeric complex with the TGFβ type II receptor. Cell 1993; 75:681–692.
34. Ebner R, Chen R-H, Shum L *et al.* Cloning of a type I TGFβ receptor and its effect on TGFβ binding to the type II receptor. Science 1993; 260:1344–1348.
35. Wrana JL, Attisano L, Wieser R *et al.* Mechanism of activation of the TGF-β receptor. Nature 1994; 370:341–347.
36. Lopez-Casillas F, Wran JL, Massague J. Betaglycan presents ligand to the TGFβ signaling receptor. Cell 1993; 73:1435–1444.
37. Wang T, Donahoe PK, Zervos AS. Specific interaction of type I receptors of the TGFβ family with the immunophilin FKBP-12. Science 1994; 265:674–676.
38. Thompson NL, Flanders KC, Smith JM *et al.* Expression of TGFβ1 in specific cells and tissues of adult and neonatal mice. J Cell Biol 1989; 108:661–669.
39. Koyama S-y, Podolsky DK. Differential expression of transforming growth factors α and β in rat intestinal epithelial cells. J Clin Invest 1989; 83:1768–1773.
40. Takahama Y, Letterio JJ, Suzuki H *et al.* Early progression of thymocytes along the CD4/CD8 developmental pathway is regulated by a subset of thymic epithelial cells expressing TGFβ. J Exp Med 1994; 179:1495–1506.
41. Wager RE, Assosian RK. A phorbol ester-regulated ribonuclease system controlling TGFβ1 gene expression in hematopoietic cells. Mol Cell Biol 1990; 10:5983–5990.
42. Kim SJ, Park K, Koeller D *et al.* Post-transcriptional regulation of the human TGF-β1 gene. J Biol Chem 1992; 267:13702–13707.
43. Grainger DJ, Kemp PR, Liu AC *et al.* Activation of TGFβ is inhibited in transgenic apolipoprotein(a)mice. Nature 1994; 370:460–462.
44. Bascom CC, Wolfshohl JR, Coffey J *et al.* Complex regulation of TGFβ1, β2, and β3 mRNA expression in mouse fibroblasts and keratinocytes by TGFs β1 and β2. Mol Cell Biol 1989; 9:5508–5515.
45. Kim S-J, Angel P, Lafyatis R *et al.* Autoinduction of transforming growth factor β1 is mediated by the AP1 complex. Mol Cell Biol 1990; 10:1492–1497.
46. Li B, Sehajpal PK, Khanna A *et al* Differential regulation of TGFβ and IL-2 genes in human T cells: demonstration by usage of novel competitor DNA constructs in the quantitative polymerase chain reaction. J Exp Med 1991; 174:1259–1262.
47. Lafyatis R, Lechleider R, Kim S-J *et al.* Structure and functional characterization of the TGFβ3 promoter. J Biol Chem 1990; 265:19128–19136.
48. Dubinett SM, Huang M, Dhanani S *et al.* Down-regulation of macrophage TGFβ mRNA expression by IL-7. J Immunol 1993; 151:6670–6680.
49. Vlasselaer PV, Borremans P, Gorp UV *et al.* IL-10 inhibits TGFβ synthesis required for osteogenic commitment of mouse bone marrow cells. J Cell Biol 1994; 124:569–577.
50. Bristol LA, Ruscetti FW, Brody DT, Durum SK. IL-1α induces expression of active TGFβ in nonproliferating T cells via a post-transcriptional mechanism. J Immunol 1990; 145:4108–4114.
51. Kehrl JH, Wakefield LM, Roberts AB *et al.* Production of transforming growth factor β by human lymphocytes and its potential role in the regulation of T cell growth. J Exp Med 1986; 163:1037–1050.

52. Udvadia AJ, Rogers KT, Higgins PDR *et al.* Sp-1 binds promoter elements regulated by the RB protein and Sp-1 mediated transcription is stimulated by RB co-expression. Proc Natl Acad Sci USA 1993:90:3265–3269.
53. Kim S-J, Lee H-D, Robbins PD *et al.* Regulation of TGFβ expression by the product of the retinoblastoma-susceptibility gene. Proc Natl Acad Sci USA 1991; 88:3052–3056.
54. Geiser AG, Busam KJ, Kim S-J *et al* Regulation of the TGFβ1 and β3 promoters by transcription factor Sp1. Gene 1993; 129:223–228.
55. Kim S-J, Wagner S, Liu F *et al.* Retinoblastoma gene product activates expression of the human TGF-β2 gene through transcription factor ATF-2. Nature 119; 358:331–334.
56. Smeland EB, Blomhoff HK, Holte H *et al.* TGFβ inhibits G1 to S transition, but not activation of human B lymphocytes. Exp Cell Res 1987; 171:213–222.
57. Matthes T, Werner-Favre C, Tang H *et al.* Cytokine mRNA expression during an in vitro response of human B lymphocytes: kinetics of B cell TNFα, IL-6, IL-10 and TGFβ mRNAs. J Exp Med 1993; 178:521–528.
58. Kehrl JH, Roberts AB, Wakefield LM *et al.* Transforming growth factor β is an important immunomodulatory protein for human B lymphocytes. J Immunol 1986; 137:3855–3860.
59. Snapper CM, Waegell W, Beernink H, Dasch JR. TGFβ1 is required for secretion of IgG of all subclasses by LPS-activated murine B cells in vitro. J Immunol 1993; 151:4625–4636.
60. Lotz M, Ranheim E, Kipps TJ. TGFβ as endogenous growth inhibitor of chronic lymphocytic leukemia B cells. J Exp Med 1994; 179:999–1004.
61. Warner GL, Ludlow JW, Nelson DA *et al.* Anti-immunoglobulin treatment of murine B-cell lymphomas induces active TGFβ but pRB hypophosphorylation is TGFβ independent. Cell Growth and Diff 1992; 3:175–181.
62. Berg DJ, Lynch RG. Immune dysfunction in mice with plasmacytomas. I. Evidence that TGFβ contributes to the altered expression of activation receptors on host B lymphocytes. J Immunol 1991; 146:2865–2872.
63. Barrett TB, Shu GL, Draves KE *et al.* Signaling through CD19, Fc receptors or TGFβ: each inhibits the activation of resting human B cells differently. Eur J Immunol 1990; 20:1053–1059.
64. Armitage RJ, Macduff BM, Spriggs MK, Fanslow WC. Human B cell proliferation and Ig secretion induced by recombinant CD40 ligand are modulated by soluble cytokines. J Immunol 1993; 150:3671–3680.
65. Tucci A, James H, Chicheportiche R *et al.* Effects of eleven cytokines and of IL-1 and tumor necrosis factor inhibitors in a human B cell assay. J Immunol 1992; 148:2778–2784.
66. Cross D, Cambier JC. TGFβ1 has differential effects on B cell proliferation and activation antigen expression. J Immunol 1990; 144:432–439.
67. Blomhof HK, Smeland E, Mustafa AS *et al.* Epstein–Barr virus mediates a switch in responsiveness to TGFβ, in cells of the B cell lineage. Eur J Immunol 1987; 17:298–301.
68. Pietenpol JA, Stein RW, Moran E *et al.* TGFβ1 inhibition of c-myc transcription and growth in keratinocytes is abrogated by viral transforming proteins with pRB binding domains. Cell 1990; 61:777–785.
69. Gold MR, Gajewski TF, DeFranco AL. Regulation of anti-immunoglobulin-induced B lymphoma growth arrest by TGFβ1 and dexamethasone. Int Immunol 1991; 3:1091–1098.
70. Lomo J, Blomhoff HK, Beiske K *et al.* TGFβ and cyclic AMP promote apoptosis in resting human B lymphocytes. J Immunol 1995; 154:1634–1643.

71. Holder MJ, Knox K, Gordon J. Factors modifying survival pathways of germinal center B cells. Glucocorticoids and TGFβ, but not cyclosporin A or anti-CD19, block surface Ig-mediated rescue from apoptosis. Eur J Immunol 1992; 22:2725–2728.
72. Rotello RJ, Lieberman RC, Purchio AF, Gerschenson LE. Coordinated regulation of apoptosis and cell proliferation by TGFβ1 in cultured uterine epithelial cells. Proc Natl Acad Sci USA 1991; 88:3412–3415.
73. Oberhammer FA, Pavelka M, Sharma S *et al.* Induction of apoptosis in cultured hepatocytes and in regressing liver by TGFβ1. Proc Natl Acad Sci USA 1992; 89:5408–5412.
74. Selvakumaran M, Lin H-K, Sjin RTT *et al.* The novel primary response gene MyD118 and the proto-oncogenes *myb, myc,* and *bcl-2* modulate TGFβ1-induced apoptosis of myeloid leukemia cells. Mol Cell Biol 1994; 14:2352–2360.
75. Ehrhardt RO, Strober W, Harriman GR. Effect of TGFβ1 on IgA isotype expression: TGFβ1 induces a small increase in $sIgA^+$ cells regardless of the method of B cell activation. J Immunol 1992; 148:3830–3836.
76. Fischer G, Kent SC, Joseph L *et al.* Lymphoma models for B cell activation and tolerance. X. Anti-μ-mediated growth arrest and apoptosis of murine B cell lymphomas is prevented by the stabilization of myc. J Exp Med 1994; 179:221–228.
77. Laiho M, DeCaprico JA, Ludlow JW *et al.* Growth inhibition by TGFβ linked to suppression of retinoblastoma protein phosphorylation. Cell 1990; 62:175–185.
78. Furukawa Y, Uenoyama S, Ohta M *et al.* TGFβ inhibits phosphorylation of the retinoblastoma susceptibility gene product in human monocytic leukemia cell line JOSK-1. J Biol Chem 1992; 267:17121–17127.
79. Rustgi AK, Dyson N, Bernards R. Amino-terminal domains of c-myc and N-myc proteins mediate binding to the retinoblastoma gene product. Nature 1991; 352:541–544.
80. Goodrich DW, Lee W-H. Abrogation by c-myc of G1 phase arrest induced by RB protein but not by p53. Nature 1992; 360:177–179.
81. Pietenpol JA, Munger K, Howley PM *et al.* Factor-binding element in the human c-myc promoter involved in transcriptional regulation of TGFβ1 and by the retinoblastoma gene product. Proc Natl Acad Sci USA 1991; 88:10227–10231.
82. Zentella A, Weis FMB, Ralph DA *et al.* Early gene responses to TGFβ in cells lacking growth-suppressive RB function. Mol Cell Biol 1991; 11:4952–4958.
83. Nevins JR. E2F: a link between the Rb tumor suppressor protein and viral oncoproteins. Science 1992; 258:424–429.
84. Schwarz JK, Bassing CH, Kovesdo I *et al.* Expression of the E2F1 transcription factor overcomes TGFβ-mediated growth suppression. Proc Natl Acad Sci USA 1995; 92:483–487.
85. Sherr CJ. Mammalian G1 cyclins. Cell 1993; 73:1059–1065.
86. Hartwell LH, Kastan MB. Cell cycle control and cancer. Science 1994; 266:1821–1828.
87. Dowdy S, Hinds P, Louie K *et al.* Physical interaction of the retinoblastoma protein with human D cyclins. Cell 1993; 73:499–511.
88. Howe PH, Draetta G, Leof EB. TGFβ1 inhibition of $p34^{cdc2}$ phosphorylation and histone H1 kinase activity is associated with G1/S phase growth arrest. Mol Cell Biol 1991; 11:1185–1194.
89. Koff A, Ohtsuki M, Polyak K, Roberts JM. Negative regulation of G1 in mammalian cells: inhibition of cyclin E-dependent kinase by TGFβ. Science 1993; 260:536–539.

90. Hengst L, Dulic V. Slingerland JM *et al.* A cell cycle-regulated inhibitor of cyclin-dependent kinases. Proc. Natl Acad Sci USA 1994; 91:5291–5295.
91. Polyak K, Kato J, Solomon MJ *et al.* p27$^{Kip1}$, a cyclin-Cdk inhibitor, links TGFβ and contact inhibition to cell cycle arrest. Genes and Dev 1994; 8:9–22.
92. Ewen M, Sluss K, Sherr CJ *et al.* Functional interactions of the retinoblastoma protein with mammalian D-type cyclins. Cell 1993; 73:487–497.
93. Ewen ME, Oliver CJ, Sluss HK *et al.* p53-dependent repression of CDK4 translation in TGFβ-induced G1 cell-cycle arrest. Genes and Dev 1995; 9:204–217.
94. Hannon GJ, Beach D. p15$^{Ink4B}$ is a potential effector of TGFβ-induced cell cycle arrest. Nature 1994; 371:257–261.
95. Rehmann JA, LeBien TW. TGFβ regulates normal human pre-B cell differentiation. Int Immunol 1994; 6:315–322.
96. Suda T, Zlotnik A. *In vitro* induction of CD8 expression on thymic pre-T cells. I. TGFβ and TNFα induce CD8 expression on CD8$^-$ thymic subsets including the CD25$^+$ CD3$^-$ CD4 –CD8$^-$ pre-T cell subset. J Immunol 1992; 148:1737–1745.
97. Inge TH, McCoy KM, Susskind BM *et al.* Immunomodulatory effects of TGFβ on T lymphocytes. Induction of CD8 expression in the CTLL-2 cell line and in normal thymocytes. J Immunol 1992; 148:3847–3856.
98. Briskin M, Kuwabara MD, Sigman DS, Wall R. Induction of κ transcription by interferon-γ without activation of NF-κB. Science 1988; 242:1036–1037.
99. Kehrl JH, Thevenin C, Rieckmann P, Fauci AS. TGFβ suppresses human B lymphocyte Ig production by inhibiting synthesis and the switch from the membrane form to the secreted form of Ig mRNA. J Immunol 1991; 146:4016–4023.
100. Eckmann L, Morzycka-Wroblewska E, Smith JR, Kagnoff MF. Cytokine-induced differentiation of IgA B cells: studies using an IgA expressing B-cell lymphoma. Immunology 1992; 76:235–241.
101. Lebman DA, Lee FD, Coffman RL. Mechanism for transforming growth factor β and Il-2 enhancement of IgA expression in lipopolysaccharide-stimulated B cell cultures. J Immunol 1990; 144:952–959.
102. Pertovaara L, Sistonen L, Bos TJ *et al.* Enhanced *jun* gene expression is an early genomic response to TGFβ stimulation. Mol Cell Biol 1989; 9:1255–1262.
103. Li L, Hu J-S, Olson EN. Different members of the *jun* proto-oncogene family exhibit distinct patterns of expression in response to TGFβ. J Biol Chem 1990; 265:1556–1562.
104. Kerr LD, Millier DB, Matrisian LM. TGFβ inhibition of transin/stromelysis gene expression is mediated through a Fos binding sequence. Cell 1990; 61:267–278.
105. Miller CL, Feldhaus AL, Rooney JW *et al.* Regulation and possible stage-specific function of Oct-2 during pre-B-cell differentiation. Mol Cell Biol 1991; 11: 4885–4894.
106. Staudt LM, Lenardo MJ. Immunoglobulin gene transcription. Annu Rev Immunol 1991; 9:373–398.
107. Hagman J, Rudin CM, Haasch D *et al.* A novel enhancer in the immunoglobulin λ locus is duplicated and functionally independent of NFκB. Genes and Dev 1990; 4:978–992.
108. Blomberg BB, Rudin CM, Storb U. Identification and localization of an enhancer for the human λ light chain immunoglobulin gene complex. J Immunol 1991; 147:2354–2358.
109. Bendall AJ, Sturm RA, Danoy PAC, Molloy PL. Broad binding-site specificity and affinity properties of Octamer 1 and brain Octamer-binding proteins. Eur J Biochem 1993; 217:799–811.

110. Roberts SB, Segil N, Heintz N. Differential phosphorylation of the transcription factor Oct1 during the cell cycle. Science 1991; 253:1022–1026.
111. LaBella F, Sive HL, Roeder RG, Heintz N. Cell-cycle regulation of a human histone H2b gene is mediated by the H2b subtype-specific consensus elements. Genes and Dev 1988; 2:32–39.
112. Corcoran LM, Karvelas M. Oct-2 is required early in T cell-independent B cell activation for G1 progression and for proliferation. Immunity 1994; 1:635–645.
113. Kim P-H, Kagnoff MF. TGFβ1 is a costimulator for IgA production. J Immunol 1990; 144:3411–3416.
114. Kim P-H, Kagnoff MF. Transforming growth factor β1 increases IgA isotype switching at the clonal level. J Immunol 1990; 145:3773–3778.
115. Bergstedt-Lindqvist S, Moon H-B, Persson U *et al.* Interleukin 4 instructs uncommitted B lymphocytes to switch to IgG1 and IgE. Eur J Immunol 1988; 18:1073–1077.
116. Savelkoul HFJ, Lebman DA, Benner R, Coffman R. Increase of precursor frequency and clonal size of murine IgE secreting cells by IL-4. J Immunol 1988; 141:749–755.
117. Lebman D, Coffman R. Interleukin 4 causes isotype switching to IgE in T cell-stimulated clonal B cell cultures. J Exp Med 1988; 168:853–862.
118. Snapper CM, Finkelman FD, Stefany D *et al.* IL-4 induces co-expression of intrinsic membrane IgG1 and IgE by murine B cells stimulated with lipopolysaccharide. J Immunol 1988; 141:489–498.
119. Cebra JJ, George A, Kerlin RL. A cautionary note concerning the possibility that TGFβ is a switch factor that acts on primary B cells to initiate IgA expression. Immunol Res 1991; 10:404–406.
120. DeFrance T, Vanbervliet B, Brière F *et al.* Interleukin 10 and transforming growth factor β cooperate to induce anti-CD40-activated naive human B cells to secrete immunoglobulin A. J Exp Med 1992; 175:671–682.
121. Kitani A, Strober W. Differential regulation of Cα1 and Cα2 germ-line and mature mRNA transcripts in human peripheral blood B cells. J Immunol 1994; 153:1466–1477.
122. McIntyre TM, Kehry MR, Snapper CM. A novel *in vitro* model for high-rate IgA class switching. J Immunol 1995; 154:3156–3161.
123. Whitmore AC, Prowse DM, Haughton G, Arnold LW. Ig isotype switching in B lymphocytes. The effect of T cell-derived interleukins, cytokines, cholera toxin, and antigen on isotype switch frequency of a cloned B cell lymphoma. Int Immunol 1991; 3:95–103.
124. Shockett P, Stavnezer J. Effect of cytokines on switching to IgA and α germline transcripts in the B lymphoma I.29μ: transforming growth factor-β activates transcription of the unrearranged Cα gene. J Immunol 1991; 147:4374–4383.
125. Shockett P. Regulation of IgA class switch recombination in the I.29μ B cell lymphoma by cytokines and inhibitors of poly(ADP-ribose) polymerase. PhD thesis, University of Massachusetts Graduate School of Biomedical Sciences, 1993.
126. Matsuoka M, Yoshida K, Maeda T *et al.* Switch circular DNA is formed in cytokine-treated mouse splenocytes: evidence for intramolecular DNA deletion in immunoglobulin class switching. Cell 1990; 62:135–142.
127. Shockett P, Stavnezer J. Inhibitors of poly(ADP-ribose) polymerase increase antibody class switching. J Immunol 1993; 151:6962–6976.
128. Islam KB, Nilsson L, Sideras P *et al.* TGF$\beta_1$ induces germ-line transcripts of both IgA subclasses in human B lymphocytes. Int Immunol 1991; 3:1099–1106.
129. Wakatsuki Y, Strober W. Effect of downregulation of germline transcripts on immunoglobulin A isotype differentiation. J Exp Med 1993; 178:129–138.

130. Lutzker S, Rothman P, Pollock R *et al.* Mitogen- and IL-4-regulated expression of germline Ig$\gamma$2b transcripts: evidence for directed heavy chain class switching. Cell 1988; 53:177–184.
131. Stavnezer J, Radcliffe G, Lin Y-C *et al.* Immunoglobulin heavy-chain switching may be directed by prior induction of transcripts from constant-region genes. Proc Natl Acad Sci USA 1988; 85:7704–7708.
132. Rothman P, Lutzker S, Cook W *et al.* Mitogen plus interleukin 4 induction of C$\epsilon$ transcripts in B lymphoid cells. J Exp Med 1988; 168:2385–2389.
133. Berton MT, Uhr JW, Vitetta E. Synthesis of germline $\gamma$1 immunoglobulin heavy-chain transcripts in resting B cells: induction by interleukin 4 and inhibition by interferon $\gamma$. Proc Natl Acad Sci USA 1989; 86:2829–2833.
134. Esser C, Radbruch A. Rapid induction of transcription of unrearranged S$\gamma$1 switch regions in activated murine B cells by interleukin 4. EMBO J 1989; 8:483–488.
135. Severinson E, Fernandez C, Stavnezer J. Induction of germ-line immunoglobulin heavy chain transcripts by mitogens and interleukins prior to switch recombination. Eur J Immunol 1990; 20:1079–1084.
136. Gauchat J-F, Lebman DA, Coffman RL *et al.* Structure and expression of germline $\epsilon$ transcripts in human B cells induced by interleukin 4 to switch to IgE production. J Exp Med 1990; 172:463–473.
137. Jung S, Rajewsky K, Radbruch A. Shutdown of class switch recombination by deletion of a switch region control element. Science 1993; 259:984–987.
138. Zhang J, Bottaro A. Li S *et al.* A selective defect in $IgG_{2b}$ switching as a result of targeted mutation of the $I_{\gamma 2b}$ promoter and exon. EMBO J 1993; 12:3529–3537.
139. Bottaro A, Lansford R, Xu L *et al.* I region transcription (*per se*) promotes basal IgE class switch recombination but additional factors regulate the efficiency of the process. EMBO J 1994; 13:665–674.
140. Collins JT, Dunnick WA. Germline transcripts of the murine immunoglobulin $\gamma_{2a}$ gene: structure and induction by IFN-$\gamma$. Int Immunol 1993; 5:885–891.
141. Lutzker S, Alt FW. Structure and expression of germline immunoglobulin $\gamma$2b transcripts. Mol Cell Biol 1988; 8:1849–1852.
142. Sideras P, Mizuta T-R, Kanamori H *et al.* Production of sterile transcripts of C$\gamma$ genes in an IgM-producing human neoplastic B cells line that switches to IgG-producing cells. Int Immunol 1989; 1:631–642.
143. Radcliffe G, Lin Y-C, Julius M *et al.* Structure of germline immunoglobulin $\alpha$ heavy-chain RNA and its location on polysomes. Mol Cell Biol 1990; 10:382–386.
144. Lebman DA, Nomura DHY, Coffman RL, Lee FD, Molecular characterization of germ-line immunoglobulin A transcripts produced during transforming growth factor type $\beta$-induced isotype switching. Proc Natl Acad Sci USA 1990; 87:3962–3966.
145. Rothman P, Chen Y-Y, Lutzker S *et al.* Structure and expression of germline immunoglobulin heavy chain $\epsilon$ transcripts: interleukin-4-plus lipopolysaccharide-directed switching to C$\epsilon$. Mol Cell Biol 1990; 10:1672–1679.
146. Gerondakis S. Structure and expression of murine germ-line immunoglobulin $\epsilon$ heavy chain transcripts induced by interleukin 4. Proc Natl Acad Sci USA 1990; 87:1581–1585.
147. Xu M, Stavnezer J. Structure of germline immunoglobulin heavy-chain $\gamma$1 transcripts in interleukin 4 treated mouse spleen cells. Dev Immunol 1990; 1:11–17.
148. Nilsson L, Islam KB, Olafsson O *et al.* Structure of TGF-$\beta$1 induced human immunoglobulin C$\alpha$1 and C$\alpha$2 germ-line transcripts. Int Immunol 1991; 3:1107–1115.

149. Stavnezer-Nordgren J, Sirlin S. Specificity of immunoglobulin heavy chain switch correlates with activity of germline heavy chain genes prior to switching. EMBO J 1986; 5:95–102.
150. Rothman P, Li SC, Gorham B *et al.* Identification of a conserved LPS/IL-4 responsive element located at the promoter of germline ϵ transcripts. Mol Cell Biol 1991; 11:5551–5561.
151. Berton MT, Vitetta ES. Interleukin 4 induces changes in the chromatin structure of the γ1 switch region in resting B cells before switch recombination. J Exp Med 1990; 72:375–378.
152. Schmitz J, Radbruch A. An interleukin 4-induced DNase I hypersensitive site indicates opening of the γ1 switch region prior to switch recombination. Int Immunol 1989; 1:570–575.
153. Lebman DA, Park MJ, Hansen-Bundy S, Pandya A. Mechanism for TGFβ regulation of α mRNA in LPS-stimulated B cells. Int Immunol 1993; 6:113–119.
154. Lin Y-CA, Stavnezer J. Regulation of transcription of the germline Igα constant region gene by an ATF-element and by novel transforming growth factor-β1-responsive elements. J Immunol 1992; 149:2914–2925.
155. Nilsson L, Paschalis S. The human $I_\alpha 1$ and $I_\alpha 2$ germline promoter elements: proximal positive and distal negative elements may regulate the tissue specific expression of $C_\alpha 1$ and $C_\alpha 2$ germline transcripts. Int Immunol 1993; 5:271–282.
156. Rossi P, Roberts AB, Roche NS *et al.* A nuclear factor I binding site mediates the transcriptional activation of a type I collagen promoter by TGFβ. Cell 1988; 52:405–414.
157. Riccio A, Pedone PB, Lund LR *et al.* TGFβ1-responsive element: closely associated binding sites for USF and CCAAT-binding transcription factor-NF-I in the type I plasminogen activator inhibitor gene. Mol Cell Biol 1992; 12:1846–1855.
158. Keeton MR, Curriden SA, Zonneveld A-Jv, Loskutoff DJ. Identification of regulatory sequences in the type I plasminogen activator gene responsive to TGFβ. J Biol Chem 1991; 266:23048–23052.
159. Sandler MA, Zhang J-N, Westerhausen J *et al.* A novel protein interacts with the major TGFβ responsive element in the plasminogen activator inhibitor type-1 gene. J Biol Chem 1994; 269:21500–21504.
160. Geiser AG, Kim S-J, Roberts AB, Sporn MB. Characterization of the mouse TGFβ1 promoter and activation by the Ha-ras oncogene. Mol Cell Biol 1991; 11:84–91.
161. Weinstein PD, Cebra JJ. The preference for switching to IgA expression by Peyer's patch germinal center B cells is likely due to the intrinsic influence of their microenvironment. J Immunol 1991; 147:4126–4135.
162. Santos LMB, Al-Sabbagh A, Londono A, Weiner HL. Oral tolerance to myelin basic protein induces regulatory TGFβ-secreting T cells in Peyer's patches of SJL mice. Cell Immunol 1994; 157:439–447.
163. Islam KB, Baskin B, Nilsson L *et al.* Molecular analysis of IgA deficiency. Evidence for impaired switching to IgA. J Immunol 1994; 152:1442–1452.
164. Sonoda E, Hitoshi Y, Yamaguch N *et al.* Differential regulation of IgA production by TGFβ and IL-5: TGFβ induces IgA-positive cells bearing IL-5 receptors, whereas IL-5 promotes their survival and maturation into IgA-secreting cells. Cell Immunol 1992; 140:158–172.
165. Gauchat J-F, Aversio JG, de Vries JE. Modulation of IL-4 induced germline ϵ RNA synthesis in human B cells by tumor necrosis factor-α, anti-CD40 monoclonal antibodies or transforming growth factor-β correlates with levels of IgE production. Int Immunol 1992; 4:397–406.

166. Ichiki T, Takahashi W, Watanabe T. The effect of cytokines and mitogens on the induction of Cε germline transcripts in a human Burkitt lymphoma B cell line. Int Immunol 1992; 4:747–754.

# 13 Interferon-Gamma

**CLIFFORD M. SNAPPER**
*Uniformed Services University of the Health Sciences, Bethesda, Maryland, USA*

## INTRODUCTION

Interferon-gamma (IFN-γ) is a cytokine released predominantly by CD4+ T cells of the Th1 and Th0 type, CD8+ T cells, and natural killer (NK) cells. IFN-γ plays a major role in cell-mediated immune responses by: (1) directing differentiation of naive, uncommitted CD4+ T cells towards a Th1 phenotype; (2) activating macrophages for enhanced killing of intracellular pathogens, in part through induction of nitric oxide (NO) synthesis; and (3) enhancement and/or induction of MHC class I and class II molecules on a variety of cell types (reviewed in reference 1). As discussed in this chapter, the role of IFN-γ in humoral immunity appears to be somewhat more complex. Thus, depending upon the activational milieu of the responding B cell, IFN-γ: (1) strongly stimulates B-cell maturation to immunoglobulin (Ig) secretion and (2) induces class switching to the murine IgG3 and IgG2a subclasses; or (3) inhibits class switching to other Ig isotypes, including murine IgG1/human IgG4, IgE and IgA; and (4) inhibits B-cell proliferation and Ig secretion. IFN-γ also regulates the expression of a number of B-cell membrane molecules and affects the capacity of B cells to function as antigen-presenting cells (APCs). In this chapter I will develop the hypothesis that IFN-γ has a dual role in humoral immunity: (1) to complement its effects on cell-mediated immunity to viruses and intracellular pathogens; and (2) to down-modulate immediate hypersensitivity responses and the response of the host to infections with nematode parasites. At the level of the B cell, the effect of IFN-γ will depend on both the manner by which the B cell becomes activated and the nature of the cytokine milieu.

## GENERAL CONSIDERATIONS

### MOLECULAR NATURE OF MURINE AND HUMAN IFN-γ

Both humans and mice contain a single gene for IFN-γ, located on chromosome 12 and 10, respectively[2,3]. Both genes were cloned in 1982[4–6]. The

*Cytokine Regulation of Humoral Immunity: Basic and Clinical Aspects.* Edited by Clifford M. Snapper.

human gene generates a 1.2-kb mRNA which encodes for a polypeptide of 166 amino acids. Proteolytic cleavage of the N-terminal hydrophobic signal sequence leads to a mature 143 amino acid polypeptide with a predicted molecular mass of 17 kDa. Two IFN-γ polypeptides non-covalently associate into a homodimer[7]. Only the dimeric form of IFN-γ displays biological activity, presumably through its ability to crosslink two IFN-γ receptors[8,9]. The murine IFN-γ gene generates a 1.2-kb mRNA that encodes a mature protein of 134 amino acids with a predicted molecular mass of 15.4 kDa that also dimerizes non-covalently. Human and murine IFN-γ activate cells with strict species specificity consistent with their modest homologies at the cDNA and protein levels (60 per cent and 40 per cent respectively). Both human and murine IFN-γ have two *N*-linked glycosylation sites which are not required for biological activity but which may influence circulatory half-life *in vivo*. Differential glycosylation at these *N*-linked sites gives rise to heterogeneity in the actual weight of the IFN-γ molecule (30–50 kDa). The X-ray crystallographic structure of human IFN-γ has revealed a dimeric molecule with a compact globular structure that is primarily helical (62 per cent) and without β-sheet structure[10]. Each polypeptide consists of 6 α-helices held together by short nonhelical regions. IFN-γ is sensitive to extremes of temperature and pH[11,12], with denaturation occurring at a temperature above 56°C and at a pH below 4.0 or above 9.0.

## THE IFN-γ RECEPTOR AND SIGNAL TRANSDUCTION

The IFN-γ receptor is now known to consist of at least two subunits, α and β, both of which have been cloned in human and mouse[13–17]. An α subunit is responsible for a high-affinity binding of IFN-γ ($Ka = 10^9–10^{10}\ M^{-1}$) in a strict species-specific manner. The genes for the human and murine α receptors are located on chromosomes 6 and 10, respectively[18–20]. Both genes are approximately 30 kb in size and give rise to a 2.3-kb mRNA transcript encoding mature proteins of 472 (human) and 451 (murine) amino acids with predicted molecular masses of 52.5 and 48.5 kDa, respectively. The sequence homology between the human and murine α receptors is 52 per cent. The α receptor must be fully glycosylated in order to be expressed at the cell surface and displays molecular masses between 80 and 95 kDa due to cell type-specific differences in glycosylation. Glycosylation of the receptor is not, however, necessary for IFN-γ binding. The human and murine α receptors belong to a new family of cytokine receptors termed the type II cytokine receptor family[21]. The β chains for the human and murine IFN-γ receptors have recently been cloned and are shown to be necessary for mediating the functional response of IFN-γ upon α receptor binding[22,23]. The human and murine β chains are located on chromosomes 21 and 16, respectively.

IFN-γ mediates its functional effects through the Jak–STAT family signaling pathway, a mechanistic paradigm employed by many other cytokines[24]. IFN-γ binding to its receptor is known to promote the tyrosine phosphorylation of a protein, p91, which is a member of a newly identified family of cytoplasmic signaling proteins, the signal transducers and activators of transcription (STAT)[25–27]. Phosphorylation of p91 enables its translocation from the cytoplasm to the nucleus, where it binds to and activates a γ activation site (GAS) located within the transcriptional control elements of many genes that then mediate at least some of IFN-γ's effects in the cell. Phosphorylation of p91 is mediated by the Janus kinases, Jak-1 and Jak-2, which associate with the IFN-γ receptor[28–31]. Activation of the Janus kinases is associated with their own phosphorylation on tyrosine residues. IFN-γ employs both a receptor and signaling pathway which is distinct from that utilized by IFN-α or IFN-β.

### INDUCTION OF IFN-γ SYNTHESIS

The primary cellular sources of IFN-γ are $CD4^+$ Th0 and Th1 cells, $CD8^+$ T cells and NK cells (reviewed in reference 1), although IFN-γ production from B cells[32] and macrophages[33] has been reported. The parameters which regulate the production of IFN-γ from these cell types are similar, in many ways, to those that apply to the synthesis of other cytokines, and are covered more fully in Chapter 6. However, it is worthy of note here that three cytokines, IL-12, transforming growth factor beta (TGF-β) and IL-10, are particularly relevant to the regulation of IFN-γ synthesis during immune responses. IL-12, a product of B cells and macrophages, induces IFN-γ gene expression in T and NK cells by a cyclosporin-resistant mechanism[34–36], and is a key parameter in directing T cells towards a Th1 pathway of differentiation, in part by a mechanism which is independent of IFN-γ itself[37]. TGF-β, synthesized by numerous cell types, most notably macrophages and platelets, has also been implicated in promoting differentiation of naive $CD4^+$ T cells into IFN-γ producing Th1 cells[38,39]. By contrast, IL-10, which is synthesized by macrophages, B cells and $CD4^+$ T cells of the Th2 type, was initially identified by its ability to inhibit IFN-γ production by T cells (reviewed in reference 40). This effect of IL-10 was shown to be indirect, and mediated at the level of the antigen-presenting cell[41]. IL-10 and IFN-γ are often induced concomitantly during immune responses, perhaps reflecting an IL-10 mediated negative feedback loop that limits the synthesis of IFN-γ.

## IFN-γ AND B-CELL FUNCTION

### REGULATION OF Ig CLASS SWITCHING

Ig class switching is a process whereby B cells initially expressing membrane (m)IgM and/or mIgD switch, upon activation, to the expression of IgE, IgA or one of four IgG subclasses. Through this mechanism, discussed in detail in

Chapter 5 (also reviewed in reference 42), a B cell expresses Ig that manifests new biological effector functions while maintaining the same specificity for antigen. Ig class switching is a directed process which is dependent upon both the nature of the B-cell activator and the pattern of stimulating cytokines (see Chapter 4). Cytokines and B-cell activators regulate Ig class switching in at least several distinct ways: (1) induction or suppression of transcription of constant heavy ($C_H$) genes prior to $C_H$ gene rearrangement — this is manifested by changes in the steady-state levels of germline $C_H$ RNA, which is believed to regulate the state of accessibility of the $C_H$ gene for binding of elements of the switch recombination machinery('accessibility model of Ig class switching'[43,44], see Chapter 5); and (2) stimulation or inhibition of additional switch regulatory factors, manifested by changes in the extent of $C_H$ gene rearrangement in the B-cell population, in the absence of associated alterations in the steady-state levels of germline $C_H$ RNA. IFN-γ is both an inducer and inhibitor of Ig class switching through mechanisms that appear to be both dependent and independent of germline $C_H$ gene transcription.

**Regulation of Murine IgG2a and IgG3 Class Switching**

Resting murine B cells stimulated *in vitro* with lipopolysaccharide (LPS) proliferate, secrete large amounts of IgM, and switch to the expression of IgG3, and to a lesser extent IgG2b. IFN-γ, although not IFN-α or IFN-β, induced LPS-activated cells to selectively secrete IgG2a[45,46]. This induction occurred in highly purified B cells, obtained by electronic cell sorting, which were membrane (m)IgM$^+$mIgG2a$^-$ at initiation of culture, and was associated with the selective appearance of germline $C_H\gamma2a$ RNA[47,48]. These data strongly suggested that IFN-γ acted directly on the B cell to promote IgG2a class switching in combination with LPS, and did so, at least in part, by making the $C_H\gamma2a$ gene accessible to the actions of the switching machinery.

IFN-γ strongly suppressed the synthesis of IgG3 and IgG2b by LPS-activated cells[45]. This was associated with a marked reduction in the percentage of mIgG3$^+$ cells, as assessed by flow cytometry (C. M. Snapper, unpublished), suggesting that IFN-γ inhibited LPS-induced IgG3 class switching. However, IFN-γ had no significant effect on the steady-state levels of germline $C_H\gamma3$ RNA, whereas it strongly inhibited germline $C_H\gamma2b$ RNA induced by LPS[49]. These data suggested at least two distinct mechanisms by which IFN-γ inhibited Ig class switching.

Many of the early studies on cytokine regulation of Ig class switching used LPS to induce B-cell activation. The role of the B-cell activator was envisioned at that time as that of a permissive stimulus allowing for the more specific actions of cytokines to become manifest. However, recent studies have emphasized a critical role for the B-cell activator in determining the pattern of Ig isotypes elicited in response to a particular cytokine(s) (reviewed in references 50 and 51). This concept was based in large part on data obtained through comparative analyses of Ig isotype production by murine B cells activated through distinct pathways of activation: (1) LPS, (2) multivalent mIg crosslinking utilizing dextran-conjugated anti-IgD antibodies (αδ-dex), and (3) activated T cells, T-cell membranes, or CD40 ligand (CD40L). These distinct signaling modalities were postulated to represent the predominant activational stimuli delivered to the B cell during immune responses to T-cell-independent type 1 (TI-1), TI-2 and T-cell-dependent (TD) antigens, respectively.

IFN-γ stimulated IgG2a secretion in concert with all three activational pathways: mitogenic (LPS), mIg crosslinking (αδ-dex)[52], and T cell activated[53] or CD40-mediated, using CD40 ligand (C. M. Snapper, unpublished). Whereas switching to IgG3 in response to LPS was strongly inhibited by IFN-γ, IgG3 was induced by IFN-γ in both αδ-dex-[52] and T-cell activated[54] B cells. The IFN-γ induction of IgG3 secretion by αδ-dex-activated cells was associated with an increased percentage of $mIgG3^+$ cells and an enhanced steady-state level of germline $C_H\gamma3$ RNA[52]. IFN-γ stimulated IgG3 secretion by highly purified αδ-dex-activated B cells, obtained by electronic cell sorting, that were $mIgM^+mIgG3^-$ at initiation of culture. These data strongly suggested that IFN-γ acted directly on the murine B cell to promote IgG3 class switching. Thus IFN-γ regulates IgG3 class switching in both a positive and negative manner, depending upon how the B cell is activated, whereas it co-stimulates IgG2a class switching independently of the nature of the activational stimulus.

The observation that IFN-γ stimulates IgG2a and IgG3 class switching *in vitro* has physiological relevance. Injection of mice with polyclonal goat anti-mouse IgD antibodies (GαMδ) induced a large T-cell-dependent polyclonal Ig secretory response dominated by the production of IgG1 and IgE and the synthesis of IL-4[55]. Administration of IFN-γ to GαMδ-injected mice resulted in a significant, selective enhancement in serum IgG2a levels[56]. Injection of mice with the heat-killed bacterium *Brucella abortus* (BA) itself induced a significant polyclonal IgG2a response that was partially inhibited by co-injection with neutralizing anti-IFN-γ monoclonal antibody (mAb). This indicated a role for endogenous IFN-γ in stimulating IgG2a synthesis. Although changes in serum IgG3 levels were not assessed in these studies, a recent report on mice immunized with live *Brucella abortus* or *Brucella ovis*, which induce large amounts of endogenous IFN-γ, indicated that the BA-specific Ig elicited *in vivo* was predominantly of the IgG3 and IgG2a subclasses[57,58]. A preferential synthesis of IgG2a and IgG3 antibody relative to IgG1 in response to other bacterial infections, such as those caused by *Salmonella* organisms, has also been reported[59]. Injection of mice with an IFN-γ-producing $CD4^+$ Th1 clone in combination with its specific antigen also led to an antigen-specific Ig secretory response dominated by the IgG3 and IgG2a subclasses[60].

Viruses, like certain bacteria, are also effective inducers of IFN-γ *in vivo*.

Many antiviral Ig isotype responses have been found to be dominated by Ig of the IgG2a subclass[61–64]. In addition, viruses have been found to modulate the Ig isotypic response to simultaneous challenge with soluble protein antigen, leading to a shift from protein-specific IgG1 to IgG2a[63]. Injection of virus-infected mice with an anti-IFNγ mAb has been shown to preferentially reduce the virus-specific IgG2a response[64]. The reduction in serum IgG2a levels after treatment with anti-IFN-γ mAb, however, was not complete, suggesting that IFN-γ was not completely neutralized by the anti-IFN-γ mAb and/or that IFN-γ-independent pathways for eliciting IgG2a responses also exist *in vivo*. Similar findings were reported for mice immunized with BA[56]. The selective, viral-induced synthesis of IgG2a required live virus, suggesting that a particular aspect of the virus life cycle and not simply the expression of unique antigenic epitopes accounted for this phenomenon[64].

Both IFN-γ-dependent and -independent pathways for eliciting IgG2a and/or IgG3 responses is also evident from studies using IFN-γ receptor (IFN-$\gamma R^{-/-}$) and IFN-γ (IFN-$\gamma^{-/-}$) knockout mice, respectively. Thus, IFN-$\gamma R^{-/-}$ mice had decreased total serum IgG2a concentrations relative to IFN-$\gamma R^{+/+}$ controls[65]. Immunization of IFN-$\gamma R^{-/-}$ mice with the TD antigen, TNP-ovalbumin, led to decreased IgG2a, and to a lesser extent IgG3 anti-TNP antibody responses[65]. Immunization of IFN-$\gamma R^{-/-}$ mice with a pseudorabies virus (PRV) led to a 6.5-fold and 7.5-fold reduction in PRV-specific IgG2a and IgG3 serum titers, respectively, with little or no change in the titers of PRV-specific IgG1 and IgG2b[66]. By contrast, immunization of IFN-$\gamma^{-/-}$ mice with type A influenza virus led to a significantly higher level of influenza-specific IgG1, consistent with the ability of IFN-γ to inhibit IgG1 responses, but little change in influenza-specific IgG2a[67]. Thus, the data suggest that the relative role of IFN-γ in regulating IgG2a and IgG3 responses to microbial challenge may depend upon the type of microbe and perhaps the nature of the immunization protocol.

Several studies have implicated NK cells as a source of IFN-γ for IgG2a production. Stimulation of LPS-activated spleen cells with IL-2 has been shown to increase *in vitro* polyclonal IgG2a secretion[68]. The IL-2-induced IgG2a response was IFN-γ-dependent and inhibited through pre-treatment of spleen cells with anti-asialo Gm-1 antibody, suggesting a role for NK cells. Likewise, co-injection of TNP-KLH-immunized mice with anti-asialo Gm-1 antibody led to a 2–3-fold reduction in serum IgG2a anti-TNP titers[69]. Addition of NK cells to LPS-activated cultures also augmented IgG2a synthesis through B-cell induction of NK cell-derived IFN-γ[70]. Injection of an NK cell activator, poly (I:C), into TNP-KLH-primed mice led to a preferential increase in antigen-specific IgG2a that was inhibited by prior depletion of NK cells through injection of anti-NK-1.1 mAb[71].

IL-12, as an inducer of IFN-γ from T cells and NK cells, can stimulate the production of IgG2a *in vivo*. Co-injection of IL-12 into mice immunized with TNP-keyhole limpet hemocyanin (KLH) led to higher anti-TNP IgG2a responses relative to mice immunized with TNP-KLH alone[69]. Similarly, injection of neutralizing anti-IL-12 antibody to TNP-KLH-immunized mice led to a reduction in serum anti-TNP IgG2a levels and an inhibition in the production of IFN-γ by antigen-stimulated T cells *in vitro*. Administration of IL-12 to unimmunized mice was shown to increase IFN-γ mRNA and protein expression and enhance serum concentrations of IgG2a[72]. In mice treated with polyclonal goat anti-mouse IgD antibodies plus anti-IFN-γ, the injection of IL-12 led to a selective increase in serum IgG2a and IgG3[72]. In this latter instance it was suggested that anti-IFN-γ *partially* neutralized the IFN-γ induced by IL-12, resulting in a selective enhancing effect of the residual IFN-γ for IgG2a and IgG3; higher levels of IFN-γ induced by IL-12 alone were inhibitory for all Ig isotypes, perhaps through inhibition of B-cell proliferation and/or maturation to Ig secretion.

Evidence to date has failed to implicate IFN-γ as a positive regulator of human Ig isotype switching. Although IFN-γ has been shown to selectively increase germline Cγ2 RNA in resting $mIgM^{+}mIgG^{-}$ human B cells[73], no data on whether this correlated with increased switching to IgG2 were provided. A recent report demonstrated that IFN-γ enhanced, and anti-IFN-γ antibody reduced, spontaneous IgG2 secretion by human peripheral blood mononuclear cells *in vitro*[74]. However, this effect of IFN-γ was abrogated by depletion of $mIgG2^{+}$ cells, suggesting that IFN-γ acted selectively on B cells that had already switched to this Ig isotype and was therefore not operating as a switch factor.

A recent study using bovine B cells has implicated IFN-γ as a selective, positive regulator of IgG2 secretion[75]. Thus, highly purified $IgM^{+}$ bovine B cells stimulated with pokeweed mitogen (PWM) synthesized significantly greater amounts of IgG2 in response to IFN-γ, with little change in the secretion of IgM or IgG1. This suggested that IFN-γ promoted IgG2 class switching in bovine B cells.

### Inhibition of Ig Class Switching

Whereas IFN-γ induced class switching to IgG2a and/or IgG3 in appropriately activated murine B cells, it inhibited the production of other Ig isotypes in both murine and human systems. In LPS-activated murine B cells, IFN-γ induced IgG2a class switching, but inhibited the switch to IgG3 and IgG2b[45]. This was associated with a strong reduction in the generation of $mIgG3^{+}$ cells (C. M. Snapper, unpublished) as well as IgG3 and IgG2b secretion. The ability of IFN-γ to inhibit IgG2b secretion was correlated with its inhibition of germline $C_H\gamma2b$ RNA in LPS-activated cells[49]. However, IFN-γ had no significant effect on the steady-state levels of germline $C_H\gamma3$ RNA in lipopolysaccharide (LPS)-activated cells[49], suggesting at least a dual mechanism for its inhibitory effects on class switching, one involving suppression of germline $C_H$ transcription, and the other independent of $C_H$ gene accessibility.

IFN-γ has been shown to inhibit many of the effects of IL-4 on both murine and human B cells (see Chapter 8). In murine B cells IFN-γ inhibited the IL-4-induced increase in cell size, expression of MHC class II molecules[76], CD23 (FcεRII)[77,78], and Thy-1[79,80], and anti-Ig-mediated proliferation[81], as well as *in vitro* and *in vivo* switching to IgG1 and IgE[82]. In human B cells IFN-γ also inhibited the IL-4-stimulated expression of CD23 and the switch to IgE[83]. As discussed below for human B cells, the ability of IFN-γ to inhibit *in vitro* IL-4-mediated IgE and IgG4 production depended upon the manner in which the B cell was activated.

The ability of IL-4 to stimulate murine IgG1 and IgE class switching has been well-established[82,84,85] (see Chapter 8). IL-4 stimulated IgG1 class switching by B cells activated with LPS, αδ-dex + IL-5, or through CD40 signaling (i.e. activated T cells, T-cell membranes, CD40L (reviewed in reference 50). IL-4 also stimulated IgE class switching by LPS- and CD40-activated B cells, but not in αδ-dex-activated B cells. The induction of IgG1 and IgE class switching in response to IL-4 is correlated with the induction of germline $C_H\gamma 1$ and $C_H\epsilon$ RNA, as well as the generation of mIgG1$^+$ and mIgE$^+$ cells and secretion of IgG1 and IgE (reviewed in reference 42). This indicated that IL-4 promoted the switch to these Ig isotypes by inducing $C_H\gamma 1$ and $C_H\epsilon$ accessibility for switching.

IFN-γ inhibited the IL-4 induction of mIgG1$^+$ and mIgGE$^+$ cells and the secretion of IgG1 and IgE in LPS-activated murine B cells. This was correlated with an IFN-γ-mediated inhibition of germline $C_H\gamma 1$ and $C_H\epsilon$ RNA[47]. Utilizing a novel assay to directly measure switch (S)μ–Sε DNA rearrangement (digestion-circularization polymerase chain reaction (DC-PCR)), it was demonstrated that IL-4 induced and IFN-γ inhibited $C_H\epsilon$ gene rearrangement[86]. IFN-γ also inhibited IgG1 and IgE production in T-cell-activated B cells[87]. To determine the mechanism by which IFN-γ inhibited germline $C_H\epsilon$ RNA expression, the cloned germline $C_H\epsilon$ promoter element (Iε) was linked 5′ to a CAT reporter gene, which was then transiently transfected into an LPS + IL-4-stimulated B-lymphoma line in the presence or absence of IFN-γ[86]. Cells cultured with LPS + IL-4 contained eight times more CAT activity than unstimulated cells. Addition of IFN-γ to LPS + IL-4-activated cells almost completely repressed the induced CAT activity, strongly suggesting that IFN-γ inhibited IL-4-induced germline $C_H\epsilon$ RNA by repressing the Iε promoter. The mechanism by which IFN-γ regulated Iε promoter activity is unknown. Factors which bind to Iε, and thus are implicated in its transcriptional regulation, have been identified[88]. However, IFN-γ did not appear to alter the binding of these factors[86].

IFN-γ also inhibited IgE secretion by human peripheral blood mononuclear cells cultured with IL-4, and human B cells cultured with IL-4 plus Epstein–Barr virus (EBV) or with IL-4 plus cell membranes from activated T cells[78,89–91]. However, IFN-γ had no effect on IgE secretion by purified human B cells cultured with IL-4 plus anti-CD40 antibody[92]. IL-12, in part through induction of IFN-γ, and partly through a direct effect on the B cell, also inhibited IgE secretion by human B cells stimulated with IL-4 + cortisol[93]. The IFN-γ inhibition of IL-4 induced IgE synthesis in peripheral blood mononuclear cells (PBMCs) was correlated with an 83 per cent suppression in productive (rearranged) $C_H\epsilon$ RNA and a 57 per cent reduction in germline $C_H\epsilon$ RNA[89]. By contrast, IFN-γ had no effect on IL-4-induced germline $C_H\epsilon$ RNA expression in highly purified normal B cells or B-cell lines[89,94,95], indicating that the effect of IFN-γ on B cells contained within the PBMC population involved the participation of non-B-cell types. IFN-γ, which inhibited IgE secretion by T-cell + IL-4-activated, highly purified B cells, failed to inhibit germline $C_H\epsilon$ RNA[96]. Thus, in contrast to what has been observed in the murine system, although IFN-γ has a specific inhibitory effect on IgE synthesis by human B cells, this inhibition does not appear to occur at the level of germline transcript synthesis. This is analogous to the IFN-γ-induced inhibition of murine IgG3 class switching in response to LPS despite no alteration in the steady-state levels of germline $C_H\gamma3$ RNA.

*In vivo* studies in mice have also confirmed an inhibitory role for IFN-γ in IgG1 and IgE secretory responses. As mentioned previously, injection of mice with polyclonal goat anti-mouse IgD antibodies (GαMδ) led to large T-cell-dependent IgG1 and IgE secretory responses[55]. Injection of IFN-γ into GαMδ-treated mice resulted in a strong reduction in serum IgG1 and IgE concentrations relative to mice receiving GαMδ alone[56]. Injection of a neutralizing anti-IFN-γ mAb into GαMδ-treated mice led to an enhancement in serum IgG1 and IgE concentrations, indicating a role for endogenous IFN-γ in down-modulating IgG1 and IgE responses[56]. Immunization of mice with heat-killed BA results in an induction of serum IgG1, though not IgE. Injection of anti-IFN-γ mAb into BA-treated mice led to a significant enhancement in serum IgG1 levels, although it did not lead to induction of an IgE response[56]. Unimmunized mice treated from birth with anti-IFN-γ mAb, when bled at 12 weeks of age, showed serum IgE levels nearly 4-fold higher than those in control mice, again supporting a role for endogenous IFN-γ in IgE regulation[97].

The clinical use of IFN-γ for treatment of IgE-mediated diseases has had limited utility. Treatment of patients with atopic dermatitis and high serum IgE levels with IFN-γ failed to consistently decrease serum IgE levels but did lead to a significant decrease in the 'spontaneous' *in vitro* production of IgE by PBMCs from most of these patients[98]. Despite no significant changes in serum IgE levels in response to IFN-γ, clinical improvement was observed in approximately one-half of IFN-γ-treated patients. PBMCs obtained from patients with helminth infections secreted IgE *in vitro* upon challenge with helminth antigen. Addition of anti-IFN-γ mAb to these cultures significantly augmented helminth antigen-stimulated IgE production as well as IL-4 synthesis[99,100]. IFN-γ suppressed both the *in vivo* and *in vitro* IgE production by B cells from patients with the hyper-IgE syndrome[101,102]. However, treatment with IFN-γ did not lead to a significant clinical improvement in these patients.

## REGULATION OF Ig SECRETION

Parameters which determined whether IFN-γ exerted an inductive or suppressive effect on Ig class switching included, in part, the nature of the activational stimuli delivered to the B cell. A similar picture has emerged concerning the ability of IFN-γ to regulate Ig synthesis. As will be discussed below, IFN-γ acts either as a potent inducer or inhibitor of Ig secretion, depending upon (1) the nature of the B-cell activator(s), (2) the presence of other cytokines, and (3) its timing of action relative to the stage of the B cell along the activation pathway.

### Stimulation of Ig Secretion

IFN-γ has been shown to have maturation-inducing effects on a number of immune cell types, including upregulation or induction of MHC class I and MHC class II expression, macrophage activation and stimulation of cytotoxic T-cell and NK cell activity (reviewed in reference 1). A series of early studies in the mouse also demonstrated the ability of IFN-γ to promote B-cell maturation to Ig secretion[103–108]. In many of these studies IL-2 costimulated IFN-γ-mediated Ig secretion, B cells were cultured under conditions which allowed for antigen receptor crosslinking, and/or IFN-γ was most inductive when its action was delayed relative to the action of other stimuli.

These early murine studies initially described a complex factor requirement in supernatants (SN) from T-cell hybridomas for induction of antigen-specific, Ig-secreting cells in response to soluble protein antigens *in vitro*. Three distinct factors were subsequently identified, IL-1, IL-2 and IFN-γ, which comprised the Ig-inducing activity of the T-cell SN[103]. A similar cytokine requirement was suggested for the *in vitro* Ig secretory response to sheep red blood cells (SRBCs)[103]. These data were later confirmed in the SRBC-specific plaque-forming cell (PFC) response, using recombinant IFN-γ, in the presence of IL-1 + IL-2[104,105]. In these studies, substantial Ig secretion was observed when IFN-γ was added 1–2 days after initiation of a 4-day culture, whereas IL-1 and IL-2 were required at initiation of culture. This suggested that the former acted to promote differentiation, whereas the latter were required to promote early activation events, including cellular proliferation. Further evidence of IFN-γ induction of Ig secretion was provided through inhibition of the Ig-inducing effects of these T-cell SNs with neutralizing anti-IFN-γ antibody. IFN-γ, when injected into mice simultaneously with, but not subsequent to, immunization with a number of soluble proteins (TD antigens), induced a 2–5-fold enhancement in antigen-specific PFCs[109]. The timing of IFN-γ action for stimulating Ig secretion in these studies suggested a possible effect of this cytokine on some early step in the immune response, such as antigen presentation, as opposed to a direct B-cell maturation effect.

## Inhibition of Ig Secretion

IFN-γ has also been shown *in vitro* to be inhibitory or ineffective for induction of Ig secretion. Many of these studies employed either LPS or activated T cells, T-cell membranes, or CD40L as the primary mode of B-cell activation[110–117]. The addition of IFN-γ to LPS-activated sort-purified B cells led to a 2–3-fold reduction in IgM secretion over that seen with LPS alone[117]. This effect of IFN-γ occurred even when its addition was delayed by 2 days during a 7-day culture. IFN-γ did not significantly alter the proliferative rate of LPS-activated cells, nor did it increase B-cell apoptosis, suggesting that its effect on IgM secretion was at the level of B-cell differentiation[117]. Limiting dilution analysis indicated that the IFN-γ-mediated decrease in total IgM secretion in response to LPS was due to a reduced precursor frequency of IgM-secreting cells, but that the precursors that did respond to LPS in the presence of IFN-γ secreted similar amounts of IgM compared to that observed with LPS alone[117]. Resting B cells cultured with IFN-γ, washed, and then activated with LPS alone, secreted similar amounts of IgM relative to B cells not exposed to IFN-γ. In this regard, resting B cells were found to express small, though detectable, levels of IFN-γ receptors, but these were markedly increased following LPS activation. IgM secretion by both $CD5^+$ and $CD5^-$ B cells in response to LPS was inhibited by IFN-γ, and both populations upregulated IFN-γ receptor expression after LPS activation[116]. Thus, B-cell activation, at least with LPS, may confer sensitivity to IFN-γ inhibition of IgM secretion on the B cell, at least in part through upregulation of the IFN-γ receptor. Nevertheless, it has been shown that similar preculture of resting B cells with IFN-γ prepares them to secrete enhanced levels of IgG2a upon subsequent exposure to LPS, indicating that resting B cells can respond to IFN-γ[46]. The ability of LPS, in concert with endogenous IL-2 production, to stimulate IFN-γ by splenic non-B cells (perhaps T cells and/or NK) cells *in vitro*[118] further suggests a negative feedback loop which limits LPS-induced Ig secretion.

## IFN-γ, IL-3 and GM-CSF

In an effort to better understand the dichotomous function of IFN-γ in regulating humoral immune responses, and to determine whether these IFN-γ effects were mediated directly at the level of the B cell or through non-B-cell types, my laboratory recently studied the ability of IFN-γ to regulate Ig secretory responses in sort-purified resting murine B cells activated through the mIg signaling pathway using dextran-conjugated anti-IgD antibodies (αδ-dex) in direct comparison to B cells activated through CD40[119]. Sort-purified resting B cells activated with αδ-dex proliferated but did not secrete Ig, even in the presence of IL-1 + IL-2[119,120]. We demonstrated that as little as 1 U (77 pg)/ml of IFN-γ when added *subsequent* to B-cell stimulation with αδ-dex + IL-1 + IL-2 induced up to 100-fold enhancements in Ig secretion, and in the numbers of Ig-secreting cells[119]. Maximal Ig secretory responses were observed when the addition of IFN-γ was delayed by 20–24 h after initiation of culture, although a modest (~5-fold) induction was still achieved when IFN-γ was added at initiation of culture. The predominant Ig isotype secreted was IgM, with IgG3 and IgG2a comprising the majority of non-IgM antibody. IFN-γ stimulated Ig secretion only in concert with IL-2, in both small resting and large *in vivo* preactivated B cells; neither cytokine alone was effective on αδ-dex-activated cells.

My laboratory also recently reported that both IL-3 and granulocyte-macrophage colony stimulating factor (GM-CSF), like IFN-γ, stimulated large Ig secretory responses in sort-purified resting B cells activated with αδ-dex + IL-1 + IL-2[121]. Since IL-3 and GM-CSF act synergistically with IFN-γ, have not hitherto been appreciated as direct-acting, murine B-cell maturation factors, and are not covered in separate chapters in this book, I will briefly describe our findings at this juncture. We showed that either IL-3 or GM-CSF caused 10–50-fold enhancements in Ig secretion by sort-purified B cells treated with αδ-dex + IL-1 + IL-2, and that the combined actions of IL-3 and GM-CSF were synergistic. Both IL-3 and GM-CSF acted primarily as B-cell differentiation factors, although IL-3 induced a modest enhancement in cellular outgrowth. The enhancing effects of IL-3 and GM-CSF required multivalent antigen receptor crosslinkage, mediated by αδ-dex, since neither cytokine induced Ig secretion in the presence of unconjugated anti-IgD antibodies. Although both αδ-dex and IL-1 + IL-2 were required for optimal IL-3 and GM-CSF-mediated Ig secretion, both IL-3 and GM-CSF stimulated a modest Ig secretory response by cells activated with αδ-dex alone. In this regard, SNs from activated $CD4^+$ Th1 or Th2 clones potently induced Ig secretion by αδ-dex + IL-1 + IL-2-activated B cells, and this was due, in large part, to the presence in these SNs of either IL-3 and/or GM-CSF[122]. IFN-γ synergized with IL-3 + GM-CSF for induction of Ig synthesis, in B cells activated with αδ-dex + IL-1 + IL-2. Although IFN-γ induced optimal Ig secretory responses only when added 20–24 h after initiation of culture, both IL-3 and GM-CSF were optimally inductive when added at initiation of culture[121].

As discussed, IFN-γ was shown to be an ineffective costimulus, and indeed, inhibitory, for T-cell-mediated, as well as LPS-induced, Ig secretion. Recent studies have demonstrated that the T-cell-inducible membrane protein, CD40 ligand (CD40L), also referred to as gp39 or T-BAM, is a key mediator of B-cell activation, subsequent to T-cell–B-cell contact (see Chapters, 2, 4 and 5). Thus we tested whether IFN-γ, as well as IL-3 and GM-CSF, could stimulate Ig secretion by sort-purified resting B cells activated with CD40L, in the presence of either IL-1 + IL-2 or IL-4. Neither IFN-γ, IL-3 nor GM-CSF stimulated significant Ig secretion by B cells activated through the CD40 signaling pathway alone. However, the combination of CD40 and mIg signaling, in the presence of IL-1 + IL-2, was synergistic for IFN-γ, as well as IL-3 + GM-CSF-mediated Ig synthesis. The demonstration that IFN-γ, IL-3 and GM-CSF acted directly as differentiation factors for B cells activated through their antigen receptor established a novel cytokine pathway for induction of humoral immunity, distinct from that previously described for IL-4 + IL-5.

Since αδ-dex is a model for mIg-induced signaling in response to TI-2 antigens[123,124], and since IL-3, GM-CSF and IFN-γ can be secreted by non-T cells, as well as T cells, these data suggest mechanisms for induction of humoral immunity in response to TI-2 antigens, and further delineate potential pathways by which T cells can enhance these responses. Indeed, the ability of B cells themselves to synthesize GM-CSF[125] also suggests the possibility of autocrine pathways for induction of Ig secretion.

In this regard we previously reported that NK cells induced Ig secretion by αδ-dex-activated B cells through release of a soluble factor(s), and suggested that NK cells could form a cellular basis for induction of TI-2 immunity[120,126]. Work in other laboratories has also demonstrated a stimulatory role for NK cells in both murine and humoral immune responses[127–130]. Preliminary work from our laboratory, using cytokine-specific ELISAs, has demonstrated the presence of GM-CSF, as well as IFN-γ, although no detectable IL-3, IL-4 or IL-5, in the conditioned medium from pure NK cell cultures (NKSN). Anti-IFN-γ or anti-GM-CSF were each found to significantly inhibit NKSN-induced IgM secretion by αδ-dex-activated B cells, suggesting a basis on which NK cells could regulate Ig secretory responses in a positive manner.

These data also help to clarify certain conflicts concerning the ability of $CD4^+$ Th1 clones to stimulate Ig secretory responses. Thus, a number of *in vitro* studies failed to demonstrate significant induction of Ig secretion in response to activated Th1 clones, which make IL-3, GM-CSF and IFN-γ, or the combination of Th1 SN + activated T-cell membranes[110,131]. The ability of activated T-cell membranes from Th1 clones to stimulate Ig secretion in the presence of exogenous IL-4 + IL-5 indicated that such membranes were effective B cell activators and that the Th1-derived cytokines accounted for the ineffective Ig secretory response. In these studies mIg-mediated signaling of the B cell was either bypassed entirely or elicited through bivalent anti-Ig antibodies, which, as we have shown, fail to costimulate Ig secretion in response to IL-3, GM-CSF and IFN-γ. Thus, the predominant mode of B-cell activation was through CD40, which we demonstrated was an ineffective costimulus for Ig secretion in response to Th1 SN. By contrast, injection of cells from a Th1 clone into mice, in combination with their specific antigen, led to substantial induction of antigen-specific serum Ig[60]. *In vivo*, antigen may become multivalent, either through formation of complement-fixing immune complexes or through binding to dendritic cell membranes, and thus be potentially capable of eliciting effective mIg signaling for induction of Ig secretion in response to IL-3, GM-CSF and/or IFN-γ, cytokines synthesized by Th1 clones.

### REGULATION OF B-CELL PROLIFERATION

IFN-γ can inhibit murine B-cell proliferation, especially in response to anti-Ig plus IL-4 or T-cell-mediated signals[81,132]. In human B cells, IFN-γ has been shown to promote the growth of anti-Ig-activated cells, and this IFN-γ induction could be upregulated by IL-2[133–135]. Perhaps the differences observed between the proliferative responses of murine and human B cells to IFN-γ reflected either the tissue from which the B cells were obtained, the general activation state of the B cell upon isolation, or species differences in B-cell responsiveness to IFN-γ.

## OVERVIEW OF THE ROLE OF IFN-γ IN HUMORAL IMMUNITY

An important role for IFN-γ in inducing as well as mediating cell-mediated immunity is widely appreciated. However, what role does IFN-γ play in humoral immunity? As indicated above, IFN-γ can be both inductive or inhibitory for B-cell maturation to Ig synthesis and for Ig class switching. Whether the IFN-γ effect will be negative or positive appears to depend upon: (1) the manner in which the B cell becomes activated, which depends upon the nature of the antigenic stimulus; (2) the profile of other cytokines and cell types in the milieu; (3) the particular $C_H$ gene in question; and (4) the timing of action of IFN-γ. Given these observations, we can put forth a reasonable hypothesis on the physiological role of IFN-γ in humoral immunity.

The ability of IFN-γ to selectively induce IgG2a and IgG3 class switching in the mouse as well as promote the secretion of these Ig isotypes may shed some light on its role in the humoral immune response. Thus many viral, as well as a number of bacterial, infections selectively elicit IgG2a and/or IgG3 responses. IgG2a is efficient at fixing complement and binds selectively to a high-affinity Fc receptor on monocytes (FcγR1) which is upregulated by IFN-γ. IFN-γ is a potent macrophage activation factor, and in concert with IgG2a is particularly effective at mediating antibody-dependent cellular cytotoxicity (ADCC). Thus, IgG2a synthesis during a viral infection could serve to augment the antiviral cell-mediated immune response, in which macrophages play a key role (reviewed in reference 136).

IgG3 also fixes complement and is unique in its ability to self-aggregate, presumably making it an effective opsonin. IgG2a and IgG3 were found to be most efficient among the IgG subclasses at mediating NK cell ADCC, through binding to the NK cell Fc receptor for IgG, CD16. NK cells are believed to play an important role in cell-mediated immune responses, in part by mediating ADCC and as a rich source of IFN-γ during viral and bacterial infections. The ability of NK cells to release cytokines such as IFN-γ and GM-CSF implicates them in T-cell independent pathways for induction of Ig secretion and/or class switching. Thus, IFN-γ may be important in engaging a qualitatively distinct arm of the humoral immune system that synergizes with the cell-mediated immune network to optimize host protection against certain types of microbial infections. Through its ability to inhibit differentiation of $CD4^+$ T cells towards IL-4 production and suppress a number of IL-4-mediated effects on B cells, IFN-γ may also serve as a key down-modulator of immediate hypersensitivity responses in which IL-4-induced IgE plays an important role. More generally, given the cross-inhibitory properties of IFN-γ producing (Th1) and IL-4-producing (Th2) T cells, IFN-γ may serve to limit induction of an immune network unsuited, and even counterproductive, for an effective response to a particular microbial challenge.

## REFERENCES


1. Farrar MA, Schreiber RD. The molecular cell biology of interferon-γ and its receptor. Annu Rev Immunol 1993; 11:571–611.
2. Naylor SL, Sakaguchi AY, Shows TB *et al.* Human immune interferon gene is located on chromosome 12. J Exp Med 1983; 157:1020–1027.
3. Naylor SL, Gray PW, Lalley PA. Mouse immune interferon (IFNγ) gene is on murine chromosome 10. Somat Cell Mol Genet 1984; 10:531–534.
4. Gray PW, Leung DW, Pennica D *et al.* Expression of human immune interferon cDNA in *E. coli* and monkey cells. Nature 1982; 295:503–508.
5. Gray PW, Goeddel DV. Structure of the human immune interferon gene. Nature 1982: 298:859–863.
6. Gray PW, Goeddel DV. Cloning and expression of murine immune interferon cDNA. Proc Natl Acad Sci USA 1983: 80:5842–5846.
7. Nagata K, Izumi T, Kitagawa T, Yoshida N. Oligomeric structure of recombinant human and murine immune interferons by means of sedimentation equilibrium. J Interferon Res 1987; 7:313–320.
8. Greenlund AC, Wenner CA, Schreiber RD. Analysis of IFNγ receptor binding to IFNγ. J Interferon Res 1992; 12:S103.
9. Fountoulakis M, Zulauf M, Lustig A, Garotta G. Stoichiometry of interaction between interferon-γ and its receptor. Eur J Biochem 1992; 209:781–787.
10. Ealick SE, Cook WJ, Vijay-Kumar S *et al.* Three-dimensional structure of recombinant human interferon-gamma. Science 1991; 252:698–702.
11. Hsu YR, Arakawa T. Structural studies on acid unfolding and refolding of recombinant human interferon gamma. Biochemistry 1985; 24:7959–7963.
12. Mulkerrin MG, Wetzel R. pH dependence of the reversible and irreversible thermal denaturation of gamma interferons. Biochemistry 1989; 28:6556–6561.

13. Aguet M, Dembic Z, Merlin G. Molecular cloning and expression of the human interferon-γ receptor. Cell 1988; 55:273–280.
14. Gray PW, Leong S, Fennie EH *et al.* Cloning and expression of the cDNA for the murine interferon gamma receptor. Proc Natl Acad Sci USA 1989; 86:8497–8501.
15. Kumar CS, Mulhukumaran G, Frost LJ *et al.* Molecular characterization of the murine interferon-γ cDNA. J Biol Chem 1989; 264:17939–17946.
16. Munro S, Maniatis T. Expression and cloning of the murine interferon-γ receptor cDNA. Proc Natl Acad Sci USA 1989; 86:9248–9252.
17. Hemmi S, Peghini P, Metzler M *et al.* Cloning of murine interferon gamma receptor cDNA: expression in human cells mediates high-affinity binding but is not sufficient to confer sensitivity to murine interferon gamma. Proc Natl Acad Sci USA 1989; 86:9901–9905.
18. Pfizenmaier K, Wiegmann K, Scheurich P *et al.* High affinity human IFN-gamma-binding capacity is encoded by a single receptor gene located in proximity to c-ros on human chromosome region 6q16 to 6q22. J Immunol 1988; 141:856–860.
19. Mariano TM, Kozak CA, Langer JA, Pestka S. The mouse immune interferon receptor gene is located on chromosome 10. J Biol Chem 1987; 262:5812–5814.
20. Kozak CA, Peyser M, Krall *et al.* Molecular genetic markers spanning mouse chromosome 10. Genomics 1990; 8:519–524.
21. Bazan JF. Structural design and molecular evolution of a cytokine receptor superfamily. Proc Natl Acad Sci USA 1990; 87:6934–6938.
22. Soh J, Donnelly RJ, Kotenko S *et al.* Identification and sequence of an accessory factor required for activation of the human interferon γ receptor. Cell 1994; 76:793–802.
23. Hemmi S, Bohni R, Stark G *et al.* A novel member of the interferon receptor family complements functionality of the murine interferon γ receptor in human cells. Cell 1994; 76:803–810.
24. Rothman P, Kreider B, Azam M *et al.* Cytokines and growth factors signal through tyrosine phosphorylation of a family of related transcription factors. Immunity 1994; 1:457–468.
25. Shuai K, Schindler C, Prezioso V, Darnell JE. Activation of transcription by IFNγ: tyrosine phosphorylation of a 91-kDa DNA binding protein. Science 1992; 258:1808–1812.
26. Schindler C, Shuai K, Prezioso V, Darnell J. Interferon-dependent tyrosine phosphorylation of a latent cytoplasmic transcription factor. Science 1992; 257:809–813.
27. Pellegrini S, Schindler C. Early events in signaling by interferons. TIBS 1993; 18:338–342.
28. Muller M, Briscoe J, Laxton C *et al.* The protein tyrosine kinase Jak-1 complements defects in the interferon-α/β and -γ signal transduction pathways. Nature 1993; 366:129–135.
29. Shuai K, Ziemiecki A, Wilks AF *et al.* Polypeptide signaling to the nucleus through tyrosine phosphorylation of Jak and Stat proteins. Nature 1993; 366:580–585.
30. Silvennoinen O, Ihle J, Schlessinger J, Levy DE. Interferon-induced nuclear signaling by JAK protein tyrosine kinases. Nature 1993; 366:583–585.
31. Watling D, Gushin D, Muller M *et al.* Complementation by the tyrosine kinase Jak2 of a mutant cell line defective in the interferon-γ signal transduction pathway. Nature 1993; 366:166–170.
32. Pang Y, Norihisa Y, Benjamin D *et al.* Interferon-γ gene expression in human B-cell lines: induction by interleukin-2, protein kinase C activators, and possible effect of hypomethylation on gene regulation. Blood 1992; 80:724–732.

33. Fultz MJ, Barber, SA, Dieffenbach CW, Vogel SN. Induction of IFN-γ in macrophages by lipopolysaccharide. Int Immunol 1993; 5:1383–1392.
34. Stern AS, Podlaski FJ, Hulmes JD *et al.* Purification to homogeneity and partial characterization of cytotoxic lymphocyte maturation factor from human B-lymphoblastoid cells. Proc Natl Acad Sci USA 1990; 87:6808–6812.
35. Wolf SF, Temple PA, Kobayashi M *et al.* Cloning of cDNA for natural killer cell stimulatory factor, a heterodimeric cytokine with multiple biologic effects on T and natural killer cells. J Immunol 1991; 146:3074–3080.
36. Chan SH, Kobayashi M, Santoli D *et al.* Mechanisms of IFN-gamma induction by natural killer cell stimulatory factor (NKSF/IL-12): role of transcription and mRNA stability in the synergistic interaction between NKSF and IL-2. J Immunol 1992; 148:92–98.
37. Manetti R, Parronchi P, Giudizi MG *et al.* Natural killer cell stimulatory factor (interleukin 12 [IL-12]) induces T helper type 1 (Th1)-specific immune responses and inhibits the development of IL-4-producing Th cells. J Exp Med 1993; 177:1199–1204.
38. Fargeas C, Wu CY, Nakajima T *et al.* Differential effect of transforming growth factor β on the synthesis of Th1- and Th2-like lymphokines by human T lymphocytes. Eur J Immunol 1992; 22:2173–2176.
39. Nagelkerken L, Gollob KJ, Tielemans M, Coffman RL. Role of transforming growth factor-β in the preferential induction of T helper cells of type I by staphylococcal enterotoxin B. Eur J Immunol 1993; 23:2306–2310.
40. Moore KW, O'Garra A, Malefyt RW *et al.* Interleukin-10. Annu Rev Immunol 1993; 11:165–190.
41. Fiorentino DF, Zlotnik A, Vieira P *et al.* IL-10 acts on the antigen-presenting cell to inhibit cytokine production by Th1 cells. J Immunol 1991; 146:3444–3451.
42. Snapper CM, Finkelman FD. Immunoglobulin class switching. In: Paul W (ed.) Fundamental Immunology, 3rd edn. 1993, pp. 837–863, Raven Press, New York.
43. Stavnezer-Nordgren J, Sirlin S. Specificity of immunoglobulin heavy chain switch correlates with activity of germline heavy chain genes prior to switching. EMBO J 1986; 5:95–102.
44. Yancopoulos GD, DePinho RA, Zimmerman KA *et al.* Secondary genomic rearrangement events in pre-B cells: $V_HDJ_H$ replacement by a LINE-1 sequence and directed class switching. EMBO J 1986; 5:3259–3266.
45. Snapper CM, Paul WE. Interferon-γ and B cell stimulatory factor-1 reciprocally regulate Ig isotype production. Science 1987; 236:944–947.
46. Snapper CM, Peschel C, Paul WE. IFN-γ stimulates IgG2a secretion by murine B cells stimulated with bacterial lipopolysaccharide. J Immunol 1988; 140:2121–2127.
47. Severinson E, Fernandez C, Stavnezer J. Induction of germ-line immunoglobulin heavy chain transcripts by mitogens and interleukins prior to switch recombination. Eur J Immunol 1990; 20:1079–1084.
48. Collins JT, Dunnick WA. Germline transcripts of the murine immunoglobulin γ2a gene: structure and induction by IFN-γ. Int Immunol 1993; 5:885–891.
49. Zelazowski P, Collins JT, Dunnick W, Snapper CM. Antigen receptor cross-linking differentially regulates germ-line $C_H$ ribonucleic acid expression in murine B cells. J Immunol 1995; 154:1223–1231.
50. Snapper CM, Mond JJ. Towards a comprehensive view of immunoglobulin class switching. Immunol Today 1993; 14:15–17.
51. Mond JJ, Lees A, Snapper CM. T cell-independent type 2 antigens. Annu Rev Immunol 1995; 13:655–692.
52. Snapper CM, McIntyre TM, Mandler R *et al.* Induction of IgG3 secretion by interferon γ: a model for T cell-independent class switching in response to T cell-independent type 2 antigens. J Exp Med 1992; 175:1367–1371.

53. Stevens TL, Bossie A, Sanders VM *et al.* Regulation of antibody isotype secretion by subsets of antigen-specific helper T cells. Nature 1988; 334:255–258.
54. Croft M, Swain SL. B cell response to T helper cell subsets. II. Both the stage of T cell differentiation and the cytokines secreted determine the extent and nature of helper activity. J Immunol 1991; 147:3679–3689.
55. Finkelman FD, Katona IM, Urban JR *et al.* Suppression of in vivo polyclonal IgE responses by monoclonal antibody to the lymphokine B-cell stimulatory factor 1. Proc Natl Acad Sci USA 1986; 83:9675–9678.
56. Finkelman FD, Katona IM, Mosmann T and Coffman RL. IFN-γ regulates the isotypes of Ig secreted during *in vivo* humoral immune responses. J Immunol 1988; 140:1022–1027.
57. Elzer PH, Jacobson RH, Nielsen KH *et al.* BALB/c mice infected with *Brucella abortus* express protracted polyclonal responses of both IgG2a and IgG3 isotypes. Immunol Lett 1994; 42:145–150.
58. de Bagues MPJ, Elzer PH, Blasco JM *et al.* Protective immunity to *Brucella ovis* in BALB/c mice following recovery from primary infection or immunization with subcellular vaccines. Infect Immun 1994; 62:632–638.
59. Thatte J, Rath S, Val V. Immunization with live versus killed Salmonella typhimurium leads to the generation of an IFN-γ-dominant versus an IL-4-dominant immune response. Int Immunol 1993; 5:1431–1436.
60. Rizzo LV, DeKruyff RH, Umetsu DT. Generation of B cell memory and affinity maturation. Induction with Th1 and Th2 T cell clones. J Immunol 1992; 148:3733–3739.
61. Coutelier JP, van der Logt JTM, Heessen FWA. IgG subclass distribution of primary and secondary immune responses concomitant with viral infection. J Immunol 1991; 147:1383–1386.
62. Coutelier JP, van der Logt JTM, Heessen FWA *et al.* IgG2a restriction of murine antibodies elicited by viral infections. J Exp Med 1987; 165:64–69.
63. Coutelier JP, van der Logt JTM, Heessen FWA *et al.* Virally induced modulation of murine IgG antibody subclasses. J Exp Med 1988; 168:2373–2378.
64. Nguyen L, Knipe DM, Finbert RW. Mechanism of virus-induced Ig subclass shifts. J Immunol 1994; 152:478–484.
65. Huang S, Hendriks W, Althage A *et al.* Immune response in mice that lack interferon-γ receptor. Science 1993; 259:1742–1745.
66. Schijns VECJ, Haagmans BL, Rijke EO *et al.* IFN-γ receptor-deficient mice generate antiviral Th1-characteristic cytokine profiles but altered antibody responses. J Immunol 1994; 153:2029–2037.
67. Graham MB, Dalton DK, Giltinan D *et al.* Response to influenza infection in mice with a targeted disruption in the interferon γ gene. J Exp Med 1993; 178:1725–1732.
68. Amigorena S, Bonnerot C, Fridman WH, Teillaud J-L. Recombinant interleukin 2-activated natural killer cells regulate IgG2a production. Eur J Immunol 1990; 21:1781–1787.
69. McKnight AJ, Zimmer GJ, Fogelman I *et al.* Effects of IL-12 on helper T cell-dependent immune responses in vivo. J Immunol 1994; 152:2172–2179.
70. Michael A, Shao A, Yuan D. Productive interactions between B and natural killer cells. Nat Immun Cell Growth Regul 1991; 10:71–82.
71. Yuan D, Koh CY, Wilder JA. Interactions between B lymphocytes and NK cells. FASEB J. 1994; 8:1012–1018.
72. Morris SC, Madden KB, Adamovicz JJ *et al.* Effects of IL-12 on in vivo cytokine gene expression and Ig isotype selection. J Immunol 1994; 152:1047–1056.
73. Kitani A, Strober W. Regulation of Cγ subclass germ-line transcripts in human peripheral blood B cells. J Immunol 1993; 151:3478–3488.

74. Kawano Y, Noma T, Yata J. Regulation of human IgG subclass production by cytokines: IFN-γ and IL-6 act antagonistically in the induction of human IgG1 but additively in the induction of IgG2. J Immunol 1994; 153:4948–4958.
75. Estes DM, Closser NM, Allen GK. IFN-γ stimulates IgG2 production from bovine B cells costimulated with anti-μ and mitogen. Cell Immunol 1994; 154:287–295.
76. Mond JJ, Carman J, Sarma C *et al.* Interferon-γ suppresses B cell stimulation factor (BSF-1) induction of class II MHC determinants on B cells. J Immunol 1986; 137:3534–3537.
77. Conrad DH, Waldschmidt TJ, Lee WT *et al.* Effect of B cell stimulatory factor-1 (interleukin 4) on Fcε and Fcγ receptor expression on murine lymphocytes and B cell lines. J Immunol 1987; 139:2290–2296.
78. Pene J, Rousset F, Briere F *et al.* IgE production by normal human lymphocytes is induced by interleukin 4 and suppressed by interferons γ and α and prostaglandin E2. Proc Natl Acad Sci USA 1988; 85:6880–6884.
79. Snapper CM, Hornbeck PV, Atasoy U *et al.* Interleukin 4 induces membrane Thy-1 expression on normal murine B cells. Proc Natl Acad Sci USA 1988; 85:6107–6111.
80. Snapper CM, Hooley JJ, Barbieri S, Finkelman FD. Murine B cells expressing Thy-1 after in vivo immunization selectively secrete IgE. J Immunol 1990; 144:2940–2945.
81. Mond JJ, Finkelman FD, Sarma C *et al.* Recombinant interferon-γ inhibits the B cell proliferative response stimulated by soluble but not by sepharose bound anti-immunoglobulin antibody. J Immunol 1985; 135:2513–2517.
82. Coffman RL, Carty J. A T cell activity that enhances polyclonal IgE production and its inhibition by interferon-γ. J Immunol 1986; 136:949–954.
83. Pene J, Rousset F, Briere F *et al.* IgE production by normal human lymphocytes is induced by interleukin 4 and suppressed by interferons γ and α and prostaglandin E2. Proc Natl Acad Sci USA 1988; 85:6880–6884.
84. Isakson PC, Pure E, Vitetta ES, Krammer PH. T cell-derived B cell differentiation factor(s). Effect on the isotype switch of murine B cells. J Exp Med 1982; 155:734–748.
85. Severinson E, Bergstedt-Lindqvist S, van der Loo W, Fernandez C. Characterization of the IgG response induced by polyclonal B cell activators. Immunol Rev. 1982; 67:73.
86. Xu L, Rothman P. IFN-γ represses ε germline transcription and subsequently down-regulates switch recombination to ε. Int Immunol 1994; 6:515–521.
87. Coffman RL, Seymour BWP, Lebman DA *et al.* The role of helper T cell products in mouse B cell differentiation and isotype regulation. Immunol Rev 1988; 102:5–28.
88. Rothman P, Li SC, Gorham B *et al.* Identification of a conserved lipopolysaccharide-plus-interleukin-4-responsive element located at the promoter of germ line ε transcripts. Mol Cell Biol 1991; 11:5551–5561.
89. Gauchat J-F, Lebman DA, Coffman RL *et al.* Structure and expression of germline ε transcripts in human B cells induced by interleukin 4 to switch to IgE production. J Exp Med 1990; 172:463–473.
90. Thyphronitis G, Tsokos GC, June CH *et al.* IgE secretion by Epstein–Barr virus-infected purified human B lymphocytes is stimulated by interleukin 4 and suppressed by interferon γ. Proc Natl Acad Sci USA 1989; 86:5580–5584.
91. Thyphronitis G, Banchereau J, Heusser C *et al.* Kinetics of interleukin-4 induction and interferon-γ inhibition of IgE secretion by Epstein–Barr virus-infected human peripheral blood B cells. Cell Immunol 1991; 133:408–419.
92. Gascan H, Gauchat J-F, Aversa G *et al.* Anti-CD40 monoclonal antibodies or

CD4+ T cell clones and IL-4 induce IgG4 and IgE switching in purified human B cells via different signaling pathways. J Immunol 1991; 147:8–13.

93. Kiniwa M, Gately M, Guller V *et al.* Recombinant interleukin-12 suppresses the synthesis of immunoglobulin E by interleukin-4 stimulated human lymphocytes. J Clin Invest 1992; 90:262–266.
94. Gauchat J-F, Gascan H, de Waal Malefyt R, de Vries JE. Regulation of germline $\epsilon$ transcription and induction of $\epsilon$ switching in cloned EBV-transformed and malignant human B cell lines by cytokines and CD4+ T cells. J Immunol 1992; 148:2291–2299.
95. Ichiki T, Takahashi W, Watanabe T. The effect of cytokines and mitogens on the induction of $C\epsilon$ germline transcripts in a human Burkitt lymphoma B cell line. Int Immunol 1992; 4:747–754.
96. Gauchat J-F, Aversa G, Gascan H, de Vries JE. Modulation of IL-4 induced germline $\epsilon$ RNA synthesis in human B cells by tumor necrosis factor-$\alpha$, anti-CD40 monoclonal antibodies or transforming growth factor-$\beta$ correlates with levels of IgE production. Int Immunol 1992; 4:397–406.
97. Finkelman FD, Holmes J, Katona IM *et al.* Lymphokine control of *in vivo* immunoglobulin isotype selection. Annu Rev Immunol 1990; 8:303–333.
98. Leung DYM, Boguniewicz M, Vercelli D *et al.* Gamma interferon inhibits IgE production in patients with atopic dermatitis. Clin Res 1989; 37:239A.
99. King CL, Ottesen EA, Nutman TB. Cytokine regulation of antigen-driven immunoglobulin production in filarial parasite infections in humans. J Clin Invest 1990; 85:1810–1815.
100. King CL, Low CC, Nutman TB. IgE production in human helminth infection: reciprocal interrelationship between IL-4 and IFN-$\gamma$. J Immunol 1993; 150:1873–1880.
101. Li JTC, Yunginger JW, Reed CE *et al.* Lack of suppression of IgE production by recombinant interferon gamma: a controlled trial in patients with allergic rhinitis. J Allergy Clin Immunol 1990; 85:934–940.
102. Vercelli D, Jabara HH, Cunningham-Rundles C *et al.* J Clin Invest 1990; 85:1666–1671.
103. Roehm NW, Marrack P, Kappler JW. Helper signals in the plaque-forming cell response to protein-bound hapten. J Exp Med 1983; 158:317–332.
104. Leibson HJ, Gefter M, Zlotnik A *et al.* Role of $\gamma$-interferon in antibody-producing responses. Nature 1984; 309:799–801.
105. Brunswick M, Lake P. Obligatory role of gamma interferon in T cell-replacing factor-dependent, antigen-specific murine B cell responses. J Exp Med 1985; 161:953–971.
106. Nakagawa T, Hirano T, Nakagawa N *et al.* Effect of recombinant IL-2 and $\gamma$-IFN on proliferation and differentiation of human B cells. J Immunol 1985; 134:959–966.
107. Nakagawa T, Nakagawa N, Volkman DJ, Fauci AS. Sequential synergistic effect on interleukin 2 and interferon-$\gamma$ on the differentiation of a TAC-antigen positive B cell line. J Immunol 1986; 136:164–168.
108. Jelinek DF, Splawski JB, Lipsky PE. The roles of interleukin 2 and interferon-$\gamma$ in human B cell activation, growth and differentiation. Eur J Immunol 1986; 16:925–932.
109. Nakamura M, Manser T, Pearson GDN *et al.* Effect of IFN-$\gamma$ on the immune response in vivo and on gene expression in vitro. Nature 1984; 307:381–383.
110. Mosmann TR, Coffman RL. TH1 and TH2 cells: different patterns of lymphokine secretion lead to different functional properties. Annu Rev Immunol 1989; 7:145–173.
111. Maliszewsi CR, Grabstein K, Fanslow WC *et al.* Recombinant CD40 ligand

stimulation of murine B cell growth and differentiation: cooperative effects of cytokines. Eur J Immunol 1993; 23:1044–1049.

112. Armitage RJ, Macduff BM, Spriggs MK, Fanslow WC. Human B cell proliferation and Ig secretion induced by recombinant CD40 ligand are modulated by soluble cytokines. J Immunol 1993; 150:3671–3680.

113. Tucci A, James H, Chicheportiche R *et al.* Effects of eleven cytokines and IL-1 and tumor necrosis factor inhibitors in a human B cell assay. J Immunol 1992; 148:2778–2784.

114. Boom WH, Liano D, Abbas AK. Heterogeneity of helper/inducer T lymphocytes. II. Effects of interleukin 4- and interleukin 2-producing T cell clones on resting B lymphocytes. J Exp Med 1988; 167:1350–1363.

115. Noelle RJ, Daum J, Bartlett WC. Cognate interactions between helper T cells and B cells. V. Reconstitution of T helper cell function using purified plasma membranes from activated Th1 and Th2 helper cells and lymphokines. J Immunol 1991; 146:1118–1124.

116. Abed NS, Chace JH, Cowdery JS. T cell-dependent and T cell-dependent B cell activation increase IFN-γR expression and renders B cells sensitive to IFN-γ-mediated inhibition. J Immunol 1994; 153:3369–3377.

117. Abed NS, Chace JH, Fleming AL, Cowdery JS. Interferon-γ regulation of B lymphocyte differentiation: activation of B cells is a prerequisite for IFN-γ-mediated inhibition of B cell differentiation. Cell Immunol 1994; 153:356–366.

118. Blanchard DK, Djeu JY, Klein TW *et al.* Interferon-γ induction by lipopolysaccharide: dependence on interleukin 2 and macrophages. J Immunol 1986; 136:963–970.

119. Snapper CM, Moorman MA, Rosas F *et al.* Interferon-gamma is a potent inducer of Ig secretion by sort-purified murine B cells activated through the mIg, but not the CD40 signalling pathway. J Immunol, in press.

120. Snapper CM, Yamaguchi H, Moorman MA *et al.* Natural killer cells induce activated murine B cells to secrete Ig. J Immunol 1993; 151:5251–5260.

121. Snapper CM, Moorman MA, Rosas FR *et al.* IL-3 and GM-CSF strongly induce Ig secretion by sort-purified murine B cells activated through the membrane of Ig, but not the CD40 signalling pathway. J Immunol 1995; 154: 5842–5850.

122. Mosmann, TR, Cherwinski H, Bond MW *et al.* Two types of murine helper T cell clone. I. Definition according to profiles of lymphokine activities and secreted proteins. J Immunol 1986; 136:2348–2357.

123. Brunswick M, Finkelman FD, Highet PF *et al.* Picogram quantities of anti-Ig antibodies coupled to dextra induce B cell proliferation. J Immunol 1988; 140:3364–3372.

124. Peçanha LMT, Snapper CM, Finkelman FD, Mond JJ. Dextran-conjugated anti-Ig antibodies as a model for T cell-independent type 2 antigen-mediated stimulation of Ig secretion *in vitro*. I. Lymphokine dependence. J Immunol 1991; 146:833–839.

125. Bickel M, Amstad P, Tsuda H *et al.* Induction of granulocyte-macrophage colony-stimulating factor by lipopolysaccharide and anti-immunoglobulin M-stimulated murine B cell lines. J Immunol 1987; 139:2984–2988.

126. Snapper CM, Yamaguchi H, Moorman MA, Mond JJ. An in vitro model for T cell-independent induction of humoral immunity. A requirement for NK cells. J Immunol 1994; 152:4884–4892.

127. Yuan D, Wilder J, Dang T *et al.* Activation of B lymphocytes by NK cells. Int Immunol 1992; 4:1373–1380.

128. Rodriguez MA, Blanca I, Baroja ML *et al.* Helper activity by human large granular lympohocytes in in vitro immunoglobulin synthesis. J Clin Immunol 1987; 7:356–364.

129. Kimata H, Sherr EH, Saxon A. Human natural killer (NK) cells produce a late-acting B-cell differentiation activity. J Clin Immunol 1988; 8:381–389.
130. Brenner MK, Vyakarnam A, Reittie JE *et al.* Human large granular lymphocytes induce immunoglobulin synthesis after bone marrow transplantation. Eur J Immunol 1987; 17:43–47.
131. Noelle RJ, Daum J, Bartlett WC. Cognate interactions between helper T cells and B cells. V. Reconstitution of T helper cell function using purified plasma membranes from activated Th1 and Th2 helper cells and lymphokines. J Immunol 1991; 146:1118–1124.
132. Rabin E, Mond JJ, Ohara J, Paul WE. Interferon-$\gamma$ inhibits the action of B cell stimulatory factor (BSF-1) on resting B cells. J Immunol 1986; 137:1573–1576.
133. Defrance T, Aubry J-P, Vanbervliet B, Banchereau J. Human interferon-$\gamma$ acts as a B cell growth factor in the anti-IgM antibody costimulatory assay but has no direct B cell differentiation activity. J Immunol 1986; 137:3861–3867.
134. Romagnani S, Giudizi MG, Biagiotti R *et al.* B cell growth factor activity of interferon-$\gamma$. Recombinant human interferon-$\gamma$ promotes proliferation of anti-$\mu$ activated human B lymphocytes. J Immunol 1986; 136:3513–3516.
135. Morikawa K, Kubagawa H, Suzuki T, Cooper MD. Recombinant interferon-$\alpha$, -$\beta$ and -$\gamma$ enhance the proliferative response of human B cells. J Immunol 1987; 139:761–768.
136. Snapper CM. The regulation of B cell function by interferon-gamma. In: Baron S, Coppenhaver D, Dianzani F *et al.* (eds) Interferon: Principles and Medical Applications. Galveston TX: The University of Texas Medical Branch, 1992, pp. 373–385.

# 14 Neuropeptides

**HAJIME KIMATA**
*Kyoto University Hospital, Kyoto, Japan*

## MODULATION OF CYTOKINE SECRETION AND CELLULAR SOURCES

Initially, neuropeptides were observed in the brain and gut, where they were found to affect various responses in the central nervous system and endocrine organs[1,2]. However, it later became clear that they also have functional effects on various cell types in both the murine and human immune systems.

Neuropeptides modulate secretion of inflammatory mediators and cytokines. Vasoactive intestinal peptide (VIP) inhibits peptidoleukotriene release from rat lung, while it increases interleukin-6 (IL-6) production by rat anterior pituitary cells[3,4]. Somatostatin (SOM) induces histamine secretion from rat peritoneal mast cells[5]. Substance P (SP) enhances production of interferon gamma (IFN-$\gamma$), IL-1, IL-2, IL-6 and tumor necrosis factor alpha (TNF-$\alpha$) by human peripheral blood mononuclear cells (PBMNCs), monocytes and T cells[6–9]. SP also enhances the secretion of TNF-$\alpha$ from rat neuroglial cells[10]. Neuropeptides are synthesized by various cells which participate in immune and inflammatory responses. Thus, VIP, SOM and SP are present in human neutrophils, eosinophils and mononuclear cells (MNCs)[11,12]. VIP is also present in rat anterior pituitary tissues, human nasal mucosa and lung[13–15].

## NEUROPEPTIDE RECEPTORS ON LYMPHOCYTES

Neuropeptide receptors are expressed on lymphocytes and monocytes. VIP receptors are expressed on mouse lymphocytes from mesenteric lymph nodes, subcutaneous lymph nodes, spleen, Peyer's patches and thymus[16]. VIP receptors are also present on human peripheral blood T cells, B cells and natural killer (NK) cells, human lymphoblastoid B-cell lines, T-cell lines and a myeloma cell line[17–21]. SOM receptors are expressed on mouse spleen and Peyer's patch T and B lymphocytes[22], and on a mouse plasmacytoma line[23]. SOM receptors are also present on human peripheral blood lymphocytes, monocytes, T cells and T-cell lines[24–26]. SP receptors are present on a mouse

*Cytokine Regulation of Humoral Immunity: Basic and Clinical Aspects.* Edited by Clifford M. Snapper.

B-lymphoma cells line, and human T cells and a plasma cell line, and within arterioles and lymph nodules[27–30].

## CELL PROLIFERATION

Neuropeptides modulate proliferation or infiltration of many cell types. VIP inhibits proliferation of mouse T cells stimulated with concanavalin A (Con A) or phytohemagglutinin (PHA)[16]. VIP also inhibits human T-cell proliferation stimulated with mercuric chloride[31]. By contrast, we have reported that VIP enhances spontaneous proliferation of human B-cell lines (Figure 14.1b and Table 14.1)[32]. SOM inhibits proliferation of rat thymocytes stimulated with Con A[33], while SOM enhances spontaneous proliferation of mouse spleen lymphocytes and of a plasmacytoma line[23,34]. In addition, SOM inhibits proliferation of human hepatoma cells stimulated with insulin and of breast cancer cells stimulated with insulin and/or estradiol[35,36]. By contrast, SOM enhances proliferation of human T cells stimulated with mercuric chloride[31], while SOM fails to stimulate proliferation of a human B-cell line (Figure 14.1b)[32]. SP inhibits human T-cell proliferation stimulated with mercuric chloride[31] and fails to stimulate proliferation of a human B-cell line (Figure 14.1b)[32]. SP also stimulates mouse eosinophil and neutrophil infiltration[37].

## IMMUNOGLOBULIN PRODUCTION

Neuropeptides have differential effects on Ig production. VIP enhances Con A-induced IgA production by MNCs from mouse spleen and mesenteric

**Table 14.1** Effects of VIP on CBL and IM-9 cells

| | CBL | | IM-9 | |
|---|---|---|---|---|
| Factors | IgM (ng/ml) | Thymidine (ct/min) | IgG (ng/ml) | Thymidine (ct/Min) |
| Medium | 13.2 | 850 | 9.2 | 341 |
| VIP $10^{-11}$M | 17.1 (30)* | 2014 (137) | 11.3 (23) | ND |
| VIP $10^{-10}$M | 31.0 (135)* | 2185 (157) | 15.6 (70) | 648 (90) |
| VIP $10^{-9}$M | ND | ND | 22.6 (146) | 1028 (216) |

CBL and IM-9 cells were cultured with increasing concentrations of VIP. After 3 days of culture, immunoglobulin production and thymidine uptake were determined. Results are the means of triplicate cultures. s.d. were <15%.
*Percentage on enhancement of control is indicated in parentheses.
ND, not done.

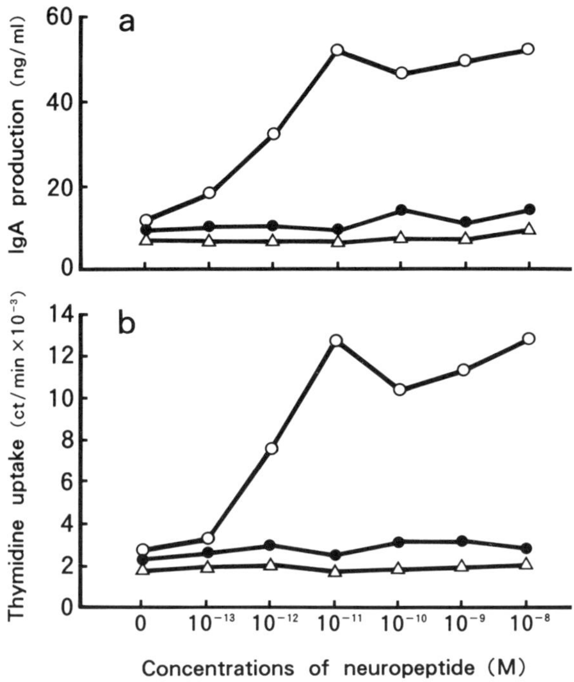


**Figure 14.1** Effect of VIP on IgA production and thymidine uptake by GM-1056 cells. (a) GM-105 cells are cultured with increasing concentrations of VIP (○), SOM (△) or SP (●). After 3 days of culture, IgA production is measured. (b) GM-1056 cells are cultured with increasing concentrations of VIP (○), SOM (△) or SP (●). After 3 days of culture, thymidine uptake is measured. Results are the means of triplicate cultures. SD <15 per cent. Reproduced by permission of Blackwell Scientific Publications Ltd

lymph nodes, while VIP inhibits IgA production by MNCs from Peyer's patches. In contrast, VIP enhances IgG production by MNCs from Peyer's patches, but not from the spleen or mesenteric lymph nodes[38]. In humans, VIP enhances pokeweed mitogen (PWM)-induced production of IgG, IgM and IgA by PB MNCs[39]. VIP also enhances spontaneous production of IgM, but not of IgG or IgA, by normal donors' PB MNCs[40]. Moreover, high concentrations of VIP *in vivo* increased serum IgM, but not IgG and IgA levels[40]. In contrast, VIP inhibits PWM-induced production of IgG and IgM but not IgA, while VIP enhances IL-4-induced IgE production by PB MNCs[41].

SOM either enhances or inhibits spontaneous IgA production by a mouse plasmacytoma line, depending on the concentration of SOM[23]. SOM also inhibits IgA production by mouse MNCs from spleen and Peyer's patches, but not from mesenteric lymph nodes, while SOM has no effect on IgG and

IgM production from the spleen, Peyer's patch or mesenteric lymph node[38]. In contrast, SOM selectively inhibits *schistosome* soluble egg antigen-induced IgG2a production by spleen MNCs in mice infected with *Schistosoma mansoni*[42].

SP enhances IgA and IgM production by a mouse B-lymphoma cell line and stimulates production of IgM and IgG, particularly IgG3, by mouse spleen MNCs stimulated with lipopolysaccharide (LPS)[27,43]. SP also enhances schistosome soluble egg antigen-induced IgG2a production by spleen MNCs in mice infected with *Schistosoma mansoni*[42]. Further, in Con A-stimulated cultures, SP enhances IgA production by MNCs from the spleen, mesenteric lymph nodes and Peyer's patches, enhances IgM production by MNCs from the spleen but not from mesenteric lymph nodes or Peyer's patches, and has no effect on IgG production by MNCs from these organs[38]. Moreover, *in vivo* exposure to SP in mice increases *in vitro* IgG, IgM and IgA production by MNCs from spleen and Peyer's patch[44]. In humans, SP enhances IgG production by peripheral blood B cells stimulated with *Staphylococcus aureus* protein A or Epstein–Barr virus (EBV), while SP has no effect on IgM and IgA production[45]. SP also enhances production of IgG, IgM and IgA by human duodenal mucosa stimulated with PWM[46].

## IMMUNOGLOBULIN PRODUCTION AND DIFFERENT CULTURE SYSTEMS

Taken together, these results indicate that VIP, SOM and SP can differentially modulate Ig production, depending on the culture system. We have previously reported that nerve growth factor, a neurotrophic protein, specifically induces IgG4 production by human B cells[47] and stimulates Ig production by human lymphoblastoid B-cell lines[48]. Erythropoietin, an erythroid cell growth and differentiation cytokine, enhances spontaneous and IL-4-induced IgE production[49]. IL-8, a chemokine for neutrophils, inhibits IL-4-induced IgE and IgG4 production[50]. Therefore, we studied the effects of VIP, SOM and SP on (1) human B-cell lines, (2) IL-4-induced Ig production, and (3) spontaneous IgE and IgG4 production.

### HUMAN B-CELL LINES

As shown in Figure 14.1a, VIP enhanced IgA production by the lymphoblastoid B-cell line GM-1056 in a dose-dependent fashion, while SOM and SP fail to do so[32,51]. VIP also enhances production of IgM by the lymphoblastoid line CBL and IgG by the plasma cell line IM-9 (Table 14.1). As mentioned, VIP enhances thymidine uptake by these B-cell lines (Figure 14.1b and Table 14.1). Further, VIP enhances production of IgM and IgG by the lymphoblastoid cell lines SKW and CESS, respectively[52]. The VIP-induced enhancement of IgA production in GM-1056 cells is specific, since it is blocked by the VIP antagonist [D-*p*-chloro-Phe6,Leu17]-VIP, while the addition of the VIP antagonist did not affect spontaneous IgA production[32]. Moreover, VIP receptors were demonstrated on the SKW cell line[53]. These results indicate that VIP enhances spontaneous Ig production by activated B cells. Indeed, our subsequent study revealed that VIP also enhances (50–300 per cent enhancement) spontaneous IgA production by tonsillar activated B cells[32].

## IL-4-INDUCED Ig ISOTYPE PRODUCTION

Our previous results have demonstrated that IL-4-induced IgE and IgG4 production in non-atopic donors is modulated by many factors, including erythropoietin, and the antiallergic drugs disodium cromoglycate and nedocromil sodium[49,54,55]. We studied the effects of VIP, SOM and SP on IgE and IgG subclass production in IL-4-stimulated cultures of MNCs, and by B cells in the presence or absence of T cells and/or monocytes[56].

### Effects of VIP, SOM and SP on IL-4-induced Ig Production

As shown in Figure 14.2, in cultures of MNCs from non-atopic donors, VIP and SOM (10 pM to 10 nM) inhibit IL-4-induced IgE production, while SP (0.1 pM to 1 μM) fails to do so. In contrast to IgE production, IL-4 does not induce IgM or IgA production, and neither VIP, SOM or SP inhibits IgM or IgA production at any of the concentrations tested (Figures 14.2B,C). In the absence of IL-4, none of the neuropeptides affect production of IgE (<0.15 ng/ml), IgM or IgA (Figure 14.2). As shown in Figure 14.3A,B and C, IL-4 does not affect production of IgG1, IgG2 or IgG3. In contrast, IL-4 induces IgG4 production (100–200 per cent enhancement) (Figure 14.3D). In IL-4-stimulated cultures. VIP, SOM and SP fail to affect IgG1 production (Figure 14.3A), while all of the neuropeptides at concentrations from 1 pM to 10 nM enhance IgG2 production (Figure 14.3B). In contrast, VIP and SP (10 pM to 1 nM) inhibit IgG3 production, while SOM has no effect at any concentrations tested (Figure 14.3C). On the other hand, SOM (10 pM to 100 nM) and SP (100 pM to 100 nM) enhance IgG4 production, while VIP does not affect it (Figure 14.3D). In the absence of IL-4, none of the neuropeptides affect IgG subclass production (Figures 3A–D).

### Specificity of the Effects of Neuropeptides

The specificity of action of each neuropeptide is demonstrated in Table 14.2. None of the antagonists by themselves affect Ig production. However, the VIP antagonist blocks the VIP-induced inhibition of IgE and IgG3

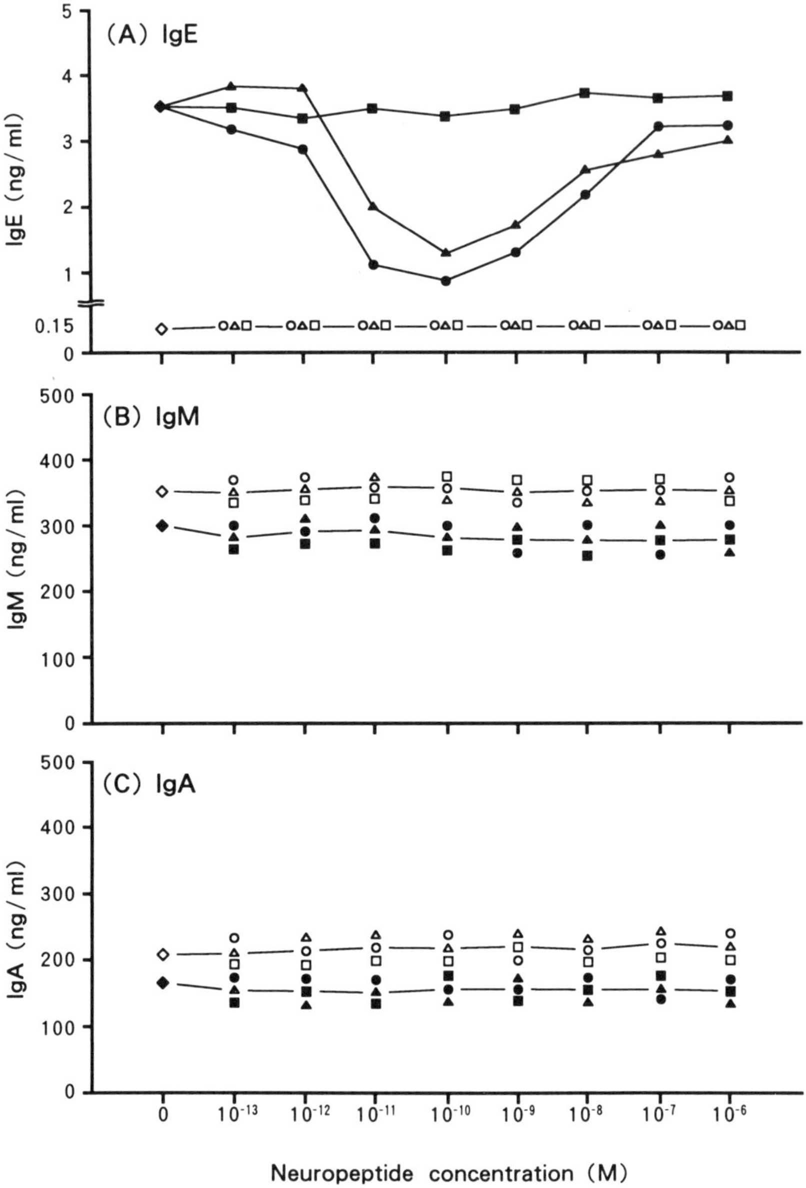


**Figure 14.2** Effects of neuropeptides on IgE, IgM and IgA production[56]. MNCs are cultured with IL-4 (◆), and various concentrations of VIP (●), SOM (▲) or SP (■) are added. MNCs are also cultured with medium (◇), and VIP (○), SOM (△) or SP (□) are added. On day 14 of culture, IgE (A), IgM (B) and IgA production (C) are measured. Values are the mean of triplicate cultures. SD were <15 per cent. Reproduced by permission of Academic Press Inc, Florida

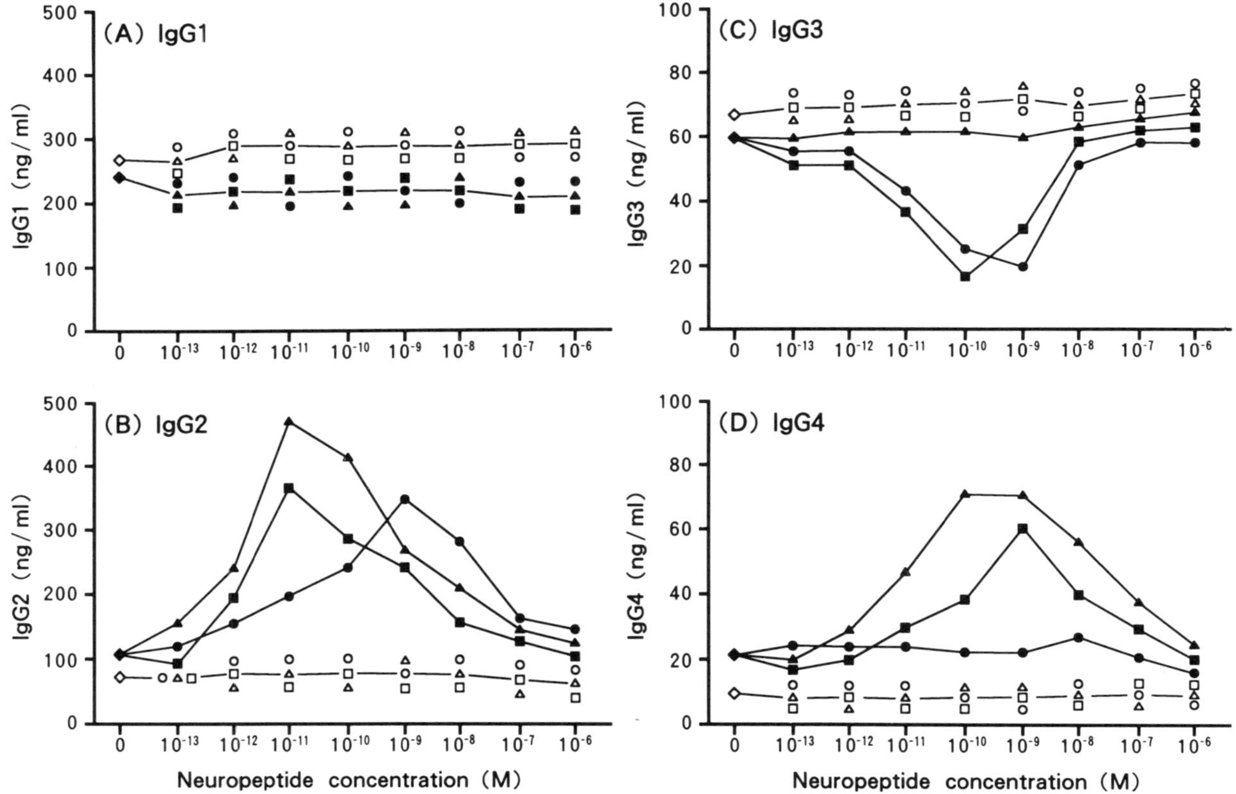


**Figure 14.3** Effects of neuropeptides on IgG subclass production[56]. MNCs are cultured with IL-4 (◆), and various concentrations of VIP (●), SOM (▲) or SP (■) are added. MNCs are also cultured with medium (◇), and VIP (○), SOM (△) or SP (□) are added. On day 14 of culture, IgG1 (A), IgG2 (B), IgG3 (C) or IgG4 (D) production are measured. Values are the mean of triplicate cultures. SD were $<$15 per cent. Reproduced by permission of Academic Press Inc, Florida

production and enhancement of IgG2 production. In contrast, the SOM antagonist and the SP antagonist had no effect on VIP-induced modulation of Ig production. Similarly, inhibition of IgE production by SOM and enhancement of IgG2 and IgG4 production are blocked by the SOM antagonist, but not by the VIP antagonist or the SP antagonist (data not shown). Likewise, enhancement of IgG2 and IgG4 production and inhibition of IgG3 production by SP are blocked by the SP antagonist, but not by other antagonists (data not shown).

### Kinetic Analysis of the Effects of Neuropeptides

We analyzed the time-course of the effects of the neuropeptides on IgE and IgG subclass production. First, neuropeptides were added daily on days 0–5 of culture. As shown in Figure 14.4A and B, VIP must be added at initiation of culture, i.e. day 0, since it does not affect IgE, IgG2 or IgG3 production if added after day 1. In contrast, VIP has no effect on IgG4 production irrespective of the time of the VIP addition. Secondly, MNCs were preincubated with VIP in the absence of IL-4, and then cultured with IL-4 in the absence of VIP. Alternatively, MNCs were incubated with VIP for various periods in the presence of IL-4, washed and then cultured with IL-4 in the absence of VIP. As shown in Figure 14.5, preincubation with VIP has no effect. Moreover, VIP has to be present during the entire 14 days of culturing for modulation of IgE, IgG2 and IgG3 production to be maximized.

**Table 14.2** Specificity of the effects of neuropeptides. Reproduced by permission of Academic Press Inc, Florida

| Factors | Ig production (ng/ml) | | | | | | |
|---|---|---|---|---|---|---|---|
| | IgE | IgG1 | IgG2 | IgG3 | IgG4 | IgM | IgA |
| Medium | 3.7 | 297 | 113 | 64 | 26 | 232 | 182 |
| VIP | 1.9* | 290 | 424** | 31* | 28 | 249 | 175 |
| VIP antagonist | 3.8 | 280 | 118 | 69 | 29 | 256 | 180 |
| VIP + VIP antagonist | 3.4 | 285 | 123 | 61 | 30 | 245 | 192 |
| VIP + SOM antagonist | 2.0* | 300 | 413** | 33* | 34 | 231 | 164 |
| VIP + SP antagonist | 1.8* | 275 | 434** | 28* | 25 | 262 | 167 |
| SOM | 2.2* | 302 | 501** | 60 | 93** | 248 | 174 |
| SOM antagonist | 3.3 | 275 | 108 | 68 | 22 | 201 | 186 |
| SOM + SOM antagonist | 3.4 | 299 | 125 | 66 | 31 | 237 | 195 |
| SP | 3.9 | 283 | 362** | 35* | 83** | 246 | 187 |
| SP antagonist | 3.5 | 305 | 134 | 58 | 30 | 225 | 177 |
| SP + SP antagonist | 3.6 | 311 | 123 | 62 | 28 | 249 | 181 |

VIP is used at 1 nM, VIP antagonist at 100 nM, SOM at 0.1 nM, SOM antagonist at 10 nM, SP at 1 nM, and SP antagonist at 100 nM.
*Significant inhibition ($P < 0.01$) compared to medium.
**Significant enhancement ($P < 0.01$) compared to medium.

Again, VIP does not affect IgG4 production. Similarly, VIP does not affect IgG1, IgM or IgA production (data not shown). Similar results were observed with the addition of SOM and SP, i.e. SOM and SP have to be added at the start of culturing and be present throughout the entire culture

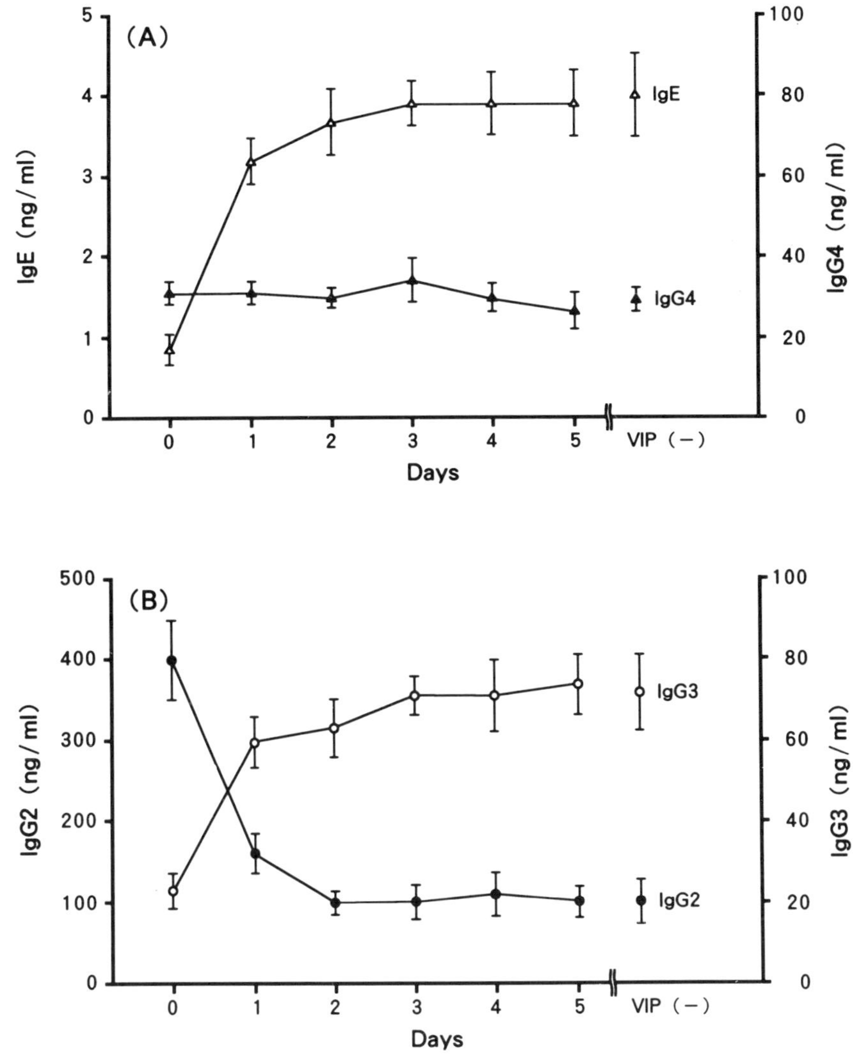


**Figure 14.4** Kinetic analysis of VIP addition[56]. MNCs are stimulated with IL-4, and VIP (1 nM) is added to the cultures on days 0–5. As controls, IL-4-stimulated MNCs are cultured with medium alone, i.e. VIP (−). On day 14 of culture, IgE (△) and IgG4 production (▲) in (A), and IgG2 (●) and IgG3 production (○) in (B) are measured. Values are the mean of triplicate cultures. SD were $<15$ per cent. Reproduced by permission of Academic Press Inc, Florida

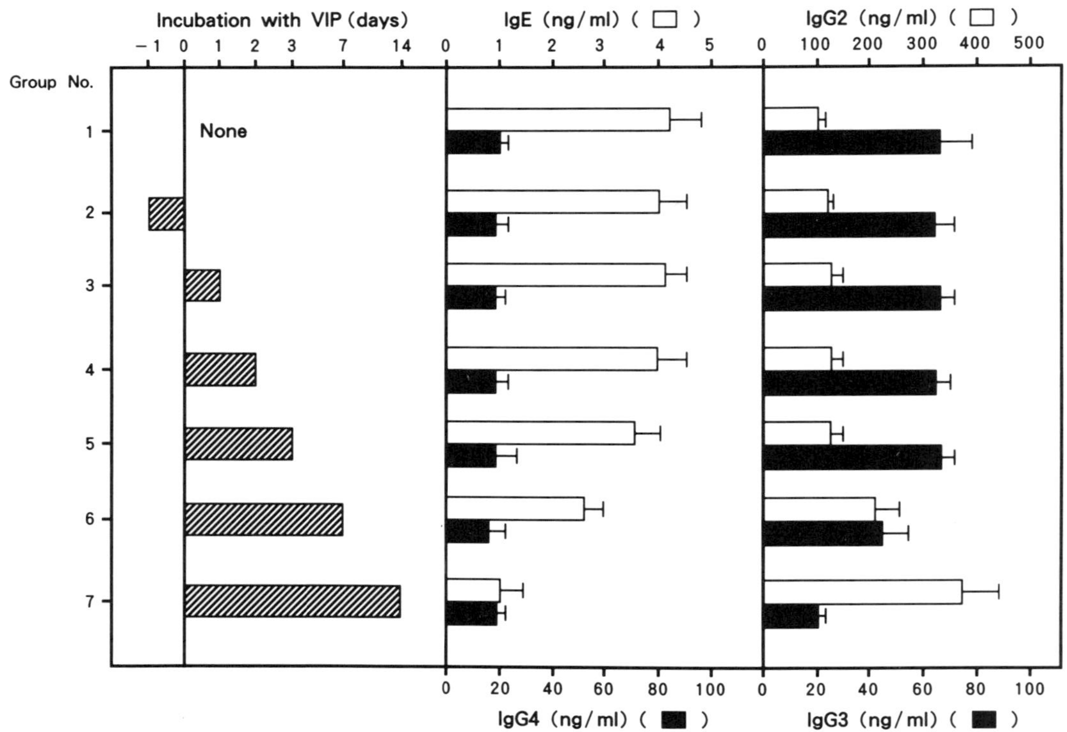


**Figure 14.5** Effect of incubation with VIP[56]. MNCs are divided into the following experimental groups: group 1, MNCs are cultured with IL-4 for 14 days in the absence of VIP; group 2, MNCs are preincubated with VIP (1 nM) for 1 day, washed and then cultured with IL-4 for 14 days; groups 3–6, MNCs are stimulated with IL-4 and incubated with VIP for the indicated numbers of days, washed and then cultured with IL-4 in the absence of VIP; group 7, MNCs are stimulated with IL-4 and VIP for 14 days. On day 14 of culture, Ig production is measured. Values are the mean ± 1 SD of triplicate cultures. Reproduced by permission of Academic Press Inc, Florida

period to achieve the optimal modulation of Ig production (data not shown).

**Effects of Endogenous Factors**

We next studied whether neuropeptides affected IgE and IgG4 production via various known factors[56–58]. To do so, MNCs were cultured with IL-4, and various factors were added. As shown in Table 14.3, IL-5 and IL-6 enhanced IgE and IgG4 production, while they had no effect on the synthesis of IgG2 or IgG3. IFN-α and IFN-γ inhibited IgE and IgG4 production, while they had no effect on the synthesis of IgG2 or IgG3. Platelet-activating factor (PAF), transforming growth factor beta (TGF-β) and prostaglandin $E_2$ ($PGE_2$) inhibited IgE production without affecting the synthesis of the various IgG subclasses, while nerve growth factor (NGF) enhanced IgG4 production without affecting the synthesis of IgE or other IgG subclasses. Except for inhibition of IgM production by TGF-β, these factors had no effect on IgG1, IgM or IgA production. These results indicate that the observed modulation of IgG2 and IgG3 production by neuropeptides is unique.

In this regard addition of a neutralizing anti-IFN-γ monoclonal antibody (mAb) or the prostaglandin inhibitor indomethacin had no effect on the inhibition of IgE production by VIP or SOM. Similarly, these agents had no effect on the enhancement of IgG4 production by SOM or SP, inhibition of

**Table 14.3** Effects of various factors on Ig production in IL-4-stimulated mononuclear cells from normal donors[56]. Reproduced by permission of Academic Press Inc, Florida

| Factors | Ig production (ng/ml) | | | | | | |
|---|---|---|---|---|---|---|---|
| | IgE | IgG1 | IgG2 | IgG3 | IgG4 | IgM | IgA |
| Medium | 4.4 | 297 | 123 | 53 | 29 | 203 | 169 |
| IL-1β | 4.8 | 312 | 136 | 57 | 31 | 225 | 180 |
| IL-2 | 4.6 | 272 | 149 | 51 | 35 | 239 | 165 |
| IL-3 | 3.9 | 321 | 118 | 60 | 34 | 208 | 185 |
| IL-5 | 6.2* | 312 | 133 | 59 | 45* | 249 | 176 |
| IL-6 | 6.5* | 335 | 153 | 68 | 56* | 260 | 198 |
| IFN-α | 0.4** | 311 | 109 | 61 | 9** | 239 | 151 |
| IFN-γ | 0.2** | 278 | 114 | 62 | 7** | 232 | 182 |
| PAF | 1.3** | 247 | 107 | 50 | 11** | 214 | 152 |
| TGF-β | 1.2* | 270 | 109 | 49 | 6** | 62** | 146 |
| $PGE_2$ | 1.8** | 269 | 102 | 50 | 16** | 237 | 181 |
| NGF | 4.1 | 299 | 123 | 55 | 99* | 248 | 197 |

IL-1β is used at 100 U/ml, IL-2 at 100 U/ml, IL-3 at 100 U/ml, IL-5 at 100 ng/ml, IL-6 at 100 U/ml, IFN-α at 100 U/ml, IFN-γ at 100 U/ml, PAF at 10 μM, TGF-β at 1 ng/ml, GM-CSF at 1000 U/ml, prostaglandin $E_2$ ($PGE_2$) at 1 μM, and nerve growth factor (NGF) at 100 ng/ml.
*Significant enhancement ($P < 0.01$) compared to medium.
**Significant inhibition ($P < 0.01$) compared to medium.

IgG3 production by VIP or SP, or enhancement of IgG2 production by VIP, SOM or SP (data not shown)[56]. Thus, the neuropeptides do not appear to work through modulation of well-described factors known to affect Ig isotype production.

### Effects of Neuropeptides Require T cells and Monocytes

IL-4 induces IgE and IgG4 production by purified B cells when acting in concert with anti-CD40 antibody[57–59]. As shown in Figure 14.6A, none of the neuropeptides affected IgE production by purified B cells stimulated with IL-4 plus anti-CD40. Further, addition of either T cells or monocytes did not modulate IgE production either in the presence or absence of neuropeptides. However, in the presence of both T cells and monocytes, VIP and SOM, but not SP, inhibited IgE production. Similarly, only in the presence of both T cells and monocytes did SOM and SP enhance IgG4 production (Figure 14.6B), all of the neuropeptides enhanced IgG2 production (Figure 14.6C), and VIP and SP inhibited IgG3 production (Figure 14.6D). These results indicate that modulation of IgE and IgG subclass production by neuropeptides requires the presence of T cells and monocytes.

### Do Neuropeptides Regulate Ig Class Switching?

To determine the mechanism(s) by which neuropeptides regulate IgE and IgG subclass production, we utilized populations of B cells in which subpopulations expressing various surface(s) Ig isotypes were selectively depleted. Such cultures were then stimulated with IL-4 in the presence of both T cells and monocytes. As shown in Figure 14.7A, IL-4 induced IgE production by sIgE$^-$ cells. This induction was inhibited by both VIP and SOM to the same extent as that observed for control B cells or by sIgG4$^-$ B cells which were used as controls in the panning process employed for depletion. On the other hand, SOM and SP enhanced IgG4 production by sIgG4$^-$ B cells to a similar extent as that observed for control B cells or for sIgE$^-$ B cells (Figure 14.7B). By contrast, VIP, SOM and SP failed to enhance IgG2 production by sIgG2$^-$ B cells, while all of the neuropeptides enhanced IgG2 production by sIgG3$^-$ B cells to a similar extent as that observed for control B cells (Figure 14.7C). Likewise, none of the neuropeptides affected IgG3 production in sIgG3$^-$ B cells, while VIP and SP inhibited IgG3 production by control B and sIgG2$^-$ B cells (Figure 14.7D).

To exclude any negative effects on IgG2 or IgG3 synthesis that could potentially be mediated by the anti-IgG2 or anti-IgG3 antibody itself, which was used for panning, control B cells were incubated with anti-IgG2 or anti-IgG3 antibody without panning, washed and cultured with VIP, SOM or SP. All of the neuropeptides enhanced IgG2 production, and VIP and SP inhibited IgG3 production to the same extent as that observed for non-

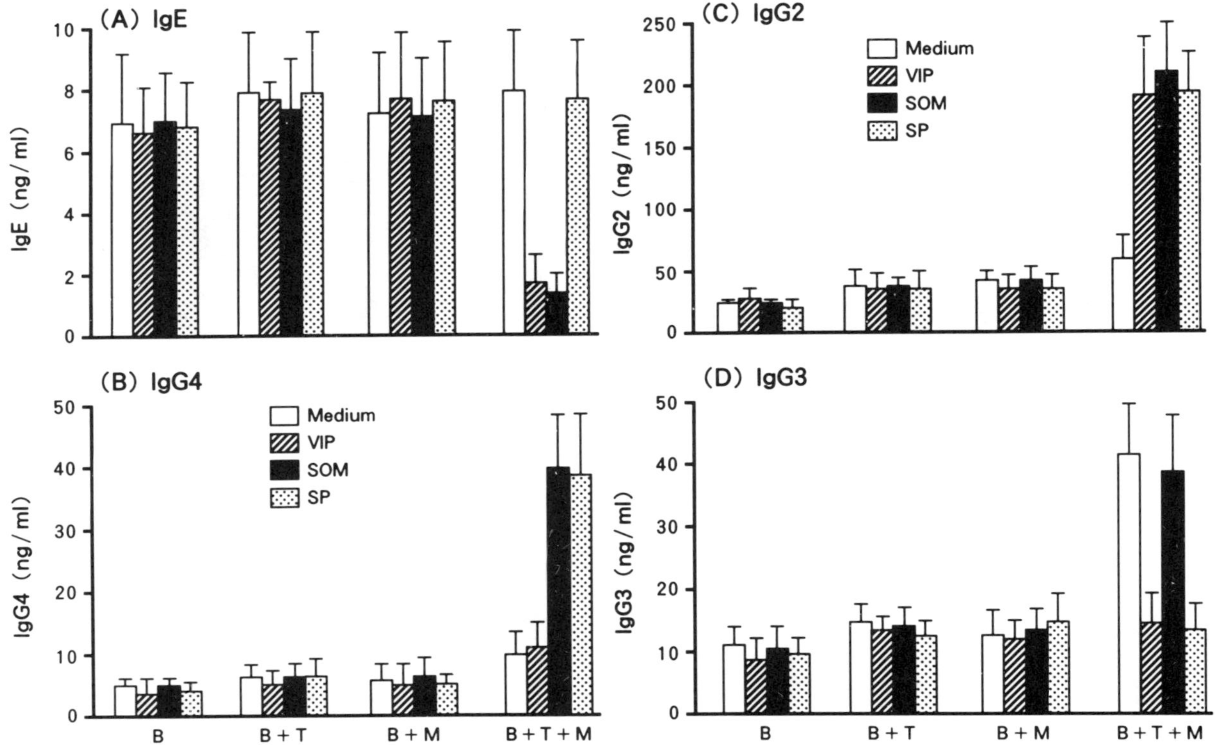


**Figure 14.6** Effect of T cells and/or monocytes on modulation of Ig production by neuropeptides in cultures of IL-4 plus anti-CD40 antibody[56]. Purified B cells are cultured with IL-4 plus anti-CD40 mAb, and T cells and/or monocytes are added. They are cultured with medium (open), VIP (1 nM, hatched bar), SOM (0.1 nM, closed) or SP (1 nM, dotted). On day 14 of culture, IgE (A), IgG4 (B), IgG2 (C) and IgG3 production (D) are measured. Values are the mean ± 1 SD of triplicate cultures. Reproduced by permission of Academic Press Inc, Florida

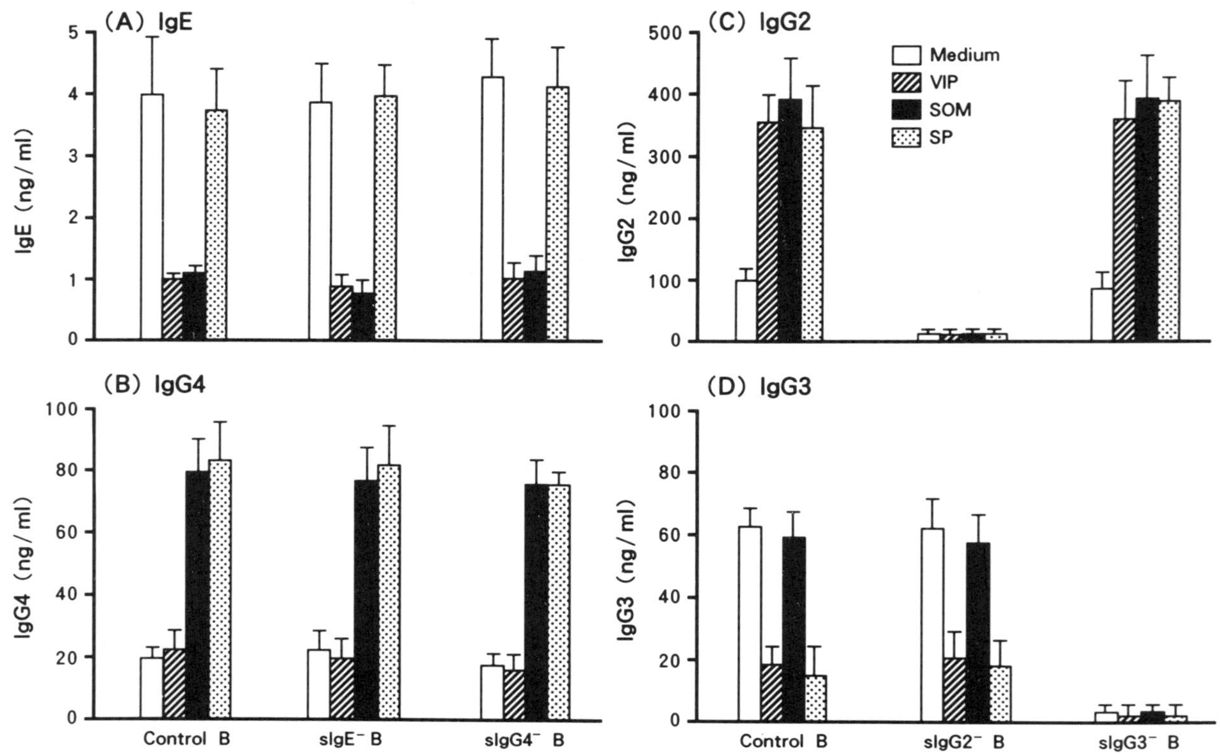


**Figure 14.7** Effect of depletion of $sIg^+$ cells[56]. Purified control B cells or various $sIg^-$ B-cell populations are cultured with T cells and monocytes as indicated. They are stimulated with IL-4, and medium (open), VIP (1 nM, hatched bar), SOM (0.1 nM, closed) or SP (1 nM, dotted) are added. On day 14 of culture, IgE (A), IgG4 (B), IgG2 (C) and IgG3 production (D) are measured. Values are the mean ± 1 SD of triplicate cultures. Reproduced by permission of Academic Press Inc, Florida

treated B cells (data not shown). In the absence of IL-4, neuropeptides had no effect on IgG2 and IgG3 production by $sIgG2^-$ and $sIgG3^-$ B cells, respectively (data not shown). These results indicate that *neuropeptides modulate IgE and IgG4 production by affecting IL-4-induced switching, while they modulate IgG2 and IgG3 production by affecting $sIgG2^+$ B and probably $sIgG3^+$ B cells.* The effects of VIP, SOM, and SP on IL-4-induced Ig production are summarized in Table 14.4.

## EFFECTS OF VIP, SOM AND SP ON SPONTANEOUS IgE AND IgG4 PRODUCTION IN ATOPIC PATIENTS

We and others have reported that spontaneous IgE production by MNCs from atopic patients is enhanced by IL-4 and erythropoietin[49,60–62], while it is inhibited by disodium cromoglycate, IFN-γ, IFN-α and $PGE_2$[54,60–63]. Moreover, we have also reported that NK cells and anti-CD23 antibodies each directly inhibit spontaneous IgE production by purified B cells from atopic patients[64,65]. Correspondingly, spontaneous IgG4 production by MNCs from atopic patients is enhanced by disodium cromoglycate and IL-4[54–62], while it is inhibited by IFN-γ and IFN-α[61,63].

### Role of non-B Cells Types in Neuropeptide Modulation of Spontaneous Ig Production in Atopic Patients

In the above studies it was not determined whether these factors acted directly at the level of the B cell to modulate IgG4 and IgE production, and/or through non-B cells, such as monocytes and T cells present in the starting population. However, in regard to the effects of neuropeptides, we studied the effects of VIP, SOM and SP on spontaneous IgE and IgG4 production by MNCs, as well as by B cells and T cells/or monocytes in atopic patients[63].

As shown in Figure 14.8A, in tonsil MNCs from atopic patients, VIP and SOM (10 pM to 10 nM) inhibited spontaneous IgE production, while SP (0.1 pM

**Table 14.4** Summary of the effects of VIP, SOM and SP on IL-4-induced Ig production in non-atopic donors[56]. Reproduced by permission of Academic Press Inc, Florida

| Factors | Ig production | | | | | | |
|---|---|---|---|---|---|---|---|
| | IgE | IgG1 | IgG2 | IgG3 | IgG4 | IgM | IgA |
| VIP | ↓ | → | ↑ | ↓ | → | → | → |
| SOM | ↓ | → | ↑ | → | ↑ | → | → |
| SP | → | → | ↑ | ↓ | ↑ | → | → |

MNCs from non-atopic donors are cultured with IL-4 (800 U/ml), and neuropeptides are added. Arrows indicate inhibition (↓), enhancement (↑), or no effect (→).

to 1 μM) failed to do so. By contrast, neither VIP, SOM nor SP inhibited IgM or IgA production at any concentrations tested (Figure 14.8B,C). Furthermore, VIP and SP (10 pM to 10 nM), but not SOM (0.1 pM to 1 μM), each inhibited IgG4 production without affecting that of IgG1, IgG2 or IgG3 (Figure 14.9). Identical results were obtained in PB MNCs from atopic patients (Table 14.5).

## Kinetic Analysis

The time-course of the effect of neuropeptide incubation on IgE and IgG4 production was studied. MNCs were preincubated with neuropeptides for 1 day, washed and then cultured with medium in the absence of neuropeptides.

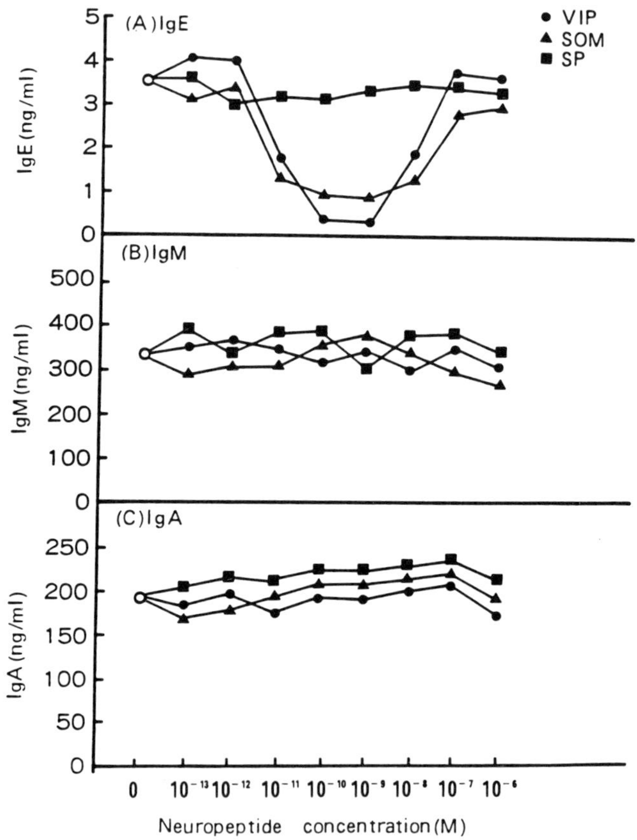


**Figure 14.8** Effects of neuropeptides on spontaneous production of IgE, IgM and IgA[63]. Tonsil MNCs from atopic patients were cultured with medium (○), and various concentrations of VIP (●), SOM (▲) or SP (■) are added. On day 14 of culture, production of IgE (A), IgM (B) and IgA (C) is determined. Values are the means of results of triplicate cultures from one experiment, representative of 10. SD were <15 per cent. From reference 63 © 1994, Journal of Immunology, with permission

**Table 14.5** Effect of neuropeptides on Ig production by peripheral blood MNC

| | Ig production (ng/ml) | | | | | | |
|---|---|---|---|---|---|---|---|
| Expt. | IgE | IgM | IgA | IgG1 | IgG2 | IgG3 | IgG4 |
| 1. Medium | 5.4 | 428 | 259 | 328 | 154 | 83 | 17.9 |
| VIP | 1.2 | 412 | 238 | 345 | 137 | 81 | 3.8 |
| SOM | 1.0 | 451 | 249 | 348 | 160 | 79 | 18.2 |
| SP | 5.3 | 415 | 220 | 323 | 145 | 72 | 3.0 |
| 2. Medium | 7.2 | 247 | 152 | 278 | 102 | 53 | 22.9 |
| VIP | 2.3 | 262 | 135 | 270 | 106 | 51 | 4.7 |
| SOM | 2.0 | 250 | 142 | 256 | 112 | 45 | 21.5 |
| SP | 7.8 | 231 | 159 | 292 | 100 | 59 | 3.8 |
| 3. Medium | 2.6 | 210 | 178 | 319 | 178 | 32 | 10.2 |
| VIP | 0.5 | 236 | 182 | 301 | 192 | 28 | 3.1 |
| SOM | 0.6 | 204 | 162 | 328 | 165 | 35 | 11.2 |
| SP | 2.8 | 225 | 191 | 313 | 171 | 27 | 4.7 |
| 4. Medium | 1.0 | 349 | 114 | 267 | 121 | 64 | 6.3 |
| VIP | 0.4 | 367 | 121 | 251 | 130 | 57 | 1.3 |
| SOM | 0.3 | 321 | 105 | 248 | 112 | 60 | 5.8 |
| SP | 1.2 | 342 | 101 | 280 | 126 | 71 | 1.7 |

Peripheral blood MNC from atopic patients are culturedd with VIP (0.1 nM), SOM (0.1 nM) and SP (0.1 nM).

Neuropeptides were also added daily from days 0 through day 2 of culture. As shown in Figure 14.10, in the case of VIP, preincubation had no effect in MNCs both from tonsil and peripheral blood. In order to obtain maximal inhibition of IgE and IgG4 production, VIP had to be present from the initiation of culture. Similar results were observed using SOM and SP, i.e. SOM and SP had to be added at the start of culture to achieve optimal inhibition of IgE or IgG4 production in MNCs from tonsil and peripheral blood (data not shown).

### Role of Endogenous IFN-$\alpha$, IFN-$\gamma$ or $PGE_2$

We determined whether neuropeptides inhibited IgE and IgG4 production via the known inhibitory factors IFN-$\alpha$, IFN-$\gamma$ and/or $PGE_2$[63]. Tonsil MNCs were cultured with neuropeptides in the presence or absence of neutralizing anti-IFN-$\alpha$ or anti-IFN-$\gamma$ antibodies, or indomethacin. As shown in Figures 14.11A and B, none of these factors overcame the inhibition by neuropeptides of IgE and IgG4 production. Similar results were observed using PB MNCs (Figure 14.11C,D). These results suggest that the inhibitory effect of neuropeptides on IgE and IgG4 production was not mediated by IFN-$\alpha$, IFN-$\gamma$ or $PGE_2$.

### Role of T Cells and Monocytes

The effect of T cells and monocytes on neuropeptide inhibition of IgE and IgG4 production was determined. As shown in Figure 14.12A, none of the

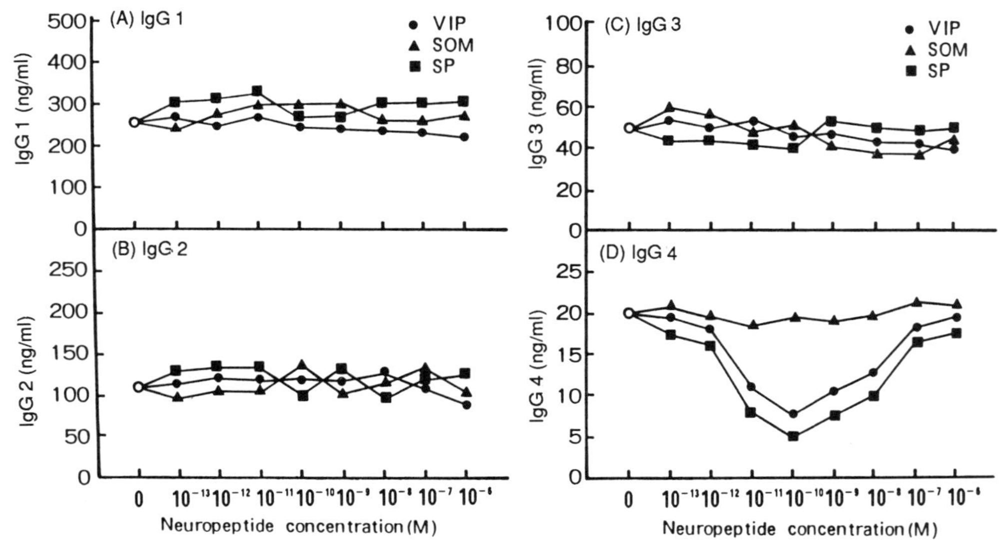


**Figure 14.9** Effects of neuropeptides on spontaneous production of IgG subclass[63]. Tonsil MNCs from atopic patients are cultured with medium (○), and various concentrations of VIP (●), SOM (▲) or SP (■) are added. On day 14 of culture, production of IgG1 (A), IgG2 (B), IgG3 (C) and IgG4 (D) is determined. Values are the means of results of triplicate cultures from one experiment, representative of 10. SD were <15 per cent. From reference 63 © 1994, Journal of Immunology, with permission

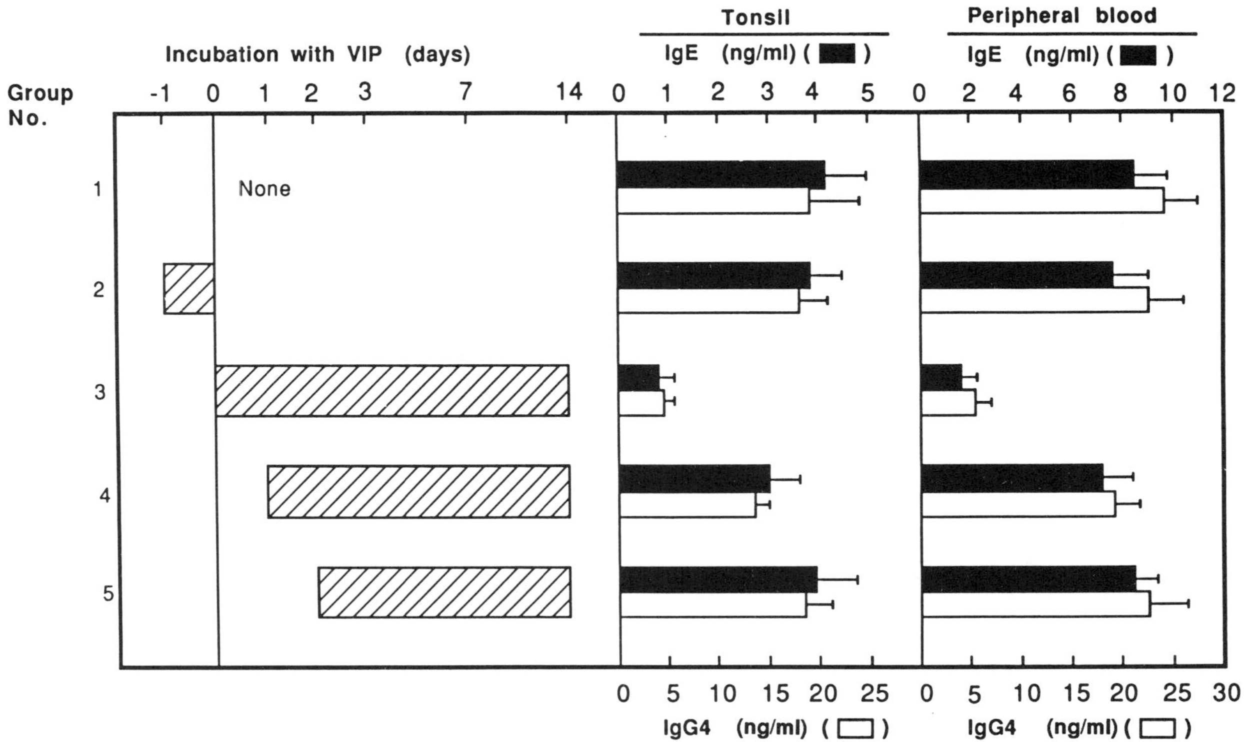


**Figure 14.10** Kinetic analysis of incubation with VIP.[63] The following experimental groups were considered in tonsil and PB MNCs from atopic patients: group 1, MNCs are cultured with medium for 14 days in the absence of VIP; group 2, MNCs are preincubated with VIP (0.1 nM) for 1 day, washed and then cultured with medium for 14 days; group 3, MNCs are incubated with VIP for 14 days; groups 4 and 5, MNCs are cultured with medium, and VIP is added on day 1 or day 2 as indicated. On day 14 of culture, IgE (■) and IgG4 (□) production are determined. Values are the mean ± 1 SD of results of triplicate cultures from one experiment, representative of four. From reference 63 © 1994, Journal of Immunology, with permission

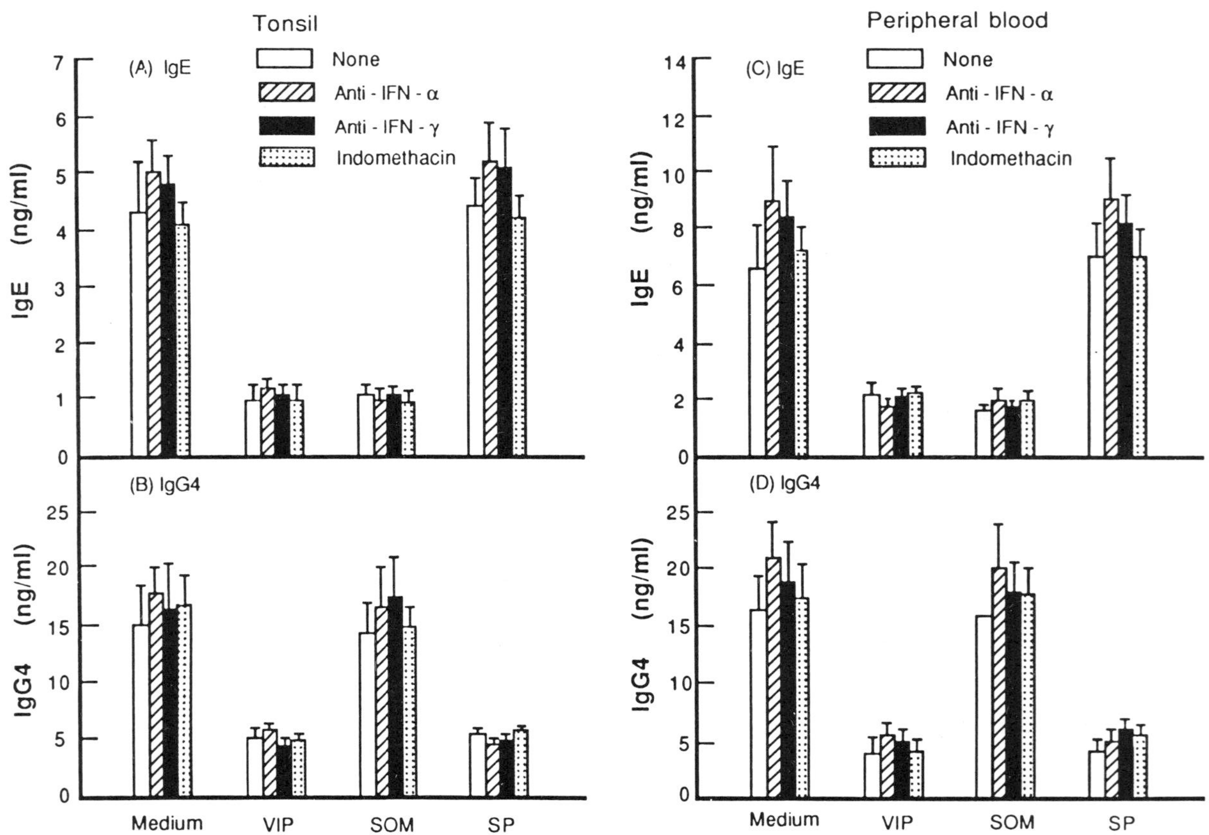


**Figure 14.11** Effect of anti-IFN-α, anti-IFN-γ or indomethacin on inhibition of IgE and IgG4 production by neuropeptides[63]. Atopic patients' MNCs from tonsil (A and B) and peripheral blood (C and D) are incubated with medium, VIP (0.1 nM), SOM (0.1 nM) or SP (0.1 nM). They are cultured with no additional agents (open), anti-IFN-α (10 μg/ml, hatched bar), anti-IFN-γ (10 μg/ml, closed) or indomethacin (0.1 μM, dotted). On day 14 of culture, IgE (A and C) and IgG4 (B and D) production are determined. Values are mean ± 1 SD of results of triplicate cultures from one experiment, representative of four. From reference 63 © 1994, Journal of Immunology, with permission

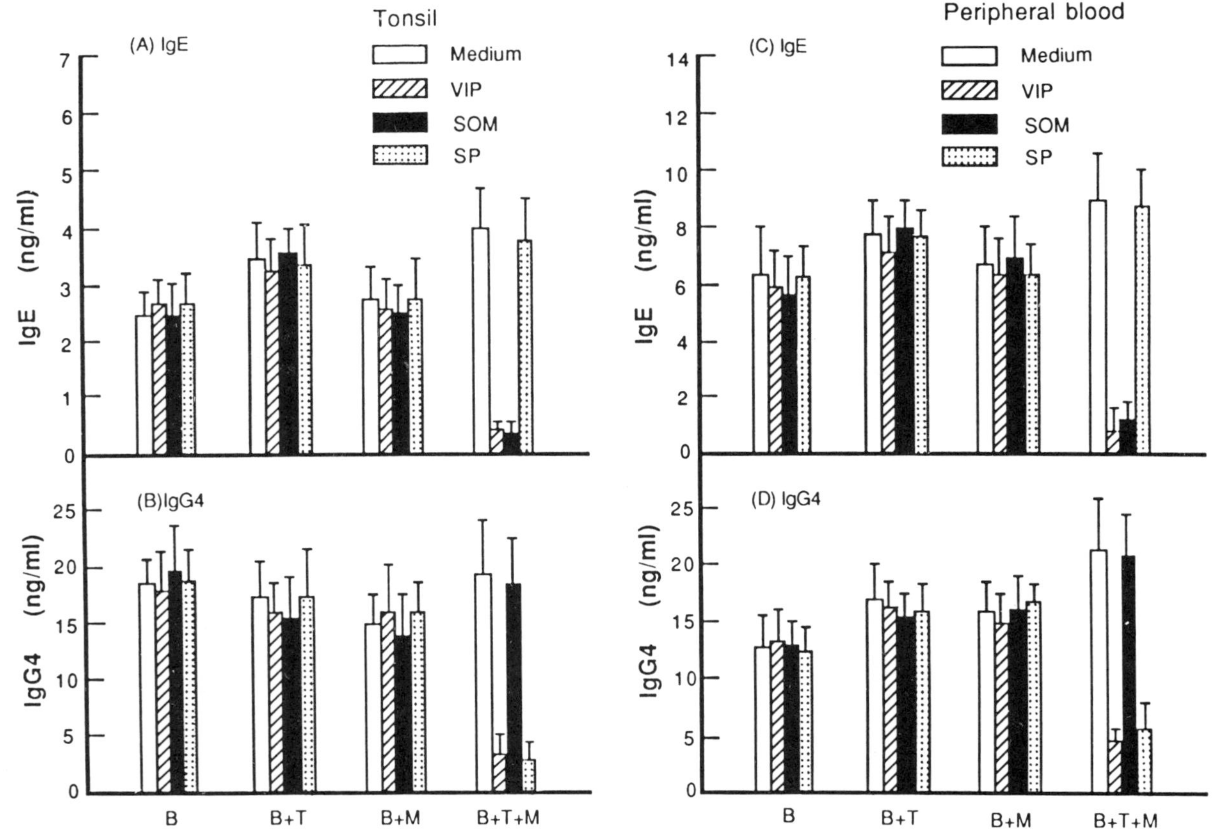


**Figure 14.12** T cells and monocytes are required for the inhibition of spontaneous production of IgE and IgG4 by neuropeptides[63]. Atopic patients' B cells from tonsil (A,B) and peripheral blood (C,D) are incubated with medium (open), VIP (0.1 nM, hatched bar), SOM (0.1 nM, closed) or SP (0.1 nM, dotted). They were co-cultured with T cells and/or monocytes. On day 14 of culture, IgE (A,C) and IgG4 (B,D) production are determined. Values are the mean ± 1 SD of results of triplicate cultures from one experiment, representative of four. From reference 63 © 1994, Journal of Immunology, with permission

neuropeptides tested inhibited IgE production by purified tonsil B cells or by B cells cultured with either T cells or monocytes, but not both. However, VIP and SOM, but not SP, inhibited IgE production when B cells were cultured with both T cells and monocytes. Similarly, VIP and SP, but not SOM, inhibited IgG4 production when B cells were cultured with both T cells and monocytes (Figure 14.12B). Identical results were observed using peripheral blood B cells (Figure 14.12C,D).

### Effects on Ig Class Switching

The mechanisms of inhibition of IgE and IgG4 production by neuropeptides were studied in B cells depleted of $sIgE^+$ cells ($sIgE^-$ B cells) or $sIgG4^+$ cells ($sIgG4^-$ B cells). As a control for the panning, a B-cell population was also prepared that was depleted of $sIgG3^+$ cells ($sIgG3^-$ B cells). These cells were cultured with neuropeptides in the presence of both T cells and monocytes. As shown in Figures 14.13A and D, $sIgE^-$ B cells from both tonsil and peripheral blood failed to spontaneously produce significant amounts of IgE (<0.15 ng/ml), and none of the neuropeptides affected this. In contrast, $sIgG4^-$ and $sIgG3^-$ B cells each spontaneously produced IgE in quantities similar to those produced by control B cells, and VIP and SOM each inhibited this production. On the other hand, $sIgG4^-$ B cells failed to produce significant amounts of IgG4 (<0.3 ng/ml), and none of the neuropeptides affected this. However, VIP and SP inhibited IgG4 production from $sIgE^-$ and $sIgG3^-$ B cells (Figure 14.13B,E). In contrast, none of the neuropeptides tested affected IgG3 production from $sIgE^-$ B cells, $sIgG4^-$ B cells or $sIgG3^-$ B cells (Figure 14.13C,F). As in $sIgG3^-$ B cells, VIP and SOM inhibited IgE production, while VIP and SP inhibited IgG4 production from $sIgG1^-$ or $sIgG2^-$ B cells (data not shown). A summary of the effects of VIP, SOM and SP on spontaneous IgE and IgG4 production is shown in Table 14.6.

**Table 14.6** Summary of the effects of VIP, SOM and SP on spontaneous IgE and IgG4 production in atopic patients[56]. From reference 63 © 1994, Journal of Immunology, with permission

| Factors | Ig production | | | | | | |
|---|---|---|---|---|---|---|---|
| | IgE | IgG1 | IgG2 | IgG3 | IgG4 | IgM | IgA |
| VIP | ↓ | → | → | → | ↓ | → | → |
| SOM | ↓ | → | → | → | → | → | → |
| SP | → | → | → | → | ↓ | → | → |

MNCs from atopic patients are cultured with medium alone, and neuropeptides are added. Arrows indicate inhibition (↓) or no effect (→).

## CONCLUSIONS

Our results demonstrate that VIP directly stimulates Ig production by human activated B cells and B-cell lines. In contrast, VIP, SOM and SP differentially modulate IL-4-induced IgE and IgG subclass production while they inhibit spontaneous IgE and/or IgG4 production in atopic patients. The exact mechanisms of the differential effects of neuropeptides remain to be elucidated. However, this is not surprising, since neuropeptides not only have different effects on isotypes of Ig production, but their effects are also organ specific[38]. Moreover, the effects of neuropeptides are also dependent on the method of stimulation[39].

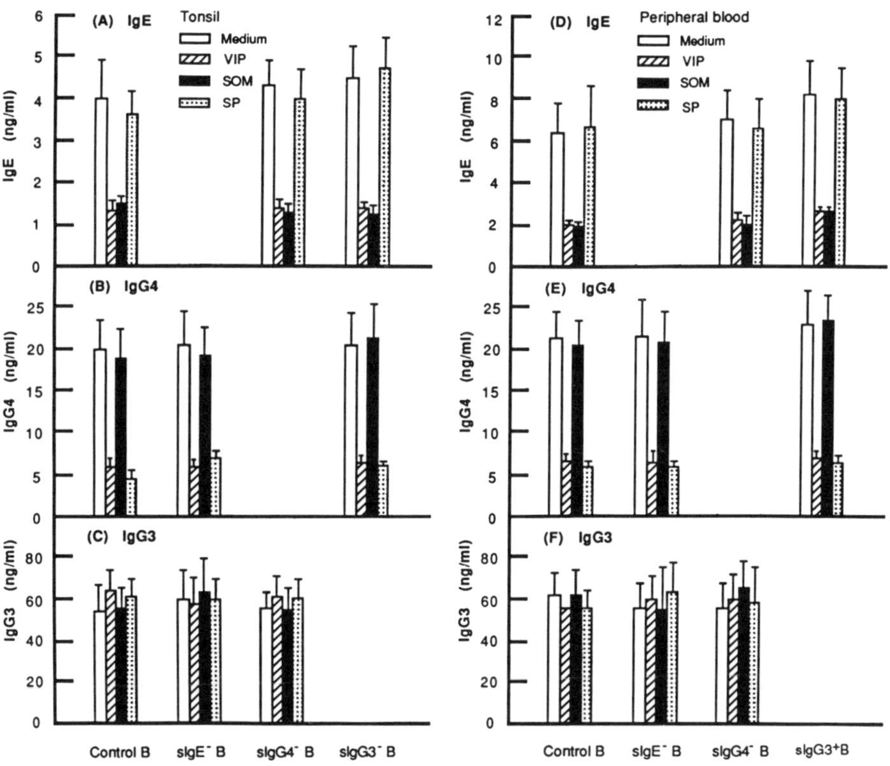


**Figure 14.13** Effect of depletion of sIg+ cells[63]. Atopic patients' control B cells or various sIg+ B-cell populations from tonsil (A,B,C) and peripheral blood (D,E,F) are incubated with medium (open), VIP (0.1 nM, matched bar), SOM (0.1 nM, closed) or SP (0.1 nM, dotted) in the presence of T cells and monocytes. On day 14 of culture, IgE (A,D), IgG4 (B,E) and IgG3 (C,F) production are determined. Values are the mean ± 1 SD of results of triplicate cultures from one experiment, representative of four. From reference 63 © 1994, Journal of Immunology, with permission.

In our culture system, VIP directly affects B-cell lines and enhances Ig production by them. These results indicate that some neuropeptides may have B-cell-stimulatory activities *per se*. On the other hand, in IL-4-stimulated cultures, neuropeptide effects require T cells and monocytes. This is not surprising, since receptors for VIP, SOM or SP have been demonstrated on many cells, including B cells, T cells and monocytes[18,25,26]. It therefore seems possible that VIP, SOM or SP affect the nature of physical contact between cells, in turn inhibiting the production of IgE and IgG subclass expression. Neuropeptides modulate IL-4-induced IgE and IgG4 production in $sIgE^-$ and $sIgG4^-$ cells, respectively. These results indicate that neuropeptides modulate IL-4-induced IgE and IgG4 switching. In contrast, IL-4 does not induce IgG2 or IgG3 production in $sIgG2^-$ or $sIgG3^-$ B cells, respectively. Neuropeptides do not modulate IgG2 or IgG3 production in $sIgG2^-$ or $sIgG3^-$ B cells, respectively, suggesting that the effects of neuropeptides on IgG2 and IgG3 expression may be on the $sIgG2^+$ and $sIgG3^+$ B cells, respectively, but not on switching of $sIgG2^-$ and $sIgG3^-$ B cells to these respective Ig isotypes[58].

In atopic patients neuropeptides inhibit spontaneous production of IgE and/or IgG4, but not of IgG2 or IgG3. The exact mechanism for the difference of IL-4-induced IgE and IgG4 production in normal donors versus spontaneous IgE and IgG4 production in atopic patients is not known. However, T cells from atopic patients are found to have IgE-inducing activity, not blocked completely by anti-IL-4 antibody[66]. It has recently been reported that IL-13 also induces IgE and IgG4 production[67] (see Chapter 8). It is possible that in addition to IL-4 some other factors may be involved in spontaneous IgE and IgG4 production in atopic patients. In atopic patients, effects of neuropeptides also require T cells and monocytes. Our results, using double-chamber wells, indicate that if atopic patients' B cells were cultured in one chamber while T cells and monocytes were cultured in another, VIP, SOM and SP each failed to inhibit IgE and/or IgG4 production. However, if B cells, T cells and monocytes were cultured together in the same chamber, VIP, SOM and SP inhibited IgE and/or IgG4 production to the same extent as for MNCs from atopic patients[63]. Therefore, the neuropeptide effects on IgE and IgG4 production might not be mediated by secondary factor(s). Nevertheless, we cannot exclude the possibility that unknown factor(s) are produced upon interaction of B cells, T cells and monocytes, which in turn inhibit the spontaneous production of IgE and IgG4.

There are at least two possible ways of accounting for the inhibition of spontaneous production of IgE and/or IgG4 by VIP, SOM and SP: (1) these neuropeptides affect $sIgE^-$ and/or $sIgG4^-$ B cells by prevention of switching *in vitro*, and (2) these neuropeptides inhibit $sIgE^+$ and/or $sIgG4^+$ B cells from proliferating and/or differentiating. We have shown that removal of $sIgE^+$ and $sIgG4^+$ B cells results in abrogation of IgE and IgG4 production, respectively. These results indicate that $sIgE^+$ and $sIgG4^+$ B cells produce IgE and IgG4 spontaneously, and VIP, SOM or SP may be acting on $sIgE^+$ and $sIgG4^+$ B cells as maturation–inhibitory factors in the presence of T cells and monocytes.

Taken together, VIP, SOM and SP can modulate IL-4-induced switching of IgE and/or IgG4 production, while they can also inhibit spontaneous production of IgE and/or IgG4 in atopic patients. The *in vivo* influence of these neuropeptides on IgE and IgG4 production remains to be elucidated. However, these peptides play many roles in allergic and inflammatory responses. It has been reported that there is a loss of VIP from pulmonary nerve fibers in patients with asthma[15]. SOM induces histamine secretion from mast cells[5], and SP induces eosinophil infiltration[37]. It is tempting to speculate that these neuropeptides also affect IgE and IgG4 production locally, and that they may modulate allergic and inflammatory responses. Finally, VIP, SOM and SP seem to be excellent reagents for the study of IgE and IgG subclass regulation.

## REFERENCES


1. Payan DG, Levine JD, Goetzel EJ. Modulation of immunity and hypersensitivity by sensory neuropeptides. J Immunol 1984; 132:1601–1604.
2. Nagy G, Mulchahey JJ, Neill JD. Autocrine control of prolactin secretion by vasoactive intestinal peptide. Endocrinology 1988; 122:364–366.
3. Di Marzo V, Tippins JR, Morris HR. The role of cyclic AMP in the inhibition of leukotriene biosynthesis by neuropeptides. Eur. J. Pharmacol 1988; 162:115–121.
4. Spangelo BL, Iskason PC, Macleod RM. Production of interleukin-6 by anterior pituitary cells is stimulated by increased intracellular adenosine 3′,5′-monophosphate and basoactive intestinal peptide. Endocrinology 1990; 127:403–409.
5. Theoharides TC, Douglas WW. Somatostatin induces histamine secretion from rat peritoneal mast cells. Endocrinology 1978; 102:1637–1640.
6. Wagner F, Fink R, Hart R, Dancygier H. Substance P enhances interferon-γ production by human peripheral blood mononuclear cells. Regul Peptides 1987; 19:355–364.
7. Lotz M, Vaughan JH, Carson DA. Effect of neuropeptides on production of inflammmatory cytokines by human monocytes. Science 1988; 241:1218–1221.
8. Laurenzi MA, Persson MAA, Dalsgaard C-J, Haegerstrand A. The neuropeptide substance P stimulates production of interleukin 1 in human blood monocytes: activated cells are preferentially influenced by the neuropeptide. Scand J Immunol 1990; 31:519–533.
9. Calvo C-F, Chavanel G, Senik A. Substance P enhances IL-2 expression in activated human T cells. J. Immunol 1992; 148:3498–3504.
10. Luber-Narod J, Kage R, Leeman SE. Substance P enhances the secretion of tumor necrosis factor-α from neuroglial cells stimulated with lipopolysaccharide. J Immunol 1994; 152:819–824.
11. Lygren I, Revhaug, A, Burhol PG *et al.* Vasoactive intestinal polypeptide and somatostatin in leukocytes. Scand J Clin Lab Invest 1984; 44:347–351.

12. Aliakbari J, Sreedharan SP, Turck CW, Goetzl EJ. Selective localization of vasoactive intestinal peptide and substance P in human eosinophils. Biochem Biophys Res Commun 1987; 148:1440–1445.
13. Arnaout MA, Garthwaite TL, Martinson DR, Hagen TC. Vasoactive intestinal polypeptide is synthesized in anterior pituitary tissue. Endocrinology 1986; 119:2052–2057.
14. Baraniuk JN, Lundgren JD, Okayama M *et al.* Vasoactive intestinal peptide in human nasal mucosa. J Clin Invest 1990; 86:825–831.
15. Ollerenshaw S, Jarvis D, Woolcock A *et al.* Absence of immunoreactive vasoactive intestinal polypeptide in tissue from the lungs of patients with asthma. N Engl J Med 1989; 320:1244–1248.
16. Ottaway CA, Greenberg GR. Interaction of vasoactive intestinal peptide with mouse lymphocytes: specific binding and the modulation of mitogen responses. J Immunol 1984; 132:417–423.
17. Danek A, O'Dorisio MS, O'Dorisio TM, George JM. Specific binding sites for vasoactive intestinal polypeptide on nonadherent peripheral blood lymphocytes. J Immunol 1983; 131:1173–1177.
18. Ottaway CA, Lay TE, Greenberg GR. High affinity specific binding of vasoactive intestinal peptide to human circulating T cells, B cells and large granular lymphocytes. J. Neuroimmunol 1990; 29:149–155.
19. Beed EA, O'Dorisio SM, O'Dorisio TM, Gaginella TS. Demonstration of a functional receptor for vasoactive intestinal polypeptide on Molt 4b T lymphoblasts. Regul Peptides 1983; 6:1–12.
20. O'Dorisio MS, Shannon BT, Fleshman DJ, Campolito LB. Identification of high affinity receptors for vasoactive intestinal peptide on human lymphocytes of B cell lineage. J Immunol 1989; 142:3533–3536.
21. Finch PJ, Sreedharan SP, Goetzel EJ. High-affinity receptors for vasoactive intestinal peptide on human myeloma cells. J Immunol 1989; 142:1977–1981.
22. Scicchitano R, Dazin P, Bienenstock J *et al.* Distribution of somatostatin receptors on murine spleen and Peyer's patch T and B lymphocytes. Brain Behav Immun 1987; 1:173–184.
23. Scicchitano R, Dazin P, Bienenstock J *et al.* The murine IgA-secreting plasmacytoma MOPC-315 expressed somatostatin receptors. J Immunol 1988; 141:937–941.
24. Bhathena SJ, Recant L. Somatostatin receptors on circulating human blood cells. Horm Metab Res 1980; 12:277–278.
25. Bhathena SJ, Louie J, Schechter GP *et al.* Identification of human mononuclear leukocytes bearing receptors for somatostatin and glucagon. Diabetics 1981; 30:127–131.
26. Payan DG, Hess CA, Goetzel EJ. Inhibition by somatostatin of the proliferation of T-lymphocytes and Molt-14 lymphoblasts. Cell Immunol 1984; 84:433–438.
27. Pascual DW, Xu-Amano J, Kiyono H *et al.* Substance P acts directly upon cloned B lymphoma cells to enhance IgA and IgM production. J Immunol 1991; 146:2130–2136.
28. Payan DG, Brewster DR, Missirian-Bastian A, Goetzel EJ. Substance P recognition by a subset of human T lymphocytes. J Clin Invest 1984; 74:1532–1539.
29. Payan DG, Brewster DR, Goetzel EJ. Stereospecific receptors for substance P on cultured human IM-9 lymphoblasts. J Immunol 1984; 133:3260–3265.
30. Mantyh CR, Gates TS, Zimmerman RP *et al.* Receptor binding sites for substance P, but not substance K or neuromedin K, are expressed in high concentrations by arterioles, venules, and lymph nodules in surgical specimens

obtained from patients with ulcerative colitis and Crohn disease. Proc Natl Acad Sci USA 1988; 85:3235–3239.
31. Nordlind K, Mutt V. Influence of beta-endorphin, somatostatin, substance P and vasoactive intestinal peptide on the proliferative response ot human peripheral blood T lymphocytes to mercuric chloride. Int Arch Allergy Appl Immunol 1986; 80:326–328.
32. Ishioka C, Yoshida A, Kimata H, Mikawa H. Vasoactive intestinal peptide stimulates immunoglobulin production and growth of human B cells. Clin Exp Immunol 1992; 87:504–508.
33. Mascardo RN, Barton RW, Sherline P. Somatostatin has an antiproliferative effect on concanavalin A-activated rat thymocytes. Cell Immunol 1984; 33:131–138.
34. Pawlikowski M, Stepien H, Kunert-Radek J, Schally AV. Effect of somatostatin on the proliferation of mouse spleen lymphocytes *in vitro*. Biochem Biophys Res Commun 1985; 129:52–55.
35. Chou C-K, Ho L-T, Hu C-P *et al.* Selective suppression of insulin-induced proliferation of cultured human hepatoma cells by somatostatin. J Clin Invest 1987; 79:175–178.
36. Styono-Han B, Henkelman MS, Foekens JA, Klijin JG. Direct inhibitory effects of somatostatin (analogues) on the growth of human breast cancer cells. Cancer Res 1987; 47:1566–1570.
37. Matsuda H, Kawakita K, Kiso Y *et al.* Substance P induces granulocyte infiltration through degranulation of mast cells. J Immunol 1989; 142:927–931.
38. Stanisz AM, Befus D, Bienstock J. Differential effects of vasoactive intestinal peptide, substance P, and somatostatin on immunoglobulin synthesis and proliferation by lymphocytes from Peyer's patches, mesenteric lymph nodes, and spleen. J Immunol 1986; 136:152–156.
39. Drew PA, Sherman DJC. Vaso-active intestinal peptide: a neurotransmitter which reduces human NK cell activity and increases Ig synthesis. Aust J Exp Biol Med Sci 1985; 63:313–318.
40. Annibale B, Fais S, Boirivant M *et al.* Effects of high *in vivo* levels of vasoactive intestinal polypeptide on function of circulating lymphocytes in humans. Gastroenterology 1990; 98:1693–1698.
41. Hassner A, Lau MS, Goetzl EJ, Adelman DC. Isotype-specific regulation of human lymphocyte production of immunoglobulins by sustained exposure to vasoactive intestinal peptide. J Allergy Clin Immunol 1993; 92:891–901.
42. Blum AM, Metwail A, Mathew RC *et al.* Substance P and somatostatin can modulate the amount of IgG2a secreted in response to Schistosome egg antigens in murine Schistosomiasis mansoni. J Immunol 1993; 151:6994–7004.
43. Pascual DW, McGhee JR, Kiyono H, Bost KL. Neuroimmune modulation of lymphocyte function—I. Substance P enhances immunoglobulin synthesis in lipopolysaccharide activated murine splenic B cell cultures. Int Immunol 1991; 3:1223–1229.
44. Scicchitano R, Biennenstock J, Stanisz AM. *In vivo* immunomodulation by the neuropeptide substance P. Immunology 1988; 63:733–735.
45. Laurenzi MA, Persson MAA, Dalsgaard C-J, Ringden O. Stimulation of human B lymphocyte differentiation by the neuropeptides substance P and neurokinin A. Scand J Immunol 1989; 30:695–701.
46. Hart R, Dancygier H, Wagner F *et al.* Effect of substance P on immunoglobulin and interferon-gamma secretion by cultured human duodenal mucosa. Immunol Lett 1990; 23:199–204.
47. Kimata H, Yoshida A, Ishioka C *et al.* Nerve growth factor specifically induces human IgG4 production. Eur J Immunol 1991; 21:137–141.

48. Kimata H, Yoshida A, Ishioka C, Midawa H. Stimulation of Ig production and growth of human lymphoblastoid B-cell lines by nerve growth factor. Immunology 1991; 72:451–452.
49. Kimata H, Yoshida A, Ishioka C, Midawa H. Effect of human recombinant erythropoietin on human IgE production *in vitro*. Clin Exp Immunol 1991; 83:483–487.
50. Kimata H, Yoshida A, Ishioka *et al.* Interleukin 8 (IL-8) selectively inhibits immunoglobulin E production induced by IL-4 in human B cells. J Exp Med 1992; 176:1227–1231.
51. Kimata H, Saxon A. Subset of natural killer cells is induced by immune complexes to display Fc receptors for IgE and IgA and demonstrate isotype regulatory function. J Clin Invest 1988; 82:160–167.
52. Jiang Y, Yoshida A, Ishioka C *et al.* Parathyroid hormone inhibits immunoglobulin production without affecting cell growth in human B cells. Clin Immunol Immunopathol 1992; 65:286–293.
53. Cheng PP-J, Sreedharan SP, Kishiyama JL, Goetzel EJ. The SKW 6.4 line of human B lymphocytes specifically binds and responds to vasoactive intestinal peptide. Immunology 1993; 79:64–68.
54. Kimata H, Yoshida A, Ishioka C, Mikawa H. Disodium cromoglycate (DSCG) selectively inhibits IgE production and enhances IgG4 production by human B cells *in vitro*. Clin Exp Immunol 1991; 84:395–399.
55. Kimata H, Mikawa H. Nedocromil sodium selectively inhibits IgE and IgG4 production in human B cells stimulated with IL-4. J Immunol 1993; 151:6723–6732.
56. Kimata H, Yoshida A, Ishioka C, Mikawa H. Differential effect of vasoactive intestinal peptide, somatostatin and substance P on human IgE and IgG subclass production. Cell Immunol 1992; 144:429–442.
57. Jabara HH, Fu SM, Geha RS, Vercelli D. CD40 and IgE: synergism between anti-CD40 monoclonal antibody and interleukin 4 in the induction of IgE synthesis by highly purified human B cells. J Exp Med 1990; 172:1861–1864.
58. Zhang K, Clark EA, Saxon A. CD40 stimulation provides an IFN-$\gamma$-independent and IL-4-dependent differentiation signal directly to human B cells for IgE production. J Immunol 1991; 146:1836–1842.
59. Gascan H, Gauchat J-F, Aversa G *et al.* Anti-CD40 monoclonal antibodies or $CD4^+$ T cell clones and IL-4 induce IgG4 and IgE switching in purified human B cells via different signalling pathways. J Immunol 1991; 147:8–13.
60. Yang X-D, De Weck AL, Stadler BM. Effect of recombinant human interleukin 4 on spontaneous *in vitro* human IgE synthesis. Eur J Immunol 1988; 18:1699–1704.
61. Rousset F, Robert J, Andary M *et al.* Shifts in interleukin-4 and interferon-$\gamma$-production by T cells of patients with elevated serum IgE levels and the modulatory effects of these lymphokines on spontaneous IgE synthesis. J Allergy Clin Immunol 1991; 87:58–69.
62. Nüsslein HG, Winter M, Träg T, Kalden JR. Interleukin-4-induced IgG subclass and IgE secretion by mononuclear cells from atopic donors. Int Arch Allergy Appl Immunol 1991; 95:257–260.
63. Kimata H, Yoshida A, Fujimoto A, Mikawa H. Effect of vasoactive intestinal peptide, somatostatin, and substance P on spontaneous IgE and IgG4 production in atopic patients. J Immunol 1993; 150:4630–4640.
64. Kimata H, Shanahan F, Brogan M *et al.* Modulation of ongoing human immunoglobulin synthesis by natural killer cells. Cell Immunol 1987; 107:74–88.
65. Sherr E, Macy E, Kimata H *et al.* Binding the low affinity Fc$\epsilon$R on B cells suppress ongoing human IgE synthesis. J Immunol 1988; 142:481–489.

66. Zhang X, Polla B, Hauser C, Zubler RH. T cells from atopic individuals produce IgE-inducing activity incompletely blocked by anti-interleukin-4 antibody. Eur J Immunol 1992; 22:829–833.
67. Punnonen J, Aversa G, Cocks BG *et al.* Interleukin 13 induces interleukin 4-independent IgG4 and IgE synthesis and CD23 expression by human B cells. Proc Natl Acad Sci USA 1993; 90:3730–3734.

# Part III

# PATHOPHYSIOLOGY

# 15 IgE Regulation in Allergy and Helminth Parasite Infections

**ROBERT L. COFFMAN**
*DNAX Research Institute of Molecular and Cellular Biology, Palo Alto, California, USA*

## INTRODUCTION

Nearly all studies of the mechanism and regulation of class switching have, of necessity, taken a reductionist approach, using cell lines or simple cultures of purified B cells. However, the biological and medical implications of these studies require that they reflect accurately class switching as it occurs *in vivo*, during normal or pathological immune responses. This chapter will summarize evidence from animal and human studies concerning the regulation of IgE switching and expression as it occurs *in vivo*. The focus on IgE is appropriate, as its regulation *in vivo* has been studied in more detail than that of other isotypes in either mice or humans. There are at least two good reasons why this is so. The first is that IgE levels are regulated over the widest range within an individual and appear to be regulated rather independently of the other isotypes. Baseline serum levels are much lower for IgE than for any other isotype and can increase as much as $10^3$–$10^4$-fold in mice or humans during the course of a chronic helminth infection. The second reason is that IgE mediates a unique and potent set of effector functions that are central features of allergy and asthma.

As suggested in the title, prominent IgE responses in humans occur in two principal situations: allergic diseases and helminth parasite infections. As a consequence, nearly all *in vivo* studies in either humans or experimental animals examine IgE regulation in one of these two disease states or in model systems designed to mimic allergic-type responses. Several important generalizations emerge from such studies and suggest that *in vitro* studies have given us a reasonably clear picture of how IgE is induced and regulated. The principal pathway of cellular events leading to IgE production *in vivo* involves B-cell activation via the CD40–Cd40L (CD40 ligand) interaction and requires IL-4 for the responding B cells to switch to IgE. In humans, it is probable that either IL-4 or IL-13 are required and bind and signal through shared receptor components (see Chapter 8). In addition, Th1-like cells,

*Cytokine Regulation of Humoral Immunity: Basic and Clinical Aspects.* Edited by Clifford M. Snapper.

acting predominantly through the production of IFN-γ, are important natural inhibitors of this pathway. The remainder of this chapter will be a review of the evidence to support these generalizations.

## T-CELL REGULATION OF IgE PRODUCTION

The central roles of IL-4 as an inducer of switching to IgE and IFN-γ as an inhibitor of that switching have been well described in several previous chapters. A key to understanding IgE regulation has come from the recognition that these cytokines are, for the most part, produced by distinct subsets of CD4+ T cells (Th cells)[1]. Th subsets with different functions and cytokine synthesis patterns were first recognized in panels of clonal mouse Th cell lines. The subsets termed Th1 and Th2 were initially distinguished by the fact that activated Th1 clones make interleukin-2 (IL-2) and interferon gamma (IFN-γ), but not IL-4 or IL-5, whereas Th2 clones made IL-4 and IL-5, but not IL-2 or IFN-γ[2]. Subsequent analysis has shown additional differences in cytokines between these two subsets, as well as a number of cytokines, such as IL-3 and granulocyte/macrophage colony-stimulating factor (GM-CSF), that are made by both subsets.

Th2 cells are efficient helpers for B-cell proliferation and immunoglobulin (Ig) production but do not mediate delayed-type hypersensitivity (DTH) or other cell-mediated immune functions. As a consequence of their production of IL-4, but not IFN-γ, they can provide helper function for substantial IgE responses[3]. Th1 cells, in contrast, mediate DTH, activate macrophages and carry out many of the functions associated with cell-mediated immunity. They can provide help to B cells, but, at least *in vitro*, they do so under a limited range of conditions. They are not able to provide help for IgE, but are instead potent inhibitors of IgE production[3–6].

There is now strong evidence in the mouse that antigen-stimulated Th cells *in vivo* have discrete Th1- and Th2-like cytokine patterns. Some antigens and pathogens stimulate Th populations with cytokine patterns closely resembling those of Th1 and Th2 clones[7–11]. Furthermore, techniques for detecting cytokine expression by single cells have provided considerable evidence for distinct Th subsets among normal cells[12,13]. It is now recognized that a similar dichotomy exists in humans[14], and that Th2, but not Th1, clones provide help for IgE[15–17]. A third cytokine profile is also prominent among human Th clones and has been designated Th0. These clones secrete both IL-4 and IFN-γ in various amounts, and their ability to help an IgE response is a function of the ratio of IL-4 to IFN-γ that they produce[18,19].

Th cells are not the only cell types capable of producing IFN-γ and IL-4, of course, and other cells may be able to influence the production of IgE by production of either of these cytokines. Most CD8+ T cells produce significant amounts of IFN-γ, and there is some evidence for CD8+ inhibitors of IgE production in rodents[20–22]. CD8+ T cells with a Th2-like cytokine pattern have also been described, but their occurrence *in vivo* and their possible role in IgE regulation are not yet understood. A small subset of CD4+ T cells expressing the NK1.1 marker has recently been described[23]. These cells appear capable of producing large amounts of IL-4 within 30–90 min of activation *in vivo*, but their possible role in IgE responses has not yet been clarified. Furthermore, cells with the characteristics of mast cells and basophils have been shown to produce IL-4 and IL-13 upon Fc-receptor-mediated triggering *in vitro*[24–27], and human basophils have also been shown to express the CD40 ligand and provide help for IgE production[28].

## IL-4 REGULATION OF IgE PRODUCTION *IN VIVO*

There is now a compelling body of evidence that IL-4 is required for virtually all primary IgE responses in the mouse[7,29]. Treatment of mice with an excess of neutralizing anti-IL-4 antibody inhibited 95–99 per cent of the primary IgE response to a number of T-cell-dependent stimuli, including helminth infections[30], protein antigens[31] and anti-IgD antibodies[30,32]. These findings have been confirmed in mice that have had their IL-4 genes disrupted by homologous recombination. Only trace elements of IgE are detectable in such mice after infection with *Nippostrongylus brasiliensis*[33] or *Plasmodium chaubudii*[34]. These results also suggest that, in contrast to the human, IL-13 does not stimulate IgE switching or production in the mouse, and this has been confirmed *in vitro* with recombinant IL-13 (B.W.P. Seymour and R.L. Coffman, unpublished). Mice exposed to high levels of IL-4 either from long-term treatment with IL-4[35] or via a constitutively expressing IL-4 transgene[36] have very high levels of IgE. These results confirm the IgE-inducing activity of IL-4 and suggest that IL-4 is almost always a limiting factor in IgE responses *in vivo*. In humans, there is not yet direct evidence of the sort above that IL-4 and/or IL-13 are the major or only inducers of switching to IgE, but Th2-like responses of IL-4 expression can be demonstrated in a variety of allergic and parasitic diseases[9,16,17,37]. The induction of human IgE production *in vivo* has been shown in SCID-hu mice treated with recombinant human IL-4 (see Chapter 8).

Primary IL-4-dependent IgE responses involve switch recombination, as shown by the isolation of circular extrachromosomal DNA pieces containing the deleted intervening $C_H$ loci from mice infected with a helminth parasite[38]. Furthermore, sequential switching of B cells, first to IgG1 and then to IgE, appears to be the dominant pathway for the generation of IgE-producing cells *in vivo*, as opposed to a single-step deletion of all genes between the Sμ and Sε regions[38]. This mechanism appears not to be required, however, as

IgE responses are relatively normal in mice that cannot switch first to IgG1 because of a deletion in their Sγ1 region[39].

The major, if not the only, mechanism by which IL-4 and IL-13 are known to enhance IgE specifically is by the induction of switching to IgE. Therefore, it is of considerable interest whether secondary IgE responses become independent of these cytokines after switching has occurred. Treatment of mice with anti-IL-4 during a secondary challenge with a protein antigen inhibits the IgE response as effectively as it does during a primary response[31]. In contrast, secondary responses to helminth parasite infections are only partially inhibited by anti-IL-4[31]. Using polyclonal IgE responses stimulated *in vivo* with either anti-IgD or anti-IgE, Katona *et al.*[40,41] have shown that the fraction of secondary IgE responses that develop directly from B cells already switched to IgE is unaffected by anti-IL-4, whereas the fraction that arises from $IgD^+$ B cells, via a switch, is inhibited by anti-IL-4 treatment. Significant inhibition of secondary IgE responses to ovalbumin can be accomplished by the induction of an ovalbumin-specific Th1 response, and this inhibition is blocked with anti-IFNγ[5,6]. Ongoing IgE production in SCID-hu mice, as described in Chapter 8, can be significantly inhibited with a mutant IL-4 that acts as a competitive antagonist of IL-4 and IL-13. Thus, the available evidence suggests that continued IL-4/IL-13 dependent switching may be required to maintain IgE responses even to repeated challenges. A clearer resolution of the contribution of switching to the chronic IgE responses that characterize allergic diseases would give a clearer view of the possible clinical impact of inhibitors of IL-4.

## INHIBITION OF IgE *IN VIVO* BY IFN-γ, IFN-α AND IL-12

A number of experiments have directly addressed whether IFN-γ can inhibit switching to IgE *in vivo*, as would be predicted on the basis of its activities *in vitro*. IFN-γ, either as rIFN-γ administration, or as stimulation of endogenous IFN-γ production, can inhibit IgE responses to goat anti-mouse IgD[32], helminth infections[42], or allergenic protein antigens[5,43]. Similarly, IFN-α administration can substantially inhibit IgE responses in mice with helminth infections[42] or injected with anti-IgD[29]. In humans, the *in vivo* evidence for a similar activity is based on the reductions of IgE observed in patients with hyper-IgE syndrome treated with either IFN-α[44] or IFN-γ[45].

IL-12 has been shown to inhibit IL-4-induced IgE synthesis in cultures, possibly by a mechanism independent of its ability to induce IFN-γ production[46]. In the mouse, IL-12 was quite effective at inhibiting the primary, but not the secondary, IgE response to *N. brasiliensis*[47]. Furthermore, it caused an overall inhibition of the strong Th2 response induced by this parasite. IL-12 also inhibits the IgE response to protein antigens[48], but is somewhat less effective at inhibiting the IgE response to heterologous anti-IgD. In all of these examples, the effects of IL-12 on IgE and other isotypes, as well as on Th subset differentiation, appear to be largely or completely inhibited by anti-IFN-γ.

## B-CELL ACTIVATION SIGNALS INVOLVED IN IgE PRODUCTION *IN VIVO*

In order for IL-4 to induce isotype switching, B cells must be activated in some way. Quite a variety of methods have been used experimentally *in vitro* to accomplish this in the absence of T cells, including lipopolysaccharide (LPS) in mice[49] and Epstein–Barr virus (EBV) in humans[50]. It appears now that the most important activation signal mediated by contact with activated Th cells involves the interaction between the B-cell surface molecule, CD40, and the CD40 ligand (CD40L) on T cells[51]. CD40L is rapidly induced upon T-cell activation and is expressed by both Th1 and Th2 clones. The addition of IL-4 to B-cell cultures stimulated via the CD40–CD40L interaction leads to substantial switching to IgE and gives results equivalent to those obtained with B cells activated with live Th clones (see Chapters 4 and 8)[52]. Several other ligand–receptor pairs, including membrane TNF–TNF receptor[53] and CD2–CD58[54], appear to have B-cell activation activities similar to those of CD40–CD40L. Not all B-cell stimuli appear to permit IL-4-mediated switching to IgE, however. For example, murine B cells activated with anti-IgD conjugated to dextran, a polyclonal surrogate for a TI-2 antigen, cannot switch to IgE in the presence of IL-4, even though they can switch to other isotypes[55].

A rare immunodeficiency syndrome in humans, hyper-IgM syndrome, provides dramatic evidence that the CD40–CD40L interaction is central to isotype switching *in vivo*, including switching to IgE. Most patients have elevated IgM, but greatly reduced levels of other isotypes and undetectable IgE[56]. Such patients have mutations that render CD40L non-functional, although CD40 expression on B cells is fairly normal and these B cells respond normally to signaling via wild-type CD40L or anti-CD40 antibodies[51]. A few hyper-IgM syndrome patients have low but detectable levels of IgE, and clones from one such patient were able to activate B cells to switch to IgE in the presence of IL-4[57]. Thus, nearly all IgE in humans originates from B cells activated through a CD40–CD40L interaction, although a small minority may arise from B cells activated by other pathways.

In the mouse, homologous recombination mutants lacking either CD40[58,59] or CD40L[60,61] have phenotypes resembling closely the hyper-IgM syndrome. In general, these mice have severe defects in switching to all isotypes, including IgE, when challenged with T-dependent protein antigens or infected with *N. brasiliensis*. Serum levels of IgM and IgG3 were normal, and in some cases, elevated: however, IgA and other IgG isotypes are quite low and IgE levels undetectable. Stimulation with TI-2 antigens, which are not known to involve the CD40–CD40L interaction, leads to good production of all isotypes except IgE.

## THE ROLE OF CD23 IN IgE REGULATION

There has been much speculation about the role of CD23 (also known as FcεRII, the low-affinity IgE receptor) in IgE regulation. In addition to binding IgE, CD23 also binds CD21, and it has been shown that the interaction of CD21 on B cells with CD23 on T cells can prime B cells for IL-4-dependent IgE production *in vitro*[28]. Furthermore, the soluble forms of CD23 in humans have B-cell growth activity in some *in vitro* culture systems[62]. Antibodies to CD23 cause modest inhibition of IgE responses in rats[63], but not in mice[64]. Somewhat paradoxically, mice with transgenic overexpression of CD23 have reduced IgE responses to parasite infection and anti-IgD stimulation[65]. Mice with deletions introduced into the CD23 gene have essentially normal IgE responses to *N. brasiliensis* infection, but had either sustained[66] or relatively normal responses to protein antigens[67,68]. Thus, these transgenic and 'knockout' experiments fail to confirm the proposed IgE-regulatory activities of CD23 and suggest that CD21–CD23 interactions are not required for normal murine B-cell responses.

CD23 and IgE are, however, clearly involved in an IgE-mediated enhancement of IgE, as well as IgM, IgG1 and IgG2a responses. This is an indirect consequence of the IgE/FcεRII-enhanced uptake and presentation of antigens by B cells to Th cells[64,69]. This process requires IgE specific for the challenge antigen and is blocked by antibodies to mouse CD23. This IgE/FcεRII-mediated enhancement of Th activation and antibody expression is also absent in the CD23 knockout mice[67]. This activity may account for some of the IgE-enhancing activities proposed for CD23 and, if it also can lead to the activation of T cells with inhibitory activities (such as Th1 cells), may also account for examples of IgE inhibition ascribed to CD23.

## SUMMARY

There is now a significant body of literature on the regulation of switching and expression of IgE *in vivo*, in humans and in rodents, and a relatively consistent view has emerged from these studies. Some types of antigens, such as allergens and helminth parasites, stimulate $CD4^+$ T-cell responses dominated by Th2 cells, although the reasons for this are not yet well understood. Th2 cells stimulate the production of the three hallmark features of allergic diseases and helminth infections: mast cells, oesinophils and IgE antibodies. The cytokines responsible for these activities are IL-4 for IgE production[30,49], IL-5 for eosinophilia[70], and the combination of IL-3, IL-4 and IL-10 for mast cell production[71]. Virtually all of the IgE produced during primary responses to either class of antigens originates from B cells activated directly by Th2 cells via the CD40–CD40L interaction. The activated B cells are induced to switch the IgE, and then mature to IgE-producing cells. Subsequent challenges of the same antigen stimulate higher IgE responses both from memory cells that have already switched to IgE and from a continuing process of IL-4-mediated switching. IgE responses are tightly controlled *in vivo*, however, and the principal mediators of this control are cytokines associated with Th-1 like responses, principally IFN-γ, IFN-α and IL-12. This control is exerted at several levels, including IFN-γ and IFN-α-mediated inhibition of switching to IgE and the inhibition of the development and persistence of Th2 responses by all three cytokines.

## ACKNOWLEDGEMENT

The DNAX Research Institute is supported by the Schering-Plough Corporation.

## REFERENCES

1. Mosmann TR, Coffman RL. Two types of mouse helper T cell clone: implications for immune regulation. Immunol Today 1987; 8:223–227.
2. Mosmann TR, Coffman RL. Heterogeneity of cytokine secretion patterns and functions of helper T cells. Adv Immunol 1989; 46:111–147.
3. Coffman RL, Seymour BW, Lebman DA *et al.* The role of helper T cell products in mouse B cell differentiation and isotype regulation. Immunol Rev 1988; 102:5–28.
4. DeKruyff RH, Ju S-T, Hunt AJ *et al.* Induction of antigen-specific antibody responses in primed and unprimed B cells: functional heterogeneity among TH1 and TH2 T cell clones. J Immunol 1989; 142:2575–2582.
5. Hayglass KT, Stefura BP. Anti-interferon-gamma treatment blocks the ability of glutaraldehude-polymerized allergens to inhibit specific IgE responses. J Exp Med 1991; 173:279–285.
6. Yang X, Gieni RS, Mosmann TR, Hayglass KT. Chemically modified antigen preferentially elicits induction of Th1-like cytokine synthesis patterns in vivo. J Exp Med 1993; 178:349–353.
7. Urban J, Madden K, Svetic A *et al.* The importance of Th2-cytokines in protective immunity to nematodes. Immunol Rev 1992; 127:205–220.
8. Finkelman FD, Pearce EJ, Urban JF Jr, Sher A. Regulation and biological function of helminth-induced cytokine responses. Immunol Today 1991; 12:A62–A66.
9. Sher A, Coffman RL. Regulation of immunity to parasites by T cells and T cell-derived cytokines. Annu Rev Immunol 1992; 10:385–409.
10. Locksley RM, Scott P, Helper t-cell subsets in mouse leishmaniasis induction expansion and effector function. Immunol Today 1991; 12:A58–A61.

11. Coffman RL, Varkila K, Scott P, Chatelain R. The role of cytokines in the differentiation of CD4+ T cell subsets *in vivo*. Immunol Rev 1991; 123:189–207.
12. Carding SR, West J, Woods A, Bottomly K. Differential activation of cytokine genes in normal CD4-bearing T cells is stimulus dependent. Eur J Immunol 1989; 19:231–238.
13. Taguchi T, McGhee JR, Coffman RL *et al.* Analysis of Th1 and Th2 cells in murine gut-associated tissues. Frequencies of CD4+ and CD8+ T cells that secrete IFN-gamma and IL-5. J Immunol 1990; 145:68–77.
14. Romagnani S. Human TH1 and TH2 subsets; doubt no more. Immunol Today 1991; 12:256–257.
15. Del Prete G, Maggi E, Parronchi P *et al.* IL-4 is an essential factor for the IgE synthesis induced in vitro by human T cell clones and their supernatants. J Immunol 1988; 140:4193–4198.
16. Yssel H, Johnston KE, Schneider PV *et al.* T cell activation-inducing epitopes of the house dust mite allergen Der pI. Proliferation and lymphokine production patterns by Der pI-specific CD4+ T cell clones. J Immunol 1992; 148:783–745.
17. Romagnani S. Lymphokine production by human T cells in disease states. Annu Rev Immunol 1994; 12:227–257.
18. Maggi E, Del Prete G, Macchia D *et al.* Profiles of lymphokine activities and helper function for IgE in human T cell clones. Eur J Immunol 1988; 18:1045–1050.
19. Pene J, Rousset F, Briere F *et al.* IgE production by normal human B cells induced by alloreactive T cell clones is mediated by IL-4 and suppressed by IFN-gamma. J Immunol 1988; 141:1218–1224.
20. Kemeny DM, Noble A, Holmes BJ, Diaz-Sanchez D. Immune regulation: a new role for the CD8+ T cell. Immunol Today 1994; 15:107–110.
21. Diaz-Sanchez D, Lee TH, Kemeny DM. Ricin enhances IgE responses by inhibiting a subpopulation of early-activated IgE regulatory CD8+ T cells. Immunology 1993; 78:226–236.
22. McMenamin C, Holt PG. The natural immune response to inhaled soluble protein antigens involves major histocompatibility complex (MHC) class I-restricted CD8+ T cell-mediated but MHC class II-restricted CD4+ T cell-dependent immune deviation resulting in selective suppression of immunoglobulin E production. J Exp Med 1993; 178:889–899.
23. Yoshimoto T, Paul WE. CD4pos, NK1.1pos T cells promptly produce interleukin 4 in response to in vivo challenge with anti-CD3. J Exp Med 1994; 179:1285–1295.
24. Seder RA, Plaut M, Barbieri S *et al.* Purified Fc epsilon R+ bone marrow and splenic non-B, non-T cells are highly enriched in the capacity to produce IL-4 in response to immobilized IgE, IgG2a, or ionomycin. J Immunol 1991; 147:903–909.
25. Paul WE, Seder RA, Plaut M. Lymphokine and cytokine production by Fc epsilon RI+ cells. Adv Immunol 1993; 53:1–29.
26. Dvorak AM, Seder RA, Paul WE *et al.* Ultrastructural characteristics of Fc epsilon R-positive basophils in the spleen and bone marrow of mice immunized with goat anti-mouse IgD antibody. Lab Invest 1993; 68:708–715.
27. Brunner, T, Heusser CH, Dahinden CA. Human peripheral blood basophils primed by interleukin 3 (IL-3) produce IL-4 in response to immunoglobulin E receptor stimulation. J Exp Med 1993; 177:605–611.
28. Gauchat JF, Henchoz S, Mazzei G *et al.* Induction of human IgE synthesis in B cells by mast cells and basophils. Nature 1993; 365:340–343.
29. Finkelman FD, Holmes J, Katona IM *et al.* Lymphokine control of in vivo immunoglobulin isotype selection. Annu Rev Immunol 1990; 8:303–333.
30. Finkelman FD, Katona IM, Urban JF Jr *et al.* Suppression of in vivo polyclonal

IgE responses by monoclonal antibody to the lymphokine B-cell stimulatory factor 1. Proc Natl Acad Sci USA 1986; 83:9675–9678.

31. Finkelman FD, Katona IM, Urban JF Jr *et al.* Interleukin-4 is required to generate and sustain in vivo IgE responses. J Immunol 1988; 141:2335–2341.
32. Finkelman FD, Katona IM, Mosmann TR, Coffman RL. IFN-gamma regulates the isotypes of Ig secreted during in vivo humoral immune responses. J Immunol 1988; 140:1022–1027.
33. Kuhn R, Rajewsky K, Muller W. Generation and analysis of interleukin-4 deficient mice. Science 1991; 254:707–710.
34. von der Weid T, Kopf M, Kohler G, Langhorne J. The immune response to Plasmodium chabaudi malaria in interleukin-4-deficient mice. Eur J Immunol 1994; 24:2285–2293.
35. van Ommen R, Vredendaal AE, Savelkoul HF. Prolonged in vivo IL-4 treatment inhibits antigen-specific IgG1 and IgE formation. Scand J Immunol 1994; 40:1–9.
36. Tepper RI, Levinson DA, Stanger BZ *et al.* IL-4 induces allergic-like inflammatory disease and alters T cell development in transgenic mice. Cell 1990; 62:457–467.
37. Wierenga EA, Snoek M, de Groot C *et al.* Evidence for compartmentalization of functional subsets of CD2+ T lymphocytes in atopic patients. J Immunol 1990; 144:4651–4656.
38. Yoshida K, Matsuoka M, Usuda S *et al.* Immunoglobulin switch circular DNA in the mouse infected with *Nippostrongylus brasiliensis*: Evidence for successive class switching from $\mu$ to $\epsilon$ via $\gamma 1$. Proc Natl Acad Sci USA 1990; 87:7829–7833.
39. Jung S, Siebenkotten G, Radbruch A. Frequency of immunoglobulin E class switching is autonomously determined and independent of prior switching to other classes. J Exp Med 1994; 179:2023–2026.
40. Katona IM, Urban JF Jr, Kang SS *et al.* IL-4 requirements for the generation of secondary in vivo IgE responses. J Immunol 1991; 146:4215–4221.
41. Thyphronitis G, Katona IM, Gause WC, Finkelman FD. Germline and productive C epsilon gene expression during in vivo IgE responses. J Immunol 1993; 151:4128–4136.
42. Urban JF Jr, Madden KB, Cheever AW *et al.* IFN inhibits inflammatory responses and protective immunity in mice infected with the nematode parasite, Nippostrongylus brasiliensis. J Immunol 1993; 151:7086–7094.
43. Hayglass KT, Stefura W. Isotype-selective abrogation of established IgE responses. Clin Exp Immunol 1990; 82:429–434.
44. Souillet G, Rousset F, de Vries JE. Alpha-interferon treatment of patient with hyper IgE syndrome. Lancet 1989; 1:1384.
45. King CL, Gallin JI, Malech HL *et al.* Regulation of immunoglobulin production in hyperimmunoglobulin E recurrent-infection syndrome by interferon gamma. Proc Natl Acad Sci USA 1989; 86: 10085–10089.
46. Kiniwa M, Gately M, Gubler U *et al.* Recombinant interleukin-12 suppresses the synthesis of immunoglobulin E by interleukin-4 stimulated human lymphocytes. J Clin Invest 1992: 90:262–266.
47. Morris SC, Madden KB, Adamovicz JJ *et al.* Effects of IL-12 on in vivo cytokine gene expression and Ig isotype selection. J Immunol 1994; 152:1047–1056.
48. Germann T, Bongartz M, Dlugonska H *et al.* Interleukin 12 profoundly up-regulates the synthesis of antigen-specific complement-fixing IgG2a, IgG2b and IgG3 antibody subclasses *in vivo*. Eur J Immunol 1995; 25:823–829.
49. Coffman RL, Carty J. A T cell activity that enhances polyclonal IgE production and its inhibition by interferon-gamma. J Immunol 1986; 136:949–954.
50. Thyphronitis G, Tsokos GC, June CH *et al.* IgE secretion by Epstein-Barr virus-

infected purified human B lymphocytes is stimulated by interleukin 4 and suppressed by interferon gamma. Proc Natl Acad Sci USA 1989; 86:5580–5584.

51. Banchereau J, Bazan F, Blanchard D *et al.* The CD40 antigen and its ligand. Annu Rev Immunol 1994; 12:881–922.
52. Spriggs MK, Armitage RJ, Strockbine L *et al.* Recombinant human CD40 ligand stimulates B cell proliferation and immunoglobulin E secretion. J Exp Med 1992; 176:1543–1550.
53. Aversa G, Punnonen J, de Vries JE. The 26-kD transmembrane form of tumor necrosis factor alpha on activated CD4+ T cell clones provides a costimulatory signal for human B cell activation. J Exp Med 1993; 177:1575–1585.
54. Diaz-Sanchez D, Chegini S, Zhang K, Saxon A. CD58 (LFA-3) stimulation provides a signal for human isotype switching and IgE production distinct from CD40. J Immunol 1994; 153:10–20.
55. Snapper CM, Pecanha LM, Levine AD, Mond JJ. IgE class switching is critically dependent upon the nature of the B cell activator, in addition to the presence of IL-4. J Immunol 1991; 147:1163–1170.
56. Notarangelo LD, Duse M, Ugazio AG. Immunodeficiency with hyper-IgM (HIM). Immunodefic Rev 1992; 3:101–121.
57. Life P, Gauchat JF, Schnuriger V *et al.* T cell clones from an X-linked hyper-immunoglobulin (IgM) patient induce IgE synthesis in vitro despite expression of nonfunctional CD40 ligand. J Exp Med 1994; 180:1775–1784.
58. Castigli E, Alt FW, Davidson L *et al.* CD40-deficient mice generated by recombination-activating gene-2-deficient blastocyst complementation. Proc Natl Acad Sci USA 1994; 91:12135–12139.
59. Kawabi T, Naka T, Yoshida K *et al.* The immune responses in CD40-deficient mice: impaired immunoglobulin class switching and germinal center formation. Immunity 1994; 1:167–178.
60. Renshaw BR, Fanslow WC, Armitage RJ *et al.* Humoral immune responses in CD40 ligand-deficient mice. J Exp Med 1994; 180:1889–1900.
61. Xu J, Foy TM, Laman JD *et al.* Mice deficient for the CD40 ligand. Immunity 1994; 1:423–431.
62. Gordon J, Cairns JA, Liu YJ *et al.* Role of membrane and soluble CD23 in lymphocyte physiology. Monogr Allergy 1991; 29:156–168.
63. Flores-Romo L, Shields J, Humbert Y *et al.* Inhibition of an in vivo antigen-specific IgE response by antibodies to CD23. Science 1993; 261:1038–1041.
64. Gustavsson S, Hjulstrom S, Liu T, Heyman B. CD23/IgE-mediated regulation of the specific antibody response in vivo. J Immunol 1994; 152:4793–4800.
65. Texido G, Eibel H, Le Gros G, van der Putten H. Transgene CD23 expression on lymphoid cells modulates IgE and IgG1 responses. J Immunol 1994; 153:3028–3042.
66. Yu P, Kosco-Vilbois M, Richards M *et al.* Negative feedback regulation of IgE synthesis by murine CD23. Nature 1994; 369:753–756.
67. Fujiwara H, Kikutani H, Suematsu *et al.* The absence of IgE antibody-mediated augmentation of immune responses in CD23-deficient mice. Proc Natl Acad Sci USA 1994; 91:6835–6839.
68. Stief A, Texido G, Sansig G *et al.* Mice deficient in CD23 reveal its modulatory role in IgE production but no role in T and B cell development. J Immunol 1994; 152:3378–3390.
69. Kehry MR, Yamashita LC. Low-affinity IgE receptor (CD23) function on mouse B cells; role in IgE-dependent antigen focusing. Proc Natl Acad Sci USA 1989; 86:7556–7560.
70. Sanderson CJ, O'Garra AO, Warren DJ, Klaus GG. Eosinophil differentiation

factor also has B-cell growth factor activity: proposed name interleukin 4. Proc Natl Acad Sci USA 1986; 83:437–440.

71. Thompson-Snipes L, Dhar V, Bond MW *et al.* Interleukin 10: a novel stimulatory factor for mast cells and their progenitors. J Exp Med 1991; 173:507–510.

# 16 Regulation of Mucosal Immunity

**K. W. BEAGLEY and C. A. BLACK**
*University of Newcastle, Newcastle, NSW, Australia* and
*Australian Institute for Mucosal Immunology, Newcastle, Australia*
**M. L. DUNKLEY**
*Australian Institute for Mucosal Immunology, Newcastle, Australia*
and
**J. R. McGHEE**
*University of Alabama at Birmingham, Birmingham, Alabama, USA*

## INTRODUCTION

The mucosa-associated lymphoreticular tissues (MALT) are major inductive sites for IgA responses in higher mammals and consist of gut-associated, nasal-associated and bronchus-associated lymphoreticular tissues, which are usually abbreviated as GALT, NALT and BALT, respectively. In addition, lymphoid aggregates also occur in the large intestine and are termed rectal-associated (or RALT). Sections of the reproductive tract are also considered to be part of the mucosal immune system, although systematic immunity also contributes to protection of this site. Collectively, the MALT comprise approximately 65–75 per cent of organized lymphoid tissues in humans and in experimental animals (mice, rats, rabbits and primates). As we will emphasize throughout this chapter, the MALT supplies immune B and T cells to all mucosal tissues, which in humans represent a surface area greater than 400 $m^2$, which is more than 200 times larger than that covered by the squamous epithelial surfaces such as the skin.

When one considers that most microorganisms invade through or cohabitate these mucosal surfaces as normal flora, it becomes clear that higher mammals require a large investment from the mucosal immune system for host protection. The protection at mucosal surfaces is due in part to the local production of antibodies, largely of the IgA isotype, and IgA-producing plasma cells in lamina propria and glandular ascinar regions fulfill this task. The greatest collection of immunocompetent cells occur in the gastrointestinal (GI) tract, where GALT provides the precursor B and T cells destined for lamina propria (LP) regions which contain more than $10^{10}$ IgA-producing plasma cells per meter of human intestine[1,2]. Large numbers of T

*Cytokine Regulation of Humoral Immunity: Basic and Clinical Aspects.* Edited by Clifford M. Snapper.

cells of both CD4-positive ($CD4^+$) and $CD8^+$ phenotypes also populate these same mucosal tissues. Thus, T cells and cytokines regulate IgA synthesis in mucosal tissues, where 3–4 g of IgA is secreted daily into the human GI tract[3].

Early studies comparing IgA responses in athymic or thymectomized animals with their euthymic counterparts have demonstrated the essential requirement for T lymphocytes in the regulation of IgA responses[4–7]. The regulatory function of T cells is due largely to the secretion of soluble regulatory molecules (cytokines) into the local microenvironment[8]. These cytokines bind to high-affinity receptors on other immune cells and regulate their activation, proliferation and differentiation. In this chapter, we will review the cell types that make up the various compartments of the mucosal immune system, with emphasis on the GI tract and the mechanisms whereby T cells and cytokines regulate IgA production in the gut.

## MUCOSAL INDUCTIVE AND EFFECTOR TISSUES

GALT are organized lymphoid aggregates which occur frequently in small intestine as well as at the ileocecal junction, and the major lymphoid nodules are termed Peyer's patches (PP), although numerous smaller, solitary lymphoid nodules (SLN) also occur. It is useful to consider the GALT as inductive sites where mature B and T cells, and antigen-presenting cells (APCs), first encounter foreign antigens, and the effector regions such as the LP where B and T cells which leave GALT take up final residence for provision of mucosal immunity[8]. In this network, one may also consider the intraepithelial lymphocytes (IELs) which populate the epithelial cell layer, and our limited knowledge of this important effector population is briefly summarized below.

### INDUCTIVE SITES

The PP of the small intestine and the lymphoid follicles associated with the large bowel constitute the major inductive sites in the GI tract. The PP consist of three anatomically and functionally distinct regions: (1) a specialized dome epithelium; (2) the follicular B-cell zone; and (3) the parafollicular T-cell-enriched area[8]. The dome epithelium consists of specialized antigen-sampling cells termed microfold (M) cells or follicle-associated epithelial (FAE) cells which pinocytose lumenal antigen and transport it into the underlying PP[9–16] (Figure 16.1). It was thought that M cells do not express MHC class II; however, HLA-DR antigen has been detected by some investigators but not by others. Whether M cells can present antigen in the classical sense is not known. It is presently thought that M cells transfer antigen intact to APCs and lymphocytes which are closely associated with the M cell basolateral surface. It may be that discrimination between food antigen and potential pathogens occurs at the level of the M

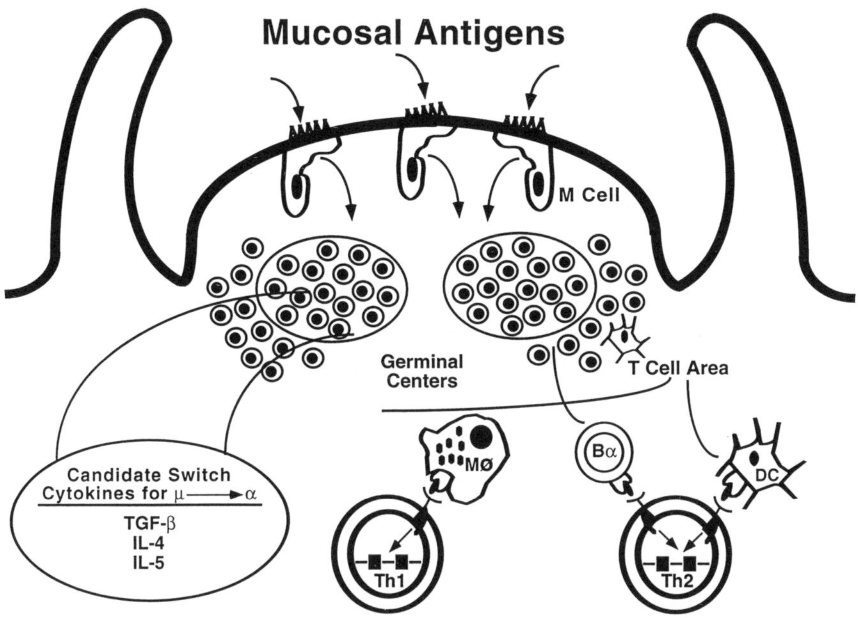


**Figure 16.1** Functional regions of Peyer's patches involved in mucosal antigen uptake, presentation and possible pathways for Th1 or Th2 cell induction. B-cell switches to IgA are thought to occur in germinal centers, perhaps under the influence of T cells and cytokines such as TGF-β. Three potential antigen-presenting cells may regulate induction of Th1 (macrophages; MØ) or Th2 ($sIgA^+$ B cells/dendritic cells (DC)) cells in these mucosal inductive sites

cell, where the former remain unprocessed while the latter are processed as foreign. Antigens taken up by M cells include soluble proteins[10–12], viruses such as reovirus types 1 and 3[13], poliovirus[14], HIV[15], and rotavirus and enterobacteria species such as *Salmonella, Escherichia coli* and *Shigella.*

T cells present in the parafollicular regions are predominantly (>95 per cent) αβ $TCR^+$ T cells. Of these T cells, 50–60 per cent are $CD4^+$, $CD8^-$ T-helper (Th) cells, with the remainder being $CD4^-$, $CD8^+$ T cells which include precursors of cytotoxic T lymphocytes (CTLs)[8,17]. B-cell follicles are found beneath the dome region and these contain active germinal centers (GCs). It is in these GCs that $\mu \rightarrow \alpha$ switching is thought to occur (Figure 16.1), and 60–70 per cent of surface IgA-positive ($sIgA^+$) B cells are within the GC itself[18]. All three major types of APCs, i.e. macrophages, dendritic cells (DC) and class II MHC-positive (class $II^+$) B cells, are associated with the PP[8,19] (Figure 16.1). Macrophages are found in significant numbers in the dome region and in the GC, while DCs are more predominant in the T-cell zones. In addition, large numbers of activated, class $II^+$ B cells are found in PP, which could serve as APCs for T-cell activation.

Delivery of antigen into the PP by M cells results in stimulation of antigen-specific B and T lymphocytes[16], which then leave the PP and migrate through the systemic immune system to finally home back to mucosal effector sites, including the LP of the GI tract[3,8,17]. This induction followed by migration to multiple effector sites is often referred to as the common mucosal immune system[3,8,17].

## MUCOSAL EFFECTOR SITES

### Lamina Propria Lymphocytes (LPLs)

The LP of the GI tract is the only tissue where large numbers of plasma cells are found under normal physiological conditions[17]. Seventy to ninety per cent of these plasma cells are of the IgA isotype[17,20,21] and daily IgA production in the human adult is estimated at 3–4 g per day. In the mouse, the average lifespan of these plasma cells is approximately 5–9 days[22], and thus these cells must be continuously replaced by PP-derived precursors. It is generally assumed that migrating, sIgA$^+$ B cells rapidly differentiate into IgA plasma cells in the presence of T-cell and cytokine help.

Estimates of T-cell numbers in the LP range from 40 to 90 per cent in different studies[1,23]. This wide range is most likely due to the different techniques used to identify cells (*in situ* immunohistochemical staining versus analysis of cells prepared by enzymatic digestion). The majority of CD3$^+$ T cells in the LP (65–80 per cent) are CD4$^+$, again consistent with the observation that the LP is the major site of T-cell-dependent IgA synthesis. The LP T cells demonstrate lower proliferative responses to T-cell mitogens when compared to T cells from lymphoid tissues or the peripheral blood. However, these T cells proliferate spontaneously when cultured in the presence of IL-2, and LP T cells spontaneously secrete cytokines. These observations are consistent with the hypothesis that LP T cells are activated *in vivo* (reviewed in reference 24). More studies are needed to fully characterize the lymphoid cells present in the LP of the GI tract. The role of class II$^+$ B cells and macrophages in activation of CD4$^+$ T cells in this region should receive more emphasis. Further, the mechanisms whereby T cells provide help for the terminal differentiation events for B cells is another area for study. In spite of the difficulties in enzymatic isolation of functional cells and in triggering T cells, this will no doubt be a major focus of future studies in the mucosal immune system.

### Intraepithelial Lymphocytes (IELs)

The lymphoid cells resident between intestinal epithelial cells are the first cells to contact lumenal antigen that crosses the mucosa in an M cell-independent manner. This heterogeneous population of mainly T cells is estimated to be more than half as numerous as all T cells in peripheral organs; however, their function remains poorly understood. The majority of murine IELs (80 per cent) are CD3+, and over 75 per cent of these also express CD8[25–28]. In mice and chickens, significant numbers of γδ TCR+ IEL are found (40–60 per cent)[29,30] in addition to αβ TCR+ cells; however, this number varies with mouse strain, age and housing conditions. The γδ TCR+ IELs represent a minor component of human IELs (~15 per cent) under normal conditions[31], but significantly increase in numbers in conditions such as celiac disease.

In mice, CD4+ (single positive), CD4−, CD8− (double negative) and CD4+, CD8+ (double positive) IELs all constitute minor fractions (~5–10 per cent) of CD3+ IELs[32]. IELs are greatly reduced in athymic animals, but are not totally absent—an observation that provided the first evidence that some IELs can develop in the absence of a functional thymus, an idea that was first suggested by Fichtelius in 1968[33]. Recent studies suggest that both γδ TCR+ and αβ TCR+ IELs can develop extrathymically. The evidence for this will not be presented in this chapter and the reader is referred to recent reviews of IEL development[34,35]. A distinguishing feature for some IEL T cells which may have developed extrathymically is the expression of CD8 in the form of an αα homodimer whereas CD8 expressed by thymus-derived IELs (and conventional CD8 T cells) is an αβ CD8 heterodimer[34]. As is the case in murine thymus, the γδ TCR+ IELs also develop first in ontogeny[36,37]. The αβ TCR+ IELs represent only a minor fraction at birth, but this subset increases in number during early adult life. This increase in αβ TCR+ IELs appears to be driven by exposure to lumenal antigens, as this increase is not observed in mice maintained in a germ-free environment[38]. The absolute number of IELs increases 5–16-fold between 6 and 20 weeks of age, due to expansion of αβ TCR+ IELs, but within individual strains of mice the absolute numbers of γδ TCR+ IELs remain relatively constant during this period.

The physiological role of IELs is poorly understood; however, several functions for these cells have been described and this diversity is consistent with their phenotypic heterogeneity. IELs have been shown to mediate antigen-specific delayed-type hypersensitivity (DTH) responses, to exhibit virus-specific CTL function, to express natural killer (NK)-like activity and to produce a local graft-versus-host reaction (GVHR) when transferred to semiallogeneic hosts (reviewed in reference 31). IELs respond poorly to conventional T-cell mitogens when compared to splenic T cells; however, there is evidence that human IELs are induced to proliferate via a CD2 pathway rather than through stimulation of the CD3–T-cell receptor (TCR) complex[39,40]. Proliferation of both γδ and αβ TCR+ mouse IELs can be induced by the 70-kDa heat shock protein (HSP) from *Mycobacterium tuberculosis*[41], an observation consistent with an immune surveillance function. With regard to regulation of humoral immunity, IELs have been shown to abrogate the induction of oral tolerance and to contain helper T cells which can enhance secretion of IgA[42–44]. Interestingly, feeding of cholera toxin (CT) to mice causes a transient deletion of IELs[45]. This observation suggests a role for IELs in maintenance of oral tolerance, since it is well known that CT prevents the induction of systemic unresponsiveness to co-orally administered proteins, which when given alone readily induce oral tolerance. IELs can be induced to produce a variety of cytokines which are characteristically produced by Th1- and Th2-type cells[31,32,41,46]. Studies from our group have shown that αβ TCR$^+$ IELs can exhibit help for B-cell responses[43,44].

## REGULATION OF MUCOSAL IgA RESPONSES

T-cell regulation of IgA synthesis can be considered to occur at two distinct levels. First, T cells and more recently cytokines have been shown to be involved in $\mu \rightarrow \alpha$ isotype switching and, second, both T cells and cytokines regulate the terminal differentiation of post-switched B cells into IgA-secreting plasma cells.

### T-CELL REGULATION OF IgA RESPONSES

A role for T cells in isotype switching to IgA emanated from studies by Kawanishi, Strober and colleagues[47,48], who showed that T-cell clones derived from PP T cells, when added to cultures of lipopolysaccharide (LPS)-stimulated splenic B cells, increased the frequency of sIgA$^+$ B cells in these cultures. Similar clones of splenic T cells did not cause an increase in numbers of sIgA$^+$ B cells. These switch T cells appeared to require cognate interactions with B cells, since the isotype switching to IgA could not be induced by soluble factors, and nor did the switch T cells induce IgA secretion. The switch T cells were shown to be autoreactive and probably arose in the unique PP microenvironment[49].

A second type of T-helper (Th) cell was also identified and antigen-specific Th cell clones induced IgA responses[50,51]. In these latter studies, sheep red blood cell (SRBC)-specific T-cell clones were isolated from the PP of mice fed SRBCs, and these Th cell clones preferentially supported IgA anti-SRBC antibody responses[50,51]. Cloned Th cells supported IgA responses in B-cell cultures containing sIgA$^+$ but not sIgA$^-$ B cells, suggesting the provision of help to post-switched, mature sIgA$^+$ B cells. The actions of these Th cells could be replaced with cell-free supernatants, suggesting that terminal differentiation was due to soluble factors (Fc receptors and possibly cytokines)[52].

Another cell type resident in the PP, the dendritic cell (DC), has also been shown to regulate B-cell switching to IgA. A co-culture technique was used where clusters of periodate-activated T cells and DCs from PP with either spleen or PP B cells resulted in production of large amounts of IgA, whereas T-cell–DC clusters from spleen induced secretion of 10–100-fold less IgA[53].

In subsequent studies, these T-cell–DC clusters from PP were shown to induce isotype switching to IgA in a pre-B-cell line, while similar clusters from spleen could not mediate this effect[54]. These studies suggested that with regard to IgA it was the source of the DCs rather than the T cells that was critical for switching to and secretion of this isotype[54]. Further studies have now suggested that the DCs may mediate their effects by activating T cells to secrete a particular subset of cytokines which favor IgA production[55], and this concept will be discussed in more detail in subsequent sections.

## ISOTYPE SWITCHING TO IgA

Isotype switching involves the recombination between DNA segments (switch or S regions) that are located 2 kb 5′ (upstream) of the respective $C_H$ genes (see Chapter 5). These segments are composed of multiple repeats of short (~5 bp) sequences. Recombination occurs when upstream and downstream S regions join such that a DNA loop is formed which contains the intervening $C_H$ genes to be deleted. For switching to occur, the S regions must first become accessible to recombinase(s). Such switch circles have now been shown in B-cell populations undergoing isotype switching[56,58]. In addition to the isotype switching induced by switch T cells, which required cognate interaction with B cells[47,48], isotype switching can also be induced by cytokines in combination with 'non-cognate' activational signals. The best studied example is interleukin-4 (IL-4)-induced switching to IgG1 and IgE in cultures of LPS-stimulated mouse splenic B cells[59,60].

Cytokine-induced switching is preceded by the induction of germline transcripts corresponding to the Ig isotype to which the B cell will switch. Thus, IL-4 will induce IgG1 and IgE germline transcripts prior to the expression of either IgG1 or IgE in LPS-stimulated splenic B cells. Interferon gamma (IFN-γ) has also been shown to induce isotype switching in mouse splenic B cells to IgG2a[61] if LPS is used as the primary stimulus and to IgG3 as well as IgG2a[62] when the stimulus is anti-IgD coupled to dextran.

Studies using LPS-stimulated mouse splenic B cells have shown that transforming growth factor beta (TGF-β) can induce isotype switching to IgA[63,64] (see Chapter 12). TGF-β was shown to act on $sIgM^+$, $sIgA^-$ B cells, thus ruling out an effect on the terminal differentiation of post-switched B cells, and to induce Cα germline transcripts[65], a prerequisite for switching to IgA. TGF-β could induce human $sIgD^+$ B cells to secrete IgA (in combination with IL-10) if the primary stimulus was anti-CD40 monoclonal antibody (mAb) presented by Fc receptor-positive CDW32L cells[66,67], but not if the B cells were stimulated by crosslinking of surface IgD. Likewise, TGF-β induced germline transcripts for both IgA1 and IgA2 in human splenic B-cell cultures stimulated with *Branhamella catarrhalis*[68] (a bacterium associated with the upper respiratory tract), and switching to IgA by human splenic B cells activated with $CD4^+$ T cells and pokeweed mitogen (PWM)[69].

Recent data, however, have suggested that the isotype switch-inducing effects of TGF-β may not be exclusive for IgA[70], since TGF-β has been shown to selectively stimulate IgG2b secretion by LPS-activated (but not anti-IgD-dextran activated) splenic B cells from −BALB/c mice. TGF-β1 selectively stimulated an increase in steady-state germline $C_H\gamma 2b$ RNA levels and stimulated IgG2b secretion by $IgM^+$, $IgG2b^-$ B cells indicating that TGF-β induced switching to IgG2b and enhanced secretion when B cells were activated with LPS. Highly purified splenic B cells from DBA mice were shown to release biologically active TGF-β when stimulated with LPS, and neutralization of this TGF-β reduced secretion of all IgG subclasses—an effect independent of class switching. These data demonstrate that following activation with the appropriate B-cell activator, TGF-β induces isotype switching to both IgG2b and IgA and enhances secretion of all IgG subclasses. TGF-β-induced switching to IgA is consistent with the finding that the TGF-β response element (TGF-β-RE)[71,72] is located 5′ of the Iα gene segment on the I.29 B-cell line; however, this gene sequence is not exclusively associated with the α heavy chain gene but is also found upstream of other $C_H$ genes[73]. Thus, while TGF-β appears to be essential for isotype switching to IgA *in vitro*, this does not occur with all B-cell mitogens, leaving open the possibility that the primary stimulus may also influence isotype switching. As already mentioned, human B cells stimulated through CD40 or via CD4 T cells plus PWM can be induced by TGF-β to switch to and secrete IgA[66,67,69] (in the presence or absence of IL-10); however, this does not occur if the primary stimulus is provided by *Staphylococcus aureus* Cowen I (SAC), anti-Ig, or PWM alone[66,74]. It could thus be argued that TGF-β can induce germline transcripts for multiple isotypes but the specificity is determined by the primary stimulus which selectively makes certain $C_H$ genes accessible. Thus, Cα accessibility may be induced by LPS and anti-CD40 but not by anti-IgD-dextran or PWM, in which case isotype determination is not due to TGF-β but rather to the nature of the primary B-cell stimulus.

A second issue relating to the role of TGF-β for *in vivo* switching to IgA is the tissue-specific nature of switching to, and secretion of, IgA. TGF-β is produced by both lymphoid and non-lymphoid cells in many tissues, and this is difficult to reconcile with the fact that IgA B-cell development occurs only in PP germinal centers, and in similar structures in NALT, BALT and the large intestine. In PP germinal centers, it has been estimated that up to 60–70 per cent of B cells are $sIgA^+$[18], while in most *in vitro* studies the frequency of switching to IgA is only of the order of 2–3 per cent[63,75]. This point has been recently addressed by McIntyre and associates, who showed that TGF-β together with IL-4 and IL-5 induced $sIgA^+$ B-cell populations of up to 15–20 per cent[76]. It is unfortunate in this regard that the TGF-β gene knockout mouse dies from a generalized lymphoproliferative disease at 2–3 weeks after birth, a fact which makes it difficult to use this mouse to investigate the role of TGF-β in IgA regulation *in vivo*. It should be remembered, however, that prior to studies of TGF-β-induced isotype switching, this cytokine was shown to have profound suppressive effects on the proliferation of both B and T cells, as well as IgA secretion[77–79], and it is possible that loss of mucosal immunity in these mice contributes to their early death.

## CYTOKINES FOR TERMINAL IgA B-CELL DIFFERENTIATION

Earlier studies have shown that addition of culture supernatants from DC–T cell clusters, T-cell clones or T-cell hybridomas to cultures of PP or splenic B cells resulted in enhanced secretion of IgA. One factor responsible for this activity was subsequently shown to be IL-5[80–85]. Removal of $sIgA^+$ B cells from PP B-cell cultures abrogated the effect of IL-5, demonstrating that the effect of this cytokine was on post-switched IgA-committed B cells[83]. When the target B-cell population was PP B cells, no *in vitro* stimulus was required, and IL-4 did not further enhance the effect of IL-5[83]. If splenic B cells were used, these cells first needed to be stimulated with LPS before increased IgA secretion could be shown. Using LPS-stimulated splenic B cells, the IgA-enhancing effect of IL-5 could be further increased by addition of IL-2 or IL-4. Taken together, these results suggest that IL-5 induces $sIgA^+$ B cells which are in cell cycle (blasts) to differentiate into IgA-producing cells. Interestingly, another B-cell population that has been shown to contain precursors of LP IgA B cells comprises peritoneal cavity B1 cells (see Chapter 3)[86]. This population also contains cells that can be induced by IL-5 to secrete IgA.

Human IL-5 is thought to act mainly as an eosinophil differentiation factor and thus may have little effect on B-cell isotype switching and differentiation. It has been reported, however, that human B cells, when stimulated with the bacterium *Branhamella catarrhalis*, can be induced by IL-5 to secrete IgA, and also to possibly undergo isotype switching to IgA[87]. This effect could not be demonstrated using other more conventional B-cell mitogens, a finding which once again demonstrates the important role of the primary *in vitro* activation signal for B-cell switching.

IL-6, when added to PP B cells in the absence of any *in vitro* stimulus, causes a marked increase in IgA secretion with little effect on either IgM or IgG synthesis[88]. In these studies, IL-6 induced 2–3-fold more IgA secretion than IL-5[88]. The removal of $sIgA^+$ B cells abolished the effect of IL-6, demonstrating that this cytokine, like IL-5, also acted on post-switched B cells. In mice where the IL-6 gene has been inactivated (IL-6 knockout), the numbers of $IgA^+$ B cells in the LP is markedly reduced, and local antibody responses following mucosal challenge with ovalbumin or vaccinia virus are greatly diminished, demonstrating the *in vivo* importance of IL-6 for mucosal IgA responses[89]. B cells isolated from human appendix are also induced to secrete both IgA1 and IgA2 by IL-6 in the absence of any *in vitro* activation[90]. This effect was also shown to be on IgA-committed B cells, again demonstrating the importance of IL-6 for terminal differentiation of IgA plasma cells.

## T-CELL SUBSETS AND MUCOSAL IMMUNE RESPONSES

The T-cell dependence of IgA responses has been well established and cells which induce isotype switching (Tsw) and Th cells which induce terminal differentiation of IgA-committed B cells have been summarized above. The recent description of two mutually exclusive subsets of CD4 helper T cells/clones defined by their pattern of cytokine secretion has been important for understanding mucosal and systemic immune responses[91,92]. Th1 cells secrete IL-2, IFN-$\gamma$ and tumor necrosis factor beta (TNF-$\beta$) and provide help for cell-mediated immunity (CMI) against intracellular bacteria such as *Mycobacterium tuberculosis* via activation of macrophages. The Th2 cells secrete IL-4, IL-5, IL-6, IL-10 and IL-13 and provide help for Ig (IgG1, IgE and IgA) synthesis. The cytokine milieu in which primary T-cell activation and subsequent differentiation occurs are key factors in determining the ultimate T-cell phenotype (reviewed in reference 93). Thus, the cytokines IL-12 and IL-4 may direct naive T cells down the Th1 or Th2 pathways, respectively, when present during primary activation. Later in development, IFN-$\gamma$ and IL-10 reinforce the expansion of Th1 and Th2 cells, respectively. Development down either of these pathways is also influenced by the type of APC, with class II$^+$ B cells reinforcing an established Th2 phenotype, while macrophages and liver Küppfer cells favor Th1 cell development. For stimulation of virgin T cells, DCs comprise the most effective (and perhaps only) APC.

From the above description, one could hypothesize that Th2 cells would predominate at mucosal sites and that immunization protocols and adjuvants that favor the induction of IgA responses should preferentially activate Th2 rather than Th1 cells. The importance of the cytokines IL-5 and IL-6 for IgA responses has already been described, providing support for this contention.

Using SRBCs as antigen, it has been shown that oral immunization of mice induced a predominant Th2 cell response in PP, while systemic immunization produced a mixed Th1 and Th2 cell response[94]. When mice were immunized orally with tetanus toxoid (TT) together with CT, an adjuvant known to prevent induction of oral tolerance and promote mucosal S-IgA responses[95], significant IgA responses in both fecal extracts and serum were induced[96,97]. If PP and splenic CD4$^+$ T cells were isolated at the peak of the S-IgA response and restimulated *in vitro* with TT or the B subunit of CT (CT-B), high numbers of IL-4 and IL-5 spot-forming cells (SFCs) (Th2) were seen while IFN-$\gamma$ and IL-2 SFCs (Th1) were the same as background. These studies demonstrate that induction of a mucosal IgA response is coincident with predominant activation of CD4$^+$ Th2 cells in PP. Infection of mice with an intestinal helminth (*Heligmosomoides polygyrus*) also resulted in an increase in mRNA for Th2-type cytokines in PP and mesenteric lymph nodes (MLN)[98], a finding consistent with the hypothesis that stimulation of GALT results in preferential activation of Th2 cells. In support of this concept, recent studies in IL-4 deficient (knockout) mice, which are defective in Th2 cytokine responses, failed to respond to orally administered proteins even when CT was used as adjuvant[99].

Interestingly, a Th2-like cell has recently been isolated from the mesenteric lymph nodes of mice fed myelin basic protein (MBP). These cells secreted IL-4, IL-10 and TGF-β[100] and could prevent or ameliorate the severity of experimental autoimmune encephalomyelitis (EAE) induced by immunization of SJL mice with MBP. Suppression of induction of EAE was abrogated by anti-TGF-β mAb. These mucosally derived CD4 T-cell clones resembled MBP-specific encephalitogenic T-cell clones in their epitope specificity, TCR usage and MHC restriction but differed only in cytokine secretion patterns. These cells may be important, therefore, in the maintenance of oral tolerance to food antigens via secretion of immunosuppressive cytokines such as TGF-β. The fact that both suppressive and disease-inducing CD4 T-cell clones utilize the same TCR and recognize the same MBP-derived peptide suggests that it is something in the mucosal microenvironment that preferentially induces cells of this phenotype. As already noted, TGF-β, at least *in vitro*, has also been demonstrated to play a role in switching to IgA.

Recent studies suggest that distinct populations of CD8 T cells may also exist at mucosal sites; these T cells provided help for B cells[101]. Others have demonstrated that lymph node $CD8^+$ T cells, when cultured *in vitro* with phorbol ester, ionomycin, IL-2 and IL-4 become non-cytotoxic, lose expression of surface CD8 and assume a Th2-like phenotype (with secretion of IL-4, IL-5 and IL-10)[102]. These T cells could also provide help for Ig secretion by B cells. $CD8^+$ T cells have recently been isolated from mouse PP, which secreted IL-5 and IL-10 as well as IFN-γ, expressed message for IL-4 and also provided help for Ig secretion by PP B cells. Further, $CD8^+$ T cells that promote humoral immunity have been demonstrated in human lepromatous leprosy[103]. These T cells secrete IL-4, suppress *M. leprae*-specific CMI responses and enhance antibody production, which in the case of leprosy results in a chronic non-resolving infection. The recent demonstration that bacterial antigens can be processed by macrophages and presented to $CD8^+$ T cells in the context of MHC class I[104] may be significant for mucosal immune responses if these CD8 cells become Th2-like and promote IgA secretion via production of cytokines such as IL-4, IL-5 and IL-10.

## SUMMARY

Rapid strides have been made during the past decade in our understanding of regulatory modes for development of mucosal immunity. For example, early work with PP T-cell clones revealed that T cells and soluble factors mediate $\mu \rightarrow \alpha$ B-cell switches as well as provide help for preferential IgA responses. Clearly, the APCs in PP, e.g. DCs, MØ and class $II^+$ B cells, help provide unique microenvironments for initial activation of T cells as well as triggering Th cell subsets for mucosal and systemic immunity. Cytokines such as TGF-β (and possibly IL-4 and IL-5) clearly promote $\mu \rightarrow \alpha$ switching in appropriately triggered B cells, while Th2-type cytokines such as IL-5, IL-6 and IL-10 support B-cell differentiation into IgA-producing plasma cells which characterize mucosal effector sites. Recent evidence also indicates that mucosal antigens and adjuvants which promote brisk mucosal IgA responses, do so by induction of $CD4^+$ Th2-type cells. These studies have strong implications for mucosal vaccine development, and future studies may allow the delivery of vaccines, adjuvants and appropriate cytokines for optimization of mucosal and systemic immune responses.

## ACKNOWLEDGMENTS

We thank our colleagues in the Mucosal Immunization Research Group and the Immunobiology Vaccine Center for positive criticisms of this review and the ideas expressed. We also thank Ms Sheila D. Shaw for preparation of the manuscript. The studies briefly described were supported by DMID-NIAID Contract AI 15128 and NIH grants AI 18958, DE 04217, DK 44240, DE 09837, AI 35544, AI 35932 and DE 08228.

## REFERENCES

1. Brandtzaeg P, Baklien K. Immunohistochemical studies of the formation and epithelial transport of immunoglobulins in normal and diseased human intestinal mucosa. Scand J Gastroenterol 1976; 11 (Suppl 36):1–45.
2. Brandtzaeg P. Overview of the mucosal immune system. Curr Top Microbiol Immunol 1989; 146:13–25.
3. Mestecky J. The common mucosal immune system and current strategies for induction of immune responses in external secretions. J Clin Immunol 1987; 7:265–276.
4. Crewther P, Warner NL. Serum immunoglobulins and antibodies in congenitally athymic (nude) mice. Aust J Exp Biol Med Sci 1972; 50:625–635.
5. Pritchard H, Riddaway J, Micklem HS. Immune responses in congenitally thymus-less mice. II. Quantitative studies of serum immunoglobulins, the antibody response to sheep erythrocytes, and the effect of thymus allografting. Clin Exp Immunol 1973; 13:125–138.
6. Clough JD, Mims LH, Strober W. Deficient IgA antibody responses to arsanilic acid bovine serum albumin (BSA) in neonatally thymectomized rabbits. J Immunol 1971; 106:1624–1629.
7. Ebersole JL, Taubman MA, Smith DJ. The effect of neonatal thymectomy on the level of salivary and serum immunoglobulins in rats. Immunology 1979; 36:649–657.
8. McGhee JR, Mestecky J, Elson CO, Kiyono H. Regulation of IgA synthesis and immune response by T cells and interleukins. J Clin Immunol 1989; 9:175–199.

9. Bockman DE, Cooper MD. Pinocytosis by epithelium associated with lymphoid follicles in the bursa of Fabricius, appendix, and Peyer's patches. An electron microscopic study. Am J Anat 1973; 136:455–477.
10. Owen RL, Jones AL. Epithelial cell specialization within human Peyer's patches: an ultrastructural study of intestinal lymphoid follicles. Gastroenterology 1974; 66:189–203.
11. Owen RL. Sequential uptake of horseradish peroxidase by lymphoid follicle epithelium of Peyer's patch in the normal unobstructed mouse intestine: an ultrastructural study. Gastroenterology 1977; 72:440–451.
12. Neutra MR, Philips TL, Mayer EL, Fishkind DJ. Transport of membrane-bound macromolecules by M cells in follicle-associated epithelium of rabbit Peyer's patch. Cell Tissue Res 1987; 247:537–546.
13. Wolf JL, Rubin DH, Finberg R *et al.* Intestinal M cells: a pathway for entry of reovirus into the host. Science 1981; 212:471–472.
14. Sicinski P, Rowinski J, Warchol JB *et al.* Poliovirus type 1 enters the human host through intestinal M cells. Gastroenterology 1990; 98:56–58.
15. Amerongen HM, Weltzin R, Farnet CM *et al.* Transepithelial transport of HIV-1 by intestinal M cells: a mechanism for transmision of AIDS. J AIDS 1991; 4:760–765.
16. Kato T, Owen RL. Structure and function of intestinal mucosal epithelium. In: Ogra PL *et al.* (eds) Handbook of Mucosal Immunology. San Diego, CA: Academic Press 1994; pp. 11–26.
17. Mestecky J, McGhee JR. Molecular and cellular interactions involved in IgA biosynthesis and immune response. Adv Immunol 1987; 40:153–245.
18. Butcher EC, Rouse RV, Coffman RL *et al.* Surface phenotype of Peyer's patch germinal center cells: implications for the role of germinal centers in B cell differentiation. J Immunol 1982; 129:2698–2707.
19. Spalding DM, Koopman WJ, Eldridge JH *et al.* Accessory cells in murine Peyer's patch: I. Identification and enrichment of functional dendritic cells. J Exp Med 1983; 157:1646–1659.
20. Brandtzaeg P, Valnes K, Scott H *et al.* The human gastrointestinal secretory immune system in health and disease. Scand J Gastroenterol 1985; 20 (Suppl 114):17–38.
21. Brandtzaeg P, Baklien K, Bjerke K *et al.* Nature and properties of the human gastroitestinal immune system. In: Miller K, Nicklin S (eds) Immunology of the Gastrointestinal Tract, Vol 1. Boca Raton, FL: CRC Press, Inc. 1987; p. 1.
22. Mattioli CA, Tomasi TB Jr. The life span of IgA plasma cells from the mouse intestine. J Exp Med 1973; 138:452–460.
23. Selby WS, Janossy G, Goldstein G, Jewell DP. T lymphocyte subsets in human intestinal mucosa: the distribution and relationship to MHC-derived antigens. Clin Exp Immunol 1981; 44:453–458.
24. James SP, Zeitz M. Human gastrointestinal mucosal T cells. In Ogra PL *et al.* (eds) Handbook of Mucosal Immunology. San Diego, CA: Academic Press 1994; pp. 275–285.
25. Selby WS, Janossy G, Jewell DP. Immunohistological characterization of intraepithelial lymphocytes of the human gastrointestinal tract. Gut 1981; 22:169–176.
26. Selby WS, Janossy G, Bofill M, Jewel DP. Lymphocyte subpopulations in the human small intestine. The findings in normal mucosa and in the mucosa of patients with adult coeliac disease. Clin Exp Immunol 1983; 52:219–228.
27. Selby WS, Janossy G, Bofill M, Jewell DP. Intestinal lymphocyte subpopulations in inflammatory bowel disease: an analysis by immunohistological and cell isolation techniques. Gut 1984; 25:32–40.

28. Goodman T, Lefrancois L. Expression of the γδ T-cell receptor on intestinal CD8+ intraepithelial lymphocytes. Nature 1988; 333:855–858.
29. Bonneville M, Janeway CA, Ito K *et al.* Intestinal intraepithelial lymphocytes are a distinct set of γδ T cells. Nature 1988; 336:479–481.
30. Bucy RP, Chen CL, Cihak J *et al.* Avian T cells expressing γδ receptors localize in the splenic sinusoids and the intestinal epithelium. J Immunol 1988; 141:2200–2205.
31. Mowat AM. Human intraepithelial lymphocytes. Springer Semin Immunopathol 1990; 12:165–190.
32. Fujihashi K, Yamamoto M, McGhee JR, Kiyono H. Immunoregulatory function and cytokine production by αβ and γδ TCR+ T cells for mucosal immune responses. In: Kiyono H, McGhee JR (eds) Advances in Host Defense Mechanisms, Vol 9. Mucosal Immunology: Intraepithelial Lymphocytes. New York: Raven Press 1993; pp. 89–114.
33. Fichtelius KE. The gut epithelium: a first level lymphoid organ? Exp Cell Res 1968; 49:87–104.
34. Poussier P, Julius M. Thymus independent T cell development and selection in the intestinal epithelium. Annu Rev Immunol 1994; 12:521–523.
35. Guy-Grand D, Rocha B, Vassalli P. Origin and development of gut intraepithelial lymphocytes. In: Kiyono H, McGhee JR (eds) Advances in Host Defense Mechanisms, Vol 9 Mucosal Immunology: Intraepithelial Lymphocytes. New York: Raven Press 1993; pp. 21–32.
36. Havran WL, Allison JP. Origin of thy-1+ dendritic epidermal cells of adult mice from fetal thymic precursors. Nature 1990; 344:68–70.
37. Yoshikai Y, Ishida A, Murosaki S *et al.* Sequential appearence of T-cell receptor γδ- and αβ-bearing intestinal intraepithelial lymphocytes in mice after irradiation. Immunology 1991; 74:583–588.
38. Bandeira A, Mota-Santos T, Itohara S *et al.* Localization of γδ T cells to the intestinal epithelium is independent of normal microbial colonization. J Exp Med 1990; 172:239–244.
39. Ebert EC, Roberts AI, Brolin RE, Raska K. Examination of the low proliferative capacity of human jejunal intraepithelial lymphocytes. Clin Exp Immunol 1986; 65:148–157.
40. Ebert EC. Proliferative responses of human intraepithelial lymphocytes to various T cell stimuli. Gastroenterology 1989; 97:1372–1381.
41. Beagley, KW, Fujihashi K, Black CA *et al.* The *Mycobacterium tuberculosis* 71-kDa heat-shock protein induces proliferation and cytokine secretion by murine gut intraepithelial lymphocytes. Eur J Immunol 23:2049–2052.
42. Fujihashi K, Taguchi T, McGhee JR *et al.* Regulatory function for murine intraepithelial lymphocytes: two subsets of CD3+ T cell receptor-1+ IEL T cells abrogate oral tolerance. J Immunol 1990; 145:2010–2019.
43. Fujihashi K, Taguchi T, Aicher WK *et al.* Immunoregulatory functions for murine intraepithelial lymphocytes: γδ T cell receptor-positive (TCR+) T cells abrogate oral tolerance while αβ TCR+ T cells provide B cell help. J Exp Med 1992; 175:695–707.
44. Fujihashi K, Yamamoto M, McGhee JR *et al.* Function of αβ TCR bearing intraepithelial lymphocytes: Th1 and Th2 type cytokine production by CD4+, CD8− and CD4+, CD8+ T cells possess helper activity. Int Immunol 1993; 5:1473–1481.
45. Elson CO, Holland SP, Dertzbaugh MT *et al.* Morphological and functional alterations of mucosal T cells by cholera toxin and B subunit. J Immunol 1995; in press.
46. Barrett TA, Gajewski TF, Danielpur D *et al.* Differential function of intestinal intraepithelial lymphocyte subsets. J Immunol 1992; 149:1124–1130.

47. Kawanishi H, Saltzman LE, Strober W. Characteristics and regulatory function of murine Con A-induced, cloned T cells obtained from Peyer's patches and spleen: mechanisms regulating isotype-specific immunoglobulin production by Peyer's patch B cells. J Immunol 1982; 129:475–483.
48. Kawanishi H, Saltzman L, Strober W. Mechanisms regulating IgA class-specific immunoglobulin production in murine gut-associated lymphoid tissues. II. Terminal differentiation of post switch sIgA-bearing Peyer's patch B cells. J Exp Med 1983; 158:649–669.
49. Kawanishi H, Ozato K, Strober W. The proliferative response of cloned Peyer's patch switch T cells to syngeneic and allogeneic stimuli. J Immunol 1985; 134:3586–3591.
50. Kiyono H, McGhee JR, Mosteller LM *et al.* Murine Peyer's patch T-cell clones: characterization of antigen-specific helper T cells for immunoglobulin A responses. J Exp Med 1982; 156:1115–1130.
51. Kiyono H, Cooper MD, Kearney JF *et al.* Isotype-specificity of helper T cell clones. Peyer's patch Th cells preferentially collaborate with mature IgA B cells for IgA responses. J Exp Med 1984; 159:798–811.
52. Kiyono H, Mosteller-Barnum LM, Pitts AM, *et al.* Isotype-specific immunoregulation: IgA binding factors produced by Fcα receptor$^+$ T cell hybridomas regulate IgA responses. J Exp Med 1985; 161:731–747.
53. Spalding D, Williamson SI, Koopman WJ, McGhee JR. Preferential induction of polyclonal IgA secretion by murine Peyer's patch dendritic cell–T cell mixtures. J Exp Med 1984; 160:941–946.
54. Spalding DM, Griffin JA. Different pathways of differentiation of pre-B cell lines are induced by dendritic cells and T cells from different lymphoid tissues. Cell 1986; 44:507–515.
55. Everson MP, Koopman WJ, Beagley KW. Divergent T-cell cytokine-profiles induced by dendritic cells from different tissues. In: Kempered K *et al.* (eds) Dendritic Cells in Fundamental and Clinical Immunology. New York: Plenum Press 1993; pp. 44–53.
56. Iwasato T, Shimizu A, Honjo T, Yamagishi H. Circular DNA is excised by immuoglobulin class switch recombination. Cell 1990; 62:143–149.
57. Matsuoka M, Yoshida K, Maeda T *et al.* Switch circular DNA formed in cytokine-treated mouse splenocytes: evidence for intermolecular DNA deletion in immunoglobulin class switching. Cell 1990; 62:135–142.
58. Yoshida K, Matsuoka M, Usuda S *et al.* Immunoglobulin switch circular DNA in the mouse infected with *Nippostrongylus brasiliensis*: evidence for successive class switching from μ to ϵ via γl. Proc Natl Acad Sci USA 1990; 87:7829–7833.
59. Isakson PC, Puré E, Vitetta ES, Krammer PH. T cell derived B cell differentiation factor(s). Effect on the isotype switch of murine B cells. J Exp Med 1982; 155:734–748.
60. Coffman RL, Seymour BWP, Lebman DA *et al.* The role of helper T cell products in mouse B cell differentiation and isotype regulation. Immunol Rev 1988; 102:5–28.
61. Snapper CM, Paul WE. Interferon-gamma and B cell stimulatory factor-1 reciprocally regulate Ig isotype production. Science 1987; 236:944–947.
62. Snapper CM, McIntyre TM, Mandler R *et al.* Induction of IgG3 secretion by interferon γ: a model for T cell independent class switching in response to T cell independent type 2 antigens. J Exp Med 1992; 175:1367–1371.
63. Coffman RL, Lebman DA, Schrader B. Transforming growth factor β specifically enhances IgA production by lipopolysaccharide-stimulated murine B lymphocytes. J Exp Med 1989; 170:1039–1044.

64. Sonada E, Matsumoto R, Hotoshi Y *et al.* Transforming growth factor β induces IgA production and acts additively with interleukin 5 for IgA production. J Exp Med 1989; 170:1415–1420.
65. Lebman DA, Nomura DY, Coffman RL, Lee FD. Molecular characterization of germ-line immunoglobulin A transcripts produced during transforming growth factor type β-induced isotype switching. Proc Natl Acad Sci USA 1990; 87:3962–3966.
66. Defrance T, Vanbervliet B, Briére F *et al.* Interleukin-10 and transforming growth factor β cooperate to induce anti-CD40-activated naive human B cells to secrete immunoglobulin A. J Exp Med 1992; 175:671–682.
67. Rousset F, Garcia E, Banchereau J. Cytokine-induced proliferation and immunoglobulin production of human B lymphocytes triggered through their CD40 antigen. J Exp Med 1991; 173:705–710.
68. Islam KB, Nilsson L, Sideras P *et al.* TGF-β1 induces germ-line transcripts of both IgA subclasses in human B lymphocytes. Int Immunol 1991; 3:1099–1106.
69. van Vlasselaer P, Punnonen J, de Vries JE. Transforming growth factor-β directs IgA switching in human B cells. J Immunol 1992; 148:2062–2067.
70. McIntyre TM, Klinman DR, Rothman P *et al.* Transforming growth factor β1 selectively stimulates immunoglobulin G2b secretion by lipopolysaccharide-activated murine B cells. J Exp Med 1993; 177:1031–1037.
71. Stavnezer-Nordgren J, Sirlin S. Specificity of immunoglobulin heavy chain switch correlates with activity of germline heavy chain genes prior to switching. EMBO J 1986; 5:95–102.
72. Stavnezer J, Sirlin S, Abbot J. Induction of immunoglobulin isotype switching in cultured I.29 B lymphoma cells. Characterization of the accompanying rearrangements of heavy chain genes. J Exp Med 1985; 161:577–601.
73. McIntyre TM, Klinman DR, Rothman P *et al.* Transforming growth factor β1 selectively stimulates immunoglobulin G2b secretion by lipopolysaccharide-activated murine B cells. J Exp Med 1993; 177:1031–1037.
74. van den Wall Bake AWL, Black KP, Kulhavy R *et al.* Transforming growth factor-β inhibits the production of IgG, IgM and IgA in human lymphocyte cultures. Cell Immunol 1992; 144:417–428.
75. Lebman DA, Lee FD, Coffman RL. Mechanism for transforming growth factor β and IL-2 enhancement of IgA expression in lipopolysaccharide-stimulated B cell cultures. J Immunol 1990; 144:952–959.
76. McIntyre TM, Kehry MR, Snapper CM. Novel *in vitro* model for high-rate IgA class switching. J Immunol 1995; 154:3156–3161.
77. Kehrl JH, Roberts AB, Wakefield LM *et al.* Transforming growth factor beta is an important immunomodulatory protein for human B lymphocytes. J Immunol 1986; 137:3855–3860.
78. Kehrl JH, Wakefield LM, Roberts AB *et al.* Production of transforming growth factor beta by human T lymphocytes and its potential role in the regulation of T cell growth. J Exp Med 1987; 163:1037–1050.
79. Kehrl JH, Thevenin C, Rieckmann P, Fauci AS. Transforming growth factor-beta suppresses human B lymphocyte Ig production by inhibiting synthesis and the switch from the membrane form to the secreted form of Ig mRNA. J Immunol 1991; 146:4016–4023.
80. Beagley KW, Eldridge JH, Kiyono H, McGhee JR. The identification of murine Peyer's patch T cell-derived factors which enhance IgA isotype-specific responses. Adv Exp Med Biol 1987; 237:641–647.
81. Coffman RL, Shrader B, Carty J *et al.* A mouse T cell product that preferentially enhances IgA production. I. Biologic characterization. J Immunol 1987; 139:3685–3690.

82. Harriman GR, Kunimoto DY, Elliott JF *et al.* The role of IL-5 in IgA B cell differentiation. J Immunol 1988; 140:3033–3039.
83. Beagley KW, Eldridge HI, Kiyono H *et al.* Recombinant murine IL-5 induces high rate IgA synthesis in cycling IgA-positive Peyer's patch B cells. J Immunol 1988; 141:2035–2042.
84. Murray PD, McKenzie DT, Swain SL, Kagnoff MF. Interleukin 5 and interleukin 4 produced by Peyer's patch T cells selectively enhance immunoglobulin A expression. J Immunol 1987; 139:2669–2674.
85. Lebman DA, Coffman RL. The effects of IL-4 and IL-5 on the IgA response by murine Peyer's patch B cell subpopulations. J Immunol 1988; 141:2050–2056.
86. Kroese FGM, Butcher EC, Stall AM *et al.* Many of the IgA producing plasma cells in murine gut are derived from self-replenishing precursors in the peritoneal cavity. Int Immunol 1989; 1:75–84.
87. Benson EM, Bertolini JN, Brodtmann ME. T cell regulation of immunoglobulin isotypes in health and disease. Pediatr Infect Dis J 1990; 9:525–535.
88. Beagley KW, Eldridge JH, Lee F *et al.* Interleukins and IgA synthesis. Human and murine IL-6 induce high rate IgA secretion in IgA-committed B cells. J Exp Med 1989; 169:2133–2148.
89. Ramsey AJ, Husband AJ, Ramshaw IA *et al.* The role of interleukin-6 in mucosal IgA antibody responses *in vivo*. Science 1994; 264:561–563.
90. Fujihashi K, McGhee JR, Lue C *et al.* Human appendix B cells naturally express receptors for and respond to interleukin 6 with selective IgA1 and IgA2 synthesis. J Clin Invest 1991; 88:248–252.
91. Mosmann, TR, Cherwinski H, Bond MW *et al.* Two types of murine helper T cell clone. 1. Definition according to profiles of lymphokine activities and secreted proteins. J Immunol 1986; 136:2348–2357.
92. Mosmann TR, Coffman RL. Th1 and Th2 cells: different patterns of lymphokine secretion lead to different functional properties. Annu Rev Immunol 1989; 7:145–173.
93. Seder RA, Paul WE. Acquisition of lymphokine-producing phenotype by $CD4^+$ T cells. Annu Rev Immunol 1994; 12:635–673.
94. Xu-Amano J, Aicher WK, Taguchi T *et al.* Selective induction of Th2 cells in murine Peyer's patches by oral immunization. Int Immunol 1992; 4:433–445.
95. Elson CO, Dertzbaugh MT. Mucosal adjuvants. In: Ogra PL *et al.* (eds) Handbook of Mucosal Immunology. San Diego: Academic Press 1994; pp.391–402.
96. Jackson RJ, Fujihashi K, Xu-Amano J *et al.* Optimizing oral vaccines: induction of systemic and mucosal B cell and antibody responses to tetanus toxoid by use of cholera toxin as adjuvant. Infect Immun 1993; 61:4272–4279.
97. Xu-Amano J, Kiyono H, Jackson RJ *et al.* Helper T cell subsets for immunoglobulin A responses: oral immunization with tetanus toxoid and cholera toxin as adjuvant selectively induces Th2 cells in mucosa associated tissues. J Exp Med 1993; 178:1309–1320.
98. Svetic A, Madden KB, Zhou XD *et al.* A primary intestinal helminthic infection rapidly induces a gut-associated elevation of Th2-associated cytokines and IL-3. J Immunol 1993; 150:3434–3441.
99. Vajdy M, Kosco-Vilbois MH, Kopf M *et al.* Impaired mucosal immune responses in interleukin 4-targeted mice. J Exp Med 1995; 181:41–53.
100. Chen Y, Kuchroo VK, Inobe J *et al.* Regulatory T cell clones induced by oral tolerance: suppression of autoimmune encephalomyelitis. Science 1994; 265:1237–1240.
101. Lagoo AS, Eldridge JH, Lagoo-Deenadaylan S *et al.* Peyer's patch CD8 positive memory T cells secrete Th1 and Th2 cytokines and provide help for immunoglobulin secretion. Eur J Immunol 1994; 24:3087–3092.

102. Erard F, Wild MT, Garcia-Sanz JA, LeGros G. Switch of CD8 T cells to noncytolytic CD8–CD4-cells that make Th2 cytokines and help B cells. Science 1993; 260:1802–1805.
103. Modlin RL, Kato H, Mehra V *et al.* Genetically restricted suppressor T-cell clones derived from lepromatous leprosy lesions. Nature 1986; 322:459–461.
104. Pfeifer JD, Wick MJ, Roberts TL *et al.* Phagocytic processing of bacterial antigens for class I MHC presentation to T cells. Nature 1993; 361:359–362.

# 17 Abnormalities in Cytokine Production and Responsiveness in Autoimmune Disease

**ERI HAGIWARA and DENNIS M. KLINMAN**
*Center for Biologics Evaluation and Research, Food and Drug Administration, Bethesda, Maryland, USA*

## INTRODUCTION

A complex and interactive cytokine network regulates the magnitude, nature and duration of immune responses to foreign antigens and self-antigens. An animal that cannot produce normal levels of cytokine may be unable to ward off infection. Yet an animal that produces too much cytokine or has cells that hyper-respond to normal levels of cytokine may be at increased risk for developing autoimmunity. This chapter will examine the role of cytokines in the development of such autoimmune diseases.

Organ-specific autoimmune processes, such as myasthenia gravis, multiple sclerosis and Hashimoto's thyroiditis, generally involve cell-mediated or humoral responses against one or very few self-antigens expressed on a single target organ. These diseases tend to be autoantigen-driven and abnormalities in cytokine production have not been associated with the induction of autoantibodies. On the other hand, systemic autoimmune diseases, such as systemic lupus erythematosus (SLE) and rheumatoid arthritis (RA), are characterized by the production of autoantibodies against many different self-antigens. Since a diverse array of B cells are activated in these diseases, it is considered more likely that a defect in the production of (or response to) immunoregulatory cytokines contributes to their pathogenesis. This chapter will consider findings from animal models and patients with such systemic autoimmune diseases.

## EXPERIMENTAL LIMITATIONS

In only a small number of cases has a cause–effect relationship been established between abnormalities in cytokine production and the development of autoimmune diseases. In many other instances, irregularities in cytokine production have been associated with the development or

*Cytokine Regulation of Humoral Immunity: Basic and Clinical Aspects.* Edited by Clifford M. Snapper.

persistence of an autoimmune state. Such abnormalities could (1) play a critical role in the disease process, (2) be the result rather than the cause of the autoimmune process, or (3) represent an attempt by the host's immune system to re-establish homeostasis in the face of strong and persistent antigenic stimulation. In an example of the latter case autoantibodies against cytokine-producing cells (such as T lymphocytes) are common in SLE[1]. Such anti-T-cell antibodies might either induce or inhibit the production of cytokines by targeted T cells. Given these reservations and the complexity of the immunoregulatory network, caution must be exercised before concluding that a given cytokine abnormality is causally linked to the development of an autoimmune disease.

A variety of experimental approaches have been used to analyze the role of cytokines in systemic autoimmune disease. Most commonly, cells from animals or patients are cultured *in vitro* and their production of (or response to) cytokines monitored. This approach has the advantage of simplicity and has yielded important insights concerning the functional capability of immunologically active cells from patients with autoimmune disease. A drawback to this approach is the potential influence of the culture conditions used on the type and amount of cytokine produced *in vitro*. For example, mitogens that prolong cell survival during culture may induce a pattern of lymphocyte maturation and cytokine release that differs (in some cases dramatically) from that observed *in vivo*. Further complicating this approach is the fact that soluble products released by mitogen-stimulated cells may alter the activation state and rate of cytokine production by other cells in culture. Thus, unless very pure cell populations are isolated and studied, analysis of supernatant cytokine levels may be misleading. Even when pure cell populations are available, interpretation may be difficult. Some cytokines act in an autocrine fashion, in that they are consumed by the cells that produce them[2]. Thus, the amount of cytokine present in the culture supernatant may not accurately reflect levels of production. Finally, cells that were activated *in vivo* may be inhibited by conditions *in vitro*, thus obscuring their contribution to cytokine production in the living animal. The reader should bear these caveats in mind when analyzing data involving *in vitro* comparisons of normal versus autoreactive cells.

An alternative approach involves comparing the concentration of cytokine present in the serum of autoimmune versus normal animals. When differences are detected, it can reasonably be concluded that the rate of production or consumption of that cytokine is abnormal. A concern with this approach, however, is that cytokines are active primarily at or near their site of production (i.e. the lymphoid organs) and have very short half-lives *in vivo*[3,4]. Thus, a localized abnormality in cytokine production may not induce detectable abnormalities in serum cytokine levels. In addition, the physiological implications of an abnormality in the serum concentration of a given cytokine are unclear, since the blood is not normally a site of cytokine action.

It should also be noted that anti-cytokine antibodies and soluble cytokine receptors may interfere with assays designed to detect circulating cytokines, further complicating the utility of serum assay systems[5].

To overcome some of these obstacles, investigators have examined the amount of cytokine mRNA present in the lymphoid tissues of animals with autoimmune disease. This approach provides insight into the degree of cytokine activation *in vivo*, and has generated useful information concerning the rate at which cytokine mRNAs are induced when the immune system is stimulated by antigen or mitogen. Yet the correlation between mRNA levels and protein production is neither uniform nor direct, and the amount of mRNA in an organ provides little information concerning the number, phenotype or specificity of cells secreting that factor. To clarify these issues, *in situ* polymerase chain reaction (PCR) technology is currently being employed to directly identify and quantitate those cells containing cytokine mRNA.

A competing technology designed to analyze cytokine production at the single-cell level is the ELIspot assay. This approach detects single cells secreting as little as 100 molecules of cytokine per second[2]. It is a technically demanding assay requiring pairs of high-titered and anti-cytokine antibodies. Where available, cytokine ELIspot assays have provided important information concerning the number and phenotype of cells secreting specific cytokines in humans and animals with autoimmune disease.

All of the experimental approaches described above can be used to examine whether cytokine production by autoimmune animals is abnormal. The alternative possibility, that autoimmunity arises from a heightened sensitivity of immunologically active cells to normal levels of cytokine, has also been investigated.

The most straightforward experiments involved treating animals *in vivo*, or cells from those animals *in vitro*, with cytokines or anti-cytokine antibodies. Such studies provided valuable insights into the pathogenesis of autoimmune disease and useful guides for future therapies involving the manipulation of the cytokine milieu. Yet the interpretation of experiments in which autoimmune animals are treated with exogenous cytokines or anti-cytokine antibodies is more complicated than generally appreciated. Cytokines form a complex, mutally interactive network *in vivo*. When one element of that network is perturbed by the addition of a cytokine or anti-cytokine antibody (Ab), effects on other multiple elements of the immune system may ensue. Thus, it is difficult to determine whether the immediate target of a given intervention is directly or only indirectly responsible for the observed outcome.

Studies in which unfractionated lymphoid populations are treated *in vitro* with exogenous cytokines suffer from the same drawback. To eliminate this concern, purified cell subpopulations can be analyzed in culture. Such experiments have provided evidence that certain types of immunologically active cells from autoimmune animals are abnormally responsive to specific cytokines. Yet the interpretation of even these straightforward experiments is complicated, since the removal of other immunoregulatory cell types from culture may alter the responses being examined.

With these caveats in mind, the remainder of this chapter will examine the contribution of cytokines to B-cell activation and isotype switching in autoimmune diseases.

## LYMPHOCYTE ACTIVATION IN MURINE LUPUS

To understand why cytokines might be expected to play a role in systemic autoimmune diseases, it is important to appreciate the B- and T-cell defects that characterize autoimmune states. In diseases such as SLE, end-organ damage is mediated primarily by IgG autoantibodies. The serum of mice and humans with lupus characteristically contains increased levels of immunoglobin (Ig) (hypergammaglobulinemia) and there is a significantly increased number of activated B cells in major lymphoid organs of these animals. Two types of B-cell activation have been detected in mice and humans with lupus. Polyclonal B-cell stimulation (involving many different clones reactive with a variety of self-antigens and foreign antigens) is prevalent during the early stage of disease, frequently before clinically detectable symptoms develop. Subsequently, autoantigen-driven immune stimulation magnifies and perpetuates autoantibody production in animals with established disease. Whether a common set of immunoregulatory abnormalities underlie these two types of B-cell activation is unknown, although a cytokine-induced increase in B-cell activation might contribute to both polyclonal and autoantigen-specific B-cell activation.

## CYTOKINE ABNORMALITIES IN MURINE MODELS OF AUTOIMMUNE DISEASE

### (NZB × NZW)F1 MICE

(NZB × NZW)F1 mice (hereafter referred to as B/W mice) are widely considered the most representative model of human SLE. The diseases developed by B/W mice and humans have important similarities, including the following: (1) multiple genes on different chromosomes are involved in disease induction; (2) both are characterized by an age-dependent shift from IgM to IgG autoantibody production; and (3) the production of IgG anti-double-stranded DNA (dsDNA) autoantibodies act as a marker for, and contribute to the development of, life-threatening glomerulonephritis. Since the overproduction of pathogenic IgG autoantibodies is central to disease, attention has focused on whether cytokines known to augment humoral immune responses are abnormally increased in B/W mice.

Early studies examined the responsiveness of B/W B-cells to Th2 cytokines. Initially, it was shown that supernatants from Th2 cell clones could induce B cells from 2–3-month-old B/W mice to secrete over 10 times more IgM anti-DNA Ab than normal B cells[6]. Although the Th2 supernatant examined in those studies contained multiple cytokines, interleukin 5 (IL-5) was identified as the probable stimulatory factor, since antibodies against IL-5 (but not other Th2 cytokines) blocked the effect. Subsequently, it was shown that Ly-1$^+$ B cells (a subpopulation of cells known to produce IgM autoantibodies) from B/W mice were more responsive to IL-5-induced stimulation than Ly-1$^-$ B cells, although both Ly-1$^-$ and Ly-1$^+$ populations responded[7]. While instructive in terms of B/W disease, these findings have not been generalized to human or other examples of murine lupus, since B cells from other strains of autoreactive mice do not appear to be hyper-responsive to IL-5[7].

Another Th2 cytokine whose role in B/W disease has been carefully examined is IL-4. As described in Chapter 8, IL-4 is both an isotype switch factor and a B-cell maturation factor in mice. Since end-organ damage in B/W mice is mediated by IgG autoantibodies, the potential role of IL-4 in disease progression has been investigated. Although IL-4 alone has little effect on B-cell activation or IgG production in B/W mice, the combination of IL-4 plus IL-5 induced B-cell proliferation as well as IgG and IgM secretion[8,9]. Moreover, the combination of IL-4 plus IL-5 induced IgG anti-DNA Ab production[8]. It is noteworthy that lymphocytes from adult B/W mice with active disease were more susceptible to the stimulatory effects of these cytokines, in terms of the induction of IgM and IgG anti-DNA Ab production, than were B cells from young B/W mice[8]. This suggests that the observed B-cell reactivity may result from the maturation of normal lymphocytes in an abnormal (autoreactive) environment rather than an intrinsic defect in B/W B cells.

The Th2 cytokine IL-6 was also found to induce increased B-cell stimulation in B/W mice. As was true of IL-4 and IL-5, this effect was most pronounced when cells were obtained from animals with active disease. Culturing adult B/W B cells with IL-6 induced a 3–4-fold increase in the production of IgG and IgG anti-DNA autoantibodies[10–13]. The phenotype of the cells induced by IL-6 to secrete these autoantibodies was CD5$^-$, CD43$^+$, while cells induced by IL-5 to secrete IgM anti-DNA were CD5$^+$, CD43$^-$[10]. Recently, it was shown that chronic administration of anti-IL-6 (500 μg i.p. weekly starting at 3 months of age) almost completely inhibited the production of anti-dsDNA Abs, delayed the development of proteinuria, and prolonged survival[14]. This well-designed study provided clear evidence that endogenous IL-6 can contribute (either directly or indirectly) to the development of autoimmune disease in this strain.

Given the interactive nature of the cytokine network, investigators examined whether factors that regulate Th1 cytokine production might influence disease progression. IL-10 has a pronounced inhibitory effect on the production of Th1 cytokines (such as interferon gamma (IFN-γ) and IL-2; see Chapter 6). In addition, IL-10 can directly stimulate B cells to proliferate and produce IgG (see Chapter 11). Studies were undertaken to determine whether the suppression of IL-10-dependent responses (by administration of anti-IL-10 Abs) could affect disease progression in B/W mice. Results indicate that injection of 0.2–1.0 mg of anti-IL-10 two or three times a week from birth to 10 months of age decreased the production of IgG anti-DNA Abs, substantially delayed the onset of glomerulonephritis, and prolonged survival[15]. These effects were confirmed in studies showing that exogenous IL-10 could accelerate disease progression in young B/W mice[15].

Determining the mechanism(s) responsible for these *in vivo* changes has been difficult. Anti-IL-10 Abs can upregulate Th1 cytokines such as IFN-γ and proinflammatory cytokines such as tumor necrosis factor alpha (TNF-α) and IL-6. Indeed, those B/W mice with the highest levels of serum TNF-α induced by treatment with IL-10 showed the least disease[15]. When the TNF-α in these animals was neutralized by anti-cytokine Ab, autoimmunity developed rapidly. It is also interesting that anti-IL-10 Abs decreased IgG anti-DNA Ab production by B/W mice. Since anti-IL-10 can upregulate endogenous production of IL-6, and since IL-6 can promote IgG anti-DNA Ab production, it is clear that multiple (and in some case antagonistic) effects may result from treatment with a single factor.

The capacity of TNF-α to protect against the development of lupus was confirmed by treating B/W mice for 2–6 months with 10 μg per animal of that cytokine[16–18]. This intervention delayed the development of lethal nephritis. However, use of 0.2 μg of TNF-α for the same period accelerated renal disease and mortality in this strain[19]. The mechanism by which a high dose of cytokine might interfere with disease progression while a lower dose accelerates it is currently unclear. One possibility is that high doses of exogenous TNF-α might compensate for inadequate physiological levels of that cytokine. For example, peritoneal cells from B/W mice cultured *in vitro* with lipopolysaccharide (LPS) plus IFN-γ secreted less TNF-α than controls[16,17]. Yet subsequent studies suggest that TNF-α levels *in vivo* are normal in B/W mice—indeed, the kidneys of mice with active glomerulonephritis contain increased levels of TNF-α mRNA[19].

In general, it should be noted that there are no published reports of B/W mice overproducing any of the cytokines examined *in vivo*, including IL-4, IL-5, IL-10 or TNF-α. Only serum levels of soluble IL-6R were reported to be elevated in these animals[20]. Thus the effects seen in B/W mice may be due to an increased responsiveness of B cells to normal levels of cytokine, rather than to abnormalities in cytokine production/consumption.

Whether Th1-type cytokines play a role in the development of B/W disease has been less well investigated. B lymphocytes from this strain cultured *in vitro* with LPS plus IFN-γ show lower levels of proliferation and Ab production than normals[21]. However, when 6–10 × $10^4$ units of IFN-γ were administered three times per week to B/W mice for 6 months, the onset of disease was accelerated[22,33]. These two sets of data are inconsistent, and presumably reflect differences in the experimental approaches employed. However, since there is no evidence that the production of IFN-γ is abnormal in B/W mice, the role of this Th1 cytokine in murine lupus remains uncertain.

The potential contribution of IL-2 to B/W disease has also been examined. When spleen cells from adult B/W mice were stimulated *in vitro* with mitogen, their production of IL-2 was 10-fold lower than that of normal controls[24]. However, no corresponding *in vivo* defect has been detected. When B cells from young B/W mice were stimulated with IL-2, they showed increased levels of proliferation[25]. Unlike the response of B/W B cells to Th2 cytokines, the susceptibility of these B cells to IL-2 decreased with age and disease progression[25–27]. These findings imply that B cells from young B/W mice may have been activated *in vivo*, and thus are unusually responsive to further stimulation by IL-2.

On the basis of experiments reported to date, definitive conclusions cannot be drawn concerning the contribution of Th2 and Th1 cytokines to the development of lupus in B/W mice. It appears that B lymphocytes from young mice of this strain are more sensitive to IL-2 and IL-5 than are normal B cells. Thus, it is possible that IL-5 plays a role in the early polyclonal activation of B cells in this strain. Yet the increased responsiveness of lymphocytes from these animals to IL-4 and IL-6 seems to be acquired with age. The latter cytokines may thus be involved in perpetuating the proliferation or IgG secretion of B cells that were already activated. Consistent with such a possibility, IL-6 was found to facilitate the production of IgG anti-DNA Abs in adult but not young B/W mice[10–12]. At a more fundamental level, these observations suggest that abnormalities in B-cell responsiveness to most cytokines are 'acquired' during maturation in an autoimmune environment, and thus are not intrinsic cellular defects. Such an interpretation is consistent with a series of experiments showing that B cells from normal mice, when transferred into a lupus-prone environment, are activated to produce autoantibodies similar to those secreted by B cells of autoimmune origin[28,29]. Finally, these data suggest that IL-10 and TNF-α may play a more central role in regulating the production of other cytokines as well as by directly influencing immune function. Unfortunately, in the absence of definitive evidence that the production of these cytokines is abnormal *in vivo*, it cannot be definitively concluded that the cytokine abnormalities described in B/W mice are directly relevant to their disease.

## MRL-*lpr/lpr* MICE

MRL-*lpr/lpr* (hereafter MRL/*lpr*) mice provide another model of human lupus. Autoimmunity in this strain resembles human SLE with respect to the production of IgG autoantibodies and the development of life-threatening glomerulonephritis. Disease in MRL/*lpr* mice has been linked to a defect in the *lpr/fas* gene, which encodes a cell surface protein critical to the apoptotic elimination of activated lymphocytes. The defect in Fas protein expression interferes with the death of activated T cells. Thus, one might expect that cytokines produced by activated T cells would be abnormal in MRL/*lpr* mice. The defect in apoptosis also affects activated B cells, further enlarging the list of cytokines which might be associated with disease in these animals.

In MRL/*lpr* mice, elevated levels of serum IL-6 have been detected. The concentration of serum IL-6 increases with age and disease severity[30], and is accompanied by an increase in the expression of IL-6 receptor (IL-6R)[31]. In normal mice, IL-6R are expressed on $CD4^+$ T cells but not splenic B cells, whereas in adult MRL/*lpr* mice the IL-6R is absent from $CD4^+$ LN (lymph node) cells but present on splenic B cells[31]. It has also been shown that soluble IL-6R is present at increased concentrations in the serum of adult MRL/*lpr* mice[20]. This constellation of findings suggests that the overproduction of IL-6 may lead to abnormalities in the expression of IL-6R immunologically relevant cells. These disturbances in cytokine production/recognition may contribute to the immune dysfunction characteristic of this strain.

Abnormalities in the production of IFN-γ have also been detected in MRL/*lpr* mice. Serum from adult mice with active disease contains elevated concentrations of IFN-γ[32–34]. In addition, T cells from adult MRL/*lpr* mice constitutively express IFN-γ mRNA and secrete that cytokine[35]. When stimulated *in vitro* with phorbol ester (PMA) and ionomycin, the amount of IFN-γ secreted per cell was significantly increased when compared to cells from normal mice[34,36]. In addition, the ratio of IFN-γ and IL-4-producing cells in MRL/*lpr* mice is significantly increased, even at an early age[37]. This altered ratio of Th1- and Th2- secreting cells is associated with the overproduction of IgG2a autoantibodies in mice with active disease[37].

In a related series of experiments, B cells from *lpr* mice were found to be hyper-responsive to exogenous IFN-γ. When stimulated *in vitro* with IFN-γ plus LPS, for example, they undergo isotype switching from IgM to IgG2a production 5–25 times more efficiently than B cells from normal or B/W mice[38]. This increased B-cell responsiveness to IFN-γ is acquired with age; lymphocytes from young MRL/*lpr* mice do not respond abnormally to stimulation with IFN-γ. Thus, it appears that the maturation of MRL/*lpr* B cells in an environment enriched in IFN-γ (or IL-6) may result in hypersensitivity to stimulation by these cytokines.

The increased levels of IFN-γ present in MRL/*lpr* mice may also explain two additional phenomena described in this strain. The first is a relative decrease in the maturation of Th0 → Th2 (IL-4-secreting) lymphocytes. In young MRL/*lpr* mice, the number of IL-4-secreting cells is normal, while in adults the number is significantly reduced. We found that loss of IL-4-secreting cells is due to a fall-off in the absolute number of T cells capable of secreting that cytokine in animals with active disease[37]. Increased IFN-γ production may also account for the large number of cells expressing MHC class II on their surface[39].

Thus in MRL/*lpr* mice, changes in the pattern of Th1/Th2 secreting cells clearly accompany the development of active disease. The altered ratio of cytokine-producing cells was found to correlate with changes in the absolute and relative number of IgG autoantibody-secreting B cells in these animals, and with changes in the activation state of immunologically relevant cells. Thus, while a defect in the *lpr/fas* gene may be the root cause of disease in this strain, abnormalities in the production of (and response to) B-cell stimulatory cytokines appear to be responsible for specific aspects of the immune stimulation present in these animals.

## NEW ZEALAND BLACK MICE

New Zealand Black (NZB) mice (one of the two strains used as parents for B/W mice) represent another murine model of systemic autoimmune disease. Unlike those of the other strains examined, the autoantibodies produced by NZB mice are primarily of the IgM isotype. Disease in these animals, most notably hemolytic anemia and renal damage, results from the binding of IgM autoantibodies to their cellular targets. The relative absence of IgG antibodies in NZB mice appears to stem from an intrinsic resistance of their B cells to the isotype switch-inducing effects of IL-4 and IFN-γ[38]. Four-fold fewer B cells from NZB mice secrete IgG1 or IgG2A when cultured *in vitro* with LPS plus IL-4 or IFN-γ, respectively, than B cells from normal mice or other autoimmune strains (such as B/W or MRL/*lpr*)[38]. This resistance to isotype switching is present in NZB B cells of all ages, indicating that lymphocytes from this strain may be intrinsically hyporesponsive to the effects of thesc factors.

NZB B cells show other abnormalities in their responsiveness to cytokines. NZB B cells proliferate when exposed to IL-4 alone, whereas normal B cells require additional stimulatory signals[40]. In NZB.H-$2^{bm12}$ mice (a strain that develops autoimmune disease but can secrete IgG autoantibodies), an IL-4-containing Th2 supernatant was able to induce B cells to proliferate and secrete IgG anti-DNA Abs[41]. This supernatant induced a similar response in B cells from normal B6.H-$2^{bm12}$ mice. One interpretation of these results is that B cells from lupus-prone NZB mice are activated *in vivo* such that they can proceed to proliferate and/or secrete Ab in the presence of IL-4, without the need for additional T-cell or mitogenic stimulation. In experiments involving IFN-γ, the long-term administration of that cytokine to NZB mice accelerated their production of autoantibodies and resulted in the more rapid development of renal disease and hemolytic anemia[23]. In contrast, *in vitro* studies showed that IFN-γ could inhibit the LPS-induced secretion of IgM and anti-DNA autoantibodies by NZB B cells[42]. These *in vitro* studies also showed that IFN-γ reduced IgM production by LPS-stimulated but not spontaneously active NZB B cells—an effect also observed in B/W mice. At present, no abnormalities in the production of IFN-γ *in vivo* have been reported in NZB mice.

## OTHER ANIMAL MODELS

The influence of cytokines on the development of autoimmunity in several other murine models of disease has been investigated. Normal mice treated with $HgC1_2$ develop a systemic autoimmune syndrome characterized by glomerulonephritis, high-titered anti-nuclear Abs and elevated levels of serum IgE and IgG1. Treatment with anti-IL-4 Abs 1 week post-$HgC1_2$ injection abrogated the expected increase in serum IgE and partially blocked the secretion of IgG1. These animals also developed lower titers of anti-nucleolar autoantibodies[43].

Another model of autoimmunity involves the transfer of neonatal (C57BL/5 × Balb/c)F1 cells into adult Balb/c mice. When recipients were treated with an anti-IL-4 monoclonal antibody (mAb), there was a reduction in the amount of IgG1, IgE and anti-DNA autoantibodies produced[44]. These findings suggest that IL-4 may play an important role in the production of pathogenic autoantibodies in multiple murine models of lupus. Yet it would be inappropriate to conclude that abnormalities in IL-4 are associated with all systemic autoimmune diseases. Rather, IL-4 appears to contribute to diseases marked by B-cell hyperactivation (including non-autoimmune diseases such as AIDS and GVH (graft-versus-host disease))[45,46]. In autoimmune diseases characterized by cell-mediated immunity, IL-4 appears to play a protective role, perhaps downregulating Th1 cytokine production. For example, treatment with IL-4 protects against disease progression in several animal models of arthritis. When rats are injected with group A streptococcal cell wall fragments, RA is induced. Small amounts of IL-4 (100 ng i.p.) administered every 12 h for 2–4 weeks can suppress the chronic joint destruction normally associated with this form of arthritis[47]. In mice with collagen-induced arthritis, 100 μg of IL-4 administered for 4 days following the first appearance of disease was also beneficial, accelerating the rate of disease remission[48]. These two models both provide examples of cell-mediated (rather than autoantibody-mediated) autoimmune disease, in which suppression of the cellular response by IL-4 was of therapeutic benefit.

## CYTOKINE ABNORMALITIES IN HUMAN AUTOIMMUNE DISEASES

### SYSTEMIC LUPUS ERYTHEMATOSUS

SLE in humans, as in mice, is characterized by B-cell hyperactivation and the production of pathogenic autoantibodies. Since T cells and the factors they produce play a critical role in the stimulation of autoreactive B cells, considerable interest has focused on the potential contribution of B-cell tropic cytokines such as IL-1, IL-2, IL-4 IL-5, IL-6 and IFN-$\gamma$ in this disease. The two cytokines most intensively studied in SLE patients are IL-4 and IL-6, since both play well-established roles in the induction of B-cell proliferation and Ig production.

#### IL-6

As described in Chapter 10, IL-6 promotes the secretion of Ig and B lymphocytes. Despite the large number of studies on this issue, evidence implicating IL-6 in the overproduction of autoantibodies in SLE is limited. Several investigators have shown that serum levels of IL-6 are increased in patients with lupus[49,50], with elevations as high as 10-fold above normal reported for patients with active disease[51]. Other groups have not been able to reproduce these findings[52,53]. It has also been shown that IL-6 mRNA is present in the peripheral blood mononuclear cells (PBMNCs) from patients with SLE but not from normals[49]. Our laboratory has found that the number of PBMNCs spontaneously secreting IL-6 *in vivo* is increased, but that this increase is modest (approximately 50 per cent) and is unrelated to disease severity.[54]

Several studies have reported that IL-6 levels in serum are selectively increased in subsets of lupus patients with specific disease manifestations. In particular, serum IL-6 levels were elevated in patients with lymphadenopathy, nephrotic syndrome and hypogammaglobulinemia[51]. Increased IL-6 in the cerebrospinal fluid was also detected in SLE patients with central nervous system disease[55,56].

Exogenous IL-6 has been shown to stimulate SLE B cells. When IL-6 was added to cultures of SLE lymphocytes, it induced polyclonal IgG secretion as well as a selective increase in the production of IgG anti-DNA autoantibodies[49,57,58]. These effects were reversed by the addition of neutralizing anti-IL-6 Abs to culture. B cells from lupus patients are unusually sensitive to the stimulatory effects of IL-6, since resting B cells from SLE patients but not controls were induced to differentiate into Ig-producing cells by that cytokine[59]. Indeed, IL-6 was more effective than other cytokines, including IL-2 or IL-4, at inducing low-density/resting B cells to produce IgG and IgG anti-DNA Abs[59]. Despite these positive findings, not all investigators have detected a stimulatory effect of IL-6 on SLE B cells, especially when high levels of Il-6 were used[60]. This may reflect a requirement for specific *in vitro* conditions to observe the effect of IL-6.

There are several potential sources for the IL-6 detected in lupus serum. We find that most of the IL-6-producing cells in human peripheral blood are $CD14^+$ monocytes/macrophages[54]. B lymphocytes also secrete IL-6, but at low frequency. During *in vitro* culture, B cells from SLE patients secrete 5 to over 10 times more IL-6 than normal lymphocytes[57,58]. They can also constitutively express IL-6R on their surface[57,58]. This series of findings suggests that a positive feedback loop might exist in which lupus cells activated by IL-6 secrete IL-6 in an autocrine manner and thereby maintain their activated state (see also Chapter 10).

## IL-4

IL-4 can stimulate human B lymphocytes to proliferate and differentiate to Ig-secreting cells. Several laboratories have reported that PBMNCs from lupus patients produce more IL-4 than those in normal controls[61]. Early reports on this issue indicated that SLE T cells were the primary *in vivo* source of B-cell growth factor (BCGF) (in those experiments, BCGF included both IL-4 and IL-5), and that active lupus T cells produced two to three times more of this factor than controls following mitogen stimulation[62,63]. It was subsequently shown that purified, mitogen-activated SLE T cells produced more IL-4 than normals[64]. Yet in the same study, unfractionated PBMNCs did not hypersecrete IL-4, a finding confirmed by other laboratories[54].

In early experiments involving BCGF and in subsequent studies using purified IL-4, that cytokine was found to enhance the proliferation and/or the production of IgG antibodies by SLE B cells by 2-fold when compared to normals[62,63]. It was also shown that patients with elevated serum levels of IL-4 preferentially produced IgG1 anti-DNA autoantibodies when compared to patients with normal serum IL-4 levels[65]. These findings are consistent with the ability of IL-4 to induce B-cell activation and isotype switching (as noted in the murine models above).

The contribution of other cytokines to B-cell activation in SLE patients is more controversial. One group reported that PBMNCs from lupus patients produced 30 times more IL-10 than normal PBMNCs *in vitro*[66]. *In vivo*, we found that the number of IL-10-secreting cells in the peripheral circulation of lupus patients is increased, but only 2-fold[54]. IL-10 mRNA has also been detected in the PBMNCs of most lupus patients, whereas it is only rarely present in those of normal controls. Since IL-10 is a pleiotropic cytokine that induces both IgG1 and IgG3 production from naive human B cells ($IgD^+$ B cells)[67], increased IL-10 production in SLE might be responsible for a generalized defect in immunoregulation. Indeed, such a role for IL-10 is consistent with the observation that IgG1 and IgG3 are the predominant anti-DNA Ab isotypes in SLE patients[65].

Elevated levels of IFN-γ have also been detected in the serum of lupus patients. Indeed, a positive correlation was found between IFN-γ serum levels and the presence of lymphadenopathy and nephritis[51]. It has also been shown that IFN-γ synergizes with other T-cell factors (such as IL-2) to induce IgG production by normal and SLE B cells *in vitro*[68]. Yet *in vivo* studies suggest that the number of IFN-γ-secreting mononuclear cells (MNCs) is decreased in patients with lupus, and that the loss of Th1-type cytokine-secreting cells (both IL-2 and IFN-γ) correlates with disease severity[54].

The role of TNF-α in SLE has also been examined. That cytokine was found to inhibit the spontaneous proliferation and production of IgM by lupus B cells but not controls[69]. Since hypergammaglobulinemia is common in lupus, it might be expected that lower TNF-α levels would be associated with active disease. Consistent with their expectation, the production of TNF-α by monocytes from lupus patients stimulated with SAC or LPS was 4–10 times lower than that of controls[69]. However, serum levels of TNF-α are reportedly elevated in some patients with active lupus[51], as is the absolute number of TNF-α-secreting MNCs[54,70]. These inconsistencies may be explained by differences in the patient populations being studied, since reduced TNF-α production is found in patients who are HLA-DR2$^+$, DQw1$^+$ whereas production is higher in patients with HLA-DR3$^+$[71].

Finally, a series of apparently unrelated defects in the production of, or response to, additional cytokines have been described in SLE patients. A deficiency in the production of IL-2 by SLE T cells cultured *in vitro*[72,73] and elevated levels of IL-2 in serum[74] have been documented, although these abnormalities appear to be unrelated to autoantibody production. SLE B cells were also reported to produce more IL-1 and express a greater number of IL-1R than normal B cells when cultured *in vitro*[75]. These observations, like those involving IL-6, suggest that a self-perpetuating cycle of autocrine B-cell stimulation may contribute to the persistence of active disease.

As discussed above, some of the results involving cytokine production by lupus patients are controversial, while others have been difficult to replicate. Thus, our current state of knowledge is inadequate to draw definitive conclusions concerning the role of cytokines in human SLE. Further complicating this issue is the concern that the diagnosis of lupus is applied to patients with multiple different clinical and serologic abnormalities. It is possible (perhaps even likely) that this diagnosis is carried by patients with different diseases who manifest some common symptoms. Thus, results of clinical studies will vary depending upon the patient populations being studied. Different cytokine production profiles may also arise between patients whose disease differed in duration, severity and treatment. Yet our results and those from other laboratories generally indicate that active lupus is associated with a loss of Th1-type and an increase in Th2-type cytokine-secreting cells. Such a phenotype is consistent with the abnormal activation of autoantibody-secreting lymphocytes that characterize this disease.

## RHEUMATOID ARTHRITIS

Rheumatoid arthritis (RA) is the most common systemic autoimmune disease in humans. It is characterized by chronic progressive inflammation that primarily affects the joints. Although a majority of RA patients produce autoantibodies (especially rheumatoid factor (RF)), it is unclear whether such autoantibodies play a pathogenic role in disease. Instead, it is believed that cell-mediated inflammatory reactions are primarily responsible for disease progression. This has fueled the expectation that cytokines involved in T-cell rather than B-cell activation should play a role in RA.

There is evidence that IL-6, perhaps in its role as a proinflammatory cytokine, contributes to the pathogenesis of this disease. Elevated levels of IL-6 have been detected in both the serum and synovial fluid of RA patients[51,76], although serum levels of IL-6 do not seem to vary or predict responsiveness to treatment[77,78]. The IL-6 in synovial fluid is primarily produced by synoviocytes or macrophages[79–81] rather than T cells[82]. Indeed, T cells in RA patients are not major sources of IL-6, IL-2, IL-4 or IFN-γ[82].

When the concentration of IL-6 in synovial fluid is elevated, a local increase in the concentration of IgM and IgG RF has been detected. This effect is highly localized, since increased Ig is present in the joint space but not in the serum[83]. The level of synovial IL-6 also correlates with certain clinical features of RA, such as ESR (erythrocyte sedimentation rate) and the Lansbury activity index. These findings suggest that IL-6 may play a role in supporting the inflammatory response found in RA patients and promoting the production of RF autoantibodies.

The role of IL-4 in RA has also been explored, since this cytokine can stimulate B cells and inhibit the production of inflammatory cytokines. Unlike the situation in SLE, IL-4 appeared to exert a negative effect on Ig production in RA patients. *In vitro* studies indicate that exogenous IL-4 downregulates the expression of CD5 on B cells from RA patients[84]. IL-4 also reduces the spontaneous production of Ig and IgM RF by B cells from RA patients. This inhibitory effect could be linked to the ability of IL-4 to downregulate proinflammatory cytokines (such as IL-1, IL-6 and TNF-α), resulting in a decrease in the secretion of Ig by PBMNCs[85,86]. The same inhibitory effect on Ig and cytokine production was seen when IL-4 was added to cultured fragments of rheumatoid synovium[87]. Another effect of IL-4 is its ability to suppress the production of IL-8 by synovial MNCs[88]. IL-8 is a powerful chemoattractant of neutrophils and T cells, and is believed to play a role in the joint inflammation seen in RA[89,90].

While these data suggest that IL-4 may be clinically useful in the treatment of the humoral abnormalities associated with RA, the concentration of IL-4 in rheumatoid synovium is quite low under physiological conditions[91]. Moreover, the effectiveness of IL-4 may be lower in the synovial space than in the peripheral blood. For example, IL-4 suppresses mitogen-induced TNF-α production by peripheral blood monocytes but has little effect on synovial monocytes[92]. Similarly, IL-4 was more effective at inducing CD23 expression on monocytes from the peripheral blood than on those from the synovium.

IL-10 is another cytokine with anti-inflammatory effects. It can suppress the production of proinflammatory cytokines such as TNF-α and IL-1 and has been shown to inhibit the production of IL-8[88]. The possibility that IL-10 plays a role in RA is enhanced by the finding that IL-10 mRNA and protein are present in RA synovial membrane[93]. This IL-10 expression appears to be functionally relevant, since levels of TNF-α and IL-1β in RA synovial membrane cultures increased 2–3-fold when endogenous IL-10 was neutralized by anti-IL-10 MAbs[93]. When IL-10 was added back, a 2–3-fold decrease in TNF-α and IL-1β production was induced. These findings suggest that IL-10 may be one of the regulatory components of the cytokine network in arthritic joints.

There are additional reports suggesting that abnormalities involving cytokines other than those associated with B-cell function may be present in RA. Inflammatory cytokines such as IL-1 and TNF-α are present at increased concentration in rheumatoid synovium and serum[94–97]. Some investigators have suggested that these cytokines play a role in joint destruction[94–97]. Abnormalities of T-cell tropic cytokines such as IL-2 and IFN-γ have also been reported. Serum levels of IFN-γ and IL-2 are increased in RA patients when compared to controls[51,97]. The precise role of these cytokines in disease is unknown. IL-2 was found to enhance mitogen-induced IgM synthesis by B cells, but failed to induce IgM RF[98]. Yet IFN-γ suppresses IL-8 production by RA synoviocytes *in vitro*[99], suggesting that it might interfere with disease. Thus, definitive evidence linking a particular cytokine to disease progression in RA has not yet been achieved.

## AUTOIMMUNE DISEASES CAUSED BY CYTOKINES

Irrefutable evidence that the overproduction of IL-6 can lead to autoimmune disease has been obtained in patients with cardiac myxoma (see also Chapter 10). Cardiac myxomas are tumors of the heart. In five different patients, advanced autoimmune disease (characterized by hypergammaglobulinemia and increased autoantibody production) was present in conjunction with such myxomas. In each case, the tumor cells produced high levels of IL-6. Removal of the tumors led to the rapid resolution of the autoimmune symptoms[100]. Thus, either directly or indirectly, increased IL-6 led to the production of autoantibodies and development of autoimmune disease in humans.

A similar role for IL-6 was identified in Castleman's disease. This benign lymphoproliferative disorder is commonly associated with hypergammaglobulinemia and autoantibody production. When cells from the enlarged lymph nodes of patients with Castleman's disease were placed in culture, they produced excessive amounts of IL-6 (whereas other cytokines were undetectable)[101]. Excision of the affected lymph nodes resulted in the disappearance of both clinical symptoms and serologic abnormalities. Not surprisingly, serum levels of IL-6 correlated closely with clinical and laboratory abnormalities in these patients. Thus, in two different disease states, increased production of IL-6 was linked to hypergammaglobulinemia and the development of autoimmune disease.

IL-6 and other cytokines may play a role in several additional autoimmune diseases, including Sjogren's syndrome and autoimmune thyroiditis. In both of these syndromes, abnormalities in the production of IL-6 have been detected[102]. Yet salivary gland epithelial cells from patients with Sjogren's syndrome also produced over 40-fold more IL-1a, IL-6 and TNF-α mRNA than normal cells[103]. Thus, it remains unclear which (if any) of these specific cytokines is critical to the development of these diseases.

## CONCLUSION

Our goal in writing this chapter was to provide a comprehensive and timely review of the role of cytokines in autoimmune disease. Only in the case of cardiac myxoma and Castleman's disease has such an association been irrefutably established, and in both of these instances polyclonal B-cell activation, hypergammaglobulinemia and autoantibody production resulted from an increase in the production of IL-6. These two disease states represent examples in which a single cytokine leads to immune dysregulation —a model that can be reproduced by injecting exogenous cytokine into experimental animals.

Data suggest that no single cytokine abnormality accounts for the development of disease in other autoimmune states, such as RA and SLE. Instead, perturbation of the cytokine milieu has multiple effects on the immune system. For example, patients with lupus express a generalized increase in the production of Th2-type cytokines (including IL-6, IL-10 and TNF-α), while their production of Th1-type cytokines (IL-2 and IFN-γ) is decreased[54]. This array of abnormalities could have a single common source, but more likely represents the outcome of multiple interacting immune elements, including those that lead to disease and the host's attempts to restore homeostasis.

Murine models can help to simplify and define the genetic and environmental contributions to disease. Yet in the case of cytokine production, such models only serve to underscore the complexity and pitfalls of ascribing particular disease manifestations to specific cytokine abnormalities. In MRL/*lpr* mice, for example, a single genetic defect is found in association with the dysregulation of multiple cytokines. Moreover, several of these abnormalities were present only in adult mice with active disease, presumably reflecting the maturation of otherwise normal cells in the abnormal immunoregulatory environment.

Results in other model systems, most notably involving the immune response to pathogenic organisms, indicate that the balance between Th1- and Th2-type cytokines determines the success of the response. We predict that the same paradigm will apply to autoimmune disease, and that the ratio of immunostimulatory versus immunosuppressive cytokines will prove critical to the persistence and severity of these illnesses. Moreover, as the ability to modulate the immune environment (using cytokines, cytokine analogues and anti-cytokine antibodies) grows, so should our ability to design rational therapies to treat these diseases. Considering the great strides made in cytokine research over the past decade, we expect the next few years to provide considerable insight into (1) how changes in the cytokine network influence the development of autoimmune disease, (2) the effect of these changes on Ig production and class switching, and (3) the therapeutic interventions that can be used to promote a return to normal immune function.

## REFERENCES


1. Steinberg AD, Huston DP, Taurog JD *et al.* The cellular and genetic basis of murine lupus. Immunol Rev 1981; 55:121–154
2. Shirai A, Holmes K, Klinman DM. Detection and quantitation of cells secreting IL-6 under physiological conditions in BALB/c mice. J Immunol 1993; 150:793–799.
3. Oliver JC, Bland LA, Oettigner CW *et al.* Cytokine kinetics in an *in vitro* whole blood model following an endotoxin challenge. Lymphocyte Cytokine Res 1993; 12:115–120.
4. Waage A, Brandtzaeg P, Halstensen A *et al.* The complex pattern of cytokines in serum from patients with meningococcal septic shock. J Exp Med 1989; 169:333–338.
5. Bendtzen K, Svenson M, Jonsson V, Hippe E. Autoantibodies to cytokines—friends or foes? Immunol Today 1990; 5:167–169.
6. Herron L, Coffman R, Bond M, Kotzin B. Increased autoantibody production by NZB/NZW B cells in response to IL-5. J Immunol 1988; 141:842–848.
7. Umland S, Ning F, Cupp J, Howard M. Responses of B cells from autoimmune mice to IL-5. J Immunol 1989; 142:1528–1535.
8. Alarcon-Riquelme M, Moller G, Fernandez C. The effects of interleukin 4 and 5 on the differentiation of B cells from (NZB × NZW)F1 mice. Scand J Immunol 1991; 33:119–129.
9. Cabrero E, Snachez M, Gutierrez C. The requirements for growth of *in vivo* activated autoimmune B cells are similar to those of *in vitro* generated lipopolysaccharide B cell blasts and dissimilar to anti-IgM plus IL-4 induced B lymphocytes. J Autoimmunity 1992; 5:289–303.
10. Kanno K, Okado T, Abe M *et al.* Differential sensitivity to interleukins of CD5+ and CD5− anti-DNA antibody-producing B cells in murine lupus. Autoimmunity 1993; 14:205–214.
11. Mihara M, Ohsugi Y. Possible role of IL-6 in pathogenesis of immune complex-

mediated glomerulonephritis in NZB/W F1 mice: induction of IgG class anti-DNA autoantibody production. Int Arch Allergy Appl Immunol 1990; 93:89–92.
12. Alarcon-Riquelme M, Moller G, Fernandez C. Age-dependent responsiveness to interleukin-6 in B lymphocytes from systemic lupus erythematosus-prone (NZB × NZW)F1 hybrid. Clin Immunol Immunopathol 1992; 62:264–269.
13. Alarcon-Riquelme M, Moller G, Fernandez C. Macrophage depletion decreases IgG anti-DNA in cultures from (NZB × NZW)F1 spleen cells by eliminating the main source of IL-6. Clin Exp Immunol 1993; 91:220–225.
14. Finck BK, Chan B, Wofsy D. Interleukin-6 promotes murine lupus in NZB/NZW F1 mice. J Clin Invest 1994; 94:585–591.
15. Ishida H, Muchamuel T, Sakaguchi S *et al.* Continuous administration of anti-interleukin 10 antibodies delays onset of autoimmunity in NZB/W F1 mice. J Exp Med 1994; 179:305–310.
16. Jacob C, McDevitt H. Tumour necrosis factor-alpha in murine autoimmune 'lupus' nephritis. Nature 1988; 331:356–358.
17. Jacob C, Hwang F, Lewis G, Stall A. Tumor necrosis factor alpha in murine systemic lupus erythematosus disease models: implications for genetic predisposition and immune regulation. Cytokine 1991; 3:551–561.
18. Gordon C, Ranges G, Greenspan J, Wofsy D. Chronic therapy with recombinant tumor necrosis-alpha in autoimmune NZB/NZW F1 mice. Clin Immunol Immunopathol 1989; 52:421–434.
19. Brennan D, Yui M, Wuthrich R, Kelley V. Tumor necrosis factor and IL-1 in New Zealand Black/White mice. J Immunol 1989; 143; 3470–3475.
20. Suzuki H, Yasukawa K, Saito T *et al.* Serum soluble interleukin-6 receptor in MRL/lpr mice is elevated with age and mediates the interleukin-6 signal. Eur J Immunol 1993; 23:1078–1082.
21. Minoda M, Ohno M, Tomioka Y *et al.* Effects of gamma-interferon and FK506 on resting B cell proliferation on New Zealand Black/White F1 mice. Microbiol Immunol 1992; 36:885–894.
22. Adam C, Thoua Y, Ronco P *et al.* The effect of exogenous interferon: acceleration of autoimmune and renal diseases in (NZB/W)F1 mice. Clin Exp Immunol 1980; 40:373–382.
23. Heremans H, Billiau A, Hilgers J, De Somer P. Interferon treatment of NZB mice: accelerated progression of autoimmune disease. Infect Immun 1978; 21:925–930.
24. Dauphinee MJ, Kipper SB, Wofsy D, Talal N. Interleukin-2 deficiency is a common feature of autoimmune mice. J Immunol 1981; 127:2483–2487.
25. Hirose S, Nakanishi K, Yoshimoto T *et al.* Identification and characterization of IL-2 hyper-responsive NZB/WF1 CD5-B cells. J Immunol 1994; 153:1847–1857.
26. Sekigawa I, Noguchi K, Hasegawa K *et al.* B cell hyperresponsiveness to interleukin 2 and the age-associated decline in murine lupus. Clin Immunol Immunopathol 1989; 51:172–184.
27. Hasegawa K, Abe M, Okada T *et al.* Are Ly1 B cells responsible for the IL-2-hyperresponsiveness of B cells in autoimmune prone NZB × NZW F1 mice? Int Immunol 1989; 1:99–103.
28. Klinman DM, Steinberg AD. Proliferation of anti-DNA producing NZB B cells in a non-autoimmune environment. J Immunol 1986; 137:69–75.
29. Klinman DM, Steinberg AD. Similar in vivo expansion of B cells from normal DBA/2 and autoimmune NZB mice in xid recipients. J Immunol 1987; 139:2284–2289.
30. Tang B, Matsuda T, Akira S *et al.* Age-associated increase in interleukin 6 in MRL/lpr mice. Int Immunol 1991; 3:273–278.
31. Kabayashi I, Matsuda T, Saito T *et al.* Abnormal distribution of IL-6 receptor in

aged MRL/lpr mice: elevated expression on B cells and absence on CD4+ cells. Int Immunol 1992; 4:1407–1412.

32. Davidson W, Calkins C, Hugin A *et al.* Cytokine secretion by C3H-lpr and -gld T cells. J Immunol 1991; 146:4138–4148.
33. Murray LJ, Lee R, Martens C. In vitro cytokine gene expression in T cell subsets of the autoimmune MRL/Mp-lpr/lpr mouse. Eur J Immunol 1990; 20:163–170.
34. Budd R, Schumacher J, Winslow G, Mosmann T. Elevated production of interferon-gamma and interleukin 4 by mature T cells form autoimmune lpr mice correlates with Pgp-1 (CD44) expression. Eur J Immunol 1991; 21:1081–1084.
35. Mori K, Kobayashi S, Inobe M *et al.* In vivo cytokine gene expression in various T cell subsets of the autoimmune MRL/Mp-lpr/lpr mouse. Autoimmunity 1994; 17:49–57.
36. Manolios N, Schnieber L, Nelson M, Geczy CL. Enhanced interferon-gamma (IFN) production by lymph node cells from autoimmune (MRL/1, MRL/n) mice. Clin Exp Immunol 1989; 76:301–306.
37. Shirai A, Conover J, Klinman DM. Increased activation and altered ratio of IFN-$\gamma$: IL-4 secreting cells in MRL/lpr mice. Autoimmunity 1995; in press.
38. Klinman D. IgG1 and IgG2a production by autoimmune B cells treated in vitro with IL-4 and IFN-$\gamma$. J Immunol 1990; 144:2529–2534.
39. Jacob CO. TNF and IFN-gamma: relevance for immune regulation and genetic predisposition to autoimmune disease. Semin Immunol 1992; 3:147–154.
40. Gutierrez C, Howard M, Gasper L, Raveche E. Differential proliferative responses of B cells from BALB/c and autoimmune NZB mice to B-cell growth factor(s). Clin Immunol Immunopathol 1986; 39:319–328.
41. Cawley D, Chiang B, Naiki M *et al.* Comparison of the requirement for cognate T cell help for IgG anti-double-stranded DNA antibody production in vitro: T helper-derived lymphokines replace T cell cloned lines for B cells from NZB.H-2bm12 but not B6.H-2bm12 mice. J Immunol 1993; 150:2467–2477.
42. Chace J, Abed N, Adel G, Cowdrey J. Regulation of differentiation in CD5+ and conventional B cells. Clin Immunol Immunopathol 1993; 68:327–332.
43. Ochel M, Vohr H, Pfeiffer C, Gleichmann E. IL-4 is required for the IgE and IgG1 increase and IgG1 autoantibody formation in mice treated with mecuric chloride. J Immunol 1991; 143:3006–3011.
44. Schurmans S, Heusser C, Qin H *et al.* In vivo effects of anti-IL-4 monoclonal antibody on neonatal induction of tolerance and on an associated autoimmune syndrome. J Immunol 1990; 145:2465–2473.
45. Clerici M, Hakim F, Venzon D *et al.* Changes in interleukin-2 and interleukin-4 production in asymptomatic, human immunodeficiency virus-seropositive individuals. J Clin Invest 1993; 91:759–765.
46 De Wit D, Van Mechelen M, Zanin C *et al.* Preferential activation of the Th2 cells in chronic graft-versus-host reaction. J Immunol 1993; 150:361–366.
47. Allen J, Wong H, Costa G *et al.* Suppression of monocyte function and differential regulation of IL-1 and IL-1ra by IL-4 contribute to resolution of experimental arthritis. J Immunol 1993; 151:4344–4351.
48. Marcelletti J, Ohara J, Katz D. Collagen-induced arthritis in mice. J Immunol 1991; 147:4185–4191.
49. Linker-Israeli M, Deans R, Wallace D *et al.* Elevated levels of endogenous IL-6 in systemic lupus erythematosus. J Immunol 1991; 147:117–123.
50. Spronk P, Ter Borg E, Limburg P, Kallenberg C. Plasma concentration of IL-6 in systemic lupus erythematosus; an indicator of disease activity? Clin Exp Immunol 1992; 90:106–110.
51. Al-Janadi M, Al-Balla S, Al-Dalaan A, Raziuddin S. Cytokine profile in

systemic lupus erythematosus, rheumatoid arthritis, and other rheumatic diseases. J Clin Immunol 1993; 13:58–67.

52. Metsarinne K, Nordstrom D, Konttinen Y *et al.* Plasma interleukin-6 and renin substrate in reactive arthritis, rheumatoid arthritis and systemic lupus erythematosus. Rheumatol Int 1992; 12:93–96.
53. Swaak AJG, van Rooyen A, Aarden LA. Interleukin-6 and acute phase proteins in the disease course of patients with systemic lupus erythematosus. Rheumatol Int 1989; 8:263–268.
54. Hagiwara E, Gourley M, Klinman DM. Cytokine abnormalities in SLE. J Clin Invest 1995; in press.
55. Hirohata S, Miyamoto T. Elevated levels of interleukin-6 in cerebrospinal fluid from patients with systemic lupus erythematosus and central nervous system involvement. Arthritis Rheum 1990; 33:644–649.
56. Tsai C, Wu T, Tsai S *et al.* Cerebrospinal fluid interleukin-6, prostaglandin E2 and autoantibodies in patients with neuropsychiatric systemic lupus erythematosus and central nervous system infections. Scand J Rheumatol 1994; 23:57–63.
57. Kitani A, Hara M, Hirose T *et al.* Autostimulatory effects of IL-6 on excessive B cell differentiation in patients with systemic lupus erythematosus: analysis of IL-6 production and IL-6R expression. Clin Exp Immunol 1992; 88:75–83.
58. Nagafuchi H, Suzuki N, Mizushima Y, Sakane T. Constitutive expression of IL-6 receptors and their role in the excessive B cell function in patients with systemic lupus erythematosus. J Immunol 1993; 151:6525–6534.
59. Kitani A, Hara M, Hirose T *et al.* Heterogeneity of B cell responsiveness to interleukin 4, interleukin 6 and low molecular weight B cell growth factor in discrete stages of B cell activation in patients with systemic lupus erythematosus. Clin Exp Immunol 1989; 77:31–36.
60. Pekton B, Speckmaier M, Hylton W *et al.* Cytokine-independent progression of immunological production in vitro by B lymphocytes from patients with systemic lupus erythematosus. Clin Exp Immunol 1991; 83:274–279.
61. Tanaka Y, Saito K, Shirakawa F *et al.* Production of B cell-stimulating factors by B cells in patients with systemic lupus erythematosus. J Immunol 1988; 141:3043–3049.
62. Ueda Y, Sakane T, Tsunematsu T. Hyperreactivity of activated B cells to B cell growth factors in patients with systemic lupus erythematosus. J Immunol 1989; 143:3988–3993.
63. Martinez-Cordero E, Alcocer-Varela J, Alarcon-Segovia D. Stimulating and differentiation factors for human B lymphocytes in systemic lupus erythematosus. Clin Exp Immunol 1986; 65:598–604.
64. Ogawa N, Itoh M, Goto Y. Abnormal production of B cell growth factor in patients with systemic lupus erythematosus. Clin Exp Immunol 1992; 89:26–31.
65. Dueymes M, Barrier J, Besancenot J *et al.* Relationship of interleukin-4 to isotype distribution of anti-double-stranded DNA antibodies in systemic lupus erythematosus. Int Arch Allergy Appl Immunol 1993; 101:408–415.
66. Llorente L, Richaud-Patin Y, Wijdenes J *et al.* Spontaneous production of interleukin-10 by B lymphocytes and monocytes in systemic lupus erythematosus. Eur Cytokine Network 1993; 4:421–430.
67. Briere F, Servet-Delprat C, Bridon J *et al.* Human interleukin 10 induces naive surface immunoglobulin D+ (sIgD+) B cells to secrete IgG1 and IgG3. J Exp Med 1994; 179:757–762.
68. Funauchi M, Sugishima H, Minoda M, Horiuchi A. Effect of interferon-gamma on B lymphocytes of patients with systemic lupus erythematosus. J Rheumatol 1991; 18:368–372.
69. Mitamura K, Kang H, Tomita Y *et al.* Impaired tumour necrosis factor-alpha

(TNF-alpha) production and abnormal B cell response to TNF-alpha in patients with systemic lupus erythematosus (SLE). Clin Exp Immunol 1991; 85:386–391.

70. Malave I, Searles RP, Montano J, Williams RCJR. Production of TNF/cachectin by peripheral blood mononuclear cells in patients with systemic lupus erythematosus. Int Arch Allergy Appl Immunol 1989; 89:355–361.
71. Jacob C, Fronek Z, Lewis G *et al.* Heritable major histocompatibility complex class II-associated differences in production of tumor necrosis factor alpha: relevance to genetic predisposition to systemic lupus erythematosus. Proc Natl Acad Sci USA 1990; 87:1233–1237.
72. Kroemer G, Martinez AC. Cytokines and autoimmune disease. Clin Immunol Immunopathol 1991; 61:275–295.
73. Goldman M. Cytokines in the pathogenesis of systemic lupus erythematosus. Autoimmunity 1990; 8:173–179.
74. Huang YP, Perrin LH, Miescher PA, Zubler RH. Correlation of T and B cell activities in vitro and serum IL-2 levels in systemic lupus erythematosus. J Immunol 1988; 141:827–833.
75. Tanaka Y, Saito K, Suzuki H *et al.* Inhibitory effect of anti-class II antibody on the spontaneous activation of B cells in patients with systemic lupus erythematosus. J Immunol 1989; 143:1584–1590.
76. Hirano T, Matsuda T, Turner M *et al.* Excessive production of interleukin 6/B cell stimulatory factor-2 in rheumatoid arthritis. Eur J Immunol 1988; 18:1797–1801.
77. Wascher T, Hermann J, Brezinschek R *et al.* Serum levels of the interleukin-6 and tumour-necrosis-factor-alpha are not correlated to disease activity in patients with rheumatoid arthritis after treatment with low-dose methotrexate. Eur J Clin Invest 1994; 24:73–75.
78. Crilly A, McInnes I, Capell H, Madhok R. The effect of azathioprine on serum levels of interleukin 6 and soluble interleukin 2 receptor. Scand J Rheumatol 1994; 23:87–91.
79. Harigai M, Kitani A, Hara M *et al.* Rheumatoid adherent synovial cells produce B cell differentiation factor activity neutralizable by antibody to B cell stimulatory factor-2/interleukin 6. J Rheumatol 1988; 15:1616–1622.
80. Field M, Chu C, Feldman M, Maini R. Interleukin-6 localisation in the synovial membrane in rheumatoid arthritis. Rheumatol Int 1991; 11:45–50.
81. Guerne P, Zuraw B, Vaughan J *et al.* Synovium as a source of interleukin 5 in vitro. J Clin Invest 1989; 83:585–592.
82. Chen E, Keystone E, Fish E. Restricted cytokine expression in rheumatoid arthritis. Arthritis Rheum 1993; 36:901–910.
83. Sawada T, Hirohata S, Inoue T, Ito K. Correlation between rheumatoid factor and IL-6 activity in synovial fluids from patients with rheumatoid arthritis. Clin Exp Rheumatol 1991; 9:363–368.
84. Hidaka T, Kitani A, Harigai M *et al.* IL-4 down-regulates the surface expression of CD5 on B cells and inhibits spontaneous immunoglobulin and IgM-rheumatoid factor production in patients with rheumatoid arthritis. Clin Exp Immunol 1992; 89:223–229.
85. Chomarat P, Briolay J, Banchereau J, Miossec P. Increased production of soluble CD23 in rheumatoid arthritis, and its regulation by interleukin-4. Arthritis Rheum 1993; 36:234–242.
86. Briolay J, Dechanet J, Blanchard D *et al.* Interleukin 4 inhibits polyclonal immunoglobulin secretion and cytokine production by peripheral blood mononuclear cells from rheumatoid arthritis patients. J Clin Immunol 1992; 12:36–44.
87. Miossec P, Briolay J, Dechanet J *et al.* Inhibition of the production of

proinflammatory cytokines and immunoglobulins by interleukin-4 and an ex vivo model of rheumatoid synovitis. Arthritis Rheum 1992; 35:874–883.

88. Deleuran B, Iversen L, Kristensen M *et al.* Interleukin-8 secretion and 15-lipoxygenase activity in rheumatoid arthritis: in vivo anti-inflammatory effects by interleukin-4 and interleukin-10, but not by interleukin-1 receptor antagonist protein. Br J Rheumatol 1994; 33:520–525.
89. Deleuran B, Lemche P, Kristensen M *et al.* Localisation of interleukin-8 in the synovial membrane, cartilage–pannus junction and chondrocytes in rheumatoid arthritis. Scand J Rheumatol 1994; 23:2–7.
90. Beaulieu A, McColl S. Differential expression of two major cytokines produced by neutrophils, interleukin-8 and interleukin-1 receptor antagonist, in neutrophils isolated from the synovial fluid and peripheral blood of patients with rheumatoid arthritis. Arthritis Rheum 1994; 37:855–859.
91. Miossec P, Naviliat M, Dupuy-D *et al.* Low levels of interleukin-4 and high levels of TGF-b in rheumatoid arthritis. Arthritis Rheum 1990; 33:1180.
92. Hart P, Ahern M, Jones C *et al.* Synovial fluid macrophages and blood monocytes differ in their responses to IL-4. J Immunol. 1993; 151:3370–3380.
93. Katsikis P, Chu C, Brennan F *et al.* Immunoregulatory role of interleukin 10 in rheumatoid arthritis. J Exp Med 1994; 179:1517–1527.
94. Feldman M, Brennan FM, Chantry D *et al.* Cytokine assays: role in evaluation of the pathogenesis of autoimmunity. Immunol Rev 1991; 119:105–123.
95. Firestein GS, Alvaro-Gracia J, Maki R. Quantitative analysis of cytokine gene expression in rheumatoid arthritis. J Immunol 1990; 144:3347.
96. Miyasaka N, Sato K, Goto M. Augmented interleukin-1 production and HLA-DR expression in the synovium of rheumatoid arthritis patients: possible involvement in joint destruction. Arthritis Rheum 1988; 31:480.
97. Fong K, Boey M, Koh W, Feng P. Cytokine concentration in the synovial fluid and plasma of rheumatoid arthritis patients: correlation with bony erosions. Clin Exp Rheumatol 1994; 12:55–58.
98. Callaghan M, Whelan A, Feighery C, Bresnihan B. IL-2 enhances polyclonal IgM but not IgM-rheumatoid factor synthesis by activated human peripheral blood B cells. Clin Exp Immunol 1993; 93:212–217.
99. Seitz M, Loetscher P, Dewald B *et al.* Production of interleukin-1 receptor antagonist, inflammatory chemotactic proteins, and prostaglandin E by rheumatoid and osteoarthritic synoviocytes—regulation by IFN-gamma and IL-4. J Immunol 1994; 152:2060–2065.
100. Hirano T, Taga T, Yasukawa K *et al.* Human B-cell differentiation factor defined by an anti-peptide antibody and its possible role in autoantibody production. Proc Natl Acad Sci USA 1987; 84:228–231.
101. Yoshizaki K, Matsuda T, Nishimoto N *et al.* Pathogenic significance of interleukin-6 (IL-6/BSF-2) in Castleman's disease. Blood 1989; 74:1360–1367.
102. Yoshizaki K, Kuritani T, Kishimoto T. Interleukin-6 in autoimmune disorders. Semin Immunol 1992; 4:155–166.
103. Fox R, Kang H, Ando D *et al.* Cytokine mRNA expression in salivary gland biopsies of Sjogren's syndrome. J Immunol 1994; 152:5532–5539.

# Index


activation markers, net effect of expression, 53
αδ-dex, *see* dextra-conjugated anti-IgD antibodies
adaptive response, 145–9
ADCC, *see* antibody-dependent cellular cytotoxicity
agammaglobulinemia, X-linked, 234
AIDS, 274, 418
allergic diseases, IgE regulation, 379–85
antibodies
  anti-CD23, 361
  anti-IL-10, 274
  class switching, 109–25, 307–15
antibody responses
  cytokine expression during, 60–1
  roles of cytokines, 42
  TI-2 antigen, 35
antibody-dependent cellular cytotoxicity, 338–9
antibody-forming cells
  localization of, 62–3
  responses, peripheral B-cell responses, 84
antigen-presenting cells, 27
  role of, 54
antigen-specific suppression, 105
antigens
  administration, 33–9
  B-cell proliferation, 57–8
  complement-activating capacity, 37
  dose, 34–6
  food, oral tolerance to, 401
  memory formation, 59–60
  mIg characteristics, 44–6
  mucosal, 402
  particulate, 37–8
  phagocytosis of, 28
  protein, 27
  receptor complex, membrane Ig, 100–1
  soluble versus particulate, 36–7
  T-cell-dependent, 23–64, 27–8
    adjuvants, 34
    B-cell activation, 44–57, 172
    CD14, 55
    soluble, 39
    *in vitro*, 57–60
  T-cell-independent, 23–64, 26–7
    B-cell activation, 40–1
    CD14, 43–4
    class II major histocompatibility complex, 39–40
    crosslinking mIg receptor, 40
    lymph nodes, 43
    natural killer cells, 42
    soluble, 38
    spleen, 43
    T cell contributions to, 41–3
    type 1, 27
    type 2, 27, 102, 169
    *in vitro*, 57–60
  thymus-dependent, 24, 25
  thymus-independent, 24, 25
  TNP-BSA, 39
  TNP-KLH, 34, 39
  TNP-SRBC, 31
AP-1
  binding activity, 304
  TGF-b effects on, 304
apoptosis, TGF-β induced, 297–8
asthma, 371
autoantibody production, 412
autoimmune disease
  abnormalities in cytokines, 409–25
  IL-6, 260–1
  murine models of, 412–18

B cells (B lymphocytes)
  activation, 83, 329
    CD19, 47
    CD40 ligand, 4, 36–7
    incomplete, 52–3
    lymphoid organs, 77–8
    polyclonal, 278
    primary antibody response, 103–4
    signals, 103–5, 383–4
    T-cell independent, 39–44
    T-cell-dependent, 44–57, 177

B cells (B lymphocytes) (*cont.*)
antibody class switching, 109–25
stimulatory factor, *see* interleukins, IL-4
subsets
functional characteristics of, 88–92
receptor ligation, 105
bovine, 331
*Branhamella catarrhalis*-activated, 281
CD40 antigen activated, 276–7
CD40L, 53
CD45, 40
$CD5^+$, 81–3, 273, 276
chronic lymphocytic leukemias, IL-2 receptor expression, 165
common variable immunodeficiencies, 283
cytokine response regulation, 169
development
CD5, 40–1
differentiation, 251, 256, 276–8
regulation, 219–20
TGF-b, 302–15
differentiation factors, 264
Epstein–Barr virus, 218, 259–60, 276
IgE production, 200
follicular, 78–9, 90
growth factors, 217, 251, 420
hIL-10, 275–6
IFN-γ, 325 , 327–38
Ig secretion, 237
IL-2 role, 8, 163–4, 166–75
IL-4 role, 198–201, 207, 339
IL-5 role, 11, 217–40, 234–8
IL-6 role, 13, 256–9
IL-10 derived from, 143
IL-13 role, 198–201, 207
immature, 80, 88–9, 205–6
isotype switching, 397
Ly-1–positive, 236
lymph node, 33
lymphoma, 53, 297
marginal zone, 79–80, 90–1
markers, 76, 77
maturation, 74, 275–6
maturational subsets, 73–7, 89–92
cytoplasmic protein definitions, 75
functional responses, 89
immunoglobulin gene rearrangement, 74–5
surface marker definition, 76–7
memory, 28, 57–60, 84–5
germinal centers, 58
secondary antibody response, 104
mitogenesis, 45, 398
peritoneal, 86, 91–2
polyclonal activation of, 278, 412
progression, cytokine-dependent phase, 53–7
proliferation, 46
antigen presentation, 57–8
inhibition, 299–301
regulation, 218–19, 338
receptor expression, 302–4
responses to T-cell-dependent antigen, 172
resting subsets, lymphoid organs, 77
$sIg^+$, depletion of, 360
$sIgD^+$ tonsillar, 279
sIgM affinity, 45
specific response, 6
spleen, 29, 31, 78, 79, 81
*Staphylococcus aureus* Cowen stimulation, 171, 309
subpopulations, 73–93
peritoneal cavity, 85–8
phenotypically defined, 78–85
switch recombination
early stages, 122
systemic lupus erythematosus, 419
T-cell interaction, 27–8, 42
terminal IgA B-cell differentiation, 399
TGF-β, 289–315
developmental e, 301–2
differentiation, 302–15
inhibition, 299–301
proliferation effect, 296–301
Th2 cells, 273, 380, 413
tonsillar, 279, 292, 303
vasoactive intestinal peptide, 348
VIP, 368
B1 cells
CD40–directed stimulation, 92
derivation of, 87–8
basal Ig titers, 49
basophils, CD40 ligand, 381
BCLL, *see* lymphocytic leukemia B cells
beta glycan, 292, 293
blast formation, by B cells, 168
bovine serum albumin, 139
*Branhamella catarrhalis*, 281, 397, 399
bronchus-associated lymphoreticular tissues, 391
*Brucella abortus*, 27, 38, 43, 142, 147, 329, 333
*Brucella ovis*, 329

Bruton's tyrosine kinase
activation, 238, 240
IL-5 stimulation of, 234
mRNA, B cells, 237
Burkitt's lymphoma, 259

c-*myc*, switch recombination targeting, 123
cancer treatment, IL-6, 261
cardiac myxoma, 423, 424
IL-6, 260
Castleman's disease, 423, 424
IL-6, 260, 262
$CD4^+$ T cells, 325, 339, 384
influence on differentiation, 139–49
$CD4^+$ T-helper cells, cytokine production profiles, 195
CD5, T- and B-cell development, 40–1
$CD5^+$ B cells, 81–3
$CD8^+$ T cells, as suppressor cells, 148
CD14
T-cell-dependent antigen responses, 55
T-cell-independent antigen responses, 43–4
CD19, B-cell activation threshold, 47
CD23, 50
IgE regulation, 384
$CD23^+$ B cells, 91
anti-IgM stimulation, 90
lipopolysaccharide stimulation, 90
CD28, 49
CD28/CtLA4–Ig with B7–1/B7–2, 48–49
CD40–CD40L, 49–50, 92
gene targeting models, 52
human immune deficiency, 52
CD40L, 100
antigen-specific suppression, 105
B cells, 53
expression, 50–1
human B-cell precursors, 54
Ig isotype switching , 201–2
induced signaling, 63
memory formation, 59
T-cell expression of, 172
CD43, B-cell maturation, 76
CDKs, *see* cyclin-dependent kinases
cell-mediated immunity, 400
cellular proteins, tyrosine phosphorylation of, 227
centroblasts, germinal centers, 58
chemokine family receptors, 47
chemotherapy, IL-6, 261
class switching
BLPS-induced, 110–11
immunoglobulin, 109–25
long transcripts, 117–18
molecular mechanism of, 116–21
recombination, 116–17, 121–5
loop-out and deletion, 119–20
trans-splicing, 118–19
transcription, 116–17
common variable immunodeficiencies (CVI), 283
concanavalin A, 294, 348
conjugate stabilization, molecules involved in, 46–7
constant heavy gene, 7
corticosteroids, 263
CVI, *see* common variable immunodeficiencies
cyclin dependent kinases, 300
cyclins
activation, 300
D–Cdk4 complexes, 300
E–Cdk2 complexes, 300
cyclosporin A, 102
cysteine knot, 290–1
cytokine receptor family, type 2, 225
cytokine-producing cells, localization of, 62–3
cytoplasmic proteins, 75
cytoplasmic signaling proteins, 327
cytotoxic cells, development of, 49

dendritic cells, 396
dextra-conjugated anti-IgD antibodies, 335–6
disodium cromoglycate, IgE production, 361
DNA
recombination, IL-10 induced, 281–2
synthesis
switch recombination, 120
TGF-β, 297
DNase hypersensitive sites, 124, 312

EBV, *see* Epstein–Barr virus
encephalomyelitis, 401
endoglin, 292
endotoxin, 43
eosinophils, 217, 218
IL-5 signalling pathway, 238
infiltration, 371
XID mice, 235
epithelial cells, 33
uterine, TGF-β treatment, 298

Epstein–Barr virus, 332, 383
  B cells, 259–60, 276
  IL-10, 273
  IL-2R upregulation, 173
  substance P, 350
  switch recombination targeting, 123
  TGF-β, 297
erythrocyte sedimentation rate, 422
erythropoietin, 350
  IgE production, 361
  receptor, 229
*Escherichia coli*, 393
estrogens, 263
eukaryotic recombination systems, 125

FDC-P1 transfectants, proliferation of, 230
ficoll, 26
follicular dendritic cells, spleen, 32
Freund's complete adjuvant, 34

G-protein-coupled receptor BLR1, 47
germinal centers, 104
  cytokine production, 61
  formation of, 58–9
germlines
  α transcripts, 310
    IgA deficiency, 314
    TGF-β induced, 311, 312
  Ca RNA, 310–14
  $C_H$ RNA, 328
  $C_H\epsilon$ RNA, 332
  $C_H\gamma1$, 332
  $C_H\gamma2b$ RNA, 328, 331
  γ2b transcripts, 314–15
  ε mRNA expression, IL-4 and IL-13 induced, 204–5
glomerulonephritis, 254, 412, 414
  autoantibodies, 416
GM-CSF, *see* granulocyte-macrophage colony stimulating factor
graft-versus-host disease, 418
Gram-negative bacteria, 141, 142, 167
granulocyte colony-stimulating factor, 61
granulocyte/macrophage colony stimulating factor (GM-CSF), 61, 159, 226, 336, 337–8
growth hormone receptor, 229
guanine tetrades, 113
gut-associated lymphoreticular tissues, 391

Hashimoto's thyroiditis, 409
heavy chain isotypes, human B cell production of, 175
*Heligmosomoides polygyrus*, 144, 145, 146, 400
helminth infections, 333, 379–85
helper cytokines, 102–3
hemolytic anemia, 417, 418
*Hemophilus influenzae*, 26
hepatocytes, rat, 298
hepatoma cells, somatostatin, 348
histamine secretion, 371
HIV-1, 34, 37
  protein-specific antibody-forming cells, 62
  infected lymph nodes, 62
$HIV^+$ T cells, 202
Hodgkin's disease
  IL-10, 274
  Reed–Sternberg cells, 218
human autoimmune diseases, cytokine abnormalities in, 419–24
human immune deficiency, CD40–CD40L, 52
human immunoglobulin production, modulation of, 347–71
human peripheral blood B cells, IL-5 enhanced IgA or IgM synthesis, 220
hybridomas, switch recombination, 119, 123
hyper-IgM syndrome, 52, 201
hypergammaglobulinemia, 412, 421
hypersensitivity response, delayed-type, 49
hypogammaglobulinemia, 419

Ig-secreting plasmablasts, switch recombination inhibitor, 122
IL-, *see* interleukins
immune response
  cytokines secreted, 140
  initiation of, 140, 141–5
immune system, cells, 290
immunization route, epithelial cells, 33
immunodeficiencies, 282–3
immunoglobulins
  α chain, 311
  antigen receptor complex, 100
  Cα gene, 310
  class switching, 109–25, 368
    cellular and molecular biology of, 6
    control elements, 114–15
    induction and role of, 109–11
    inhibition, 331–4
    molecular basis of, 111–16

neuropeptide regulation, 358–61
regulation, 327–38
sequential, 110
classes
functional heterogeneity of, 109
GM-CSF, 336
in immune response, 109–10
heavy chains, 175
inhibition of synthesis, 303
IgA, 277
B-cell differentiation, 399
class switch to, 19
CVI patients, 283
deficiencies, 282–3, 314
hIL-10, 276
IL-10 as switch factor, 281
isotype switching, 397–9
mesenteric lymph nodes, 308
Peyer's patches, 308, 313, 398
switch recombination, 309
TGF-β inducing switching, 307–9
vasoactive intestinal peptide effects, 349, 350
IgD antibodies, 278, 331
IgE
atopic patients, 369
B-cells, 360, 383–4
CD23, 384
class switching *in vivo*, 379–85
helminth parasite infections, 379–85
IL-4 and, 10, 206–7, 282, 381–2
IL-6 and, 256–9
IL-10 and, 282
IL-13 and, 10, 282
inhibited switching to, 315
inhibition of, 382–3
monocytes, 367
neuropeptides on, 355, 357, 363
regulation, allergic diseases, 379–85
responses, 18
spontaneous production, 370–1
synthesis
inhibition of, 206–7
modulation by cytokines, 203–4
in SCID-hu mice, 202–3
T–B-cell interactions, 56
T cells, 367, 380–1
IgG, 279
atopic patients, 369
CVI patients, 283
hIL-10, 276
IL-10 as switch factor, 278–81
neuropeptides, 364
T-cell-dependent antigens, 28
vesicular stomatitis virus, 55
IgG2, 354
IgG2a, 328–31, 338
IgG3, 328–31, 338
IgG4, 354
monocytes, 367
neuropeptide incubation, 363
spontaneous production, 370–1
T cells, 367
IgH locus
class switching dynamics, 112
structure of, 111
IgM, 278, 279, 311, 335
hIL-10, 276
vasoactive intestinal peptide enhanced production, 351
IL-2 stimulated production, 173
IL-4–stimulated mononuclear cells, 354
IL-5, response to, 237
isotype production, IL-4 induced, 351–61
isotype selection, 220–1
isotype switching
CD40L–CD40 interaction, 201–2
multiple isotypes, in response to IL-2, 176
neuropeptides, 366, 349–50, 359
production, 349–50
culture systems, 350–68
regulation of, 334–8
sIg+ cells, depletion of, 369
spontaneous production
TGF-β inhibition, 303, 304–6
vasoactive intestinal peptide, 368
indomethacin, 357
Ig production, 366
inflammatory diseases, IL-6, 260–1
Influenza pneumonia, 147
influenza virus, type A, 330
interdigiting cells, spleen, 32
interferons
anti-IFN-α, 366
IFN-γ, 262 , 325–39, 366
B-cell differentiation, 335
B-cell function, 16, 327–38
dominant response, 141–3, 148
humoral immunity, 338–9
Ig class switching, 331–4
molecular nature of, 325–6
murine lupus, 415
polypeptides, 326

interferons (*cont.*)
  IFN-γ
    receptor, 326
    substance P, 347
    synthesis, 327
    X-ray crystallography, 326
  IgE inhibition, 382–3
  IL-6 synthesis, 252
interleukins
  IL-2, 332
    antagonistic with IL-4, 174
    as B cell growth and differentiation factor, 166–75
    B-cell functions, 8, 159–79, 170–4
    effects on isotype production, 175
    human B-cell responses to, 170–4
    Ig synthesis inhibition mechanism, 304
    induced sterile Ig transcripts, 178
    initiating intracellular signaling, 162–3
    multiple Ig isotype production, 176
    murine lupus, 415
    pleiotropic effects of, 178
    receptor, 160–2, 164–6
    source of, 160
  IL-2R, 174, 229
  IL-3, 337–8
    GM-CSF, 336
    receptor complex, molecular components for, 226
  IL-4, 195–208, 315
    B-cell proliferation, 199
    CD40L expression, 56
    dominant response, 143–7
    effects on B cells, 207
    enhanced Ig production, 174
    germline ϵ mRNA expression, 204–5
    human B-cell phenotype and function, 198–201
    IgE production, 10, 199–201, 361, 381–2
    IgE synthesis modulation, 203–4
    IgG4 production, 199–201
    immature human B cells, 205–6
    inducing Ig production, 351–4
    inducing switching, 361
    molecular characteristics of, 196
    neuropeptides, 368
    production of, 197–8
    receptor, 196–7
    stimulating cultures, 370
    stimulating mononuclear cells, 354
    systemic lupus erythematosus, 420–1
    Th2 cell development, 198
    Th2 cytokine, 413
  IL-5
    as B-cell growth and differentiation factor, 217–40
    B cell Ig secretion, 237
    B-cell proliferation, 11
    Bruton's tyrosine kinase activation, 234
    early B cell development, 219
    functional properties of, 238–9
    Jak2 activation, 233–4
    murine lupus, 413
    receptor, 217, 222–31
    SH2/SH3 domain-containing proteins, 231–3
    signalling, 12, 227–9, 230–4, 238
    structure of, 218
    tyrosine phosphorylation, 232
    XID mice, 234–8
  IL-5R, 228, 239–40
  IL-5Ra
    amino acid sequence, 223, 227
    critical cytoplasmic regions of, 227–9
    in βc dimerizations, 229–30
  IL-6, 251–64, 347
    autoimmune disease, 423
    B cells, 251, 256–9
    biological activities of, 253–4
    clinical application of, 261–3
    disease, 259–61
    identification of, 251–2
    IgE synthesis stimulation, 256–9
    myeloma, 259–60
    neutralizing activity, 262
    plasmacytomas, 259–60
    protein, 252
    receptor, 254–6
    regulation of gene expression, 252–3
    rheumatoid arthritis, 422
    role in B-cell functions, 13
    Sjögren's syndrome, 424
    synthesis of, 252
    systemic lupus erythematosus, 419–20
    transgenic mice, 254
  IL-6R, gp130 of, 229
  IL-10, 273–84
    antibodies, 274
    B cells as source, 273–4
    biological fluids, 274
    DNA recombination, 281–2

IFN-γ synthesis, 327
IgA production, 308
neutralizing, 277–8
peripheral blood mononuclear cells, 420
systemic lupus erythematosus, 14
Th1 cytokine , 414
Th2 cells, 273
IL-12, 331
IFN-γ synthesis, 327
IgE inhibition, 382–3
synergized with IL-2, 173
IL-13, 195–208
B-cell proliferation, 199
effects on B cells, 207
germline ε mRNA expression, 204–5
human B-cell phenotype and function, 198–201
IgE production, 10, 199–201
IgG4 production, 199–201
immature human B cells, 205–6
molecular characteristics of, 196
production of, 197–8
receptor, 196–7
mIL-5Rα, 224
sIL-5Rα, 224, 225
intraepithelial lymphocytes, 392, 394–6
intron enhancer, 114
ionomycin, 416
isotype production, 175–8
isotype switching, 278–82, 397–9
T cell contributions to, 41–3

Jak–STAT family signaling pathway, 326
Janus kinases, 233
IL-2 stimulation, 162
Jak2, 233–4, 240
lamina propria
lymphocytes, 394
regions, 391
Langerhans cells, 32
Lansbury activity index, 422
*Leishmania major*, 146, 147
lepromatous leprosy, 401
leukemia
70Z/3 line, 297
chronic lymphocytic, 275
lymphocytic B cells, 295
leukosialin, *see* CD43
lipopolysaccharide (LPS), 383
activated cells, 331
anti-TGF-β antibody, 306
antibody production, 415
B cells, 295
CD23+ B cells, 90
class switching, 110–11
haptenated, 27
IFN-γ, 335, 414
IL-6 synthesis, 252
RNA, 301
T-cell-independent response, 100
TGF-β effects, 301
lipopolysaccharide-binding protein, 37
*Listeria monocytogenes*, 37, 142, 147
IL-6, 253
liver
B-cell maturation, 73
Küppfer cells, 400
LPS, *see* lipopolysaccharide
lymph, veiled cells, 32
lymph nodes
functional organization of, 32–3
humoral immunity, 23
mesenteric, 308, 401
T-cell-independent antigen type 2 responses, 43
lymphadenopathy, 419, 421
lymphocytes
intraepithelial, 392, 394–6
physiological role of, 395
murine lupus, 412
neuropeptide receptors on, 347–8
lymphocytic leukemia B cells, TGF-β secretion, 295
lymphoid cells, gastrointestinal tract, 394
lymphoid follicles, 104
lymphoid organs, 410
B cells, 77–85
activated, 83
CD5+, 81–3
follicular, 78–9
immature, 80
marginal zone, 79–80
memory, 84–5
lymphoid populations, exogenous cytokines, 411
lymphoma cells, 118, 124
lymphopoiesis, 92
lymphoproliferative disorder, 423

*Macobacterium tuberculosis*, 400
α-macroglobulin, 291, 293
macrophages
marginal metallophilic, 32
peritoneal, 293
scavenging role of, 35

macrophages (*cont.*)
  spleen, 31–2, 36
major histocompatibility complex
  class II, 44, 101
    B cells, 275
    IL-10, 275
    resting B lymphocytes, 53
    T-cell receptor, 53
    TI antigen binding, 39–40
  IFN-γ, 334
MAP kinase, 256
mast cells, 371
medulla, 33
megakaryocytes, 254
  IL-6, 261
memory formation
  CD40L, role of, 59
  TI versus TD antigens, 59–60
mesangial proliferative glomerulonephritis, IL-6, 260–1
mesenteric lymph nodes, 401
*Mesocestoides corti*, 110
mitogens, 410
  induction of switch recombination, 121
monocytes
  IgE, 362, 367
  IgG4, 362, 367
  neuropeptides, 358, 363
mononuclear cells
  IFN–secreting, 421
  spontaneous IgE production, 362
  spontaneous IgG4 production, 362
*Moraxella catarrhalis*, 220
mRNA
  cytokine, 411
  trans-splicing, 118
mucosa-associated lymphoreticular tissues, 391
  structure–function relationship, 19
mucosal antibody response, 103–4
mucosal IgA responses, regulation of, 396–9
mucosal immune responses, T-cell subsets, 400–1
mucosal immunity, regulation of, 391–402
mucosal tissues
  effector sites, 394
  inductive sites, 392–4
mucosal vaccine development, 402
multiple sclerosis, 409
myasthenia gravis, 409
*Mycobacterium tuberculosis*, 395
myelin basic protein, 401
myeloid primary response gene, MyD118, 298
myeloma
  IL-6, 259–60, 262
  multiple, IL-10, 274
myelomatous disease, IL-10, 274
myelosuppression, IL-6, 261

nasal-associated lymphoreticular tissues, 391
natural killer cells, 330
  αδ-dex-activated B cells, 337
  GM-CSF, 339
  IFN-γ, 143 , 325 , 339
  Ig secretion, 337, 361
  intraepithelial lymphocytes, 395
  spleen, 32
  T-cell-independent response, 42, 100
  transforming growth factor, 289
*Neisseria meningitidis*, 26
nematode parasites, 143
nephritis, 414, 421
nephrotic syndrome, 419
neuropeptides
  B- and T-cell proliferation, 17
  Ig class switching, 358–61
  Ig production, 352, 353, 364
  kinetic analysis of effects, 355–7
  receptors, lymphocytes, 347–8
  specificity of effects, 348
  spontaneous production, 362
*Nippostrongylus brasiliensis*, 55, 117, 144, 169, 381, 382, 383, 384
  antibody responses to, 56

Oct proteins, 305
oesinophilia, 385
oligosaccharides, 46
omentum, B-cell maturation, 73
oncogenes, c-Myc, TGF-β treatment, 299
osteocalcin genes, 304–5
osteosarcoma cells, 299

p91, tyrosine phosphorylation of, 327
pan-B cell markers, 76
parasite infections, helminth, 379–85
PBMCs, *see* peripheral blood mononuclear cells
peptidoleukotriene release, 347
periarteriolar lymphocyte sheath, 30, 32, 38
  activated B-cell subsets, 77

CD40L expression, 51
germinal centers, 58
T-cell-dependent antigen, 57
peripheral blood mononuclear cells, 333
IgE high serum levels, 201
IL-4 , 200
IL-6 mRNA, 419
IL-10, 420
rheumatoid arthritis, 422
substance P, 347
peritoneal B cells, phenotypic characteristics of, 86
peritoneal cavity
B-cell subsets in, 85–8
Ly-1–positive B cells, 236
peritoneal lavage cells, 87
Peyer's patches, 33, 307, 308, 392
functional regions of, 393
germline α transcripts, 313
IgA, 313, 398
mucosal immunity, 5
T cells, 313, 396
TGF-β, 315
phorbol esters, 102, 416
phytohemagglutinin, T cells, 294, 348
plasma cells, CD40L, 54
plasmacytomas, IL-6, 259–60
plasmacytosis, 254
*Plasmodium chaubudii*, 381
platelet counts, IL-6, 261
platelet-activating factor, IgE production, 357
pokeweed mitogen, 167, 331, 350, 398
polyadenylation sites, long transcripts, 117
polymerase chain reaction
CD40L sequences, 51
cytokine mRNA, 411
polysaccharide, 26
postcapillary high endothelial venules, 33
prokaryotic recombination systems, 125
prostaglandin $E_2$, IgE production, 357
protein kinase C, 63, 102
protein tyrosine kinase, 63
IL-2 receptor, 161
IL-5 receptor, 228
proteinuria, 413
protooncogene expression, IL-5R, 230–1
pseudorabies virus, 330
pulmonary nerve fibers, 371

Ras, IL-5 stimulation of, 240
receptor–ligand pairs, 48
recombinase-associated gene products, 75
rectal-associated lymphoreticular tissues, 391
renal damage, 417
renal disease, 414, 418
retinoblastoma control elements, TGF-β, 294
rheumatoid arthritis, 409, 422–3
IL-10, 274
IL-6, 260
rheumatoid factor, 422

*Salmonella typhimurium*, 142, 144, 329, 393
*Schistosoma mansoni*, 146
substance P, 350
schistosome eggs, 46
schistosomula, 46
SCID-hu mouse, 11
serine/threonine kinases, IL-2 stimulation, 162
serum cytokine levels, 410
SH2/SH3 domain-containing proteins, IL-5–induced tyrosine phosphorylation of, 231–3
sheep red blood cells, 139
IL-2 effects, 164
plaque-forming cell response, 334
*Shigella*, 393
signal transduction mechanism, TGF-β receptors, 291–2
Sjögren's syndrome
IL-10, 274
IL-6, 424
solitary lymphoid nodules, 392
somatostatin, 347–71
spleen
B cells, 31, 81
migration patterns, 29
CD40L expression, 51
$CD4^+$ Th cells, 51
cell types in, 30–2
humoral immunity, 23
immature B cells, 80
macrophages, 31–2, 36
T cells, 30
migration patterns, 29
T-cell-independent antigen type 2 responses, 43
TNF-α, 54
vascularization of, 30
spleen cells, 82

spleen nodes, functional organization of, 28–32
*Staphylococcus aureus* Cowan (SAC), 167, 220, 398
  B cells
    activation, 171, 275, 276, 277
    memory, 279
  CD40, 278
  IL-2 stimulation, 171
  TGF-β mRNA levels, 294–5
  protein A, 350
*Streptococcus pneumoniae*, 26
substance P, 347–71
switch circles, 281–2
switch recombination
  breakpoints, 113–14
  DNA synthesis, 120
  proteins, 121
  switch transcription involvement, 125
  targeting, 122–4
switch regions, as GC-rich, 111–13
switch transcription
  control of, 124
  processing scheme, 115
synovial monocytes, 423
systemic autoimmune disease, 409
systemic lupus erythematosus (SLE), 409, 419–21
  anti-IL-10, 277
  autoimmunity, 416
  IgG autoantibodies, 412
  IL-4, 420–1
  IL-6, 419–20
  IL-10, 14, 274
  T cells, 410

T cells (T lymphocytes)
  activation, monocyte dependent, 282
  B cell interaction, 27–8, 56, 62, 64
  concanavalin A, 348
  development, CD5, 40–1
  human IL-5 mRNA, 218
  IFN-γ, 325
  Ig production, 359
  IgA responses, 396–7
  IgE, 362, 367, 380–1
  IgG4, 362, 367
  IL-2 production, 160
  IL-4 mRNA, 61
  isotype switching, 41–3
  lamina propria range, 394
  lymph node, 33
  membranes, Ig secretion, 337
  mucosal immune responses, 400–1
  naive adult B cell stimulation, 177
  neuropeptides, 358
    inhibition, 363
  Peyer's patches, 313
  phytohemagglutinin, 294, 348
  spleen, 29, 30
  substance P inhibition, 349
  systemic lupus erythematosus, 410
  T-cell-independent antigen responses, 41–3
  T-dependent pathways, 330
  transcription, 115
  *see also* $CD4^+$ T cells; $CD8^+$ T cells
T-cell help, 101–2
T-cell-dependent antigens, 23–64
  B-cell activation, 44–57
  soluble, 39
T-cell-independent antigens, 23–64
  activating B-cell subsets, 40–1
  crosslinking mIg receptor, 40
  soluble, 38
  type 2, 102
T-helper (Th) cells, 47–53
  B-cell proliferation, 298, 380
  $CD4^+$, 262
  mucosal IgA responses, 396
  subsets, 47–8, 93
  Th1 clones, stimulating Ig production, 168
  Th2
    B-cell growth, 20
    IL-4, 198, 413
    IL-10, 273
  tumor necrosis factor, 101
terminal deoxynucleotidyl transferase, 75
TGF-β, see transforming growth factor beta
thrombocytopenia, IL-6, 261
thymus
  epithelial cells, 302
  intraepithelial lymphocytes, 395
  T cell development, 302
  TGF-b development, 302
thymus-dependent antigens, 24
  properties of, 25
thymus-independent antigens, 24
  type 2, 25
tingible body macrophages, 30
TNP-Ficoll (TI-2), 36
  CD40L, 50
  murine spleen, 60
  persistence of, 35

TNP-hydroxyethyl starch, 37
TNP-KLH (TD), 36
  CD40L, 50
  murine spleen, 60–1
transforming growth factor beta (TGFβ), 289–315
  activation of, 293
  antibody class switching regulation, 307–15
  B cells, 289–315
    differentiation, 302–15
    proliferation, 296–301
    regulation, 301–2
  germline Cα RNA, 310–14
  germline γ2b transcripts, 314–15
  IFN-γ synthesis, 327
  Ig secretion, 306
  Ig synthesis, 289
    inhibition, 304–6
  IgA, switching, 307–9
  IgE production, 357
  latency-associated peptide, 290
  mRNA, 292–3
  receptors, 291–2
  responsiveness element, 315
  role of, 15
  synthesis of, 292
  T cells, 289
    regulation, 301–2
  transcription factors, 306
transin genes
  AP-1 sites, 304–5
  TGF-β transcription, 304–5
trinitrophenyl, 139
tumor necrosis factor, 101
tumor necrosis factor alpha, 414
  IL-2 responsiveness, 174
  substance P, 347
tumor necrosis factor beta, 400
tyrosine kinases
  activation, IL-2 stimulation, 162
  Janus kinase (Jak), 255–6
tyrosine phosphorylation
  HS1 proteins, 240
  IL-5–induced, 232
  IL-5R, 230–1
  Shc proteins, 240

Van der Waals forces, 39
vasoactive intestinal peptide, 347–71
  incubation, 365
veiled cells, 32
vesicular stomatitis virus, IgG responses, 55

*Index compiled by A. Campbell Purton.*